Sixth International Visual Field Symposium

Documenta Ophthalmologica Proceedings Series volume 42

Editor H. E. Henkes

Sixth International Visual Field Symposium

Santa Margherita Ligure, May 27 – 31, 1984

Edited by A. Heijl and E.L. Greve

1985 **DR W. JUNK PUBLISHERS**
a member of the KLUWER ACADEMIC PUBLISHERS GROUP
DORDRECHT / BOSTON / LANCASTER

Distributors

for the United States and Canada: Kluwer Academic Publishers, 190 Old Derby Street, Hingham, MA 02043, USA
for the UK and Ireland: Kluwer Academic Publishers, MTP Press Limited, Falcon House, Queen Square, Lancaster LA1 1RN, UK
for all other countries: Kluwer Academic Publishers Group, Distribution Center, P.O. Box 322, 3300 AH Dordrecht, The Netherlands

Library of Congress Cataloging in Publication Data

International Visual Field Symposium (6th : 1984 :
    Santa Margherita Ligure, Italy)
    Sixth International Visual Field Symposium, Santa
Margherita Ligure, May 27-31, 1984.

    (Documenta ophthalmologica. Proceedings series ;
v. 36)
    Includes bibliographies and index.
    1. Perimetry--Congresses.   2. Visual fields--
Congresses.   3. Glaucoma--Diagnosis--Congresses.
4. Neuro-ophthalmology--Congresses.   I. Heijl,
A. (Anders)   II. Greve, Erik L.   III. Title.   IV. Series.
RE79.P4I56 1984   617.7'0754   85-227

ISBN-13: 978-94-010-8932-6   e-ISBN-13: 978-94-009-5512-7
DOI:10.1007/ 978-94-009-5512-7

Copyright

CONTENTS

AUTOMATIC PERIMETRY: CARTOGRAPHY

AUTOMATIC PERIMETRY: GENERAL

THE IMPORTANCE OF PERIPHERAL VISUAL FIELDS IN NEURO-OPHTHALMOLOGY

NEURO-OPHTHALMOLOGY: GENERAL

COLOUR PERIMETRY

ERGO-PERIMETRY

GLAUCOMA

FUNDUS PERIMETRY

THE VISUAL FIELD IN STRABISMUS AND AMBLYOPIA

GENERAL TOPICS

INTRODUCTION (PROCEEDINGS 6th IPS SYMPOSIUM)

In 1972 Aulhorn, Dubois Poulsen, Greve, Jayle and Verriest met in Paris to discuss the organization of the first visual field symposium. The foundation of the International Perimetric Society took place in Marseille in 1974 on the occasion of this first symposium. Since then the International Perimetric Society has developed under the presidencies of Aulhorn and Drance into an enthusiastic and hard-working group of scientists in which valuable personal contacts were created.

The 6th International Visual Field Symposium of the International Perimetric Society, the ten-year anniversary of the Society, was held on May 27–31, 1984 at Santa Margherita Ligure, Italy. Approximately 100 IPS members and 80 guests participated in the meeting making it the largest meeting so far of the International Perimetric Society.

The main topics of the meeting were: *automated perimetry,* particularly strategies and basic knowledge, *ergo-perimetry* (practical aspects), *colour perimetry* and *neuro-ophthalmic perimetry.*

Many papers were presented on automated perimetry. Two new computerized instruments and several new automated test protocols were described and assessed. A whole group of presentations addressed the issue of threshold variability – its importance for the early recognition of visual field defects, a new method using internal inconsistencies within one test instead of double increment threshold determinations to assess subject reliability, graphic representation of areas with high threshold scatter and the variation of static as compared with kinetic testing. The difficult question of establishing visual field change over time consuming computerized perimetry (one of the main topics of the next IPS symposium) was also discussed. Several papers dealt with cartography.

No less than seven papers addressed the importance of peripheral fields. Most results were in agreement with the traditional concept that peripheral fields only rarely show defects when the central field is entirely normal. These contributions add details important to our knowledge, though, and several authors emphasized that results of peripheral field testing facilitates interpretation of test results and help in establishing topical diagnosis.

A main contribution to the proceedings is the second report on the occupational visual field concerning practical aspects. The theoretical aspects were treated in the proceedings of the 5th IVF symposium.

Colour perimetry remains of interest. Although it has not (yet) been incorporated in the daily routine of visual field examination it may well be that colour techniques can be valuable for the early detection of some diseases.

As usual there are many papers on perimetry in glaucoma. Three dealt with visual field changes after laser trabeculoplasty: one showed no regression of field defects after pressure reduction achieved through laser treatment, another even demonstrated the same rate of progression of glaucomatous field loss after laser treatment as before the operation despite considerable reduction of intraocular pressure, while the results of the third paper was considerably more positive. Other contributions shed light on the mode of progression of glaucomatous field loss and the relation between retinal nerve fibre loss and field loss.

The large number of papers ensured a rich variety of subjects and there are numerous excellent papers in these proceedings, which have not been mentioned here.

The social part of the meeting was organized in a most excellent and lavish way. This makes this ten-year anniversary of the IPS a most pleasant memory to all participants — despite the sometimes quite inhospitable weather. We want to express the sincere gratitude of the Society and to Professor Mario Zingirian and his staff for all their work in organizing the meeting. We also want to thank all authors, Mrs Els Mutsaerts, the staff at the Secretariate in Malmö and Dr. W. Junk Publishers for their effective, kind and prompt help.

We look forward to the 7th International Visual Field Symposium in the Netherlands in September 1986.

Erik Greve and Anders Heijl (Editors)

ACKNOWLEDGEMENTS

Chapters 7, 14, 22, 32, 48, 61, 66, 79, 82 and 86 were supported from a grant of the Consiglio Nazionale delle Ricerche, Progetto Finalizzato Medicina Preventiva e Riabilitativa, Sottoprogetto Malattie Degenerative, Obiettivo n. 47a, Rome, Italy.

RESULTS OF A FLUCTUATION ANALYSIS AND DEFECT VOLUME PROGRAM FOR AUTOMATED STATIC THRESHOLD PERIMETRY WITH THE SCOPERIMETER

C.T. LANGERHORST, T.J.T.P. VAN DEN BERG, R. VAN SPRONSEN
and E.L. GREVE

(*Amsterdam, The Netherlands*)

ABSTRACT

We developed a Defect Volume (DV) program with the Scoperimeter to accurately compute both fluctuation and defect volume, with the ultimate purpose to statistically evaluate progression of visual field defects. After testing glaucoma patients we were able to show that unbiased threshold selection for determining individual sensitivity is very important in computing a defect volume, that individual gradient adaptation does not seem necessary, and that use of individual versus mean fluctuation remains controversial. Normal areas in glaucomatous visual fields may not be the same as fully healthy visual fields.

INTRODUCTION

Since the beginning of the development of computerized automated perimetry, several research groups have been working on relevant software for these machines. At present many sophisticated machines and programs are available, but there is still need for good, statistical programs to accurately determine thresholds and fluctuation, to discriminate between healthy and defect visual field locations, and to detect accurately progression of visual field defects in time. Our research group in Amsterdam has also been investigating fluctuation (4, 5), and we are now developing a program which will ultimately help us in judging deterioration of the visual field. As the basic variable for such a program, we chose the Defect Volume (DV), confer Bebie et al. (1). The theoretical background and details of this program are presented by van den Berg et al. (3).

Normal visual fields are considered to be circular symmetric with a linear gradient, and totally described by I_0 (individual central sensitivity), by σ (standard deviation) and by the *gradient* of the island of vision. The DV in a patient is then defined as the total 'normal' value of the visual field (estimated on the basis of this patient's non-pathological visual field areas) minus the sum of the actually measured threshold values. We investigated the importance of the variables I_0, σ and gradient for the computation of the

Heijl, A. and Greve, E.L. (eds.), Proceedings of the 6th Int. Visual Field Symposium.
© *1985, Dr W. Junk Publishers, Dordrecht, The Netherlands. ISBN 978-94-010-8932-6*

DV. Each of these variables in isolation was judged for relevant influence on the DV. The results of this analysis are described in the present article.

PATIENT POPULATION

The first series of patients investigated with the DV program consists of nine glaucoma patients, mean age 69 years, range 62–82 and one patient of 35 years. These 9 patients were either on medical therapy or had glaucoma surgery in the past. They were selected from our glaucoma population on the basis of their having mostly relative defects of the visual field, very little maximal or absolute defects, and also some normal visual field areas at high excentricity. In each patient we investigated one eye twice. As a control group we used 15 people with a mean age of 66 years, range 61–71, who either had no complaint or visited the eye clinic for unrelated ailments such as conjunctivitis. They all had normal (below 22 mmHg) intraocular pressure, normal optic discs, and no visual field defects.

RESULTS

Correlated as they are with the rest of the method of our DV program, only one of the basic 3 variables I_0, σ and gradient was varied at the time and the effects of each of them on the DV are presented here.

1. Importance of threshold selection for I_0

To overcome the initial bias of selecting points to determine the individual central sensitivity I_0, double threshold values were determined at random for 53 locations in the visual field, and printed as series 1 (top) and series 2 (bottom) as illustrated in Fig. 1. Table 1 shows how the DV is influenced by

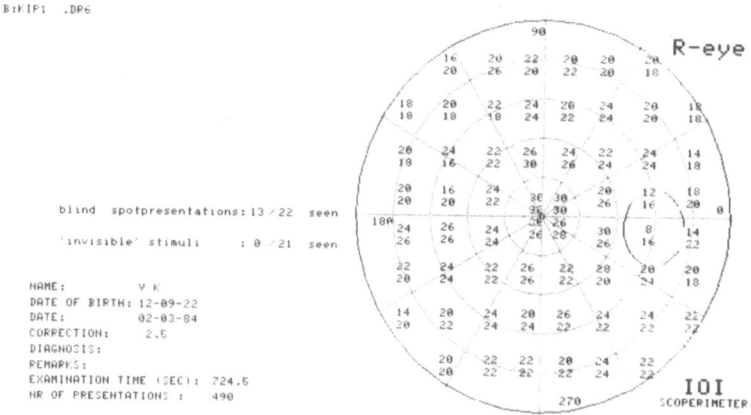

Fig. 1. Double threshold program.

2

Table 1. Influence of selection of threshold for I_0 on defect volume

patient number	$Io_1 - Io_2$	with bias (Io_1) Defect Volume	without bias (Io_2)	DV_1/DV_2
1	1.51	− 33	− 12	2.7
2	0.42	− 50	− 39	1.3
3	1.30	− 283	− 244	1.2
4	0.92	− 273	− 229	1.2
5	2.60	− 216	− 114	1.9
6	0.66	− 373	− 339	1.1
7	3.26	− 105	− 30	3.5
8	1.79	− 113	− 75	1.5
9	1.11	− 181	− 133	1.4
10	0.69	− 145	− 78	1.9
11	0.61	− 305	− 278	1.1
12	1.34	− 278	− 247	1.1
13	0.17	− 299	− 299	1.0
14	1.00	− 380	− 310	1.2
15	1.05	− 189	− 98	1.9
16	1.05	− 92	− 76	1.2
17	0.54	− 83	− 68	1.2
18	1.13	− 13	− 10	1.3

Io_1 with bias, based on highest values Series 1
Io_2 without bias, based on twin values Series 2

threshold selection. For instance when the highest thresholds are chosen from series 1 to compute the I_0, I_0 is 'artificially' high and therefore the DV artificially large, since DV is 'normal' volume (based on I_0) minus the sum of the actual threshold measurements. When I_0 is computed based on the unbiased, random twin values of series 2 the computed DV is always lower than with the series 1 points. When using a biased rather then an unbiased I_0 the DV could become up to 3.5 times as large in our patients.

2. Importance of the gradient of the correction for the island of vision

In the DV program 2 correction factors are used for the gradient of the island of vision: first the general correction of 0.25 dB/degree of excentricity, and later in the program the determination of the individual gradient of normal sensitivity by means of linear regression analysis of all healthy points. Table 2 shows the values of these individual gradients, and the resulting defect volumes with and without this extra correction used to increase accuracy in DV computation. In both cases the center of the healthy points is located on the gradient so that the effect of the gradient is studied in isolation, without influence by difference in general level of sensitivity. It is clear that the influence of the gradient correction on DV is small.

3. Influence of difference in fluctuation in normals

The point requires some extra explanation. In order to determine a DV one needs to set a criterion for which points are defect and which are not.

3

Table 2. Effect of correction for patient's individual gradient of normal sensitivity

patient number	gradients (degree^{-1})	Defect Volume (53 locations)		
		without correlation (gradient used = 0.25)	with correction (individual gradient used)	difference (%)
1	−0.24	−12	−12	0
2	−0.32	−40	−39	3
3	−0.26	−244	−244	0
4	−0.40	−231	−229	1
5	−0.32	−115	−114	1
6	−0.26	−339	−339	0
7	−0.48	−33	−30	10
8	−0.41	−76	−75	1
9	−0.48	−136	−133	2
10	−0.34	−78	−78	0
11	−0.17	−278	−278	0
12	−0.24	−247	−247	0
13	−0.33	−300	−299	0
14	−0.16	−309	−310	0
15	−0.22	−98	−98	0
16	−0.20	−76	−76	0
17	−0.22	−68	−68	0
18	−0.24	−10	−10	0

Generally points are considered defect when they fall below the 'average normal value' (in our case the central sensitivity I_0 minus the gradient correction) minus a certain standard deviation. The value of the standard deviation is a basic problem to be dealt with.

In 1976 Bebie et al. (1), measured intra-individual threshold fluctuations in 16 normal and pathological visual fields, and found an average short-term fluctuation of 1.8 dB (± 0.8 dB). They did not distinguish between fluctuation in normal and defective areas of the visual field. We did make this distinction, when we looked at fluctuation in glaucoma patients (4). In 7 'experienced' glaucoma patients we conducted the same threshold programs three times within one week, assuming that in such a short time there would be no deterioration due to glaucoma. Those patients had normal, relative defect, and absolute defect areas in their visual field. With analysis of variance techniques we found; 1) that the short-term fluctuation (Qs) within one investigation was much greater than the fluctuation (F) between sessions (Fig. 2). This finding is not dealt with in the present article. We also found; 2) that the short-term fluctuation was greatest in the relative defect areas, less in the normal areas and low in absolute defects (Fig. 2). Because of this difference in fluctuation in healthy and defect points we use the healthy fluctuation to set the limit for healthy points in our DV computation. Initially we used Bebie's σ-value and chose as criterion 2 times the fixed σ of 1.8 dB. In doing so, many of our normal controls (whose *mean* σ was also 1.8 dB) showed large 'defect volumes'. We then chose to consider all points healthy falling within $I_0 - 2\sigma$, and in this case σ is the standard deviation of healthy points determined per patient, and 2σ the patient−adapted criterion

4

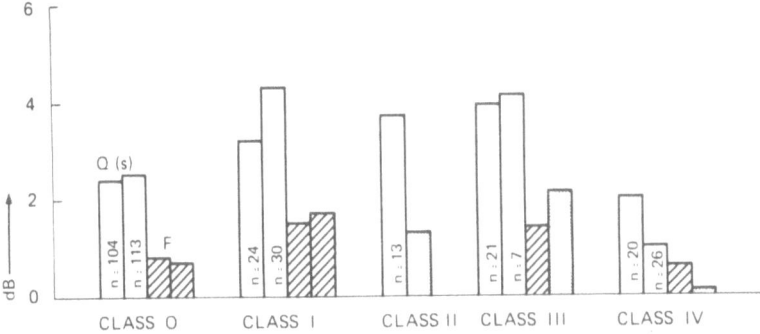

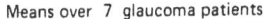

Fig. 2. Fluctuation in glaucoma patients.

for healthy points. Table 3 shows the difference in DV using the prefixed 2×1.8 dB criterion (DV fixed) or the individually determined $2 \times \sigma$ criterion (DV adapted). It is remarkable that the DV fixed is always larger than or equal to DV adapted. If the 1.8 dB would represent the mean of all standard deviations σ, one would expect to find also patients for whom DV fixed is smaller than DV adapted. This finding corresponds to the fact that the individual σ's are all larger than the mean normal value of 1.8 dB. So the mean standard deviation of a healthy population is not representative for the

Table 3. Influence of normal fluctuation on defect volume

| patient number | σ | Defect Volume | | $DV_{fixed}/DV_{adapted}$ |
		fixed criterion for healthy points	patients adapted criterion for healthy points	
1	2.47	−25	−12	2.1
2	1.78	−39	−39	1.0
3	2.29	−280	−244	1.1
4	2.16	−248	−229	1.1
5	3.49	−195	−114	1.7
6	2.43	−373	−339	1.1
7	3.30	−88	−30	2.9
8	2.69	−92	−75	1.2
9	3.03	−181	−133	1.4
10	2.40	−109	−78	1.4
11	1.77	−278	−278	1.0
12	2.25	−267	−247	1.1
13	3.76	−434	−299	1.5
14	2.05	−326	−310	1.1
15	1.70	−98	−98	1.0
16	2.13	−80	−76	1.0
17	1.95	−78	−68	1.1
18	1.78	−10	−10	1.0

mean standard deviation of the healthy areas (as determined by our program) of the visual fields of glaucoma patients.

CONCLUSIONS

Considering the strategy for DV computation we conclude:
1. Use of unbiased threshold selection for the determination of the individual sensitivity I_0 is very important. Use of biased threshold lead to an increase in DV by a factor of $1-3.5$ (mean 1.5).
2. Individual gradient adaptation gives little improvement in accuracy as it increases or decreases the DV with only $0-10\%$ (mean 1%).
3. The importance of the use of the individual fluctuation is not yet clear. Possibly, healthy visual fields and healthy areas of glaucoma fields may not be judged by the same standards.

REFERENCES

1. Bebié, H. and Fankhauser, F. Delta manual. Published by Interzeag. Schlieren, Switzerland(1981).
2. Bebié, H., Fankhauser, F. and Spahr, J. Static perimetry: accuracy and fluctuations. Acta Ophthalmologica; 54: 339–348 (1976).
3. van den Berg, T.J.T.P., van Veenendaal, W. and van Spronsen, R. Psychophysics of intensity discrimination in relation to defect volume examination on the Scoperimeter. Docum Ophthal Proc Series This volume (1984).
4. Langerhorst, C.T., van den Berg, T.J.T.P., van Veenendaal, W. and Greve, E.L. Schatting van de verschillende fluctuatiefactoren bij glaucoompatiënten. Ned. Tijdschr. v. Geneesk. 127(53): 2443 (1983).
5. Langerhorst, C.T., van den Berg, T.J.T.P. and Greve, E.L. Schätzung der verschiedene Fluktuationsfaktoren bei der Computerperimetrie von Glaukompatienten. To be published in Bücherei der Augenärztes der Enkes-Verlag (1984).

Authors' address:
The Netherlands Ophthalmic Research Institute,
P.O. Box 6411, Meibergdreef 9,
1105 AZ Amsterdam,
The Netherlands

INTERNAL INCONSISTENCIES VS ROOT MEAN SQUARE AS MEASURES OF THRESHOLD VARIABILITY

JOHN R. LYNN, ERIC P. BATSON, and RONALD L. FELLMAN

(*Dallas, Texas, USA*)

ABSTRACT

Although differences in response are permitted at the final threshold, any dimmer spots which are seen and any brighter ones not reported are considered internal inconsistencies, here called boo-boos. The root mean square (RMS) used by Octopus as a measure of intratest variability requires duplicate threshold testing in ten spots. In an effort to eliminate the time tax this implies, boo-boos were recorded during two double reversal threshold tests (4, 2, 2) at ten selected loci in eight surgically controlled glaucomatous eyes. The same 80 loci were then tested to 50% thresholds, with 2 minute rest periods after each five minutes of testing. Despite this precaution, a progressive deterioration of threshold occurred, preventing psychometric analysis in 19 of 71 valid loci. These data showed important differences from the 52 places where results were fitted to ogives. The RMS was approximately twice as effective in predicting the variable loci as the boo-boos. Since additional data for analysis of boo-boos are free of time penalty and precision increases as the square root of increase in data, this preliminary evaluation suggests boo-boo quantification may help to identify variable test loci.

INTRODUCTION

In traditional psychophysics, the reciprocal slope of the psychometric function relating stimulus intensity to frequency of seeing is the prime measure of judgmental variability. Bebie et al. (1) have described a statistical function, the root mean square or RMS, to provide a measure of variability in tests performed on the Octopus perimeter (Fig. 1). The raw data for RMS consist of pairs of independent threshold measurements at randomly chosen points in the visual field. Since RMS requires 11% to 100% extra time for testing 10 points a second time in each eye thresholded respectively at 90 to 10 different loci, an alternative measurement without this time tax would be desirable, assuming its validity were comparable to RMS. Heijl and Drance (3) have provided a special reason for saving time; the defective areas within glaucomatous fields deteriorate during prolonged testing.

Heijl, A. and Greve, E.L. (eds.), Proceedings of the 6th Int. Visual Field Symposium.
© *1985, Dr W. Junk Publishers, Dordrecht, The Netherlands. ISBN 978-94-010-8932-6*

ROOT MEAN SQUARE

$$RMS = \sqrt{\frac{\sum (X_i - Y_i)^2}{2n}}$$

Where X_i is the threshold in dB obtained
from first testing at a given point,

Y_i is the threshold in dB obtained
from second testing at the same point,

n is the number of points where at
least one of the pair of thresholds is
reported seen.

Summation proceeds over each of the n points

Fig. 1. The formula for computing RMS.

A few decades ago, an American comedian, Jerry Lewis, popularized a slang term for mistakes or slip-ups when he kept saying 'Uh oh, I made a boo-boo'. We have tracked the internal inconsistencies in our clinical perimetry, collectively referring to these data as boo-boos. The merits of counting boo-boos are the total absence of a time tax and the method's applicability to every test point in the threshold pattern.

This preliminary work involving glaucoma patients with relative defects in the visual field suggests the traditional slope of the psychometric function may need to be estimated from the 'interval of uncertainty' region where points are seen probabilistically.

MATERIALS AND METHODS

The Squid automatic perimeter was chosen because its manufacturer not only permits full access to all operational software, but encourages its users to develop their own. The computer portion of this system is an LSI-11 by DEC, its logic is programmed in Fortran IV, and its files are maintained in a language similar to COBOL.

Because of their extensive experience as subjects of perimetry and the presence of a definite glaucomatous defect in their fields, eight glaucoma patients were chosen in whom the intraocular pressures were surgically well controlled. The subjects ranged in age from 38 to 71 years. Their average RMS was 3.4 with a range from 1.2 to 5.0. A recent test of the central 28° of the visual field was used in one eye of each subject to choose five loci with relatively good thresholds, 'better points', and five with relative defects, 'worse points'. No fewer than two nor more than three tests were selected in each quadrant, and none were chosen in the blind spot area or outside 23° eccentricity (Fig. 3). Tests of 0.43° diameter (26 secs) were used on a background of 4 asb. The interest time was one-half second, and the test duration was one-tenth of a second (2). All patients had proper refractive correction finely adjusted in the perimeter.

Phase 1 and definitions

During the preliminary part of the experiment, each patient received a battery of 20 independent threshold tests, using the clinically common presentation of stimuli 4 decibels (dB) apart until a reversal of answer occurred, then steps 2 dB apart in the opposite direction to another reversal, followed by 2 dB steps in the original direction, again to reversal. This so-called 4,2,2 strategy is also known as a modified staircase method. Two of these series were performed simultaneously and independent of one another in each of the 10 chosen locations.

Threshold data from Phase 2 were recorded in two ways: first, as the mean of the two final stimuli, and second, as an occasional adjustment of that mean either up or down by one dB. The adjustment occurred when the number of boo-boos could be reduced by choosing a new threshold and ignoring any inconsistencies of response at threshold itself.

After the threshold was modified, those stimuli which had been seen during the course of the test at intensities dimmer than the adjusted threshold or had been missed at intensities brighter than the new threshold were recorded as the minimized boo-boos used in this study. The adjusted threshold was termed the boo-boo minimized threshold.

At the conclusion of the initial tests, Phase 1, each of the ten points in question had acquired a track record of stimuli presented, with responses to each, and results, including two original thresholds, as many as two boo-boo minimized thresholds, and two counts of any remaining minimized boo-boos. The difference between the two original thresholds served in each location as the basis for the root mean square (RMS) (see Fig. 2.).

Phase 2; testing to a 50% threshold

After a two or three minute rest here and following no more than five minutes of testing afterwards, 50% threshold testing began. Eleven stimuli were required at the mean of the two original thresholds. Tests were always randomly mixed with stimuli at the other nine locations. If six successive presentations were ever unseen, a 10 dB suprathreshold stimulus was delivered, and the response to this 'wake up call' did not affect the test logic.

The initial objective in 50% thresholding was to find 3 adjacent intensities which appeared to include the 50%-seen threshold without wasting time acquiring unnecessary data. The next objective was to augment the data at

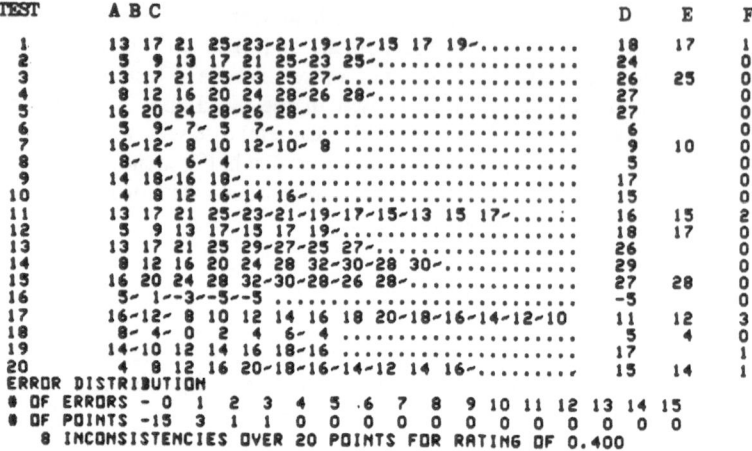

```
TEST        A B C                                                          D    E    F
  1         13  17  21  25-23-21-19-17-15  17  19-.........      18   17    1
  2          5   9  13  17  21  25-23  25-...................      24        0
  3         13  17  21  25-23  25  27-.....................      26   25    0
  4          8  12  16  20  24  28-26  28-.................      27        0
  5         16  20  24  28-26  28-.......................      27        0
  6          5   9-  7-  5   7-.........................       6        0
  7         16-12-  8  10  12-10-  8  ..................       9   10    0
  8          8-  4   6-  4  .............................       5        0
  9         14  18-16  18-...............................      17        0
 10          4   8  12  16-14  16-.......................      15        0
 11         13  17  21  25-23-21-19-17-15-13  15  17-.....:.      16   15    2
 12          5   9  13  17-15  17  19-...................      18   17    0
 13         13  17  21  25  29-27-25  27-.................      26        0
 14          8  12  16  20  24  28  32-30-28  30-..........      29        0
 15         16  20  24  28  32-30-28-26  28-..............      27   28    0
 16          5-  1-  3--5--5  .............................      -5        0
 17         16-12-  8  10  12  14  16  18  20-18-16-14-12-10      11   12    3
 18          8-  4-  0   2   4   6-  4  ..................       5    4    0
 19         14-10  12  14  16  18-16  ...................      17        1
 20          4   8  12  16  20-18-16-14-12  14  16-.........      15   14    1
ERROR DISTRIBUTION
 # OF ERRORS -  0   1   2   3   4   5  .6   7   8   9  10  11  12  13  14  15
 # OF POINTS -15   3   1   1   0   0   0   0   0   0   0   0   0   0   0   0
        8 INCONSISTENCIES OVER 20 POINTS FOR RATING OF 0.400
```

Fig. 2. An example of the type of data collected during phase one. Horizontal rows of data are the information at a single locus being tested to an independent threshold. The paired rows which are at the same loci differ in number by 10 in the vertical column labelled 'test'. Vertical column A indicates the initial intensities attempted at each location. Tildes, such as those in Column B, indicate the attempt in the preceding column was not reported as seen. Column C indicates the intensitities on the second attempt and should differ from Column A by 4 dB. The thresholding logic can thus be followed to the last two data points in this block. The mean of these two numbers is the reported threshold in Column D. If a 1 dB shift in threshold can decrease the inconsistencies, the boo-boo minimized threshold appears in Column E. After the threshold is thus minimized, the number of remaining boo-boos appears in Column F̄.

the 3 intensities which satisfied the first objective and reconfirm the threshold-bracketing level of responses, or change the intensity to provide this. The final objective was to gather at least 20 responses from the two intensities which enclosed the three contiguous peri-threshold intensities.

To minimize test time, data from the two original Phase I threshold tests were accepted as part of the required data in the 50% thresholding. After 11 tests were completed at any location, the results were analyzed, and a new requirement was set for eleven more tests, 2 dB brighter or dimmer than the first 11. When seen-unseen status changed, the intervening level of test intensity was provided with enough stimuli to total ten attempts.

A pseudorandom algorithm which rechecked for propriety of intensity then presented increasing numbers of stimuli at each location. This continued until a series of 20 or 21 stimuli were accrued at five intensities which differed from one another by 1 dB, with the 50% seen threshold among the middle three. Additional data, when collected, were retained and utilized, but not regarded as desirable because of the time required for their collection.

RESULTS

Percentages seen were calculated at each location for each stimulus intensity and computerized curve fitting was used to analyze the data. Fig. 3 shows

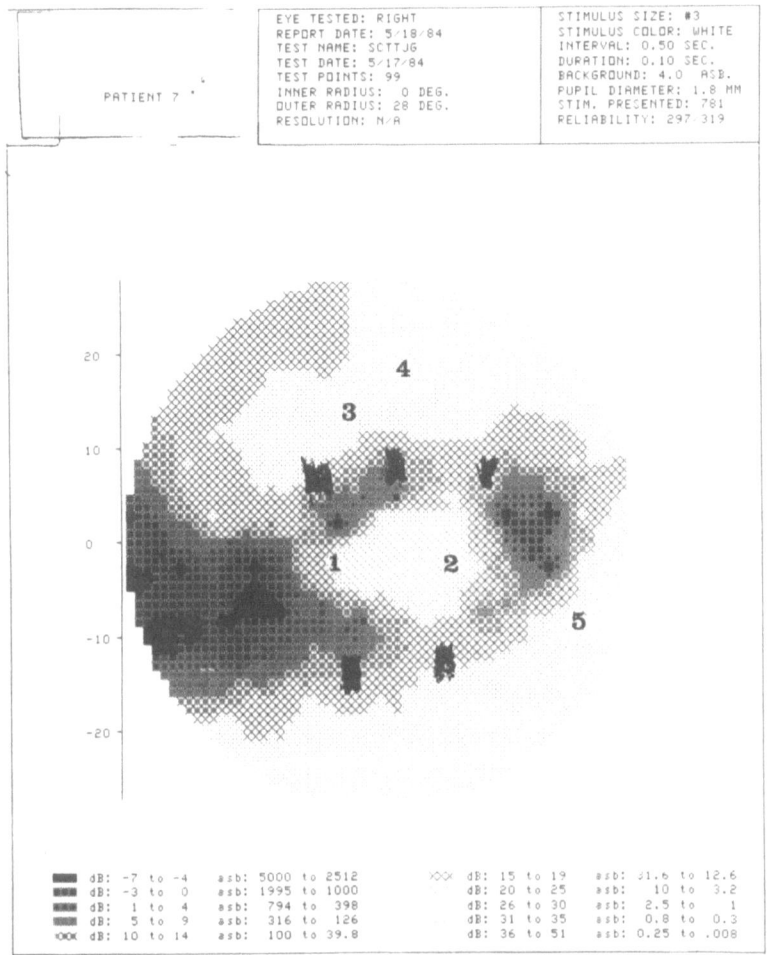

EYE TESTED: RIGHT
REPORT DATE: 5/18/84
TEST NAME: SCTTJG
TEST DATE: 5/17/84
TEST POINTS: 99
INNER RADIUS: 0 DEG.
OUTER RADIUS: 28 DEG.
RESOLUTION: N/A

STIMULUS SIZE: #3
STIMULUS COLOR: WHITE
INTERVAL: 0.50 SEC.
DURATION: 0.10 SEC.
BACKGROUND: 4.0 ASB.
PUPIL DIAMETER: 1.8 MM
STIM. PRESENTED: 781
RELIABILITY: 297/319

PATIENT 7

dB: −7 to −4	asb: 5000 to 2512	dB: 15 to 19	asb: 31.6 to 12.6
dB: −3 to 0	asb: 1995 to 1000	dB: 20 to 25	asb: 10 to 3.2
dB: 1 to 4	asb: 794 to 398	dB: 26 to 30	asb: 2.5 to 1
dB: 5 to 9	asb: 316 to 126	dB: 31 to 35	asb: 0.8 to 0.3
dB: 10 to 14	asb: 100 to 39.8	dB: 36 to 51	asb: 0.25 to .008

Fig. 3. The gray scale plot of central 28° previously tested to threshold in patient 7. Numbers 1–5 are in better-seen areas and 6–10 are in areas of relative field defects.

where 10 points were tested in an exemplary field from patient 7. Figure 4 shows the data from all points in Fig. 3. Because the percentage seen in the first row either increases with higher intensities or remains nearly the same, we describe these data as monotonic, and find they are easily fitted to an ogive, or frequency of seeing curve.

Computerized fitting of an ogive was only accomplished when the data met the following criteria: five or more adjacent intensities were tested 20 or 21 times; a normal ogive was fitted to the data and confirmed with the Kolmogorov-Smirnov one sample test; threshold was reported within the test range; and the standard deviation of the threshold was 5.5 dB or less. Although the second row of Fig. 4 shows data which are apparently less monotonic than the points on the top row, they did meet the stated criteria

11

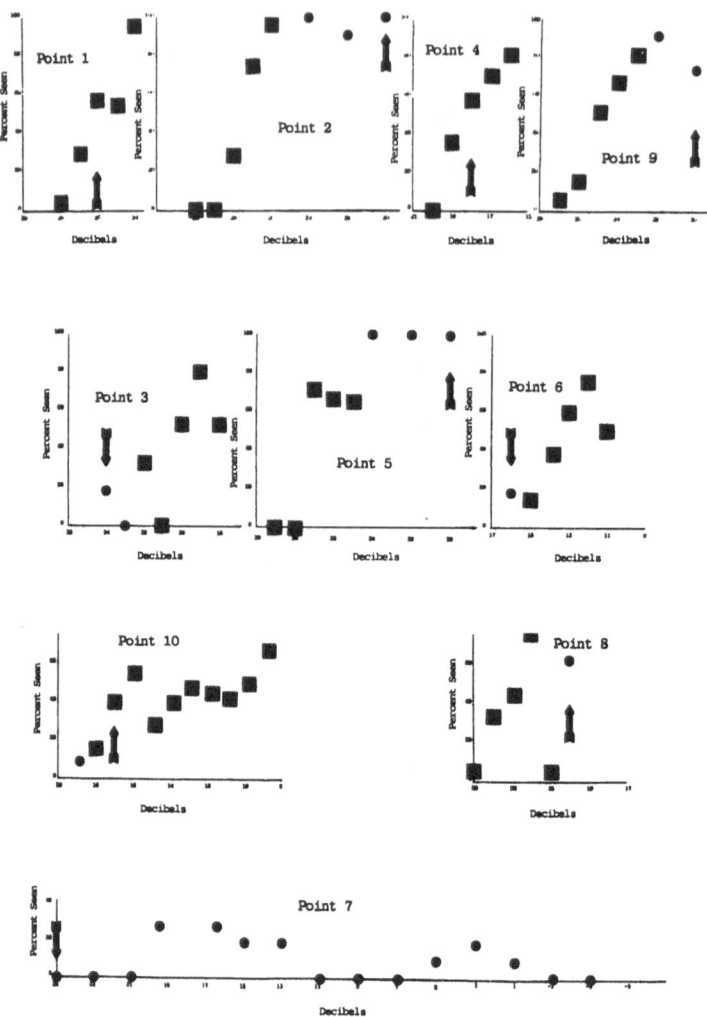

Fig. 4. The data from testing 10 points to 50% threshold in the eye whose field is shown in Fig. 3. The top row of data from points 1, 2, 4 and 9 are rather monotonically distributed so an ogive could obviously be fitted here. The second row of data from points 3, 5, and 6, though lacking perfect monotonicity, were successfully fitted with an ogive. Data from points 8 and 10 are shown in the third row and from point 7 in the fourth. These data did not meet the relatively liberal criteria for computerized ogive fitting, as detailed in the text. The arrows indicate the beginning threshold levels. Points labelled with squares were the result of 20 or more stimuli while those labelled with circles were tested only 10 or 11 times.

so they were successfully fitted. Unfittable data from points 7, 8 and 10 are shown on the last 2 rows.

Eighty locations were originally available for full threshold testing. Fifty-two met the criteria for computerized ogive fitting, including 29 which were

Table 1. Overall results of study comparing the originally better-seen Loci in each eye, 'better points', with the relatively defective areas, 'worse points'

	'Better points'	'Worse points'
Fitted by computer to Ogives	33	19
Obviously monotonic	19	4
Seen but not fittable to any psychometric function	4	15
Tested blind from beginning	1	5
Methodological failures	2	1
	40	40

Table 2. Effect of modifying threshold to minimize boo-boos

	A Loci fitted to Ogives N = 52	B Loci not fittable N = 19	A & B Loci seen & validly tested N = 71
Threshold changed toward correct result	30/104 (28.8)	11/38 (28.9)	41/142 (28.9)
Threshold changed away from correct result	16/104 (15.4)	5/38 (13.2)	21/142 (14.8)
Threshold changed: direction uncertain	0	8/38 (21.1)	8/142 (5.6)
Total thresholds changed	46/104 (44.2)	24/38 (63.2)	70/142 (49.3)
Total thresholds unchanged	58/104 (55.8)	14/38 (36.8)	72/142 (50.7)
Boo-boo location ratio (*Not* minimized)	0.442	0.632	0.493

not obviously monotonic. The 40 'better points' by prior exam could be distinguished from the 40 'worse points' in several regards, as seen in Table 1. All minimized boo-boos occurred in locations where threshold had been changed. Table 2 shows that threshold changes, all of which were only one dB in size, occurred half the time; for the better twice as often as for the worse when it was possible to decide the correct direction.

The 52 locations which could be fitted with an ogive and the 19 which could not provided 142 chances to make a boo-boo. Table 3 shows the results of these opportunities in the form of minimized boo-boo counts and ratios. The power of minimized boo-boos can be appreciated best by comparing the fitted and unfittable series in the non-minimized ratios of Table 2 with the minimized ones of Table 3, where mean RNS bases for both groups are also shown. The standard deviation of threshold averaged 2.26 ± 1.1 dB in the group of 52 ogive-fitted loci. The standard deviation would be much larger if it were computable in the 19 unfittable cases, where 3 loci were specifically rejected because their standard deviations exceeded 5.5 dB.

The lack of obvious monotonicity in more than $\frac{2}{3}$ of the valid and visualized locations led to a method of analysis which would not be required in normal subjects. The range of dB's which could include the 50% threshold was recorded for each location and correlated with its predictors, the RMS bases as well as the two boo-boo counts. Table 4 shows the results of these Pearson product moment correlations. The correlation of averaged range

Table 3. Frequency of minimized boo-boos among data fitted to ogives vs data which could not be fitted

# of minimized boo-boos per threshold (two trials per locus)	Loci fitted to ogives N = 52	Loci not fittable N = 19	Loci seen and validly tested N = 71
0	88/104 (84.6)	23/38 (60.5)	111/142 (78.2)
1	10/104 (9.6)	11/38 (29.0)	21/142 (14.8)
2	6/104 (5.8)	2/38 (5.3)	8/142 (5.6)
3	0	1/38 (2.6)	1/142 (0.7)
5	0	1/38 (2.6)	1/142 (0.7)
Minimized boo-boo location ratio	0.154	0.395	0.218
Minimized boo-boo ratio	0.212	0.605	0.317
Mean RMS base	1.74	5.00	2.62

Table 4. Correlations between predictors and the range of possible threshold values

Patient	RMS base	Boo-boo 1	Boo-boo 2
1	0.76	0	0.37
2	0.47	0.58	0.06
3	0.59	0.88	0.10
4	0.84	0	−0.24
5	0.06	0.31	−0.08
6	0.09	−0.26	−0.25
7	0.50	−0.04	0.37
8	0.97	0.63	0.06

was $+0.22$ with the RMS function and -0.18 with the averaged boo-boo count, neither being significant.

DISCUSSION

What did appear significant in Table 4 was the presence of rather good correlations between several RMS bases and some boo-boo counts with the ranges of possible threshold. Since there is twice as much data available for detecting variability in an RMS base as in a boo-boo count, it is not surprising to have RMS prove effective about twice as often as the boo-boo count. This advantage, however, is expected to disappear when the number of test points increases. If, for example, forty test locations were tested once to threshold with minimized boo-boo ratios, the four-fold increase in data is expected to produce a doubling of precision, since precision is known to increase as the square root of collected data increases.

CONCLUSIONS

The results of this study lack crisp reliability, for reasons which are not completely clear. No patient showed obvious monotonicity in more than 4 of 10 locations tested. After worrying about local adaptation and fixation shifts, we considered the temporal degradation of glaucomatous fields described by Heijl and Drance as the best prior description of this phenomenon. Unfortunetely, rest periods at intervals of five minutes between threshold determinations which lasted about one hour did not save this study from temporal degradation of sensitivity.

Root Mean Square (RMS) is an accepted, though less than perfect, measure of variability which takes extra time for duplicate testing of preselected thresholds. If only ten loci are to be tested, the time tax is 100%. If 90 are desired, the tax time is the same, but it is only 11% of this total. RMS superiority over boo-boos in individual loci is presumably based on the amount of data available to both. If one could accept the magnitude of RMS superiority over boo-boo ratios as approximately 2:1 with 10 tests performed, the boo-boo ratios should equal the RMS as a measure of variability when forty or so tests are attempted and exceed it by 50% when 90 locations are tried.

Since there is no time tax in counting internal inconsistencies, hereby dubbed boo-boos, these may be tested alone or in conjunction with RMS. Any correlation present at those 10 points allows the variability measure to be extended to the remainder of the field.

Boo-boo ratios at individual locations have been of clinical help to us when we are trying to decide whether a temporal change in threshold represents a change in visual health status.

ACKNOWLEDGEMENTS

The authors wish to express sincere gratitude to Amy Travis and Susanna Ostrov for their dedicated effots in testing the subjects and in preparation of the figures, and to Ira Bernstein, Ph.D., for his critical advice regarding the research protocol and the analysis of our psychometric data.

REFERENCES

1. Bebie, H., Fankhauser, F., and Spahr J. Static perimetry; accuracy and fluctuations. Acta Ophthalmol 54: 339–348 (1976).
2. Fellman, R. and Lynn, J. Are the larger test object size and dimmer background intensity of the Octopus improvements over standard Goldmann settings? (Poster) ARVO; May (1984).
3. Heijl, A. and Drance, S. Changes in differential threshold in patients with glaucoma during prolonged perimetry. Br J Ophthalmol 67:512 (1983).
4. Tate, G. and Lynn J. Principles of Quantitative Perimetry. New York, Grune & Stratton (1977) p 110.

Authors' address:
Glaucoma Associates of Texas,
6750 Hillcrest Plaza Drive,
Suite 104,
Dallas, Texas 75230, U.S.A.

THE FREQUENCY DISTRIBUTION OF THE DEVIATIONS IN STATIC PERIMETRY

JOSEF FLAMMER and MARIO ZULAUF

(*Berne, Switzerland*)

ABSTRACT

The outcomes of repeated measurements in quantitative static perimetry scatter around a mean value. We analysed the frequency distribution of the deviations of the single measurements from their means.

In a heterogeneous pool of data, the shape of the distribution showed a positive kurtosis but no relevant skewness. The standardized deviations, however, showed a distribution very close to normal. There was no difference between the midperiphery and the center. In a normal visual field area, the deviations were smaller and their distribution closer to normal than in relative scotomas.

INTRODUCTION

The outcome of any quantitative physical, biological and psychophysical measurement is subject to scatter. The scatter of the measurement of the threshold of the differential light sensitivity, DLS, which is measured in quantitative perimetry, is well known. Its different components as well as factors influencing their size have been described earlier (1–3).

The purpose of this study was to evaluate the shape of the distribution of the deviations of single measurements from their means. We limit ourselves here to the short-term deviations (2).

The main question is: How close can the observed distribution be approximated by a normal distribution? The normal distribution is a theoretical model based upon the idealization of the reality that the distribution is due to many mutually independent random variables. The normal frequency distribution or probability density f(x) is bell-shaped and has the following mathematical form:

$$f(x) = P(x/\mu, \sigma) = \frac{1}{\sigma\sqrt{2\pi}}\, e^{1/2 \left(\frac{x-\mu}{\sigma}\right)^2}$$

Heijl, A. and Greve, E.L. (eds.), Proceedings of the 6th Int. Visual Field Symposium.
© *1985, Dr W. Junk Publishers, Dordrecht, The Netherlands. ISBN 978-94-010-8932-6*

The cumulative normal distribution is S-shaped. Mathematically it is the integral of the probability density of a normal distribution.

$$F(X) = \int_{-\infty}^{x} f(X)\, dX$$

MATERIAL

We analyzed a pool of data consisting of 612 visual fields of 265 eyes (86 normals, 110 glaucoma suspects and 69 glaucomas) of 180 individuals. The visual fields were measured with program JO on the Octopus (4). This program measures the threshold twice at 47 test locations and at two test locations ten times. In this study we analyzed the ten measurements of the latter two test locations, one being in the midperiphery ($x = -15°$, $y = 15°$), the other at the center ($x = 0°$, $y = 0°$). We will refer to them as PTL (peripheral test location) and as CTL (central test location). There were 6120 observations at each of the two test locations in our pool.

We then eliminated all measurements of a visual field when one or more outcomes were zero (absolute scotomas). The final number of observations included was 5910 for PTL and 6010 for CTL.

METHODS

We measured and calculated the following variables for PTL and CTL separately:

— individual outcomes of the measurement of the DLS on replication i of visual field test j:

$$x_{ij}$$

— mean threshold at PTL or CTL for each visual field (n = number of replications):

$$x_{\cdot j} = \frac{\sum\limits_{i=1}^{n} x_{ij}}{n}$$

— deviation of the single outcomes from their means:

$$y_{ij} = x_{ij} - x_{\cdot j}$$

— standard deviation (S.D.) (at PTL or CTL) in visual field j:

$$\sigma_i = \frac{\sum\limits_{i=1}^{n} (x_{ij} - x_{\cdot j})^2}{n-1}$$

— standardized deviations:

$$z_{ij} = \frac{y_{ij}}{\sigma_j}$$

— S.D. of the pooled deviations (m = number of normal fields):

$$S_{(y)} = \frac{\sum\limits_{i=1}^{n} \sum\limits_{j=1}^{m} (y_{ij} - y..)^2}{n \cdot m - 1}$$

— S.D. of the pooled standardized deviations:

$$S_{(z)} = \frac{\sum\limits_{i=1}^{n} \sum\limits_{j=1}^{m} (z_{ij} - z..)^2}{n \cdot m - 1}$$

— skewness of the distribution:

$$k_{(y)} = \frac{\sum\limits_{i=1}^{n} \sum\limits_{j=1}^{m} (y_{ij} - y..)^3}{S_{(y)}^3 \cdot n \cdot m}$$

$$k_{(z)} = \frac{\sum\limits_{i=1}^{n} \sum\limits_{j=1}^{m} (z_{ij} - z..)^3}{S_{(z)}^3 \cdot n \cdot m}$$

— kurtosis of the distribution:

$$e_{(y)} = \frac{\sum\limits_{i=1}^{n} \sum\limits_{j=1}^{m} (y_{ij} - y..)^4}{S_{(y)}^4 \cdot n \cdot m} - 3$$

$$e_{(z)} = \frac{\sum\limits_{i=1}^{n} \sum\limits_{j=1}^{m} (z_{ij} - z..)^4}{S_{(z)}^4 \cdot n \cdot m} - 3$$

— maximal deviation: (Kolmogoroff-Smirnoff)

$$D_{(y)} = \text{Max}/F_N(y_{ij}) - F(y_{ij})/$$

$$D_{(z)} = \text{Max}/F_N(z_{ij}) - F(z_{ij})/$$

where y.. and z.. are the mean values of the outcomes and standardized values, respectively, averaged over all the visual fields.

The frequency distributions of y and z are represented in the form of histograms (left hand side of the figures). Superimposed are normal distributions with the same mean and SD as the corresponding histograms. This allows a visual comparison between the empirical histograms and the theoretical normal distributions.

The cumulative frequencies of y and z are drawn on normal probability paper (right hand side of the figures). The straight line represents a normal distribution calculated on the empirically found mean and S.D. In this way, the difference between the empirical distribution and the corresponding theoretical normal distribution is more easily visualized.

(To avoid too many symbols on the probability plot, only 9% of the observations – randomly selected – were used.)

To compare normal visual field areas with relative scotomas, we selected, on the one hand, all x_{ij}, if their corresponding means, $x_{\cdot j}$, were between 25 and 29 dB (Fig. 5); and, on the other hand, all x_{ij}, if their corresponding $x_{\cdot j}$ were between 14 and 20 dB.

The differences between the empirical distributions and the normal distributions were quantified on each figure by

k = skewness

e = kurtosis

D = maximal deviation by Kolmogoroff-Smirnoff

RESULTS AND DISCUSSION

There is a moderate difference between the empirical distribution and the normal distribution of the deviations (y) in PTL (Fig. 1) and CTL (Fig. 2). The standardized deviations (z), however, have a frequency distribution which is very close to normal (Figs. 3 and 4).

This indicates that the observed differences between empirical and normal distributions in Figs. 1 and 2 are due to the heterogeneity of our material.

DEVIATIONS IN THE MIDPERIPHERY

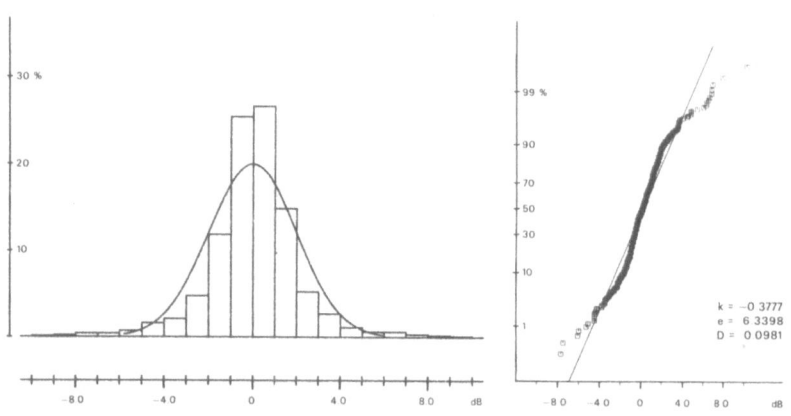

Fig. 1. Histogram and probability plot of the deviations (y) at the midperipheral test location. Number of observations: 5190: standard deviation: 1.98 dB.

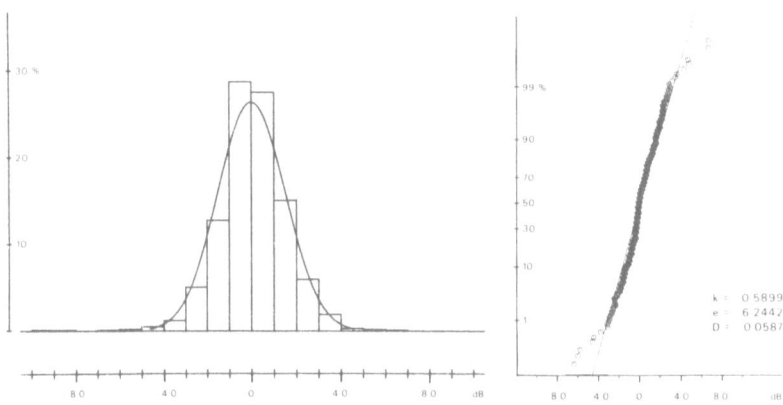

Fig. 2. Histogram and probability plot of the deviations (y) at the center. Number of observations: 6010; standard deviation: 1.51 dB.

STANDARDIZED DEVIATIONS IN THE MIDPERIPHERY

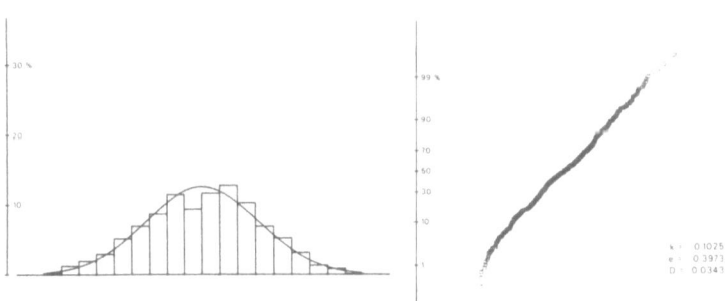

Fig. 3. Histogram and probability plot of the standardized deviations (z) in the midperiphery. Number of observations: 5910; standard deviation: 0.96 dB.

As the majority of the visual fields were normal and as normal fields have smaller scatter, a positive kurtosis results (Figs. 1 and 2) which disappears by standardization (Figs. 3 and 4). A very important finding is the fact that there is never a relevant skewness. This means that the distribution of the deviations is more or less symmetrical.

We have to emphasize, however, that absolute scotomas were excluded.

21

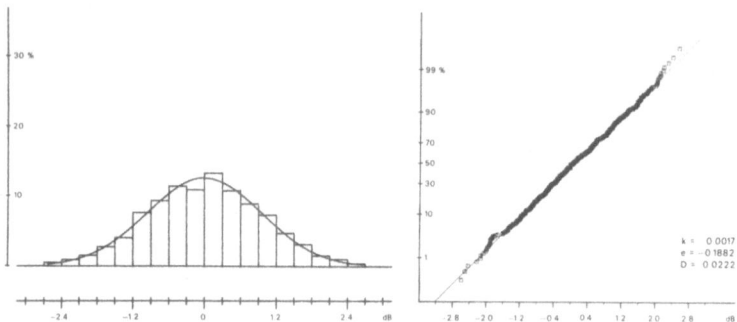

Fig. 4. Histogram and probability plot of the standardized deviations (z) at the center. Number of observations: 6010; standard deviation: 0.96 dB.

DEVIATIONS IN THE MIDPERIPHERY IN NORMAL VISUAL FIELDS

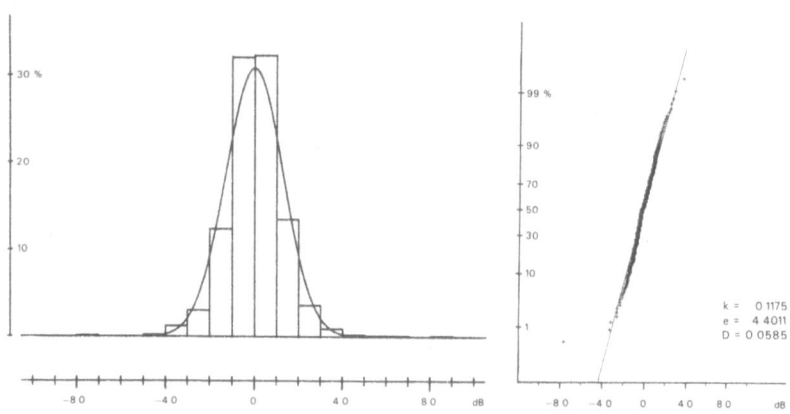

Fig. 5. Histogram and probability plot of the deviations (y) is the midperiphery in normal visual fields. Number of observations: 2740; standard deviation: 1.29 dB.

There is no relevant difference between the midperiphery of a visual field (Figs. 2 and 4) and the center (Figs. 1 and 3). Test locations lying more in the periphery were not analyzed. The deviations in normal visual field areas were smaller and their distributions were closer to normal (Fig. 5) and the deviations in relative scotomas (Fig. 6).

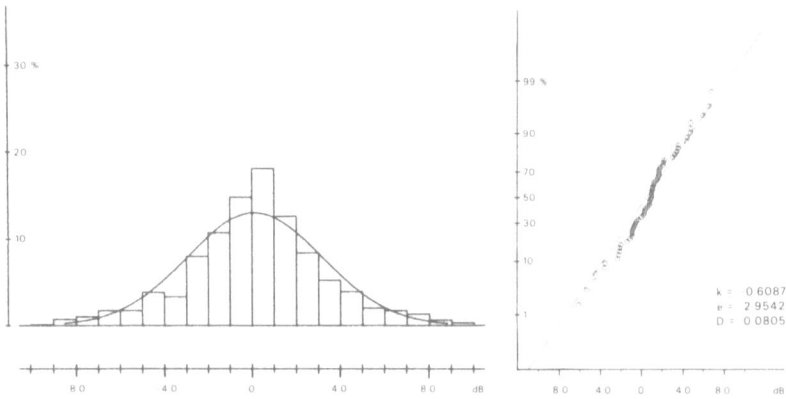

Fig. 6. Histogram and probability plot of the deviations (y) in the midperiphery in relative scotomas. Number of observations: 690; standard deviation: 3.07 dB.

CONCLUSION

The frequency distribution of the deviations of the single measurements from their means in automated static perimetry, measuring with an up and down (Octopus) bracketing strategy (5), is very close to normal. If absolute scotomas are excluded, the distribution is symmetrical (no relevant skewness).

By pooling heterogeneous material, we observe a positive or negative kurtosis. This can be avoided by taking standardized deviations. There is no substantial difference between the midperiphery and the center. The deviations in a normal area are smaller and closer to a normal distribution than the deviations in relative scotomas.

REFERENCES

1. Bebié, H., Fankhauser, F. and Spahr, J. Static perimetry: accuracy and fluctuations. Acta Ophthalmol. 54: 339–348 (1976).
2. Fankhauser, F. Problems related to the design of automatic perimeters. Doc. Ophthalmol. 47: 89–138 (1979).
3. Flammer, J., Drance, S. M. and Schulzer, M. The estimation and testing of the components of long-term fluctuation of the differential light threshold. Doc. Ophthalmol. Proc. Series 35: 383–389 (1983).
4. Flammer, J., Drance, S.M., Fankhauser, F. and Augustiny, L. Factors of the short-term fluctuation of the differential light threshold in automatic static perimetry. Arch. Ophthalmol. (in press).

5. Jenni, A., Flammer, J., Funkhouser, A. and Fankhauser, F. Special Octopus software for clinical investigation. Doc. Ophthalmol. Proc. Series 35: 351–356 (1983).

Authors' address:
University Eye Clinic
Inselspital
CH-3010 Berne, Switzerland

FLUCTUATIONS IN THRESHOLD AND EFFECT OF FATIGUE IN AUTOMATED STATIC PERIMETRY
(with the OCTOPUS 201)

P.A. RABINEAU, B.P. GLOOR* and H.J. TOBLER

(*Basle, Switzerland*)

ABSTRACT

Fluctuations in the threshold and effect of fatigue on threshold were determined by means of automated static perimetry with the Octopus in normals:

(1) In 9 persons, profiles extending from the center to 30° were examined in 12 meridians with the F_2 program. There is no age dependent increase of fluctuations over the age period from 28–42 years. *The fluctuations are higher in the central portion* than in the two other portions which is an unexpected finding.

(2) Three individuals were tested 12 times in a row with F_2 program during $2\frac{1}{2}$–$3\frac{1}{2}$ hours. Mean fluctuation of the best performing individual was 1.59, of the worst performing individual 1.95 dB. No significant increase of fluctuation over time could be demonstrated.

(3) Seven persons underwent 4 examinations by program 31 in a row. The whole examination time for each person was about 1 hour. Changes in sensitivity and fluctuations were neglegible.

For the practical test situation it may be concluded that, during a period of 1 hour, 'fatigue' influences neither the fluctuation nor the threshold determination in normals.

INTRODUCTION

In disturbed visual fields (13, 14), especially in fields of patients with glaucomatous field loss, short-term fluctuations or scatter in threshold of sensitivity are increased (3–6, 11). Recent investigations indicate that increased short-term fluctuation in a region of otherwise normal sensitivity may also be the earliest detectable changes in fields of glaucoma patients (4, 11). The same applies for decrease of sensitivity when testing is prolonged (8). To have stronger criteria by which to separate normal from diseased visual fields as

---

*Reprint requests to: Prof. B.P. Gloor, Univ.-Augenklinik, Augenspital, Mittlere Strasse 91, CH-4056 Basle/Switzerland.

Heijl, A. and Greve, E.L. (eds.), Proceedings of the 6th Int. Visual Field Symposium.
© *1985, Dr W. Junk Publishers, Dordrecht, The Netherlands. ISBN 978-94-010-8932-6*

provided by means of static threshold perimetry with the Octopus, fluctuations and influence of prolonged testing or 'fatigue' were investigated in this study.

PATIENTS AND METHODS

Criteria for admission to the study were visual acuity on both eyes 1.0 (20/20) or more with less than 1 dioptre spherical equivalent of correction, refracting media clear, I.O.P = 12–17 mm Hg measured by applanation tonometry, and cup/disc-ratio ≤ 0.3. Only right eyes have been tested.

Experiment 1. Nine normal persons 28–42 years old, 5 women and 4 men, were recruited, 4 of them familiar with Octopus testing, 5 of them not. Profiles extending 30° from the centre to the periphery were examined in 12 meridians with the F_2 program of the Octopus 201 (angle between meridians 15°, resolution 1°, diameter of the test object 0.43°, every test point tested twice). The smallest step for threshold determination was 2 dB; with the retesting logic built into the Octopus this leads to a determination in one dB steps.

In this first experiment the term 'fluctuation' in one profile is used as defined in the manual for the F program as 'RMS fluctuations' by the following formula (1)

$$\sigma^2 = \frac{1}{\Sigma\, n_i - 1} \cdot \Sigma\, (n_i - 1) \cdot \delta_i^2 \qquad n_i > 1$$

σ_i = standard deviation of the distribution of the single local results

Not more than 2 profiles were done per day. Investigation time was never longer than 30 minutes.

Experiment 2. Three of the 9 aforementioned individuals were tested 12 times in the row with the F_2 program and RMS fluctuations, as defined in experiment 1, were computed to determine a possible time-dependent change of these fluctuations.

Experiment 3. Eight of the 9 individuals mentioned in experiment 1 underwent 4 uninterrupted examinations with program 31 of the Octopus. The whole examination lasted about 1 hour. RMS fluctuations, as obtained from the 10 points with double threshold determinations, and the mean sensitivity of each individual and of the whole group in the four consecutive examinations were determined. The mean sensitivity was determined by program delta series.

RESULTS

Experiment 1. As shown in Fig. 1, when 'RMS fluctuation' is determined in the 12 meridians of each individual over a profile of 30°, 'RMS fluctuation' lies between 1.4 and 2.2 dB.

Note: there is a significant difference ($p < 0.01$; Wilcoxon-Man-Whitney test) between the performance of the 4 individuals familiar with the Octopus (3 technicians, 1 Ph.D.) with a RMS value of 0.47 dB and that of the others with a mean of 1.91 dB. This is interpreted as a learning effects. There is no age-dependent increase of fluctuations in this group of individuals 28 to 42 years old.

In Fig. 2 the sum of fluctuations, which in these calculations are the sums of the means of the differences between 2 determinations of threshold in the same point, are determined in 3 different circular portions of the visual fields (central circle 0–10°, intermediate portion 10–20°, outer portion 20–30°). Each individual shows the lowest fluctuations in the most eccentric, the highest fluctuations in the most central portion ($p < 0.01$; one-sided sign test). This is still the case if the meridians passing through the blind spot are omitted.

In Fig. 3 the sums of RMS fluctuations are analyzed with regard to the meridian of the profile and eccentricity. Again the highest fluctuations are in the central 10° circle, only exceeded by the fluctuations in the intermediate and outer portions in the meridians passing through or near the blind spot.

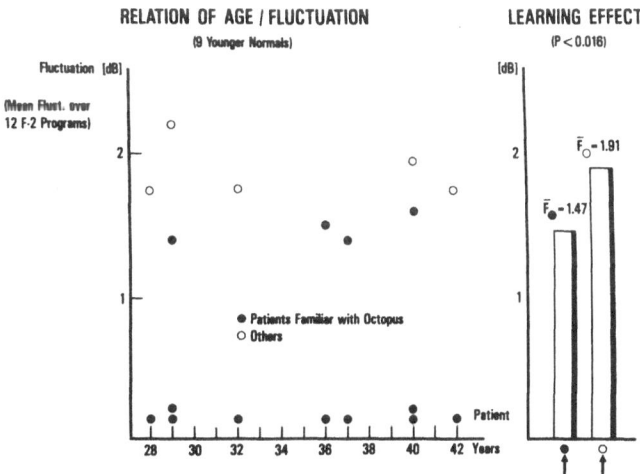

Fig. 1. Relation between age and fluctuations. Mean fluctuations over 12 F_2 programs are shown. Fluctuations do not change over the age from 28–42 years but are significantly different in the 2 groups of individuals shown, the one not, the other very familiar with Octopus testing.

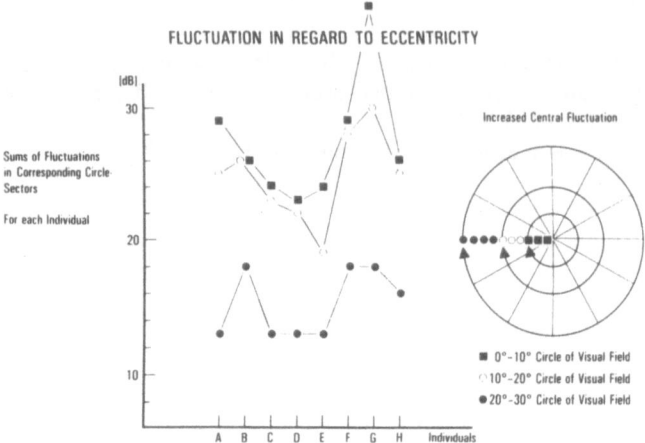

Fig. 2. Fluctuations with regard to excentricity are shown. The figure demonstrates that in each individual fluctuations are highest in the central circle somewhat lower between the 10 and 20° circles and lowest between the 20 and 30° circles.

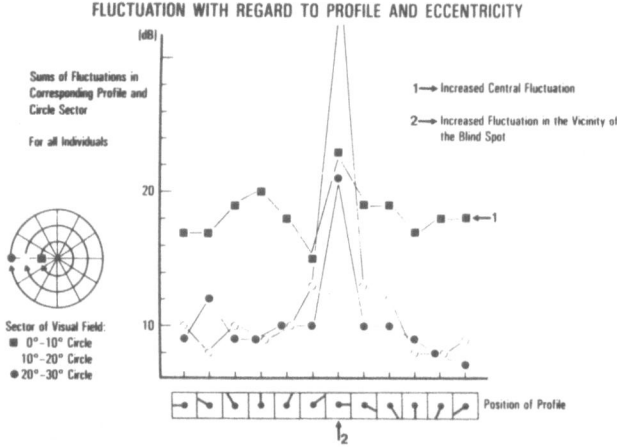

Fig. 3. The fluctuations with regard to localization of the profile in the 30° field and excentricity are shown. Independent of location of the profile, the fluctuations are highest in the innermost circle, except in the profiles passing through or near the blind spot.

Experiment 2. When in 3 individuals a 30° profile was tested 12 times in a row with the F_2 program, 2 performed the test in $2\frac{1}{4}$ hours, 1 in $3\frac{1}{2}$ hours. In Fig. 4a the results of the best-performing individual are shown. The fluctuations in the single profiles and the means in series of 3 profiles are shown.

28

The overall mean is listed. The performance is remarkably constant, the steepness of the slope is negligible, no effect of fatigue is detectable. There is no correlation between fluctuation and number of examinations ($r = 0.04$). Maximum fluctuation was 2.0 dB, minimum fluctuation in the best profile was 0.2 dB, the mean was 1.59 dB, the standard deviation 0.26 dB.

In Fig. 4b the results of the individual who used the longest period of time to perform the 12 profiles are shown. There is a slope showing a 2% increase of fluctuation over the whole period, not statistically significant ($r = 0.25$). Maximum fluctuation was 2.4, minimum fluctuation, 0.5, and mean fluctuation, 1.95 ± 0.31 dB.

In Fig. 4c the results of the worst-performing individual are shown. The slope shows a 5% increase of fluctuation over time, but again not only a statistically significant level, maximum fluctuation being 2.4, minimum fluctuation, 0.4, and mean fluctuation, 0.93 ± 0.39 dB. Note that this individual performed somewhat better in the last series than in the third series.

Experiment 3. When 8 individuals underwent 4 uninterrupted examinations with program 31 of the Octopus, the whole examination for each person lasted about 1 hour. RMS fluctuations as revealed in the 10 points with double threshold determination in program 31 and sensitivity in the 4 consecutive examinations are shown in Fig. 5. Fluctuations do not increase significantly over time, and sensitivity does not decrease if tested over a time period of 1 hour. The change of mean sensitivity for each individual is most of the time very small and every hour below 2 dB.

DISCUSSION

The aim of this study was to establish a base to separate scatter of differential light sensitivity and effect of prolonged testing (fatigue) of normal fields from that of diseased visual fields, especially if fields of glaucoma suspects and patients with glaucoma are investigated with F_2 programs and with the Octopus programs most frequently used (programs 31 and 32).

The scatter of the differential light threshold observed during a single visual field test was called short-term fluctuations (SF) by Bebie and Fankhauser (1) and Flammer et al. (3). In another publication, Flammer et al. (2) restricted the duration of the visual field examination for the definition of short-term fluctuation to approximately 20 minutes. In addition to that, Flammer et al. (3) defined the long-term fluctuation (LF) as the variation in measurements over time, when the variation due to repeated measurements at a given time, short-term fluctuation has been removed. In light of this, it has to be emphasized that when performing only 2 F programs per day in about $\frac{1}{2}$ hour, for several weeks, two new profiles were determined in every testing session. Therefore the determination of scatter in the set-up of our experiment number 1 is always the determination of another short-term fluctuation in a new profile. Then the amount of scatter or short-term fluctuations determined in this way by F_2 programs, with an amount of 1.47 dB ± 0.09 in individuals familiar with Octopus testing and 1.91 ± 0.20 in

TEST OF FATIGUE

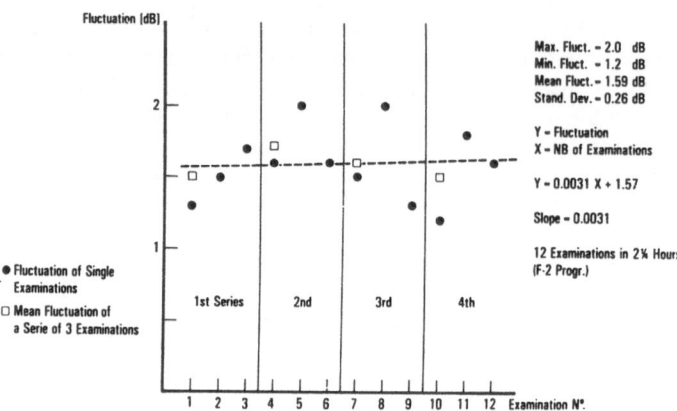

TEST OF FATIGUE

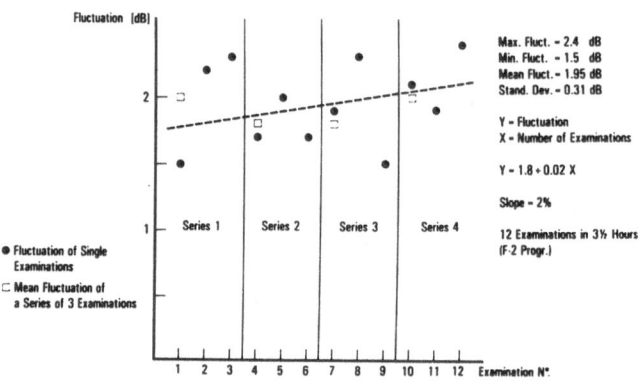

TEST OF FATIGUE

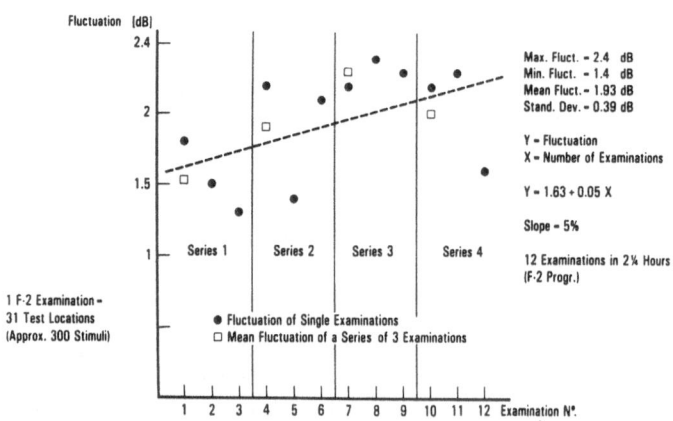

30

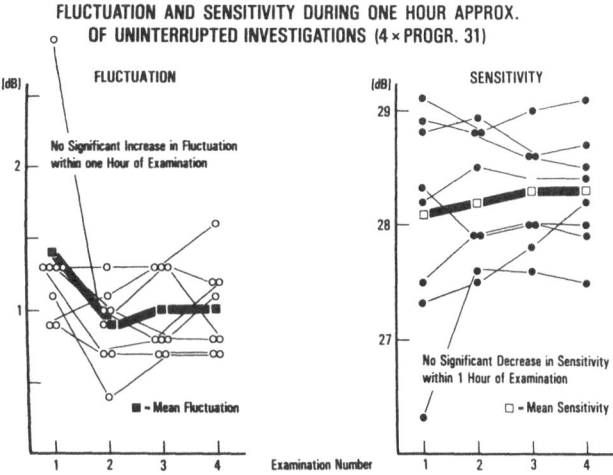

Fig. 5. The performance of the 8 individuals and the mean of all of them is shown. Mean fluctuations decrease from the first to second examination, but then remain constant and are very small. Mean sensitivity stays almost constant for all 4 examinations.

individuals not used to Octopus testing and 1.7 ± 0.26 for the whole group, differs little from the value of 1.6 dB as determined by Flammer et al. (4) with program JO (9). Our findings that differential light sensitivity threshold does not change over time during four consecutive test sessions lasting about one hour (Fig. 4) in the normal, at least in the age period from 28 to 42 years, are also in good agreement with the findings of Flammer et al. (4) and Heijl (7). It is clear that the values of normals, glaucoma suspects, and glaucomas overlap, and in an individual border-line case assignment to a certain group is difficult.

The second experiment, the test of fatigue, then shows that short-term fluctuations determined in every single field test consisting of examination of a 30° long profile with the F_2 program (lasting $11\frac{1}{4}$ to $17\frac{1}{2}$ minutes) did not grow consistently. The calculation of the slope shows an increase of 0.3 to 5%, but the regression coefficient for these slopes are extremely weak. This means that in a normal, well-motivated individual the scatter does not grow over time and does not diminish the power of the statement of the test over a time period of $2\frac{1}{2}$ to $3\frac{1}{2}$ hours. It should be noted, however, that the results

Fig. 4a–c. Twelve F_2 profiles have been tested in a row. The examinations are numbered. For each series of three examinations the mean is determined. Figure 4a: the best performing individual shows mean fluctuations of 1.59 ± 0.26 dB. The steepness of the slope is negligible (0.0031). The performance does not change considerably during the whole test period of $2\frac{1}{4}$ hours. Figure 4b shows the performance of the slowest working individual, who needed $3\frac{1}{2}$ hours to complete the test. There is a slope of 2% (not statistically significant). This also applies for the slope in figure 4c. Note that in this figure, performance at the end of the test series 4 is better than series 3.

shown in the experiments so far tell nothing about the behaviour of *sensitivity* in time. This is only the case in experiment 3, which clearly demonstrates that when program 31 was tested 4 times in a row the mean sensitivity did not decrease but rather increased slightly. In a given individual the change was never more than 1 dB per point, in most subjects approximately 0.5 dB. Also in this experiment short-term fluctuations did not increase from the first to the fourth examination.

No signs of fatigue, when testing the whole 30° field for 1 hour and during $2\frac{1}{4}$ to $2\frac{1}{2}$ hours tests along 30° profiles seems to be a characteristic feature of so-called 'normals'. Fatigue could therefore help to separate patients with glaucomatous field loss from normals, as proposed by Heijl and Drance (7). When they repeatedly tested, with the Competer, 6 points in an area close to an existing visual field defect or a suspect area close to an existing visual field defect during or in other more normals pacts of the field $\frac{1}{2}$ hour, they found that an increment of the differential light sensitivity threshold during prolonged continuous recordings is common in patients with glaucoma, and that areas in relative scotoma or immediately adjacent to it show a more pronounced deterioration of threshold than normal points far away from field defects. But caution is indicated. Time or prolongation of perimetry may not be the only cause of the findings presented by Heijl and Drance (8). In some curves it could be difficult to separate local scatter from time-dependent decrease of sensitivity, which results from some sort of exhaustion. Some of the curves found by Heijl and Drance (7) could be explained by the tremendous scatter of threshold found in relative scotomas tested with F_4 programs (5, 6, 11, 12). Nevertheless, fatigue plays an important role, as a subsequent publication will confirm (12).

With the program JO, Flammer et al. (3) could not reveal any dependence of the size of local short-term fluctuation or scatter and the location in the visual field. But if the field is tested with a much finer grid, as was done in experiment 1, an unexpected finding shows up: fluctuations are highest in the central 10° circle, lower between 10 and 20°, and even lower between the 20 and 30° circles. From our investigations with F_2 programs on glaucomatous fields (11, 12), we would agree with Flammer et al. (3) on the statement that at least in glaucomatous fields the lower the sensitivity the higher the short-term fluctuations are. This also holds true when the results are averaged, but may not be the case in a given spot (11, 12). We therefore would expect that if there are differences of scatter in circles of different eccentricity, the lowest fluctuations should be in the center. Why is this not the case? Is it due to the steepness of the threshold profile in the center of the mountain of vision, where small changes of fixation could provoke larger changes of threshold? Further investigations are necessary to clarify these findings.

The main conclusion we draw from this study is the following: because in a normal individual a test session of at least 1 hour's duration does neither considerably influence scatter of differential light sensitivity threshold (short-term fluctuations) nor sensitivity, then a test period of about $\frac{1}{2}$ hour should give reliable data from a normally attentive individual who is a glaucoma suspect or has glaucoma. If scatter above normal (more than 2.5 dB) is then found, this is most likely a sign of disease.

32

REFERENCES

1. Bebie, H., Fankhauser, F. and Spahr, J. Static perimetry: Accuracy and fluctuations. Acta Ophthal. 54: 339–348 (1976).
2. Flammer, J., Drance, S.M. and Schulzer, M. The estimation and testing of the components of long-term fluctuation of the differential light threshold. Docum. Ophthalmol. Proc. Series 35: 383–389 (1983).
3. Flammer, J., Drance, S.M. and Zulauf, M. The short- and long-term fluctuation of the differential light threshold in patients with glaucoma, normal controls and glaucoma suspects. Arch. Ophthalmol. (in print).
4. Flammer, J., Drance, S.M., Fankhauser, F. and Augustiny, L. The differential light threshold in automated static perimetry. Arch. Ophthalmol. (in print).
5. Gloor, B. Die Computerperimetrie in der langfristigen Beurteilung des Glaukoms. Krieglstein, G.K., Leydhecker, W. Medikamentöse Glaukomtherapie. J.F. Bergmann Verlag München. 59–72 (1982).
6. Gloor, B., Stürmer, J. and Vökt, B. Was hat die automatisierte Perimetrie mit dem Octopus für neue Kenntnisse über glaukomatöse Gesichtsfeldveränderungen gebracht? Klin. Mbl. Augenheilk. 184: 249–253 (1984).
7. Heijl, A. Time changes of contrast thresholds during automatic perimetry. Acta Ophthalmol. 55: 696–708 (1977).
8. Heijl, A. and Drance, S.M. Changes in differential threshold patients with glaucoma during prolonged perimetry. British Journal of Ophthal. 76: 512–516 (1983).
9. Jenni, A., Flammer, J., Funkhouser, A. and Fankhauser, F. Special Octopus Software for Clinical Investigation. Doc. Ophthalmol. Proc. Series 35: 351–357.
10. Langerhorst, Chr., van den Berg, T.J.T.P. and Greve, E.L. Schätzung der Fluktationsfaktoren bei Glaukompatienten. in 'Neuere Entwicklungen in der Ophthalmologie', ed. H.J. Merté und M. Mertz. Beihefte Klin. Mbl. Augenheilk. (in print).
11. Stürmer, J., Gloor, B. and Tobler, H.J. Wie sehen Glaukomgesichtsfelder wirklich aus? Klin. Mbl. Augenheilk. 184: (1984).
12. Stürmer, J., Gloor, B. and Tobler, H.J. The glaucomatous visual field in detail as revealed by the Octopus F-programs. Doc. Ophthalmol. Proc. Series (in print).
13. Wildberger, H. Zum Nachweis der zentralen Empfindlichkeitsminderung bei Opticus-Neuropathien mit der Computerperimetrie (Octopus) und mit den evozierten Potentialen (VEP). Klin. Nbl. Augenheilk. 1984 (in print).
14. Wildberger, H. Neuropathies of the optic nerve and visual evoked potentials with special reference to color vision and differential light threshold. Doc. Ophthalmol. (in print).

Authors' addresses:
P.A. Rabineau
B.P. Gloor
Department of Ophthalmology
University of Basle
(Chairman: Prof. B. Gloor)
H.J. Tobler
SANDOZ AG Basle, Switzerland

A SIMPLE ROUTINE FOR DEMONSTRATING INCREASED THRESHOLD SCATTER BY COMPARING STORED COMPUTER FIELDS

ANDERS HEIJL

(*Malmö, Sweden*)

ABSTRACT

It has previously been shown that before a glaucomatous visual field defect can be clearly demonstrated, the same area often shows increased variation at repeated threshold determinations. Computerized perimeters with the capability of storing visual fields can easily be programmed to compare and analyze consecutive fields from the same eye in various ways. By using a programme where the range and standard deviation of threshold values measured at consecutive examinations are printed out for all test points, areas with increased scatter can be easily identified. In early glaucoma these types of printouts may demonstrate problem areas before clearcut visual field defects are obvious.

INTRODUCTION

It has previously been shown, with manual perimetric techniques, that clearcut glaucomatous field defects often are preceded by increased threshold variation in the same area (4).

In computerized perimetry threshold values are available in a numerical format enabling statistical analysis. Several different papers have also described such analyses e.g. for determining changes in visual fields over time (2, 3) or for diagnosing hemianopsia (1). It is logical to use the data handling capabilities of the computer system of automatic, computerized perimeters to demonstrate areas of increased scatter on repeated threshold tests.

METHODS AND RESULTS

Stored threshold values from several identical tests of the same eye are retrieved from the data storage medium of the automatic perimeter. The ranges and/or standard deviations of the measured thresholds at each point are calculated by the perimeter computer. These values are printed out using the same pattern as that used for the regular field chart. In this way data from

Heijl, A. and Greve, E.L. (eds.), Proceedings of the 6th Int. Visual Field Symposium.
© *1985, Dr W. Junk Publishers, Dordrecht, The Netherlands. ISBN 978-94-010-8932-6*

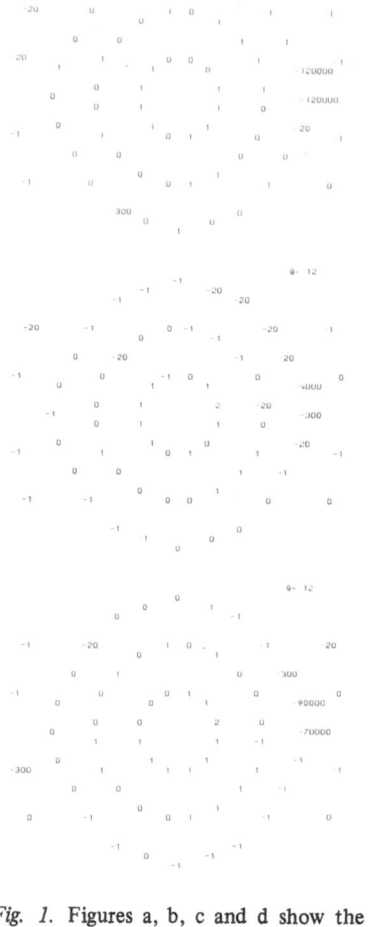

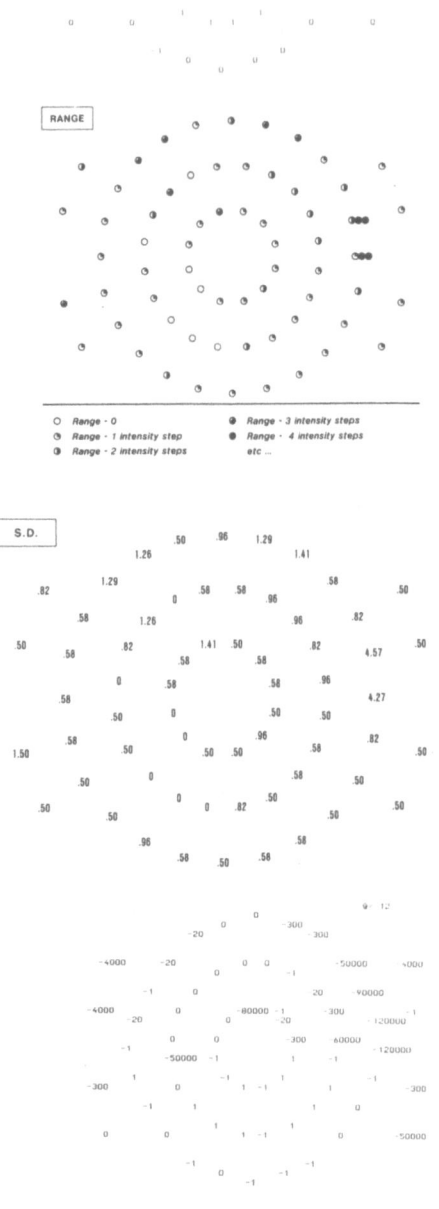

Fig. 1. Figures a, b, c and d show the results of four central Competer threshold tests of the same eye in a patient with suspect/early glaucoma (March 82, April 82, Sept 82 and Sept 83 respectively). None of the four fields is convincingly pathological. A symbol representation of the ranges of the thresholds in these four charts are displayed in e, while the standard deviations are shown in f. Ranges and standard deviations are expressed in Competer intensity steps, each unit corresponding to 0.3 log units. Variation is larger in the superior than in the inferior half of the field. A later (Dec 83), clearly pathological field is shown in g. The defects have to a large extent appeared in or in the vicinity of points previously showing high threshold variation.

36

several visual fields are summarized into one printout. The local threshold variation between consecutive tests is thus graphically displayed. In early glaucoma this may demonstrate areas of increased scatter before clearcut visual field defects are present (Fig. 1).

DISCUSSION

The number of computerized perimeters capable of storing test results on floppy discs is rapidly growing. Such instruments may easily be programmed to automatically retrieve all fields from a certain eye and to perform and print out results of the described analyses. Variation is high in relative field defects and also at the borders of absolute defects. It is of course more interesting that this technique may identify areas with high threshold scatter in cases of early glaucoma, before single field charts can be regarded as clearly pathological (Fig. 1). Obviously almost the same impression may be obtained without the described computerized analyses, by scrutinizing and comparing each individual field chart. This, however, is less exact and more time-consuming. The value and convenience of the described approach should be greatest in cases where a large number of field tests have been performed. The results might be improved further, if the result of each field test is corrected for the synchronous component of the long term fluctuation before the ranges and standard deviations are calculated. The results of the scatter analyses can be displayed in several different ways, partly depending on the capabilities of the printer of the automated perimeter. Symbol or greyscale printouts might be preferable to the numerical mode in Fig. 1f.

Even if not accepting increased scatter as a diagnostic sign of early glaucoma it is likely that directed, high-resolution perimetry performed in areas with increased threshold variation may be able to document localized field loss earlier than a standard test.

ACKNOWLEDGEMENT

This study was supported by the Järnhardt foundation.

REFERENCES

1. Bynke, H. A statistical analysis of normal visual fields and hemianopsias recorded by the computerized perimeter 'Competer'. Neuro-Ophthalmology (Amsterdam) 2: 129–137 (1983).
2. Fankhauser, F. and Jenni, A. Programs Sargon and Delta. Two new principles for the automated analysis of the visual field. Albrecht v Graefes Arch. klin. exp. Ophthalmol. 216: 41–48 (1981).
3. Holmin, C. and Krakau, C.E.T. Regression analysis of the central visual field in chronic glaucoma cases. A follow-up study using sutomatic perimetry. Acta Ophthalmol 60: 267–274 (1982).

4. Werner, E.B. and Drance, S.M. Early visual field disturbances in glaucoma. Arch. Ophthalmol. 95: 1173–1175 (1977).

Author's address:
Department of Ophthalmology
Malmö General Hospital
S-21401 Malmö, Sweden

PROBABILITY MAPS FOR EVALUATING AUTOMATED VISUAL FIELDS

BERNARD SCHWARTZ and PAUL NAGIN

(*Boston, Mass., U.S.A.*)

ABSTRACT

A computer system has been devised for the Octopus 2000R automated perimeter to transmit, analyze, display, and print statistical evaluations of visual field data. By using this system and its specific programs, three graphic displays have been devised to determine probabilities and directions of changes of visual fields. With an initial visual field, such as that using program 31, a probability contour plot is obtained in comparison to a reference population to determine by probability level whether the visual field has significant areas of abnormality. Two approaches can be used to indicate whether there is a change with visual fields over time: paired t test and regression analysis. If a paired t test is appropriate, selected areas of visual fields are compared to obtain a probability area plot. The t values and their probabilities are combined to obtain a three-dimensional plot indicating direction and significance. A similar procedure is used for a regression analysis: a contour plot of the probability values associated with the slopes of the regression lines is displayed. The slope values and their probabilities can be combined into a three-dimensional graphic display to indicate significance and direction of change. These graphic displays can provide a data analysis of visual fields that is easily visualized and clinically useful.

INTRODUCTION

The clinician evaluating a visual field faces two different tasks: to determine whether a patient's initial visual field is normal or abnormal, and to resolve whether a sequential visual field shows a significant change with time compared to one or several previous visual fields.

Unfortunately, the techniques for such clinical evaluations are somewhat limited. An initial visual field obtained from the Octopus 2000 R automated perimeter requires a judgment of abnormality based on mean normal values for each decade stored in the memory of the perimeter. The population of normal subjects is limited, however, and the subjects may not have been fully evaluated for absence of ocular disease. For a change in time of several visual

Heijl, A. and Greve, E.L. (eds.), Proceedings of the 6th Int. Visual Field Symposium.
© *1985, Dr W. Junk Publishers, Dordrecht, The Netherlands. ISBN 978-94-010-8932-6*

fields, regression techniques have been used for the sum of thresholds (4). For comparing two visual fields or the averages of several visual fields, the paired t test is used (2).

This paper describes graphic techniques to portray probability values for the degree of abnormality of an initial visual field and for significant changes in visual fields with time. The graphic display is presented on a computer terminal and can easily be evaluated for clinical purposes.

METHODS

A. Computer system

The computer system that we use for transmission, display, analysis, and printout of visual field data has been described in detail elsewhere (6). Briefly, it consists of an Octopus 2000R automated perimeter (Interzeag, Schlieren, Switzerland) transmitting to a VAX 11/780 mainframe computer (Digital Equipment Corp., Maynard, Massachusetts). An ATARI microcomputer (Atari Corp., Sunnyvale, California) instructs the VAX to transmit and analyze the data. The analysis is then displayed on the ATARI and can be printed out on a high-speed printer.

B. Probability percentile map for initial visual field

In order to obtain percentile values for the frequency distribution of thresholds for program 31 of the Octopus perimeter, the mean values as printed out on the Octopus for each decade are obtained. It is assumed that the frequency distributions for these mean values are Gaussian, or normally distributed. The standard deviation of each threshold value is ± 2.4 decibels (1). From this distribution, percentiles of 0.1, 1, 5, and 10 are calculated and stored in the computer memory. A program 31 visual field for each patient is obtained under reasonable conditions, that is, the root-mean-square (RMS) value of about 2.0 or less and the number of false positives and negatives less than 3. Each threshold value is then classified in relation to its percentile rank for normal values. Comparison of the obtained visual field with the reference values is then displayed by appropriate programs as a probability percentile map. The percentiles of probability ranges are greater than 10, 5 to 10, 1 to 4.9, 0.1 to 0.9, and less than 0.1. Values are connected by linear interpolation and the results displayed in gray scale or color with an appropriate printout.

C. Probability area map for comparison of two visual fields obtained at different times

For comparison of two visual fields taken at different times or the averages of two sets of visual fields, the thresholds obtained by program 31 are grouped into seven areas (Fig. 1). The selection arrangement of the groups is based primarily on the data by Gramer and colleagues (3) and the concepts

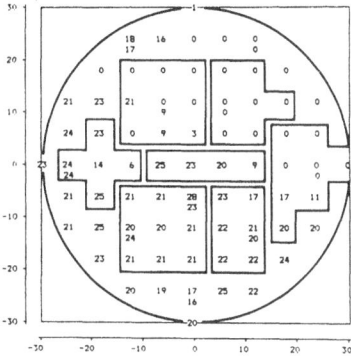

Fig. 1. Groups of thresholds obtained with program 31.

of Wirtschafter and associates (7). Based on our experience and that of others (5), peripheral values for the visual fields are excluded from the groupings since these values often show artifactual abnormalities. The nasal group is selected to detect changes in the nasal area (e.g., a nasal step); the superior and inferior areas are selected primarily for the detection of arcuate and paracentral scotomas.

For a patient with two visual fields, the first and second fields are compared using the paired t test within each area. An average of several previous fields can also be used for comparison to a recent field. The probabilities obtained using the paired t test are then displayed as a gray scale or in color for each area, and the t value, with its sign, can also be displayed. Both plots (probability area and t value area) can be combined into one three-dimensional plot to show progressive loss or improvement in an area of a visual field.

D. *Probability contour map for evaluating change of at least five visual fields with time*

When a series of five or more visual fields has been obtained, if the thresholds of the individual points can be approximated by a linear model, a linear regression analysis can be used. The linear regression models are calculated for each point in a program 31 visual field. The slopes of the regression lines are calculated, and the probability that a slope is significantly different from zero is determined. The probability values are then displayed as a gray scale or in color at each point (and the slope value with its sign can also be displayed). The probability values chosen are greater than 0.10, 0.10 to 0.05, 0.049 to 0.01, 0.009 to 0.001, and less than 0.001. The contour map can appear in color or gray scale. Finally, the two maps are combined into one three-dimensional plot to indicate the probability of a significant change in an area of a visual field as well as the direction of the change.

41

RESULTS

A. Percentile probability map for the initial visual field

Figure 2 is the gray-scale printout of a glaucomatous patient, and Fig. 3 shows the actual threshold values. There is a nasal defect, probably with superior and inferior paracentral scotomas. Figure 4 is the probability percentile plot for this visual field. This patient's RMS was 1.8, and the number of false positives was zero; there was one false negative.

B. Probability area map for comparison of two visual fields obtained at different times

Figure 5 shows the gray-scale printout of the visual field of a glaucomatous patient prior to surgery, while Fig. 6 shows the visual field of the same

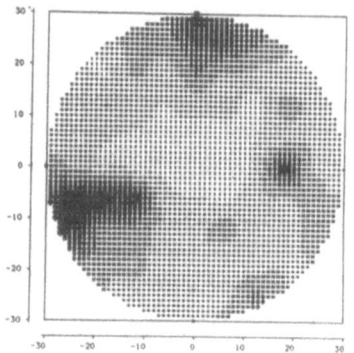

Fig. 2. Visual field, in gray scale, of a glaucomatous patient.

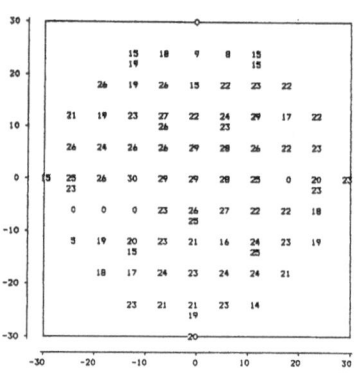

Fig. 3. Actual threshold values, same patient as in Fig. 2.

42

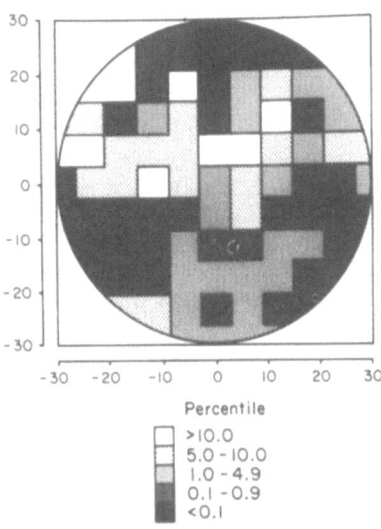

Percentile
- >10.0
- 5.0 - 10.0
- 1.0 - 4.9
- 0.1 - 0.9
- <0.1

Fig. 4. Probability percentile map for visual field (same patient as in Figs. 2 and 3).

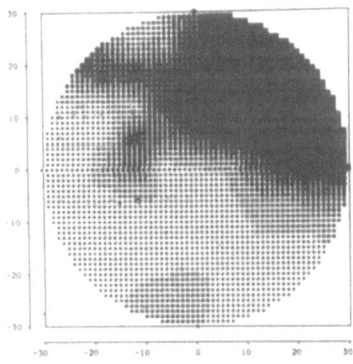

Fig. 5. This gray-scale printout of a visual field of a glaucomatous patient was obtained just before surgery.

patient after a trabeculectomy and indicates regression of the visual field loss. Figure 7 is a probability area plot comparing these two visual fields, showing significant improvement of the visual field in the superior and nasal areas. Figure 8 combines the probability are a plot and the t value plot to show the significant change and direction of the change in the visual fields.

43

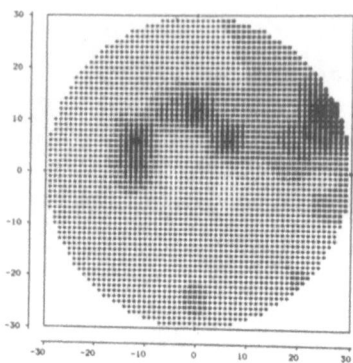

Fig. 6. Same patient as in Fig. 5; note regression of visual field loss after trabeculectomy.

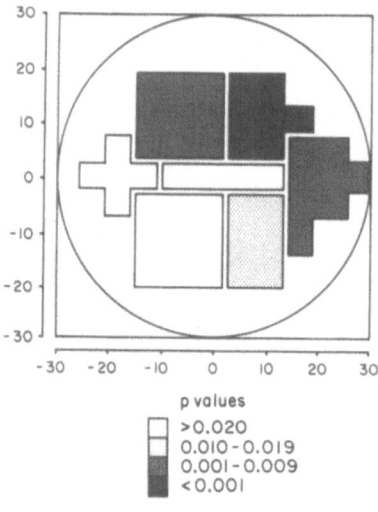

p values

□ >0.020
▨ 0.010-0.019
▦ 0.001-0.009
■ <0.001

Fig. 7. Probability area plot comparing visual fields shown in Figs. 5 and 6.

C. Probability contour map using regression analysis for evaluating change of visual fields with time

Figure 9 is a plot of the sums of the thresholds for the total visual field, versus time, for a glaucomatous patient being followed for 10 months with a series of five fields. Figure 10 is the probability contour plot based on the probability that the slope of the regression line at each point in the visual field versus time is significantly different from zero. The plot in Fig. 11 combines probability and direction of change.

44

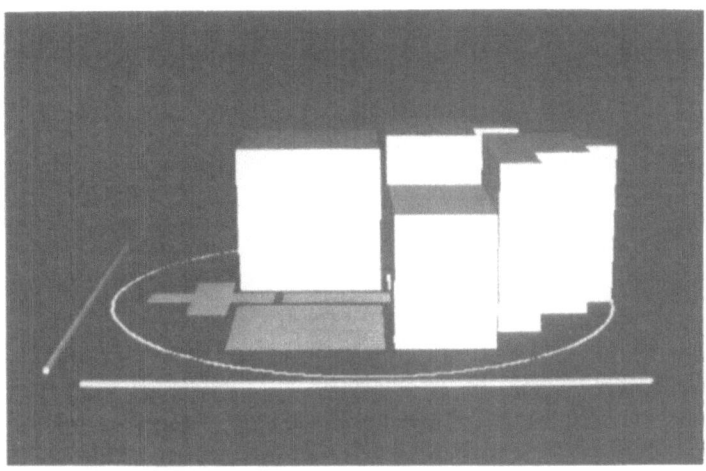

Fig. 8. Three-dimensional representation of results of paired t tests. Height above horizontal axis is inversely related to p value and represents positive t values.

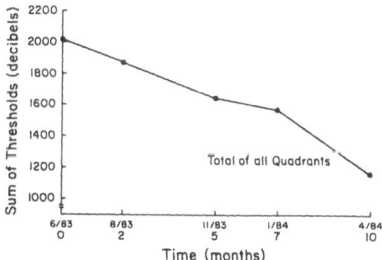

Fig. 9. Sums of thresholds for total visual field versus time, for glaucomatous patient followed for 10 months by five visual fields.

DISCUSSION

When large volumes of clinical data accumulated over a period of time require analysis, then graphic displays of significant changes are clinically more useful for interpretation than a series of numbers. If the graphic displays are appropriate, one should be able statistically to ascertain a significant abnormality based on the values of a visual field compared to a normal population or a significant change in a visual field over time. Furthermore, the graphic displays can differentiate specific areas of visual fields that are changing significantly. This paper demonstrates how graphic displays, based on statistical principles, can be formulated and used.

45

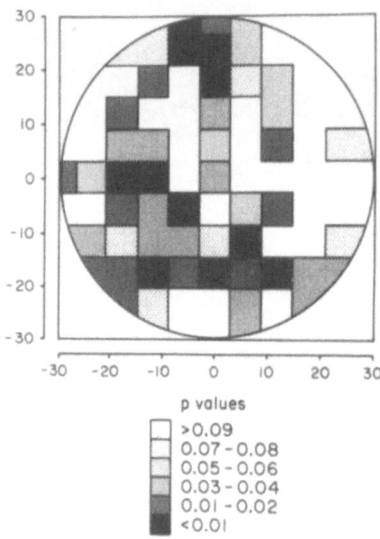

Fig. 10. Probability contour plot for patient described by Fig. 9, based on probability that slopes of regression lines are significantly different from zero.

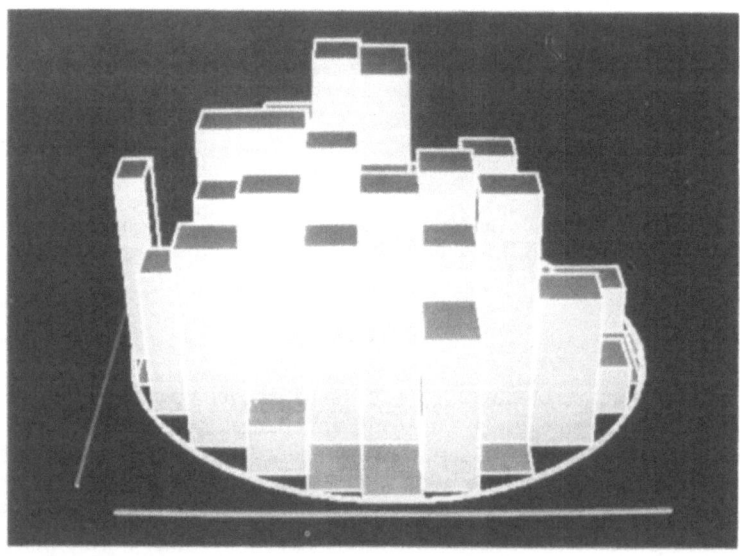

Fig. 11. Three-dimensional representation of results of linear regression analyses. Height above horizontal axis is inversely related to p values and represents negative slope values.

46

There are some limitations to the current application of this technique. For instance, for the probability percentile plot, the known statistical attributes of normal populations are limited by the small number of normal subjects that have been evaluated by decade and sex. Furthermore, it is uncertain whether these subjects are true normals, i.e., whether they have been shown by complete ocular examination to meet criteria for freedom from ocular disease. Nevertheless, when appropriate reference values for normal populations have been accumulated, they can be stored in the computer and used to obtain probability percentile plots as illustrated here. Even though the reference data may change, the clinician using this principle can quickly decide, which reference to a normal population, whether any particular area of a visual field is abnormal, suspect, or normal. The appropriate decision, based on statistical probabilities, can then be made. If the RMS value is elevated, or if there is an abnormal number of false positives or false negatives, the clinician can decide whether to use these data. In the future, there may be adequate data for comparison to a normal population with similar ranges of false positives and negatives or RMS values.

A common clinical requirement in follow-up and treatment of ocular hypertensive or glaucomatous patients is detection of visual field changes with time. The techniques that have been used to date are linear regression analysis (4) and paired t analysis (2). Both of these techniques have limitations. Linear regression analysis has been applied primarily to analysis of the total visual field, and paired t analysis has been applied to the total visual field or to quadrants. Regression analysis appears to be more powerful than a paired t analysis since more data are used to evaluate changes over time. For regression analysis, at least five independent visual fields should be obtained for an adequate estimation of the slope. The regression analysis, however, assumes linear changes with time that may not be appropriate. Our computer programs allow determination of threshold values for any point or combination of points over time to ascertain whether the plot is linear before a regression analysis is applied (Fig. 9). Once it has been determined that linear regression analysis is the appropriate statistical technique, then the probability contour plot for p values, the contour plot for slopes, and their combination can be used to detect significant changes with time. This technique assumes that each threshold point in the visual field is independent of the others; the degree of validity of this assumption must be determined in future studies.

If the changes of the visual field thresholds with time do not appear linear, then a paired t approach can be used. Probability area plots can indicate whether there are significant changes in the whole visual field or only in certain areas of the visual field.

More sophisticated statistical techniques, including polynomial regression analysis and cluster analysis, could also be developed for the analyses of visual fields.

ACKNOWLEDGEMENTS

The authors appreciate the support of Research to Prevent Blindness, New York, N.Y., and thank Judith Barton, M.S., for statistical analyses and Susan Glick, M.S., for editing the manuscript.

REFERENCES

1. Bebie, H. Compatibility of the Octopus models in view of the normal values and accuracy of the results. Proceedings of the Third Octopus Users' Society Meeting, Denver, Colo. Mar. 17 (1984).
2. Bebie, H. and Fankhauser, F. Ein statistisches Programm zur Beurteilung von Gesichtsfeldern. Klin Monatsbl Augenheilkd 177: 417–422 (1980).
3. Gramer, E., Gerlach, R., Krieglstein, G.K. and Leydhecker, W. Zur Topographie fruher glaukomatoser Gesichtsfeldausfalle bei der Computerperimetrie. Klin Monatsbl Augenheilkd 180: 515–523 (1982).
4. Holmin, C. and Krakau, C.E.T. Regression analysis of the central visual field in chronic glaucoma cases: A follow-up study using automatic perimetry. Acta Ophthalmol 60: 267–274 (1982).
5. LeBlanc, R.P. Abnormal static threshold values, in Whalen, W.R. and Spaeth, G.L. (eds): Computerized Visual Fields: What They Are – How to Use Them. Thorofare, N.J. and Charles B. Slack, in press.
6. Nagin, P. and Schwartz, B. Transmission and analysis of data on visual fields obtained with the Octopus 2000R, in Whalen, W.R. and Spaeth, G.L. (eds): Computerized Visual Fields: What They Are – How to Use Them. Thorofare, N.J. and Charles B. Slack, in press.
7. Wirtschafter, J.D., Becker, W.L., Howe, J.B. and Younge, B.R. Glaucoma visual field analysis by computed profile of nerve fiber layer function in optic disc sectors. Ophthalmology 89: 255–267 (1982).

Authors' addresses:
Department of Ophthalmology,
New England Medical Center,
Boston, Mass., U.S.A.
Tufts University School of Medicine,
Boston, Mass., U.S.A.

COMPARISON BETWEEN STATIC AND KINETIC THRESHOLD FLUCTUATIONS DETERMINED BY AUTOMATED PERIMETRY

M. ZINGIRIAN, E. GANDOLFO, P. CAPRIS, and G. CORALLO

(*Genova, Italy*)

ABSTRACT

Static threshold fluctuations have already been analyzed by other Authors. In this work, short and long term intra- and interindividual threshold fluctuations in static perimetry were compared with those obtained by kinetic perimetry under the same testing conditions. Both normal and pathological visual fields were considered. A computerized Goldmann perimeter (Perikon, Optikon) (Fig. 1) was employed to reproduce constant examination conditions and to avoid any variables due to different examiners. This investigation has demonstrated that intraindividual threshold fluctuation in

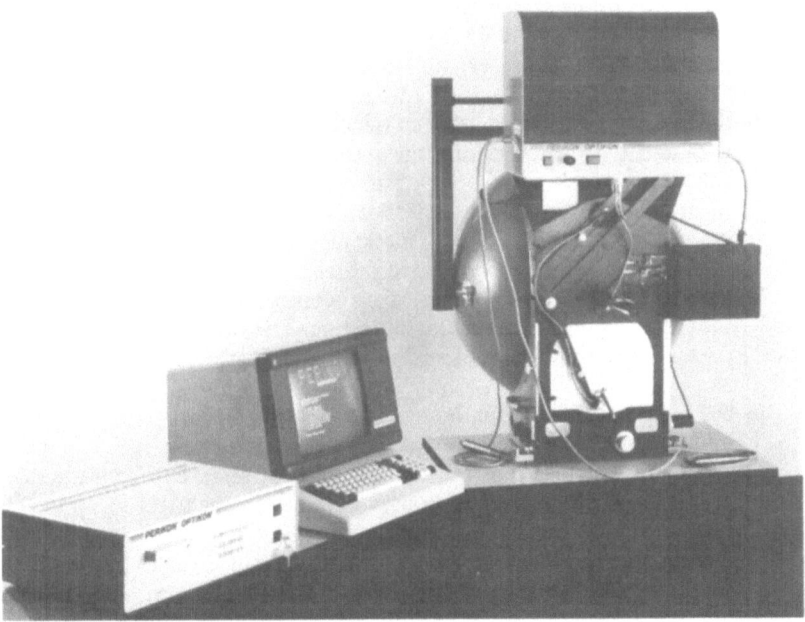

Fig. 1. The computerized Goldmann perimeter 'PERIKON'.

Heijl, A. and Greve, E.L. (eds.), Proceedings of the 6th Int. Visual Field Symposium.
© *1985, Dr W. Junk Publishers, Dordrecht, The Netherlands. ISBN 978-94-010-8932-6*

both static and kinetic procedures are not consistently correlated, however a better correlation is noted if the sensitivity gradient steepness increases. The interindividual overall average fluctuation is lower with the kinetic than the static method in both the short and long term, without any relationship to eccentricity.

INTRODUCTION

Static threshold fluctuation has been widely investigated by several Authors in the last few years (Bebie et al., Elliot et al., Fankhauser and Bebie, Flammer et al., Gloor and Vögt, Heijl, Werner and Drance).

In this paper static and kinetic threshold fluctuations were compared. A Computerized Goldmann Perimeter (Perikon, Optikon), which allows the automated execution of both the static and kinetic strategies, was used for threshold determination. This investigation's aim was to ascertain if a correlation exists between static and kinetic fluctuations either in single individual test locations, or in relationship with the overall mean responses obtained from varied ophthalmologically normal and pathological subjects.

MATERIALS AND METHODS

In 8 normal subjects static threshold measurement was automatically performed using a background luminance of 31.5 asb and the target $I(=\frac{1}{4}$ mm^2) of the Perikon at the following eccentricities on the nasal hemimeridian: 15°, 25°, 35°, and 45°. Every location was tested 5 times during the same session. The entire examination was repeated 6 times after a period of time that varied from 5 hours to 4 weeks.

In the same normal subjects 5 consecutive kinetic threshold determinations were also performed during the static session. Target $I(=\frac{1}{4}$ mm^2) was used with a luminance corresponding to the mean value obtained from the static measurements, in order to test with good approximation the same locations with both the static and kinetic methods. The entire kinetic examination, like the static test, was repeated 6 times.

6 patients with ocular disorders (4 glaucomas and 2 optic neuropathies) underwent the same static and kinetic testing. The only difference was that the locations explored were situated on the most significantly altered meridian.

In both the normal and pathological subjects the short term fluctuation (STF) and the long term fluctuation (LTF) were determined.

The STF was calculated as the Standard Deviation (S.D.) from the mean value of the 5 intraindividual responses obtained in each test location. The LTF was determined using the formula adopted by Bebie et al. (1976) where not only the spread of the average threshold obtained for each location in the 6 examinations were considered, but also the influence of short term alterations was taken into account.

The static thresholds were expressed in dB of luminance, whereas the

Table 1. Short term fluctuation (STF) and long term fluctuation (LTF) of the differential threshold in normal and pathological subjects. The minimal (min.) and the maximal (max.) values in single individual locations and the overall average values (av, ± sd) are reported in decibels for the static method and in degrees for the kinetic method.

Fluctuation types	Normal subjects		Pathological subjects	
	Static method (decibels)	Kinetic method (degrees)	Static method (decibels)	Kinetic method (degrees)
Min, STF	0.40	0.00	0.51	0.57
Max, STF	4.67	3.65	6.34	5.50
Av, STF ± sd	2.42 ± 1.63	1.12 ± 0.71	2.82 ± 1.21	1.94 ± 1.17
Min, LTF	0.36	0.51	0.39	0.49
Max, LTF	5.86	5.24	4.55	4.95
Av, LTF ± sd	2.14 ± 1.69	1.85 ± 1.29	1.90 ± 1.10	1.76 ± 1.19

kinetic thresholds were measured in angular degrees. Nevertheless the comparison between these apparently non-homogeneous measures is possible, since the kinetic angular values can be easily converted into decibels of luminance, if a mean sensitivity gradient is adopted, where 1° is approximately equal to 0.5 dB.

RESULTS

Normal subjects

The STF values of the kinetic and static threshold in single test locations of the same individual or of varied individuals belong to the same range of size, which is very similar to that of static fluctuation found by other Authors (Bebie et al., Fankhauser and Bebie). This is clearly indicated by the minimum and maximum STF obtained in our series (see Table 1). However the correlation between kinetic and static fluctuation in single individual test locations is fairly inconsistent with respect to size and direction.

All these considerations are also valid for LTF.

Considering the interindividual overall average STF and LTF values, the kinetic fluctuation is lower when compared to static vlaues. In addition only a small difference is noted between STF and LTF of static thresholds, whereas the kinetic thresholds fluctuate more widely in the long than in the short term (see Table 2).

This behaviour in the average fluctuations doesn't change if test locations with different eccentricities are considered: this means that neither the kinetic nor the static thresholds show an incremental average fluctuation toward the center or the periphery of the visual field, either in short or long term.

Pathological subjects

The results reported for normals concerning the STF and LTF in single individual locations and their interindividual average in the overall distribution of locations tested or in relationship to the eccentricity, are also valid for subjects with ocular disorders. However, some considerations are needed:

A fairly good correlation is noted between static and kinetic fluctuations in single locations according to the sensitivity gradient steepness: where the

Table 2. Average short term and long term fluctuations (STF and LTF) of static and kinetic thresholds in relationship to four different eccentricities of test location.

Fluctuation types	15°	25°	35°	45°
Static STF (decibels)	2.32	2.95	2.45	2.50
Kinetic STF (degrees)	1.30°	0.82°	1.29°	0.99°
Static LTF (decibels)	1.73	1.65	2.22	2.78
Kinetic LTF (degrees)	1.17°	2.57°	2.20°	1.79°

gradient is steeper due to pathological causes, the kinetic with respect to static fluctuation is generally smaller.

The average STF is wider in pathological than in normal subjects, but static and kinetic values are harmonically increased.

On the contrary, compared to normal individuals, the average LTF is more restricted in pathological subjects. However a harmonic relationship is always present between static and kinetic values.

Both kinetic and static average LTF is lower than the corresponding STF.

CONCLUSIONS

This study has shown that static and kinetic fluctuations are not consistently correlated in single individual test locations, but they belong numerically to the same range of size. A more consistent inverse correlation is noted if gradient steepness increases.

The interindividual average fluctuation is slightly smaller with the kinetic than the static method, in both the long and short term in normal and pathological fields, without any relationship to eccentricity.

Therefore the preference for the static or the kinetic method cannot be motivated by the influence of fluctuation on the perimetric results, because it is similar in both examination methods.

The main problem concerns how the knowledge of kinetic fluctuation can be used to evaluate the irregular shape of a single isopter or to assess changes between two corresponding isopters obtained from the same patient in two successive examinations, when automated perimetry is performed.

Our next studies will be oriented in this direction.

ACKNOWLEDGEMENTS

This study was supported from a grant of the Consiglio Nazionale delle Ricerche, Progetto Finalizzato Medicina Preventiva e Riabilitativa, Sottoprogetto Malattie Degenerative, Obiettivo n. 47a, Rome, Italy.

REFERENCES

1. Bebie, H., Fankhauser, F. and Spahr, J. Static perimetry: accuracy and fluctuations. Acta Ophthalmol. 54: 339–348 (1976).
2. Elliot, B.W., Nabil, S. and Duncan, T. Variability of static visual threshold responses. Arch. Ophthalmol. 100: 1627–1631 (1982).
3. Fankhauser, F. and Bebie, H. Threshold fluctuations, interpolations and spatial resolution in perimetry. Doc. Ophthalmol. Proc. 19: 295–310 (1979).
4. Flammer, J., Drance, S.M. and Schulzer, M. The estimation and testing of the components of long-term fluctuation of the differential light threshold. Doc. Ophthalmol. Proc. 35: 383–389 (1982).
5. Gloor, B. and Vökt, B. Long term fluctuations versus definite field loss in glaucoma patients. Invest. Ophthalmol. & Visual Sci. Suppl. 25: 103 (1983).

6.   Heijl, A. Computer test logics for automatic perimetry. Acta Ophthalmol. 55: 837–853 (1977).
7.   Werner, E.B. and Drance, S.M. Early visual field disturbances in glaucoma. Arch. Ophthalmol. 95: 1173–1175 (1977).

Authors' address:
University Eye Clinic
Viale Benedetto XV, 5
16132-Genova
Italy

THE INFLUENCE OF ARTIFICIALLY INDUCED VISUAL FIELD DEFECTS ON THE VISUAL FIELD INDICES

LOTTI AUGUSTINY and JOSEF FLAMMER

(*Berne, Switzerland*)

ABSTRACT

Visual fields of normal subjects measured with program JO on the Octopus automated perimeter were artificially changed to simulate various defects. Before and after the changes, the three visual field indices: SF (short-term fluctuation), MD (mean damage) and CLV (corrected loss variation), were calculated.

We show how these indices are influenced by different alterations of the visual field. SF is a measure of the scatter; it increases if the responses of the first and the second phase do not correspond. MD responds to any kind of change of the visual field, but is especially sensitive to diffuse alterations. CLV is increased by local deviations larger than that expected simply from the scatter.

INTRODUCTION

For the interpretation of perimetric results, there are various aids which are quite helpful. The most frequently used method is graphical data presentation. In kinetic perimetry the presentation of isopters and in static perimetry the gray scale have proved to be very useful. The three-dimensional presentation has rather an instructive character, but, for clinical use it has not yet really been proven.

Another possibility is the application of data reduction methods (1, 10–13). Here there are various possibilities as well. Reduced values allow an easier comparison with the normal values and facilitate follow-up. We have tried to reduce the visual field information (especially when concerned with perimetry in glaucoma) to three values which we call visual field indices (8). We have examined them in a group of normals and glaucoma patients (3).

The purpose of this study is to examine and to show how these visual field indices are changed if a visual field of a normal subject is artificially modified (using computer simulation). This should aid for the interpretation of these visual field indices by the clinician.

Heijl, A. and Greve, E.L. (eds.), Proceedings of the 6th Int. Visual Field Symposium.
© 1985, Dr W. Junk Publishers, Dordrecht, The Netherlands. ISBN 978-94-010-8932-6

MATERIAL AND METHODS

We used visual fields of normal subjects measured with the Octopus program JO (2, 13). This program measures up to an eccentricity of $27°$. In order to simulate various defects, some measured values of these visual fields were changed in the following way:

(a) Simulation of relative scotomas. At single test locations, the measured values of both phases were reduced.

(b) Simulation of a diffuse depression of the midperiphery. All test locations at the margin of the measured visual field area were in both phases diminished by 2 dB each.

(c) Simulation of a diffuse uniform depression. All the measured values of both phases were reduced (first by 10 dB, afterwards by 20 dB).

(d) Simulation of the nasal step. On the nasal half of the visual field the 4 test locations above $0°$ were reduced by 5 dB.

(e) Simulation of absolute scotomas in both phases. Different test locations were set to zero; first only one, then two, three and four.

(f) Simulation of absolute scotomas in only one phase. The same as in (e) but this time the simulations took place only in the first phase.

(g) The visual field was reduced by the same total amount, but this amount was differently distributed as follows: (1) reduction by 20 dB at one test location, (2) reductions by 10 dB at two test locations, (3) reductions by 5 dB at four test locations, (4) reductions by 2 dB at ten test locations.

The three indices SF (short-term fluctuation), MD (mean damage) and CLV (corrected loss variation) were calculated for all artificially induced visual field defects.

SF is calculated from the differences between the measured values of the two phases. It is influenced on the one hand by the reliability of the patient, and, on the other hand, by the character of the threshold to be measured. Changes affecting both phases in the same way have, therefore, no influence on the SF. If a value is changed in one phase only, SF increases. In our pool of normal subjects SF was 1.57 dB ± 0.69 dB. It was calculated as follows:

$$SF = \sqrt{\frac{\sum_{i=1}^{49} (x_{i1} - x_{i2})^2}{2.49}}$$

where x_{i1} and x_{i2} are the measured values at test location i in phase 1 and phase 2, respectively.

MD is the mean difference between the normal values stored in the Octopus memory and the measured values. If the sensitivity at only a few test locations is reduced, MD increases only marginally. With reductions of the whole visual field or of a great number of test locations, MD increases considerably. In our pool of normal subjects, MD was -0.22 dB ± 1.58 dB. It was calcualted as follows:

$$MD = \frac{\sum_{i=1}^{49} (z_i - x_{i.})}{49}$$

56

where z_i is the age-corrected normal value at test location i. $x_{i.}$ is the mean of the values measured in the two phases at test location i.

CLV is the component of variance of the sensitivity loss at the different test locations. It stays in the normal range if the deviations are merely due to an increased SF or if the visual field is uniformly reduced. If there are only local defects, without other changes, CLV does increase considerably, whereas SF and MD do not change much. In our pool of normal subjects, CLV was $0.95\,(dB)^2 \pm 1.20(dB)^2$. It was calculated as follows.

$$CLV = \frac{2 \cdot \sum_{i=1}^{49} (x_{i.} - z_i - MD)^2 - 48\,(SF)^2}{2.48}$$

RESULTS

The following paragraphs refer to the various simulation experiments outlined in the preceding section.

(a) Figure 1b shows the reaction of the three indices after having reduced the value of one test location by 10 dB (Fig. 1a). This artificially induced scotoma has no influence on SF and MD, whereas CLV is out of the range of our normal controls.

Figure 2b shows the influence of the reduction of the values at three different test locations by 5 dB each (Fig. 2a). Here too, SF and MD are only slightly changed; CLV, however, increases considerably.

(b) Figure 3b shows the results after having reduced the values in the margin of the measured visual field area by 2 dB (Fig. 3a). CLV amounts up to $2.44\ (dB)^2$, exceeding thereby the normal range. MD, too, lies outside of the normal range (-2.33 dB). SF remains unchanged.

(c) On a reduction of the whole visual field by 10 and 20 dB, MD increases linearly (Fig. 4). CLV and SF remain practically unchanged.

(d) Figure 5b shows the resulting values of the indices after simulation of the nasal step (Fig. 5a). CLV increases up to $3.55(dB)^2$, which is out of the range of our normal controls. MD lies with 1.80 dB at the lower limit of our normal values. SF remains unchanged.

(e) Figure 6 shows the values of the three indices after simulation of scotomas *in both phases*. CLV rapidly increases while SF remains more or less the same. MD slightly increases up to 2.2 dB when four test locations in both phases are set to zero. CLV amounts to $15(dB)^2$ as soon as one test location only is set to zero in both phases. When four test locations are set to zero, CLV rises to $59.9\ (dB)^2$.

(f) Figure 7 shows the values of the three indices after simulation of the same scotomas as in (e), but this time *in one phase only*. SF rapidly increases up to 5.6 dB, whereas MD and CLV stay in the normal range, with up to 4 points set to zero.

(g) Figure 8 shows that CLV has the highest value when only one test location is reduced by 20 dB. If this amount is distributed over different

57

One relative scotoma. Depth: 10 dB

a)

26	28	26	26	25	24	26	26
27	28	26	26	25	23	26	27
26	27	30	29	26	28	26	26
27	26	30	30	27	26	27	27

27	28 18	30	31	30			27
27	28 18	29	30 34 29				27

33 31
32 32
30
27 29 29 29 30 30 29
29 29 29 28 29 28

27	28	27	28	29	26	28	28
25	26	29	27	28	28	29	29
27	28	26	26	26	26	30	28
25	28	27	26	26	27	28	28

b)

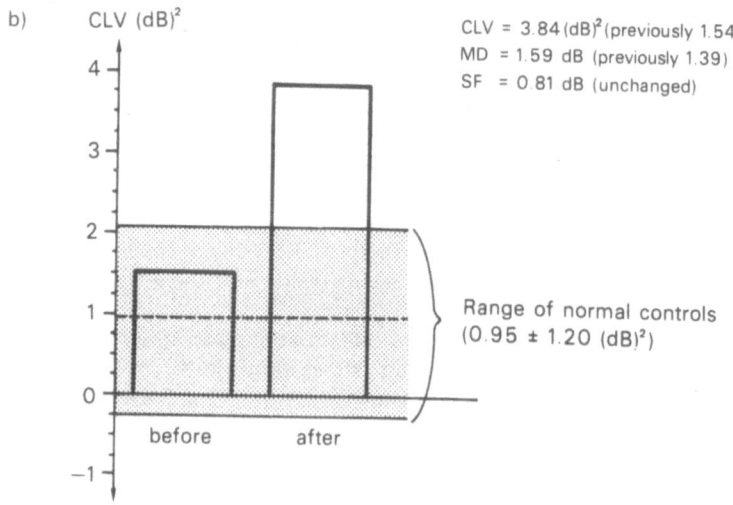

CLV = 3.84 (dB)² (previously 1.54)
MD = 1.59 dB (previously 1.39)
SF = 0.81 dB (unchanged)

Range of normal controls
(0.95 ± 1.20 (dB)²)

Fig. 1. (a) Numerical representation of the initial visual field with simulated scotoma (10 dB deep) indicated. (b) CLV calculated from the data shown in Fig. 1a before and after scotoma simulation.

58

Three shallow scotomas. Depth: 5 dB

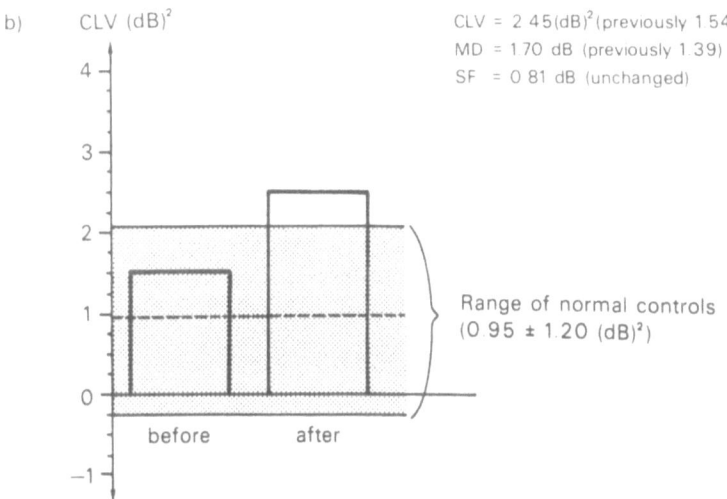

a)
```
26    28    26   |26 21|  25    24    26    26
27    28    26   |26 21|  25    23    26    27

26    27    30    29    26    28    26    26
27    26    30    30    27    26    27    27

27    28    30    31         30                27
27    28    29    30  34  29                   27
                      34
                  33     31
                  32     32
|27 22|  29    29    29  30  30                29
|29 24|  29    29    28      29                28

27    28    27    28    29    26    28   |28 23|
25    26    29    27    28    28    29   |29 24|

27    28    26    26    26    26    30    28
25    28    27    26    26    27    28    28
```

b)   CLV (dB)²

CLV = 2 45(dB)² (previously 1 54)
MD = 1 70 dB (previously 1 39)
SF = 0 81 dB (unchanged)

Range of normal controls
(0 95 ± 1 20 (dB)²)

Fig. 2. (a) Numerical representation of the initial visual field with three simulated scotomas (5 dB deep each). (b) CLV calculated from the data shown in Fig. 2a before and after scotoma simulations.

Diffuse depression of the midperiphery by 2 dB

a)
```
26 24   28      26 24   26 24   25 23   24 22   26 24   26 24
27 25   28      26 24   26 24   25 23   23 21   26 24   27 25

26 24   27      30      29      26      28      26      26 24
27 25   26      30      30      27      26      27      27 25

27 25   28      30      31         30                   27 25
27 25   28      29      30  34    29                    27 25
                            34
                        33      31
                        32      32
27 25   29      29      29  30    30                    29 27
29 27   29      29      28  30    29                    28 26

27 25   28      27      28      29      26      28      28 26
25 23   26      29      27      28      28      29      29 27

27 25   28 26   26 24   26 24   26 24   26 24   30 28   28 26
25 23   28 26   27 25   26 24   26 24   27 25   28 26   28 26
```

b)

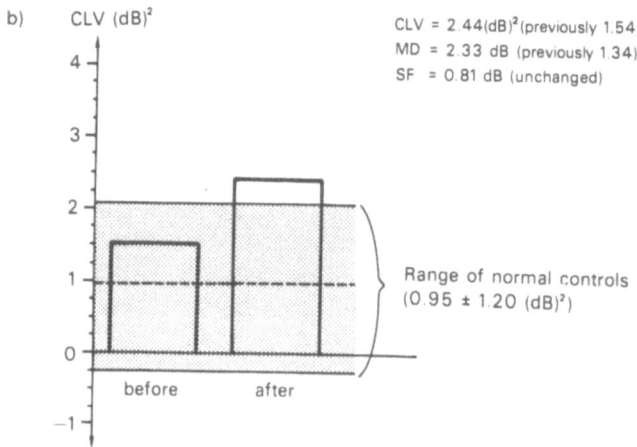

CLV = 2.44 (dB)² (previously 1.54)
MD = 2.33 dB (previously 1.34)
SF = 0.81 dB (unchanged)

Range of normal controls
(0.95 ± 1.20 (dB)²)

Fig. 3. (a) Numerical representation of the initial visual field with reductions of the values in the margin of the measured area by 2 dB (simulation of a diffuse depression of the midperiphery). (b) CLV calculated from the data shown in Fig. 3a before and after marginal reductions.

test locations, CLV decreases. The smaller the reduction per test location the smaller is CLV, even though the number of reduced test locations steadily increases.

60

Diffuse uniform depression

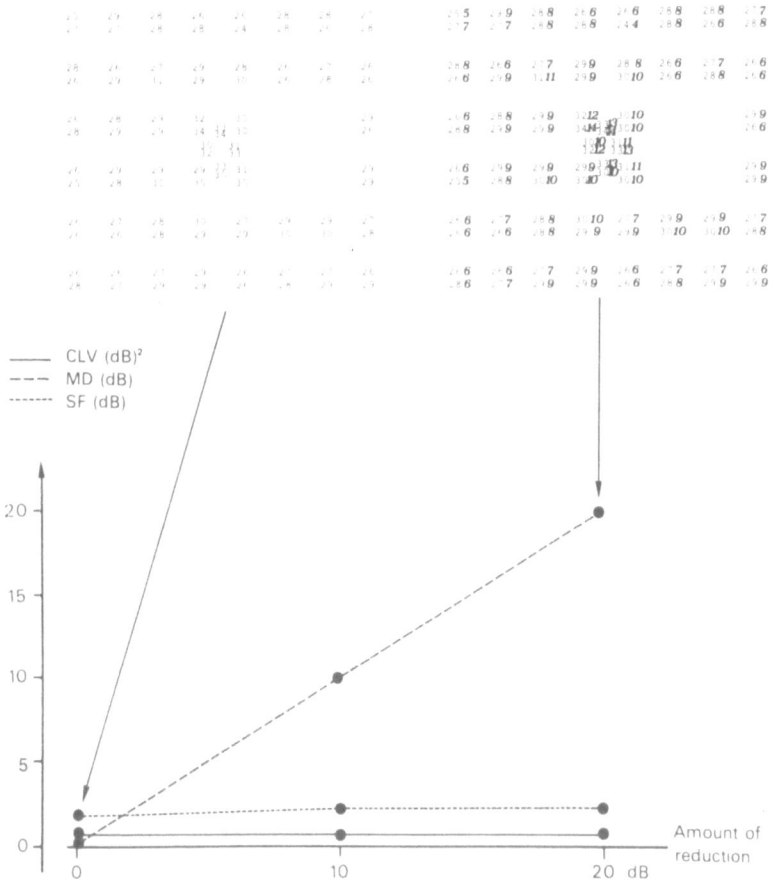

Fig. 4. Representation of SF, MD and CLV after reductions of all the measured values by 10 dB and by 20 dB.

DISCUSSION

The outcome of computer simulated changes in the visual field proves the theoretical expectations of the various possible changes of the three visual field indices. The indices allow a discrimination of diffuse and local damage, as well as a discrimination of probably present defects from deviations due to increased scatter.

An increase of the *SF* (due to differences from the first phase to the

Nasal step

a)

26	28	26	26	25	24	26	26
27	28	26	26	25	23	26	27

26	27	30	29	26	28	26	26
27	26	30	30	27	26	27	27

27 22	28 23	30 25	31 26	30			27
27 22	28 23	29 24	30 25 34	29			27
			33 32	31 32			
			30				
27	29	29	29	30 30			29
29	29	29	28	29			28

27	28	27	28	29	26	28	28
25	26	29	27	28	28	29	29

27	28	26	26	26	26	30	28
25	28	27	26	26	27	28	28

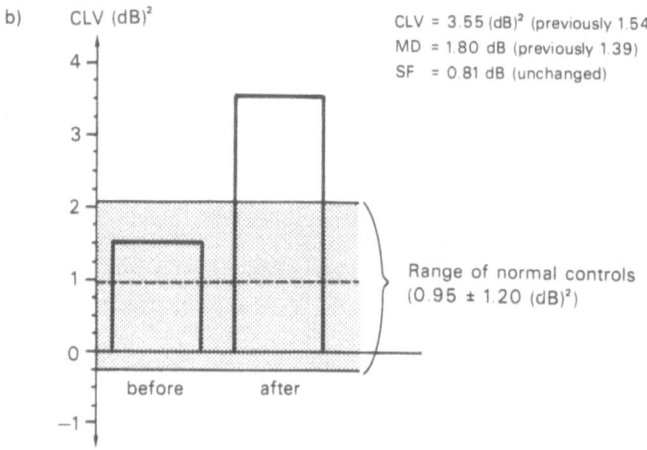

b) CLV (dB)^2

CLV = 3.55 (dB)^2 (previously 1.54)
MD = 1.80 dB (previously 1.39)
SF = 0.81 dB (unchanged)

Range of normal controls
(0.95 ± 1.20 (dB)^2)

before   after

Fig. 5. (a) Numerical representation of the initial visual field with simulated nasal step. (b) CLV calculated from the data shown in Fig. 5a before and after a simulated nasal step.

Absolute scotoma in both phases

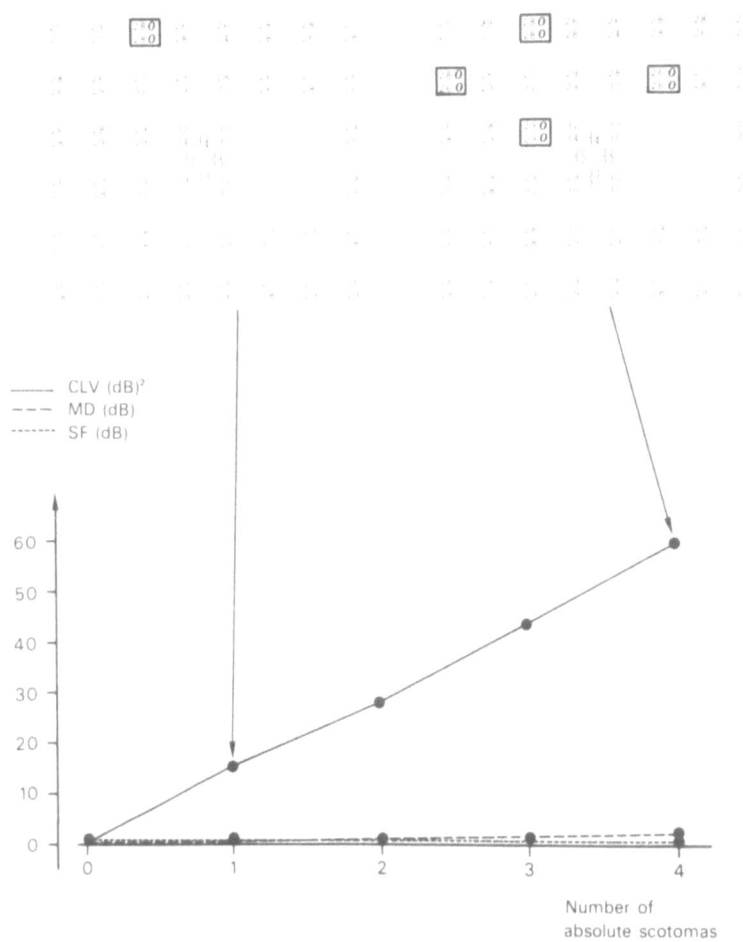

Fig. 6. Representation of SF, MD and CLV after having reduced one, two, three and finally four test locations to zero in both phases (simulation of absolute scotomas).

second (Fig. 7)) may by itself indicate pathology or a reduced ability of the patient to cooperate, or it may be due to learning (4–7).

An increase of the *MD*, while CLV remains in a normal range, indicates a uniform decrease of the whole visual field. An MD of 10 dB with a CLV of $0.6(dB)^2$ at the same time is shown in our example (Fig. 4) indicating a *uniform* decrease of the visual field by 4 dB. In Fig. 6, MD reaches 2.2 dB – which is slightly out of the range of our pool or normal subjects – while

Absolute scotoma in only one phase
(probably artefact)

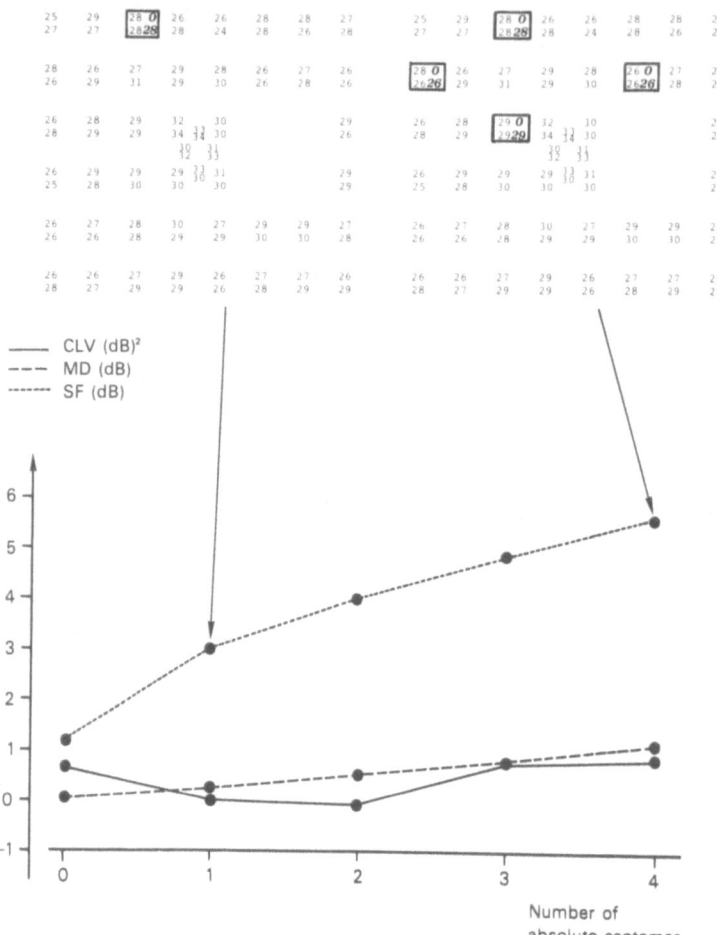

Fig. 7. Representation of SF, MD and CLV after the same simulation as in Fig. 6, but this time in the first phase only.

CLV has increased up to $59.8(dB)^2$. Such a result clearly shows that here there is not a uniform decrease of the visual field, but there are, rather, single local defects. In our example, there are 4 test locations which are set to zero.

CLV reacts very sensitively to local defects. A relative scotoma at one test location of 10 dB causes an increase of CLV out of the range of our normal

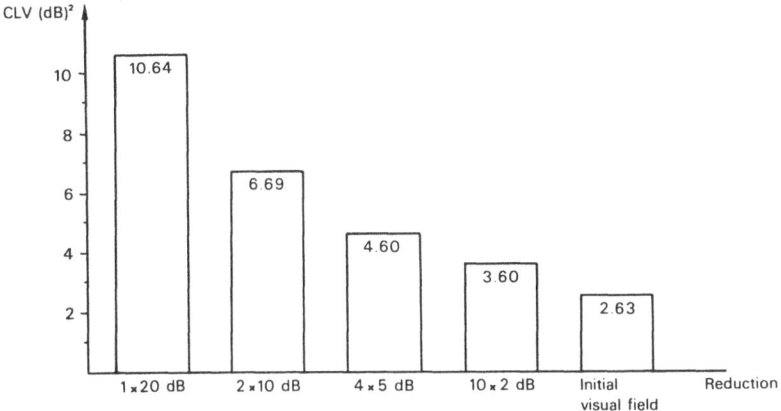

Fig. 8. Histogram representing CLV after reductions of a measured visual field by the total amount of 20 dB, distributed as follows: (1) Reduction by 20 dB at one test location. (2) Reductions by 10 dB at two test locations. (3) Reductions by 5 dB at four test locations. (4) Reductions by 2 dB at ten test locations.

controls (Fig. 1b). Equally, on the three scotomas from Fig. 2a, where three test locations were reduced by 5 dB each, CLV lies above the upper limit of the range of our normal controls (Fig. 2b). On the marginal decrease of the measured area (diffuse depression of the midperiphery, Fig. 3a/b) and on the simulation of a nasal step (Fig. 5a/b), CLV also slightly exceeds the range of our normal controls.

One must remember that the visual fields transformed by simulations are authentic visual field measurements of normal subjects. Therefore, the measured values do, obviously, not exactly correspond to the mean of our normal values. The influence of a local damage depends, therefore, on the test location. At a location having already a relatively low sensitivity (in comparison to the normal mean) a further reduction of sensitivity influences CLV more than this would be the case at another test location.

The main advantage of CLV is the fact that it allows with high probability a discrimination of real local deviations from deviations due to scatter. If deviations occur in just one phase whereas the sensitivity is normal in the other phase, we are dealing most probably with artefacts. This increases the SF, but not CLV, as shown in Fig. 7. Observing visual fields with local deviations, but CLV in the normal range, we can assume, therefore, that these are not real scotomas. These borderline situations are the major concern for the clinician.

In comparing Figs. 1a/b and 2a/b, one can state that a diminution at *one* test location by 10 dB causes a greater CLV ($3.84(dB)^2$) than diminutions at *three* test locations by 5 dB each (CLV = $2.45(dB)^2$). Both simulations are effected on the same subject so that the results can be compared. This shows that CLV is (as opposed to MD) more influenced by *the depth* than by *the extent* of the scotomas, as also shown in Fig. 8. This is explained by the fact that CLV is a squared value $(dB)^2$, while MD is an arithmetic mean (dB).

One could ask whether it would have been better to take the normal values as a basis for the simulations instead of taking real visual fields. Alterations caused by varying differences between the measured values could have been eliminated. On the other hand, this method is closer to clinical practice and the important effects of different alterations could be shown, nevertheless.

We hope that this study helps the clinician in interpreting visual field indices. These indices are useful for the detection of different types of visual field changes and their follow-up. However, they do not replace a thorough consideration of the measured values of the visual field. More specifically, they do not pay any attention to the topography of the defects, but these can be ascertained from graphic displays.

If *SF* is increased, one should check the rate of false positive and false negative responses in the catch trials. An increased SF without increased rate of false responses indicates a changed character of the threshold (4–7).

An increased *MD* — without an increase of the CLV at the same time — means that the whole visual field is more or less uniformly decreased, as it occurs in cataract patients, but also in glaucomas.

An increase of the *CLV* indicates scotomas, the location of which can be seen from graphic displays.

REFERENCES

1. Bynke, H. Statistical analysis of normal visual fields and hemianopsias recorded by a computerized perimeter. In: Greve, E.L. and Heijl, A. (eds.) Fifth International Visual Field Symposium (1983) p. 281.
2. Flammer, J., Drance, S.M., Jenni, A. and Bebie, H. JO and STATJO: programs for investigating the visual field with the Octopus automatic perimeter. Can. J. Ophthalmol. 18: 115 (1983).
3. Flammer, J., Drance, S.M., Augustiny, L. and Funkhouser, A. Quantification of glaucomatous visual field defects with automated perimetry. Investigative Ophthalmol. & Vis. Sci. (in print).
4. Flammer, J., Drance, S.M. and Zulauf, M. The short- and long-term fluctuation of the differential light threshold in patients with glaucoma, normal controls and glaucoma suspects. Arch. Ophthalmol. (in print).
5. Flammer, J. Vermehrte Fluktuation der perimeterischen Untersuchungsergebnisse bei okulaerer Hypertension. In: Krieglstein, G.K. and Leydhecker, W. Okulaere Hypertension, Bergmann-Verlag (in print).
6. Flammer, J., Drance, S.M., Fankhauser, F. and Augustiny, L. The differential light threshold in automatic static perimetry. Arch. Ophthalmol. (in print).
7. Flammer, J. Fluctuations in the visual field. In: Automated perimetry for glaucoma. Ed. by S.M. Drance and D.R. Anderson (in print).
8. Flammer, J. Methoden zur Datenreduktion in der automatischen Perimetrie. In: Neuere Entwicklungen in der Augenheilkunde. Ed. by H. Merte (in print).
9. Flammer, J. Psychophysics in glaucoma. A modified concept of the disease. In: Proceedings of the European Glaucoma Society (in print).
10. Flammer, J. and Bebie, H. The concept of visual field indices. Albrecht v. Graefes Arch. Ophthal. (submitted).
11. Gloor, B., Stuermer, J. and Voekt, B. Was hat die automatisierte Perimetrie mit

dem Octopus fuer neue Erkenntnisse ueber glaukomatoese Gesichtsfeldveraenderungen gebracht? Klin. Mbl. Augenheilk. (in print).

12. Holmin, C. and Krakau, C.E.T. Automatic perimetry in the control of glaucoma. Glaucoma 3: 154 (1981).
13. Jenni, A., Flammer, J., Funkhouser, A. and Fankhauser, F. Special Octopus Software for clinical investigations. Doc. Ophthalmol. Proc. Series 35: 351 (1983).
14. Program DELTA, Manual; Ed. by Interzeag AG, Schlieren, Switzerland, November 1981.

Authors' address:
University Eye Clinic
Inselspital
CH-3010 BERNE, Switzerland

A NEW AUTOMATIC PERIMETER

KAZUTAKA KANI, HIDEO TAGO, KATSUHIKO KOBAYASHI and
TAKASHI SHIOIRI

(*Nishinomiya, Japan/Tokyo, Japan*)

ABSTRACT

A new automatic perimeter has been developed. Light emitting diodes are mounted in a hemispheric dome and are controlled by a micro-computer. This perimeter has 8 topographical suprathreshold static programs and 4 threshold programs.

INTRODUCTION

Automatic perimeters are useful both for screening anf for precise static threshold determination. In this paper we introduce a new automatic perimeter which has been developed for clinical use.

HARDWARE

The perimeter consists of a hemisphere, light emitting diodes (LEDs), and a computer system (Fig. 1).

The specifications are as follows:

Background: hemisphere, radius 33 cm, luminance 31.5 asb automatically regulated

stimulus light source: LEDs

size: 2 mm (21') diameter

color: yellow, wavelength 585 nm

number: 257

intensity: maximum intensity 425 asb, dynamic range 25 dB in 1 dB steps

stimulus duration: 0.2–3.2 sec

stimulus interval: 0.2–3.2 sec

presentation: single or multiple stimulus, static

fixation check: television monitor system and/or blind spot check.

The location of LEDs are shown in Fig. 2. The intensity of each LED is controlled by the microcomputer.

Heijl, A. and Greve, E.L. (eds.), Proceedings of the 6th Int. Visual Field Symposium.
© *1985, Dr W. Junk Publishers, Dordrecht, The Netherlands. ISBN 978-94-010-8932-6*

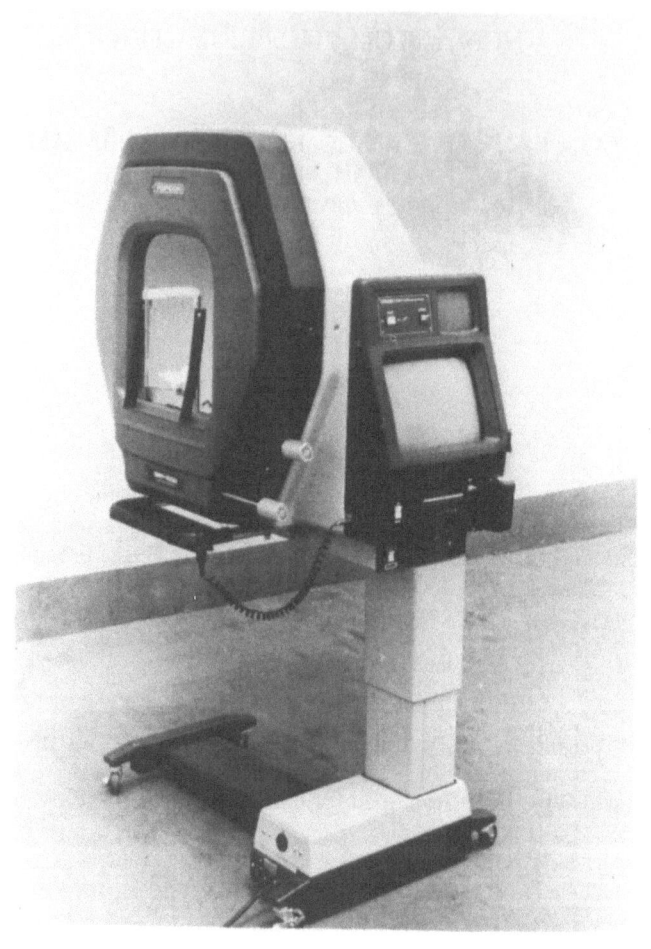

Fig. 1. Automatic perimeter.

To obtain diffuse background adaptation, all LEDs always emit light at an intensity equivalent to the background brightness.

For easy operation and for future development of software, all data or parameters are displayed on the television (CRT) screen and a communication with the perimeter is by means of a light pen.

Fixation is monitored by the perimetrist using a television display. When the perimetrist sees the subject's eye move, he can interrupt the examination by pressing the control switch. When the control switch is pressed again, the two data just before the interruption are cancelled and the examination restarts. At the same time the fixation is automatically checked by presenting the stimulus in the blind spot. If the patient responds to the stimulus in the blind spot, the preceding five data are cancelled. The automatic fixation check has three levels and can be changed during the examination.

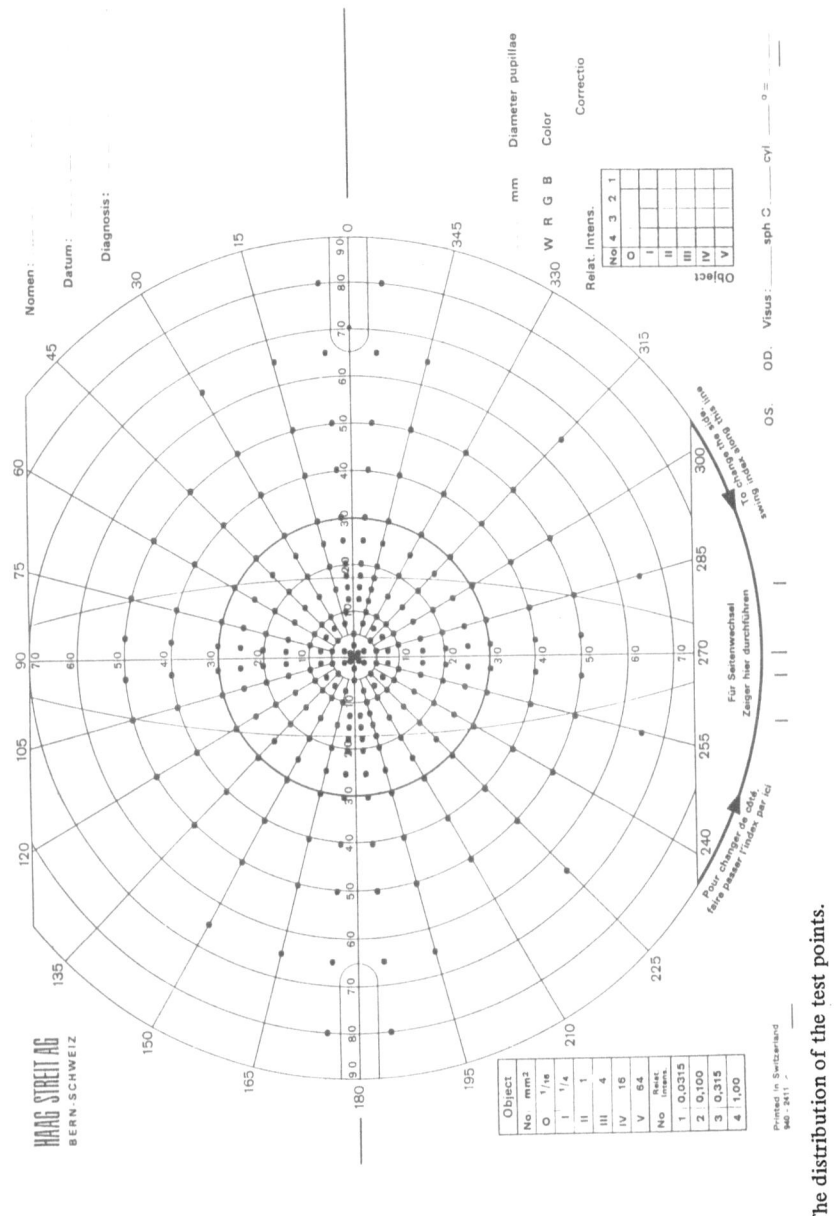

Fig. 2. The distribution of the test points.

71

SOFTWARE

1. Topographical suprathreshold programs

Eight programs are provided for topographical suprathreshold static perimetry: QUICK SCREENING (70 points), FULL SCREENING (132 points), GLAUCOMA (119 points), CENTRAL (113 points in central 30 degrees), PERIPHERAL (58 points), MACULA (31 points within 7.5 degrees), ALL POINTS (241 points) and MULTI (68 points).

Suprathreshold contour static perimetry is used in the topographical programs. The intensity level of stimuli in each latitude is classified into 4 sensitivity levels, 'normal', 'low 1', 'low 2' and 'low 3'. The 'normal' level is tested at 5 dB higher intensity than the threshold obtained from normal subjects. 'Low 1' is set 3 dB higher than 'normal', 'low 2' 3 dB higher than 'low 1' and 'low 3' is set at maximum intensity (Fig. 3).

The stimulus level is automatically selected. At the beginning of the examination, the computer measures 16 fixed points and sets the stimulus at which more than 4 of 16 points have been perceived. The level can also be set manually.

Stimuli are automatically exposed. If the patient misses a stimulus, the locus is tested at the lower sensitivity level. Thus retinal sensitivity is divided into 5 levels (normal, low 1, low 2, low 3 and not perceived).

The examination processes and the results appear on the CRT screen. The operator can interrupt, restart or end the examination at any time. If some doubtful points are found during or at the end of the examination, he can change the program to 'DIAGNOSTIC'. The location of all test points appears on on the CRT screen. Among them, the retinal sensitivity level is

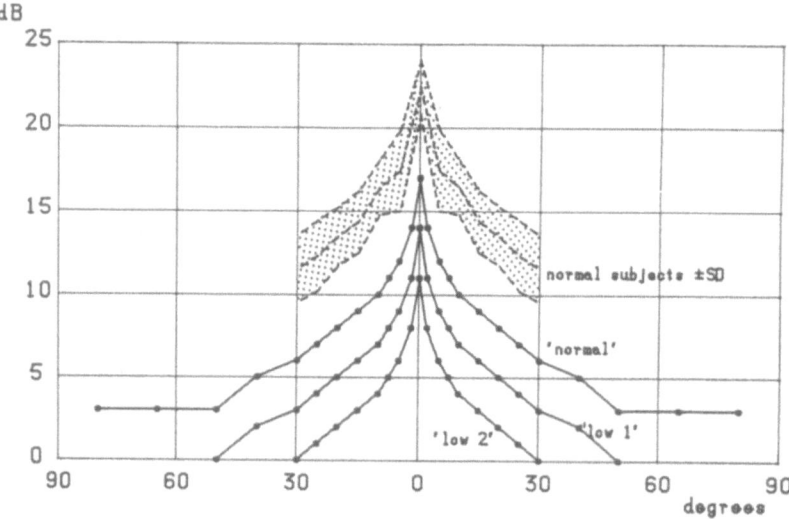

Fig. 3. Intensity of the test targets used in the topographical programs.

72

shown at previously tested points. The operator can indicate the desired points with the light pen and these points are tested. Repeating this procedure, detailed topographical results can be obtained.

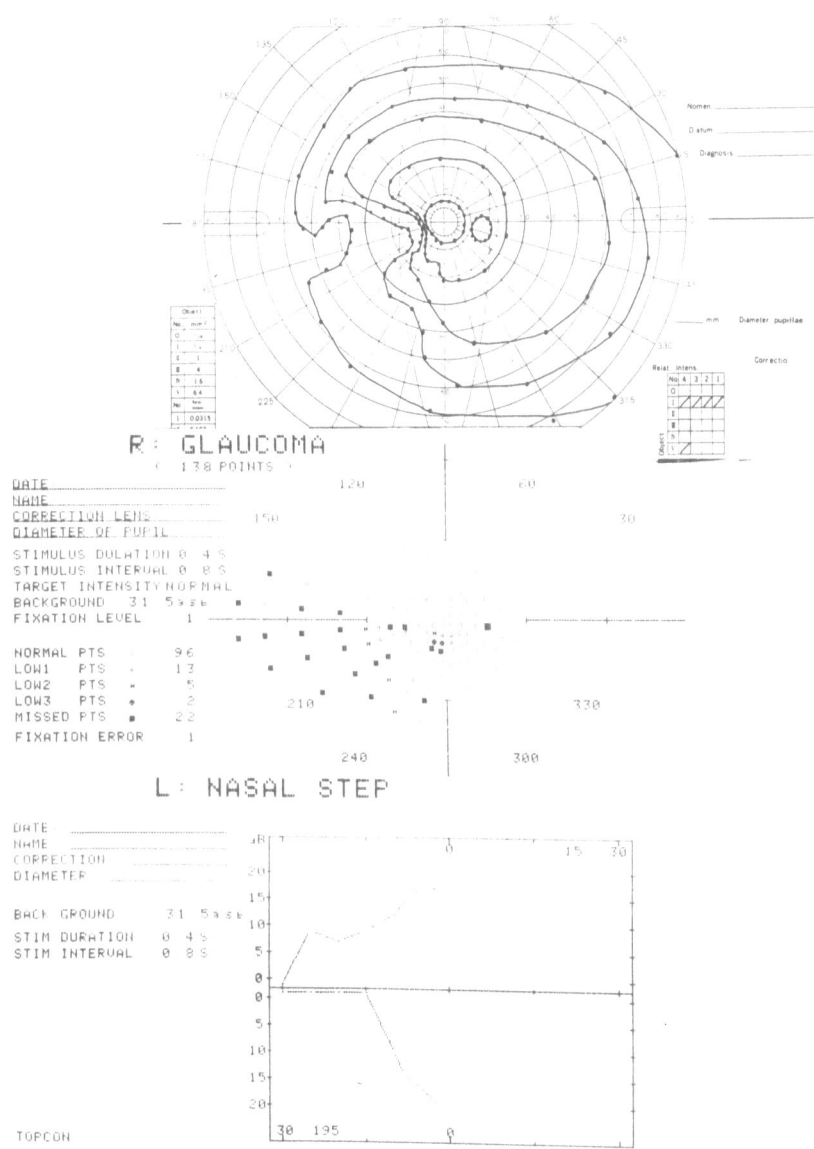

Fig. 4. Visual field of a glaucoma patient measured by Goldmann perimeter (upper part) and by the automatic perimeter (middle and lower parts).

2. Threshold programs

Four programs are provided, that is, MERIDIONAL (meridional profile), CIRCULAR (circular profile), NASAL STEP (meridional profile of the nasal meridian 15° superior and inferior to the horizontal line) and HEMIANOPSIA (meridional profile at the 45° and 135°). The threshold is tested with the up and down method and is determined in 1 dB steps. Each point is rechecked at 3 dB higher and lower intensity.

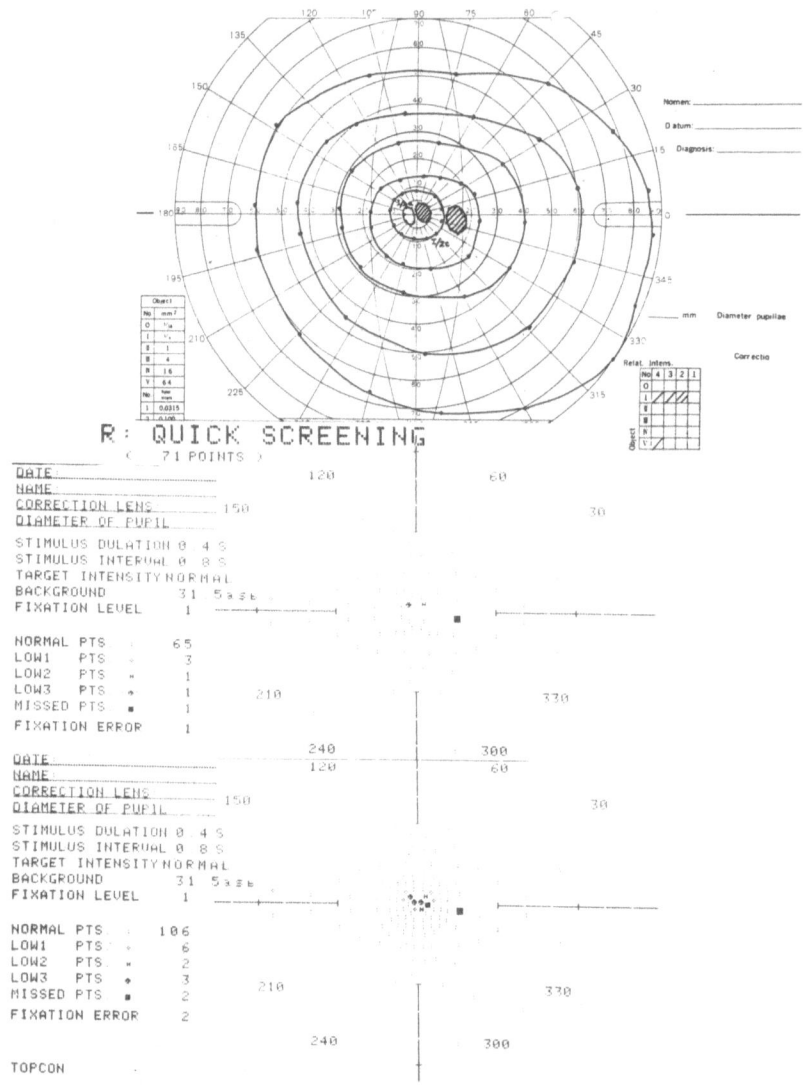

Fig. 5. Visual field of a patient with Behçet's disease.

SOME CLINICAL CASES

1. Glaucoma

A 30-year-old male with primary open angle glaucoma. The optic disc showed glaucomatous cupping. A nasal step and a spot-like defect was found by the 'GLAUCOMA' and 'NASAL STEP' program (Fig. 4).

2. Behçet's disease

A 29-year-old female had blurred vision in her right eye. A small subtle exudate was observed near the fovea. 'QUICK SCREENING' program showed two defective points in the central part and three in the periphery (Fig. 5 middle). 'DIAGNOSTIC' program was then used and a small dense scotoma was shown (Fig. 5 lower).

DISCUSSION

This perimeter has been developed for easy clinical use. Two screening programs are provided. If visual field defects or doubtful points are found, precise topographical examination can be made continuously using the 'DIAGNOSTIC' program. The sensitivity is classified into five levels. If more precise threshold determination is desired, threshold programs are available.

The target size was decided to be 2 mm. Smaller targets caused large scattering.

Using this perimeter, slight visual field defects were well detected but the remaining visual field in severe cases was hardly detected.

Authors' address:
Dr. K. Kani
Dept. of Ophthalmology
Hyogo College of Medicine
1-1, Mukogawa-cho, Nishinomiya
663 Japan

THE HUMPHREY FIELD ANALYZER, CONSTRUCTION AND CONCEPTS

ANDERS HEIJL

(*Malmö, Sweden*)

ABSTRACT

The new Humphrey Field Analyzer computerized perimeter is briefly described. The advantages and disadvantages of some of its concepts are discussed.

The Humphrey Field Analyzer is a new fully automatic, computerized projection-type perimeter manufactured by Humphrey Instruments Inc. The following presentation gives a brief description of the instrument and discusses the advantages and disadvantages of some of its concepts.

HARDWARE

The Humphrey Field Analyzer (HFA) is a single-unit instrument consisting of a stimulus generating system, a computer, a cathode ray tube (CRT) unit, a printer and a double floppy disk drive system.

Stimuli are generated through a projection system using an incandescent lamp as light source. The stimulus is projected on to a hemisphere with 33 cm radius by means of a motor-driven optical system. Background luminance is fixed at 31.5 asb, while stimulus luminance can be varied over a 5.1 log unit range (0.08–10 000 asb) through a set of fixed neutral density filters plus a filter wedge. Stimulus size is variable (0.25–64 mm^2, corresponding to Goldmann sizes I–V), as is stimulus colour. All stimuli are presented statistically in random order using a 0.2 sec exposure time.

The input unit is a cathode ray (CRT) tube. Test logics and test parameters are selected and patient ID data are entered by touching various pads on the CRT with a 'light pen'. During and after testing the CRT display is used to show the progress and the result of the test.

The computer system uses an Intel 8088 CPU. All test algorithms, input and output routines etcetera are stored in PROMs. The storage capacity of the double disk drive system is entirely reserved for results of visual field tests.

Heijl, A. and Greve, E.L. (eds.), Proceedings of the 6th Int. Visual Field Symposium.
© 1985, Dr W. Junk Publishers, Dordrecht, The Netherlands. ISBN 978-94-010-8932-6

SOFTWARE

Test strategies and printout formats

Threshold tests. At each test point the stimulus brightness is changed in a staircase fashion in 0.4 log unit steps until the first reversal (from seen to not seen or vice versa). The process then moves in the opposite direction in 0.2 log unit steps until the second reversal. The test pattern grows from four primary points and measured thresholds are used to determine starting levels for the test process in neighbouring points. If the measured threshold at a point differs by more than 0.4 log unit from the expected value (which is based on the threshold of the neighbouring point) the threshold is measured again. If the eye has been tested before, time may be saved by using previously measured thresholds, stored on disk, as starting levels for the threshold bracketing at each point. Threshold tests may be printed out numerically as actually measured threshold values, as interpolated greyscales or as a defect printout, where the defect density is numerically printed out in all points where the sensitivity is at least 0.4 log unit lower than the expected value.

A rather unusual type of test is the so called Fast Threshold test. This can be performed only when an earlier standard threshold test has been performed. Stimuli are shown slightly brighter than the threshold value from the earlier test. Only if this stimulus is not seen at a point, will the instrument perform a new threshold determination at that point. The fast threshold test can thus be regarded as an individually tailored slightly supraliminal screening, the objective of which is to see whether the field has deteriorated since the earlier examination. The instrument has eight standard test point patterns.

Screening tests. In the threshold-related suprathreshold screening programmes the instrument first measures the threshold at four points. The results in these points are then used to adjust the screening intensities to 0.6 log unit above the expected threshold. Stimulus intensities are corrected for retinal eccentricity. All missed points are retested. Three threshold screening strategies are available. In the simplest all tested points are classified as seen or not seen. Alternately the instrument can automatically measure the depth of the field defect at all missed points or divide missed points into absolute and relative defects. In the screening tests the results at the various points are thus printed out slightly differently depending on the screening mode used: 1. seen/not seen. 2. seen/relative defect/absolute defect. 3. seen/defect depth in dB (= tenths of log unit).

The HFA can also perform one-level tests, in which the operator specifies a single test brightness to be used at all test points. This is not recommended, however, and the default mode of the instrument is threshold-related, eccentricity-compensated screening as described above. The HFA has nine standard screening test point patterns.

Spatially adaptive screening. One of the test programmes, the Automatic Diagnostic Strategy, is a supraliminal test with space adaptive properties.

The testing is conducted in two phases: First an 80 point threshold-related supraliminal screening of the central visual field. In a second phase the depth of any detected defects is measured and additional points are added around missed points, thus increasing spatial resolution in pathological but not in normal areas.

Custom tests. The instrument can perform five different kinds of custom tests: meridional and circular profiles, high density grids, point clusters and single point tests. Meridional and circular profiles may be tested anywhere in the central 30° field with interstimulus interval variable between 1 and 12°. The grids can be varied in size and position. Also grid density is variable from 2 to 12° between tested points. Custom tests may be used in both in threshold and in suprathreshold screening mode.

Disk routines

The double disk drive makes it possible to store all measured fields. This is a prerequisite if a 'Fast Threshold' test shall be performed or if one wishes to save time by starting a full threshold test from the previously measured threshold values from the same eye (compare above). The storage of test results also permits merging of several different test results into one print-out. Stored perimetric data from computerized field tests are of course quite suitable for statistical analysis. Currently, the automatic analyses are limited to algebraic operations on the available data, averaging of several consecutive fields or an automated comparison where the findings from an earlier threshold test are subtracted from those of a later test. The automated comparison results in a subtraction field, quite similar to a subtraction X-ray image, where changes between the two tests are graphically illustrated. The analysis software is expected to grow considerably in the near future.

DISCUSSION OF ADVANTAGES AND DISADVANTAGES OF SOME OF THE CONCEPTS AND SOLUTIONS EMPLOYED BY THE INSTRUMENT

1. Projection system

The main advantage of projected stimuli is that they ensure flexibility in designing test point patterns — the stimulus can be projected at any desired location of the visual field. This in turn is almost a prerequisite for high-resolution custom tests, spatially adaptive strategies or any other spatially very detailed visual field examination. Using a projected stimulus the luminance of the projected spot is added to that of an evenly illuminated background and a true increment threshold is measured. In perimeters with fixed stimuli (fibre optic bundles or LEDs) this is not always the case. If the stimulus sources of fixed stimulus perimeters are not hidden, e.g. by a translucent film, each stimulus position will be visible as a 'black hole'. This will lead to changes of local retinal adaptation and the intensity of the stimulus, when lit, will not be added to an even background. Therefore a true increment threshold will not be measured. LEDs may also cause another problem. The light emission of LEDs is quite narrow and variable making their mounting critical. This can be avoided by covering them with a film as in the Computer and Tübingen Automatik-Perimeter instruments. Another problem of fixed stimulus perimeters is that all stimuli must be individually calibrated. When using projected stimuli neither of these problems exists.

Projection systems thus having large and obvious advantages they are not without problems. The light source in projection perimeters usually is an incandescent lamp. Such lamps age and must be monitored by photo cells. Their light output can be varied only over a small range and hence the stimulus intensity levels of the perimeter must be produced with the help of neutral density filters. Stimulus positioning requires a movable mirror. The position of this mirror must be checked often to prevent errors. (In the HFA, stimulus positioning is automatically checked and adjusted at the beginning of each test. Also edge detectors recheck correct mirror positioning each time the mirror passes the positions corresponding to the vertical and horizontal meridians of the visual field, i.e. between almost every stimulus presentation.) All the mechanics necessary to control the mirror, the density filters and the shutter make projection-type perimeters more complicated and costly and prevent the construction of a totally silent instrument.

2. Standard Goldmann targets and background

There is nothing controversial in using standard Goldmann-size test targets. These have been generally accepted for decades and are used in several manual and automatic perimeters.

The only problem might be that users are tempted to employ the size I target, just as they would normally do in manual kinetic perimetry. Larger stimuli offer a larger usable stimulus intensity range and less deleterious effects if incorrect lens correction is used. Although the results of one study indicate that glaucomatous field defects stand out more clearly if small targets are used (5), this finding is not in agreement with earlier investigations showing normal spatial summation in glaucoma (1). Presently we have no reason to stop recommending the use of fairly large stimuli in automated perimetry. While stimulus size is selectable in the HFA, the default mode is size III (1 mm^2).

Early computerized perimeters had rather low background luminosites (9, 13). In many instruments this was due to the fact that the stimulus light output was limited necessitating low background levels to ensure a reasonable, useful stimulus intensity range. This, however, is not a problem any more.

Therefore the HFA has adopted the standard Goldmann background, 31.5 asb, which requires less pre-adaptation and is less sensitive to stray light from ambient room lights than a lower background. It has not been shown that perimetry at lower backgrounds offers any diagnostic advantages, and e.g. the Computer instrument, which previously employed a 3.15 asb background because of the earlier limited light output of LEDs, has increased background luminosity to 31.5 asb in the new 750 model (6).

Higher stimulus intensities produce more stray light on the retina. This sets an upper limit to the stimulus intensity range that can be used in perimetry (2). It must be pointed out, however, that although higher background levels require higher maximum stimulus intensity levels producing more stray light, this no argument against the usage of higher background levels. The usable range remains the same when background luminosity is increased as long as the stimulus intensity is increased to the same degree.

3. Fixation monitoring technique

The HFA employs the blind spot monitoring technique (8). It has been employed in the Competer instrument for a decade, and is now used in automatic perimeters from at least five different manufacturers. The blind spot fixation monitoring technique simply means that the patient's fixation is sampled, at random intervals, by exposing stimuli in the blind spot of the tested eye. The advantages are that this technique is quite sensitive, even quite small deviations of fixation are detected unless the patient has large field defects in the blind spot area. It is also a technically very simple and inexpensive solution. The disadvantage, of course, is that this approach is an indirect sampling method which cannot separate between answers given when correct fixation is maintained and those given when fixation is erroneous.

Electronic solutions built on photocells or TV monitoring are continuous and might also function as blink detectors. They are therefore theoretically more attractive albeit more expensive. However, many monitors of these two complex types, may be sensitive to lateral, non-significant head movements or changes in pupillary diameter. As a consequence the sensitivity of the monitoring often must be turned down and even rather large malfixations are then missed.

4. Threshold-measuring logic

The HFA employs a repetitive staircase technique with diminishing step size (0.4, 0.2 log unit) and double crossing of the threshold. The step sizes are the same as those used in the basic Octopus threshold programmes (12) but otherwise the algorithms differ. In the Octopus the test process is always continued until the second reversal. The HFA goes further in continuing the test until the fourth reversal of the test procedure in points that are out of line with preceding points. It can be demonstrated with computer simulations that this technique is more accurate and less sensitive to patient errors than e.g. the Octopus or the Competer (9, 12) techniques, but it also requires more questions per tested point. One way of limiting the number of questions in static perimetry is to start the testing of a point close to its true threshold. The HFA takes advantage of the fact that points in the same area of the visual field usually have very similar increment thresholds by using the measured threshold of neighbouring points as starting level for the test process. This adjustment of the test process to actually measured sensitivities from the same area was first used in Competer instrument (9) and has now been adopted in test protocols of several other automated perimeters. In defective visual fields and fields with a general depression of sensitivity (e.g. due to media opacities and/or miosis) this algorithm is considerably more time-effective than the alternate method of starting from average thresholds of healthy patients from the same age group.

5. Screening techniques

The HFA screening is threshold-related and eccentricity-compensated. The compensation of eccentricity, i.e. the fact that the stimulus intensities used for the screening increase with the distance from the point of fixation, should be very non-controversial. The alternate method of conducting the test with targets of the same intensity regardless of the location in the visual field results in many false positive results (4, 10) unless the screening is repeated with stimuli of different intensities for the central and the peripheral field (11).

The HFA threshold related-screening tests are then conducted with targets supraliminal to normal parts of the actually measured field and only points with a sensitivity below this level are regarded as pathological and printed out as defects. Usually only localized field defects, and not a general reduction of sensitivity, will be printed out as defects. This concept has the advantage that the non-specific lowered sensitivity of cataract or miosis will not lead to an erroneous classification of a normal visual field as pathological. The price of this advantage, of course, is that a general depression of sensitivity, even if pathological, might escape detection unless one pays attention to the expected foveal threshold in the printout. In order to facilitate interpretation of screening results the HFA never employs screening stimuli brighter than those corresponding to an expected foveal threshold of 25 dB (with a size III stimulus) i.e. a stimulus which is approximately 1 log unit brighter than that perceived by a normal person of middle age.

6. Spatially adaptive screening

The spatial adaptive screening is a good example of a new, more patient-interactive type of programming, which will probably become more common in future computerized perimeters. The Octopus SAPRO programme (3) is another example of spatially interactive computerized field testing, but whereas SAPRO is a high-resolution mainly threshold-measuring test for small areas of the field, the HFA Automatic Diagnostic programme is a space-adaptive screening test covering the central 30° field. By increasing the number of questions and the spatial resolution in questionable areas space-adaptive algorithms mimic human perimetrists and may yield more information than a conventional computerized field test in the same test time.

7. Large selection of test programmes

Even if the custom tests are not counted the HFA has a large selection of test programmes. The variation is increased even more by the possibility of using several different modes of screening or threshold determination and by the optional fluctuation and foveal measurements of the threshold tests. This full array of test programmes makes it possible to find appropriate and effective tests for almost any clinical situation.

In perimeters offering such flexibility of test point pattern and test algorithm the selection of the most appropriate test point pattern and mode of test might become rather exacting, particularly for a user with minimal understanding of visual fields and perimetry. The multitude of test algorithms and point patterns also necessitates a certain discipline when eyes with known field defects are followed. It is always difficult to ascertain or exclude visual field changes over time. If different tests have been used at different times it might become almost impossible. It should be pointed out that the results of consecutive field tests might differ not only because different areas of the visual field have been tested, or different techniques used, but also because different tests take different time. In pathological fields longer test sessions tend to show larger and deeper field defects than shorter tests (7). Therefore pathological fields should be followed with tests using approximately the same test time on each follow-up.

One must conclude that the flexibility of the instrument is a great advantage both clinically and in experimental studies. At the same time one would hope that users of computerized perimeters with large program menus who do not understand the differences between the indications for the various test algorithms will improve their knowledge of visual field testing — at least by reading the instrument manual, and that they always use the same test when following a particular pathological field.

8. Custom tests

One of the HFA concepts is a comprehensive package of custom tests. This feature is most valuable since it permits detailed testing of virtually any area of the central visual field. The custom tests are unlikely to be used as sole tests and therefore offer the advantages of increased precision and detail without jeopardizing the necessary uniformity of one's standard clinical protocols.

9. Analyses of stored fields

The current analyses of the HFA are quite limited. The averaging and the subtraction procedure are, however, simple algebraical, quite non-controversial operations. More complex analysis programmes, where the instrument will indicate whether measured fields have statistically deteriorated or not between consecutive examinations will appear in the near future. The design of such algorithms, however, is certainly not without problems. A statistically significant decay of measured thresholds over time might well be due to e.g. increasing media opacities and lack clinical significance. In such instances a simple automatic analysis might do more harm than good. It would be a great advantage if new computerized field analyses could be designed where the changes of localized field changes are separated from a general decrease of sensitivity. The demonstration of statistically significant change of localized field defects over time would have considerable clinical importance.

SUMMARY

The HFA is a computerized perimeter with a very comprehensive set of test point patterns, strategies and custom tests. The instrument employs several solutions which have proved useful in earlier computerized perimeters and several new concepts. The construction with stimulus generation through a projection system, input through a CRT, programmes stored in PROMs and a double disc drive for storage of test results makes it simple to adapt the instrument to future needs, whether these are new test algorithms or point patterns, different input or display screens or new statistical analysis programmes. All these changes could be made without modification of actual instrument hardware.

REFERENCES

1. Dannheim, F. and Drance, S.M. Psychovisual disturbances in glaucoma. A study of temporal and spatial summation. Arch. Ophthalmol. 91: 463–468 (1974).
2. Fankhauser, F. and Häberlin, H. Dynamic range and stray light. An estimate of the falsifying effect of stray light in perimetry. Documenta Ophthalmol. 50: 143–167 (1980).
3. Fankhauser, F., Häberlin, H. and Jenni, A. Octopus programs SAPRO and F. Two new principles for the analyses of the visual field. Graefes Arch. Klin. exp Ophthalmol 216: 155–165 (1981).
4. Gramer, E. and Krieglstein, G.K. Zur Spezifität der überschwelligen Computerperimetrie. Klin. Mbl. Augenheilk. 181: 373–375 (1982).
5. Gramer, E., Kontic, D. and Krieglstein, G.K. Die computerperimetrische Darstellung glaukomatöser Gesichtsfelddefekte in Abhängigkeit von der Stimulusgrösse. Ophthalmologica 183: 162–167 (1981).
6. Heijl, A. The Competer. In print in: Computerized perimetry in glaucoma, eds D.R. Anderson and S.M. Drance, Grüne and Stratton, 1984.
7. Heijl, A. and Drance, S.M. Changes in differential threshold in patients with glaucoma during prolonged perimetry. Br. J. Ophthalmol. 67: 512–516 (1983).
8. Heijl, A. and Krakau, C.E.T. An automatic static perimeter, design and pilot study. Acta Ophthalmol. 53: 293–310 (1975).
9. Heijl, A. and Krakau, C.E.T. An automatic perimeter for glaucoma visual field screening and control. Construction and clinical cases. Albrecht v. Graefes Arch. Klin. exp. Ophthal. 197: 13–23 (1975).
10. Hong, C., Kitazawa, Y. and Shirato, S. Use of Fieldmaster automated perimeter for the detection of early visual field changes in glaucoma. Int. Ophthal. 4: 151–156 (1981).
11. Keltner, J.L. and Johnsson, C.A. Capabilities and limitations of automated suprathreshold static perimetry. Documenta Ophthalmol. Proc. Series 26: 49–55 (1981).
12. Schmied, U. Introduction to the technique and clinical application of Octopus perimetry. In: First Int. meeting on automated perimetry system Octopus, Interzeag A.G, Schlie-ren, Switzerland (1979).
13. Spahr, J. Zur Automatisierung der Perimetrie. I. Die Anwendung eines computergesteuerten Perimeters. Albrecht v. Graefes Arch. Klin. exp. Ophthalmol. 188: 323–338 (1973).

Author's address:
Department of Ophthalmology
The University of Lund
Malmö General Hospital
S-21401 Malmö, Sweden.

DEVELOPMENT OF A VISUAL FIELD SCREENING TEST USING A HUMPHREY VISUAL FIELD ANALYZER

H. DUNBAR HOSKINS, Jr. and CARL MIGLIAZZO

(San Francisco, USA)

ABSTRACT

Field test results were compared between the Octopus Perimeter and the Humphrey Automated Field Analyzer. Slopes were noted to be steeper in the superior than the inferior field. The authors found approximately 4 dB higher threshold sensitivity in the Humphrey than in the Octopus. This is probably due to variation in stimulus exposure time, 0.2 seconds in the Humphrey vs. 0.1 seconds in the Octopus. The effective development of screening devices requires characterization of slopes in normal populations.

Computerized perimetry for sophisticated threshold analysis of the visual field became clinically feasible with the introduction of the Octopus perimeter. Since that time, a variety of other instruments have become available for static threshold analysis of the visual field. Computerization has reduced operator training as well as shortening the duration of the test. Nevertheless, the test is time consuming and arduous for the patients. Routine static threshold perimetry of the central 30 degrees of the visual field using 76 points may take as long at 20 minutes in an eye with severe abnormality, and as much as 15 minutes in a normal eye. In order to expedite visual field testing, relieve patient fatigue, and more rapidly determine if the visual field is normal, screening programs have been attempted. The Humphrey Visual Field Analyzer has eleven screening programs available.

The strategy behind these screening tests uses a standard sensitivity slope with a decrease in retinal sensitivity of 0.3 decibels per degree of eccentricity from fixation for test object size III. This decision was based upon published data from Goldmann and Octopus visual fields (1, 2).

To evaluate this concept, normal patients were subjected to both Octopus static threshold perimetry and an essentially similar program on the HFA.

METHODS AND MATERIALS

Nine eyes from 5 patients, 20–35 years old, with normal ocular examinations were tested consecutively on an Octopus 201 automated perimeter and a

HFA within a two week period. Threshold sensitivities using Octopus program 31 or HFA program 30-1 were determined. A student's t-test was used to compare the mean threshold sensitivities of the 9 eyes for the Octopus and HFA.

In order to determine the slope of the hill of vision as measured by the HFA, 26 patients ranging in age from 25 to 84 years were tested with program 30-2. Only right eyes were tested. These patients were divided by age into 3 groups; less than 40 years old, 40 to 60 years old, and over 60 years old. The mean threshold sensitivity for each point in the visual field was calculated for each age group. The slope of these averaged fields was then calculated by meridian in the following manner. The difference between two points in the visual field was divided by the number of degrees separating those points. For example, the difference between the foveal threshold and the first point adjacent to the fovea along the 45 degree meridian was divided by the number of degrees that separated those two points in space. This process was repeated for every pair of points in a particular meridian. The slopes for the 45 degree, 135 degree, 225 degree and 315 degree meridians were calculated in this fashion by age group.

RESULTS

Table 1 compares the mean threshold sensitivity of all 9 eyes for the Octopus and HFA. This 4–5 dB difference was highly significant ($p < 0.001$). Figure 4 depicts a typical patient's visual field using the HFA and Octopus.

Figures 1–3 are plots of the averaged threshold sensitivities by meridian as determined by the HFA for each age group. The slope between each pair of points in each meridian for these average fields is presented in Figs. 2–4. As expected, the slope rapidly falls from fixation to 4 degrees and then gradually declines as it approaches 30 degrees. The initial steep slope from fixation is more marked in the younger age group (< 40 years old). Surprisingly, this was the main difference between the different age groups. The slopes of the 40–60 year old group and the > 60 year old group are very similar. Also, for all groups, the superior field slopes were steeper than the inferior field slopes (Figs. 1–3).

Table 1.

HUMPHREY *versus* OCTOPUS

	MEAN THRESHOLD dB	STD	N
HUMPHREY	30.1667	1.524	9
			P < .001
OCTOPUS	25.7823	1.333	9

86

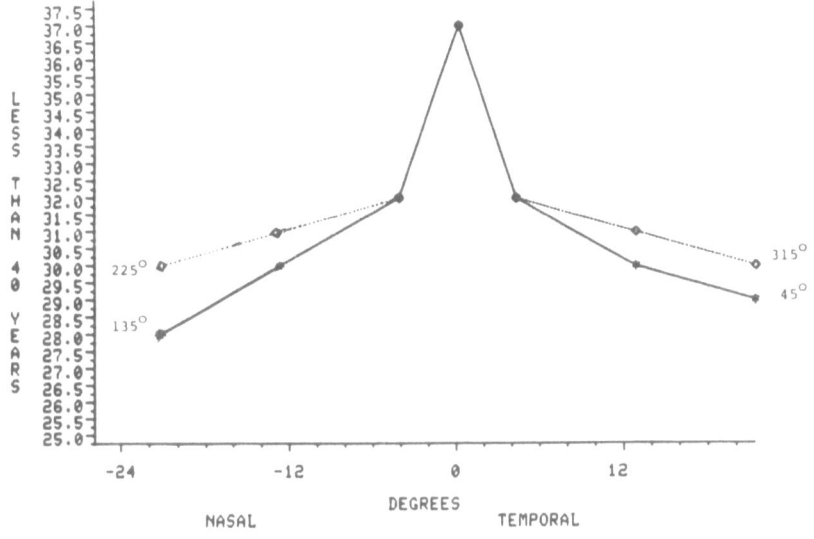

Fig. 1. Plot of average retinal sensitivities in each meridian for patients less than 40 years of age.

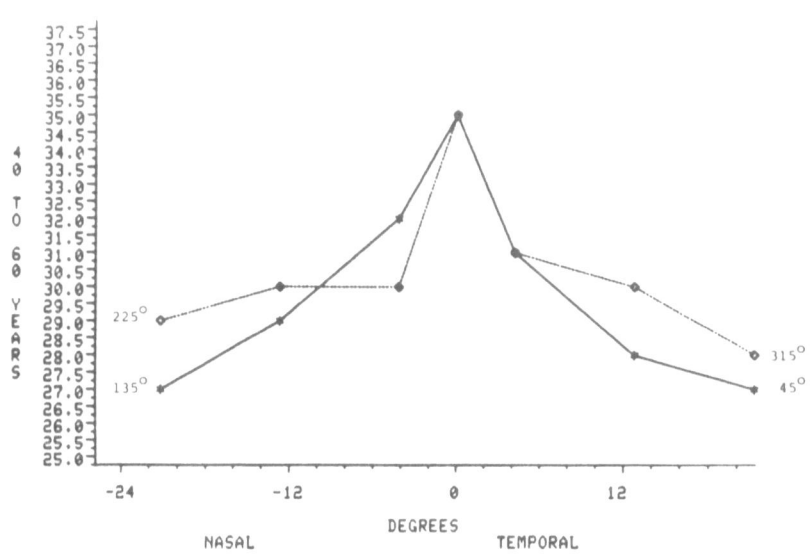

Fig. 2. Plot of average retinal sensitivities in each meridian for patients 40 to 60 years of age.

87

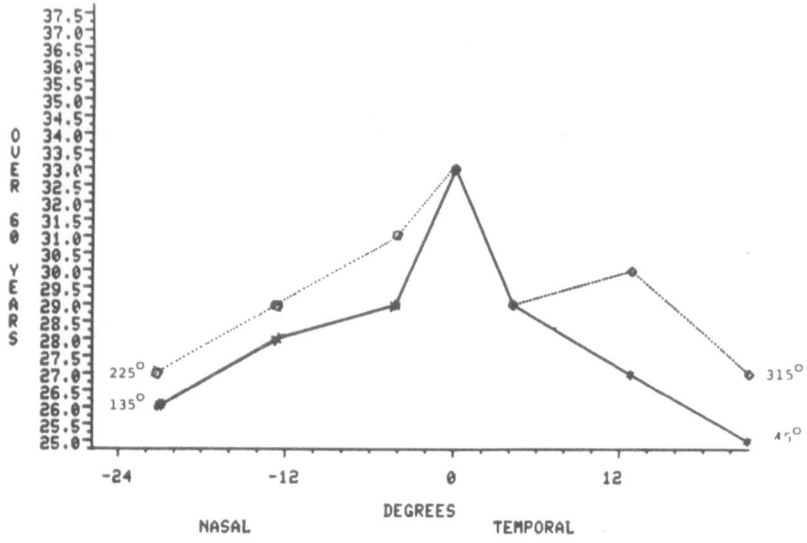

Fig. 3. Plot of average retinal sensitivities in each meridian for patients over 60 years of age.

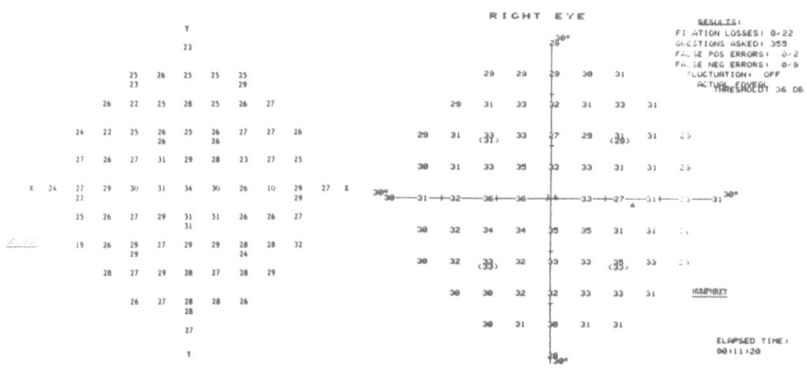

Fig. 4. Typical Octopus (left) and Humphrey (right) visual fields in the right eye of a normal patient.

DISCUSSION

Comparison of Octopus and HFA findings in the same normal subjects showed the HFA had an average higher response of approximately 4 dB per location.

The reasons for this apparent increased decibel sensitivity of the visual field when examined by the HFA are related to differences in the examination techniques.

First, the Humphrey instrument uses a background illumination of 31.5 apostilbs while the Octopus utilizes 4 apostilbs. This means that the Weber fraction which represents the ratio between absolute intensity and background intensity would be 10 000 Asb/31.5 Asb = 317 for the HFA and 1000 Asb/4 Asb = 250 for the Octopus. This difference in the Weber fraction would account for approximately 1 dB higher sensitivity registration from the HFA. Log 317 − Log 250 = 0.103 = 1.03 dB.

Secondly, the exposure time of the stimulus is different. Patients will have more sensitive threshold measurements if stimulus is left on longer below 0.5 second. The Octopus has a 100 msec exposure time and the HFA 200 msec exposure time. Aulhorn and Harms (3) indicate that temporal summation does occur for exposure times less than 0.5 sec with background luminances of less than 100 apostilbs. The difference in measured threshold between a 100 msec and a 200 msec exposure time when corrected for differences in background luminance between the two instruments is in the order of 3 dB (Fig. 5). Other factors which account for minor variation in results between the instruments may be related to patient characteristics.

Thus, due to technique it is anticipated that the HFA would register response levels at 4 dB higher than Octopus visual field. This is confirmed by our present study.

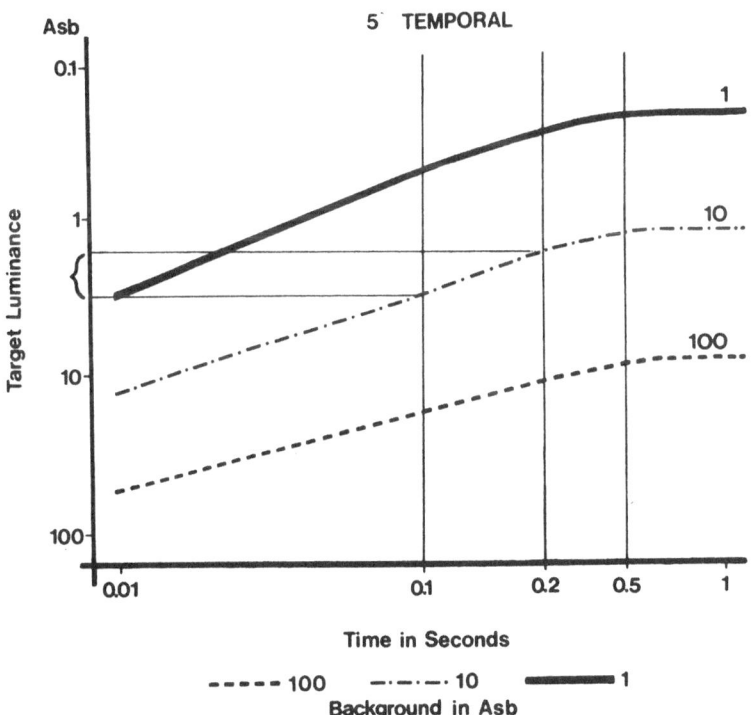

Fig. 5. Temporal summation related to background luminance redrawn from Aulhorn and Harms (3). Using the 10 dB background curve, approximately a 3 dB increase ({) can be anticipated by increasing stimulus exposure time from 0.1 to 0.2 seconds.

The slope data obtained for the HFA can be seen in Figs. 2—4. The slope is not linear, but falls off rapidly from fixation to 4.2 degrees eccentricity and then less rapidly from 4.2 degrees to 30 degrees eccentricity. Also, there is a slightly steeper slope in the upper field than in the lower fields. This is consistent with previous findings from Octopus (2) and Goldmann (1) data.

Current screening programs utilize three techniques; single stimulus intensity, arbitrary zone stimulus intensities, constantly sloping stimulus intensity. For accurate recognition of defects, threshold related analysis of the visual field in each of the quadrants is needed. The more precisely the slope can be calculated for each quadrant, the more accurate the screening method will be.

To speed and improve visual field testing, the current generation of computerized perimeters is exploring automatic diagnostic strategies which will recognize and analyze defects adequately for comparison. Careful recognition of the slope characteristic generated by each program in various areas of the visual field is essential. Diagnostic programs using these data will allow rapid detection phases of full assessment phases without unduely lengthening the procedure or inducing artifact. Work continues in this area.

REFERENCES

1. Fankhauser, F., and Schmidt, Th. Die untersuchung der raumlichen summation mit stehender and bewegter Reizmarke nach der methode der quantitativen lichtsinnperimetrie, Ophthalmologica 135: 660—666, 1958.
2. Octopus Visual Field Atlas, 2nd ed., Interzeag, Schlieren, Switzerland, 1978.
3. Aulhorn, E. and Harms, H. Visual perimetry, in Jameson, D. and Hurvich, L.M. (eds): Handbook of Sensory Physiology, Berlin, Springer-Verlag, Vol. 7 (pt 4), 1972.

Authors' address:
Dr. H. Dunbar Hoskins,
Glaucoma Research,
Clinical Eye Research Center,
UC Medical Center,
374 Parnassus Avenue,
San Francisco,
CA 94143,
U.S.A.

NEW TEST PROCEDURES FOR THE SQUID AUTOMATED PERIMETER

CHRIS A. JOHNSON, JOHN L. KELTNER and MATTHEW P. JACOB

(*Davis, CA 95616, U.S.A.*)

ABSTRACT

This paper describes two new test procedures for the Squid automated perimeter. The first method consists of a sampling routine in which thresholds are initially determined for an inner and an outer target location in each of 4 quadrants prior to testing other locations. From these evaluations, a slope is estimated for each quadrant and starting luminances for targets within individual quadrants are adjusted accordingly. This strategy, combined with smaller initial step sizes for the staircase, reduces the average testing time by 30–40%. It is most effective for eyes with moderate-to-severe visual field loss. The second method consists of automated kinetic testing of the peripheral visual field beyond 30°. Initial kinetic scans along oblique meridia are performed to determine optimal target sizes and luminances for kinetically evaluating visual field areas between 30° and 70°. Preliminary results indicate that normal peripheral visual fields can be evaluated in approximately two minutes, with an additional $\frac{1}{2}$–$1\frac{1}{2}$ minutes needed for analyzing abnormal visual fields.

INTRODUCTION

Automated threshold static perimetry is an effective method of quantitatively evaluating the visual field (1–5). However, a shortcoming of most existing techniques is that they are quite time-consuming. This paper describes two new procedures that attempt to reduce the amount of time needed to perform automated perimetric testing. The first procedure uses a sampling routine to measure thresholds at 8 predetermined locations, and estimates the slope of the visual field in each quadrant. Although it can be used for either central or peripheral threshold static tests, it is better suited for testing the central 30° visual field. The second procedure consists of kinetic testing of the peripheral visual field to generate 2 isopters between 30° and 70°. This method uses preliminary kinetic scans and decision-making to establish optimal target parameters for rapidly and accurately evaluating the peripheral visual field with an automated kinetic test strategy. Both of these procedures

Heijl, A. and Greve, E.L. (eds.), Proceedings of the 6th Int. Visual Field Symposium.
© *1985, Dr W. Junk Publishers, Dordrecht, The Netherlands. ISBN 978-94-010-8932-6*

provide substantial reductions in testing time as compared to other automated perimetric threshold procedures. Descriptions of the test strategies are presented below.

STATIC THRESHOLD SAMPLING

The sequence of operations for the threshold sampling procedure is as follows:

(1) A target pattern is selected for testing (e.g., program STD320 with 80 points in the central 30°: 6° spacing between points in a grid pattern bracketing the horizontal and vertical meridians).

(2) A starting luminance is assigned to each target location, based upon the average sensitivity values for the patient's age group (average sensitivity values are based upon 350 normal eyes, 50 in each of 7 age groups). Half of the targets are adjusted 4 dB above and half 4 dB below these average values prior to testing.

(3) Eight test points are selected from the target pattern, two from each quadrant. An inner and an outer radial point near each oblique meridian (45, 135, 225 and 315°) are chosen for the quadrants, and thresholds are obtained according to the standard staircase procedure for the 8 test points. The presentation of stimuli at these 8 locations is randomized.

(4) In each quadrant, a slope is estimated for the visual field profile on the basis of the two thresholds obtained at inner and outer radial locations. Each additional point in the quadrant is then adjusted by an appropriate amount from the average normal values to correspond to the estimated slope for that quadrant.

(5) The remaining target locations are then tested, but with smaller initial steps (4 dB intervals rather than 8 dB) and one less reversal of the staircase needed to obtain threshold (compared to the standard staircase procedure).

We have compared the results of the threshold sampling procedure to the standard static threshold staircase method in more than 100 eyes on the Squid. No meaningful differences in the quality or accuracy of the data have been noted between the two techniques. However, there is a substantial difference in the amount of time each procedure requires for completion. The threshold sampling routine requires an average of 30–40% less time than the standard threshold procedures. The differences in time are greatest when there is significant overall depression of the visual field, or when there is substantial field loss in one or two quadrants. In these cases, a time saving of 50% or more can be achieved with this procedure.

AUTOMATED KINETIC TESTING OF THE PERIPHERY

Static threshold testing of the peripheral visual field is more difficult than for the central visual field, perimarily due to the larger amount of visual field area to be tested and the greater response variability in the periphery. The amount of time required to perform automated static perimetry in the periphery is usually longer than for the central visual field. However, the incidence of visual field defects that occur solely in the periphery is much smaller than those within the central 30° visual field. Most of the visual field defects that are exclusive to the periphery conform to distinct anatomical boundaries (e.g., the vertical or horizontal meridian). Typically, these defects are not small, isolated scotomata.

With these considerations in mind, we felt that static threshold perimetry may not represent the most efficacious or appropriate method of evaluating the peripheral visual field. An automated kinetic test for the peripheral visual field was developed for the Squid as a potential alternative to threshold static testing. Since the complexity of kinetic testing is much greater in the central visual field, the present strategy was developed only for rapid evaluation of the periphery.

The basic procedure consists of kinetic testing of two isopters beyond 30°. Preliminary kinetic scans along oblique meridians (45, 135, 225 and 315°) are performed to determine the target size and luminances that will provide optimum evaluation of the peripheral visual field using a two isopter determination (greater than 30° and less than 70°, with approximately equal spacing between isopters in normal visual field regions). If the peripheral visual field is normal, testing then proceeds for the outermost isopter by performing kinetic scans along 12 meridians (30° separation between meridians, with bracketing of the horizontal and vertical borders). This is followed by a similar series of scans to define the innermost peripheral isopter. If all of the kinetic scans fall within the 95% confidence limits for local variations in curvature of normal isopters (determined from 350 normal eyes, 50 in each of 7 age groups: 5–20, 21–30, 31–40, 41–50, 51–60, 61–70 and over 70), the peripheral kinetic test stops at this point. In our preliminary studies, approximately $2-2\frac{1}{2}$ minutes are required to complete the kinetic testing for a normal peripheral visual field.

If a kinetic scan differs from one or both neighboring scans by an amount which exceeds the 95% confidence limits for curvature variations of normal isopters, it is automatically rechecked. If the second scan is within normal limits, no further evaluations are performed. However, if the second kinetic scan still exceeds the normal limits, additional kinetic scans are performed to define the boundary of the abnormality. Transitions from normal to abnormal sensitivity that bracket the vertical meridian will initiate a series of horizontal scans directed towards the vertical border at intermediate points between the initial meridional scan end points. A similar series of intermediate vertical scans are initiated for abnormalities which appear to be along the horizontal meridian. Thus, the test procedure is designed to be especially prepared to define nasal steps, vertical steps, quadrantanopic and hemianopic defects.

For abnormalities that are located at points between the horizontal and vertical meridians, the boundaries of the abnormal area are estimated by linear interpolation among the meridional scans defining the area, and kinetic scans are then performed along paths that are perpendicular to the estimated boundaries. This procedure allows the definition of localized depressions of isopters. An additional $\frac{1}{2}-1\frac{1}{2}$ minutes are needed to define areas of visual field loss with this kinetic scanning procedure.

It is possible that this procedure will provide sufficient quantitative information about peripheral visual function to be able to accurately monitor the status of the periphery in glaucoma and neuro-ophthalmology patients using this test in combination with a central 30° static test. On the other hand, this technique may only be sufficient to detect potential abnormalities in the periphery. In this case, the peripheral kinetic test would serve as a screening procedure to identify which patients need more extensive testing of the peripheral visual field. At the present time we have conducted limited clinical trials using this procedure. Further experience will be necessary to determine the overall efficacy of this type of automated peripheral visual field examination.

ACKNOWLEDGEMENTS

Supported in part by National Eye Institute Research Grants #EY-03424 (to CAJ) and #EY-01841 (to JLK).

REFERENCES

1. Bynke, H., Heijl, A. and Holmin, C. Automatic computerized perimetry in neuro-ophthalmology. Doc. Ophthalmol. Proc. Ser. 19: 319–325 (1979).
2. Fankhauser, F., Spahr, J. and Bebie, H. Three years of experience with the Octopus automatic perimeter. Doc. Ophthalmol. Proc. Ser. 14: 7–15 (1977).
3. Heijl, A. Studies on computerized perimetry. Acta Ophthalmologica (Supplementum 132) (1977).
4. Keltner, J.L. and Johnson, C.A. Preliminary examination of the Squid automated perimeter. Doc. Ophthalmol. Proc. Ser. 35: 371–378 (1983).
5. Schmied, U. Automatic (Octopus) and manual (Goldmann) perimetry in glaucoma. Albrecht von Graefe's Arch. Klin. Exp. Ophthalmol. 213: 239–244 (1980).

Authors' address:
Chris A. Johnson, Ph.D.
Department of Ophthalmology
University of California, Davis
Davis, CA 95616, U.S.A.

HISTOGRAM ADAPTION IN SPARO OPERATION

A. FUNKHOUSER and F. FANKHAUSER

(*Bern, Switzerland*)

ABSTRACT

The spatially-adaptive program, SAPRO, being developed for the Octopus 201 automated perimeter and presently undergoing clinical trials, is not only spatially adaptive, it can also adjust its measurement process according to the differential light sensitivity threshold distribution that it encounters during a visual field examination. This feature, along with related aspects of its operation are described.

INTRODUCTION

The time savings achieved by adaptive response to the visual field situation encountered as well as the higher spatial resolution made possible by the new spatially adaptive program SAPRO have been described previously in a number of publications (1 5). Its development has passed through several stages and it is presently undergoing final refinements while being used and tested in various clinical trials.

In its present form, the SAPRO program permits the operator to choose the geometrical form most suited to the examination goals while the resolution is varied dynamically and adaptively by the program itself in order to zero in on disturbed areas. Test locations which exhibit anomalous behavior in the first stage of examination are then surrounded by a finer grid of test points and such regions are investigated further. The question which needs to be discussed is: What constitutes disturbed behavior. How much must a threshold vary from the age-corrected normal value for that location before the program decides that it is worthy of more detailed investigation? The approach employed by the SAPRO program as it attempts to answer this question forms the substance of the following.

FIXED LOSS AND SENSITIVITY LIMITS

The initial grid of test locations is known as the coarse grid. There are two further grids that are employed and are used to surround and investigate

Heijl, A. and Greve, E.L. (eds.), Proceedings of the 6th Int. Visual Field Symposium.
© *1985, Dr W. Junk Publishers, Dordrecht, The Netherlands. ISBN 978-94-010-8932-6*

further suspect regions. The so-called medium grid has twice the spatial resolution of the coarse grid; and, there is even a fine grid which has twice the resolution of the medium one. As a numerical example, if one wishes to examine the circularly shaped region 0° to 30° eccentricity (equivalent to standard program 31 or 33), one can have a coarse grid with 6° between neighboring coarse grid test locations. The medium grid would then have 3° between its test locations and the fine grid 1.6° (half of 3° would be 1.5°, but the finest spatial step on the Octopus 201 is 0.2°).

In its original conception and in the initial versions, the SAPRO program was designed to be as versatile as possible. There, the operator had the possibility to determine all the loss level and sensitivity limits at which the various grids would begin their bracketing operations and also cease functioning (loss at any given test location is defined to be the difference between the age-corrected normal value for that location and the actually measured sensitivity threshold). While this is fine for those engaged in research where such 'finely tuned' operation may be of interest and even necessary, it was felt that for more routine usage, this flexibility was too cumbersome. It made program use too formidable and even confusing.

In its present form, then, the SAPRO program allows the operator to choose from a menu of 10 various possibilities a limit-combination which best suits the problem at hand. The one to be used is specified during the initial dialogue (and it appears in the printout of the examination results as the program number: H0–H9). At the moment, only six of these have been defined, leaving four available for future and custom-tailored usage.

This all may be made clearer by referring to Fig. 1. Figure 1a shows the results of a SAPRO examination: one sees a normal interpolated gray-scale representation of the visual field as determined in the measurement. In Fig. 1b, the loss values which were found are depicted located at the actual test locations where they were determined. The symbols employed to represent the loss values are now the same as those used in the Octopus CO (combination) printout. One can see where the medium grid and the fine grids surround the areas of interest and measure there with greater resolution.

Figure 1c shows a histogram of the loss levels encountered in the measurement. The loss levels at which the three grids began and ceased their operations are depicted by the letters C, M, and F (coarse, medium and fine). Usually, a loss of 3 dB or less is considered to be within tolerable fluctuation limits and one does not wish to take examining time to define such areas more carefully. At the other extreme, if a defect is absolute, exhibiting no measurable sensitivity at all, higher resolution there also represents wasted time in most cases. In this example, the medium grid upper limit was set so that it was triggered into operation around those points which exhibited loss exceeding 6 dB and it was set to desist when the sensitivity reached absolute zero. In order to make the fine grid sensitive to regions exhibiting even more loss, the upper loss limit was set to be 12 dB, and the lower limit was the same as for the medium grid. Here the results of the medium grid measurement are taken into account as well.

The current SAPRO version includes intermissions between the various grids so that the patient has a chance to rest his or her eye before continuing.

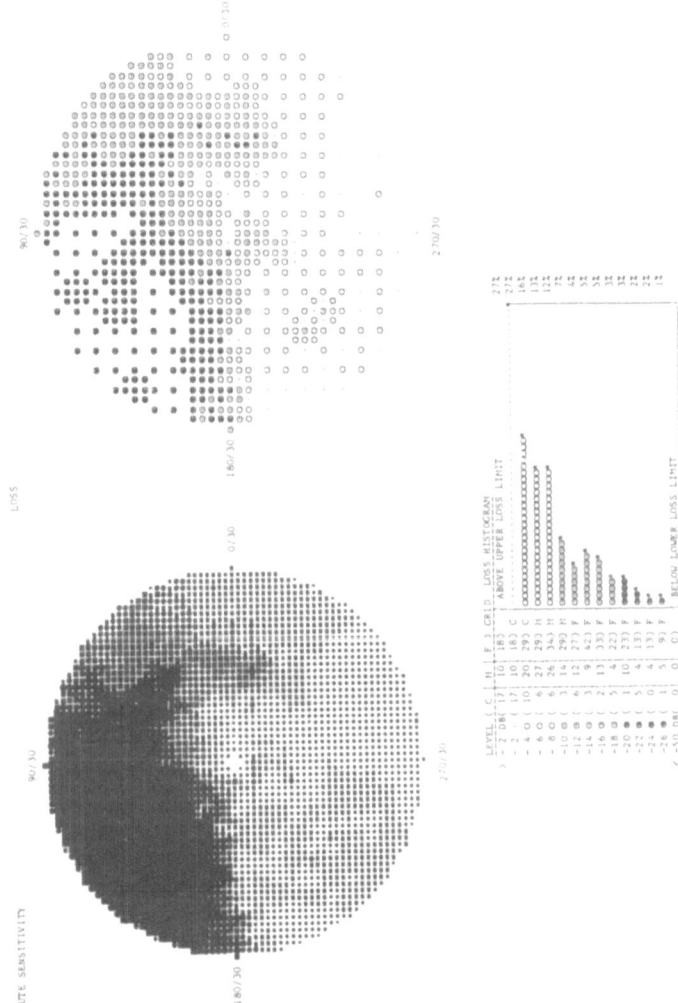

Fig. 1a. Gray-scale representation of visual field measured with fixed grid-limit boundaries. (The missing point at the center indicates that this location was not tested.) *b.* Test-locations actually measured for the visual field shown in Fig. 1a. The measured loss at each location is indicated by the same symbols used in the standard Octopus CO printout. *c.* Histogram of loss distribution encountered in the measurement shown in Figs. 1a and b. C, M, and F refer to the coarse, medium and fine grids and indicate the loss regions where they were operative.

Given the above limits, the examination required 1849 stimulus expositions and, leaving out the intermission times, the actual examination time required was 50 minutes. This was quite long and exhausting for the patient; it was decided not to even bother measuring the central region (thus the hole in the printout)! As a way of reducing this time investment and in order to make the program even more adaptive to the situation it encounters, loss-histogram adaption was introduced.

ABSOLUTE SENSITIVITY

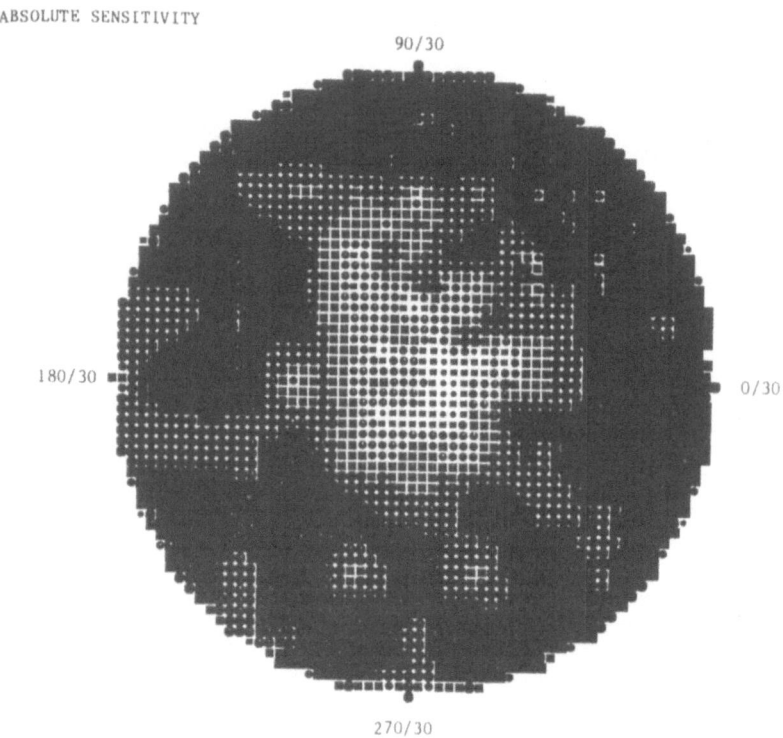

Fig. 2a. Gray-scale representation of a severely damaged visual field. *b.* Histogram of loss distribution encountered in the measurement shown in Fig. 2a. The majority of the test locations exhibit loss below the mean loss value.

98

Fig. 3a. Gray-scale representation of the same visual field shown in Fig. 1, but here measured with loss-histogram adaption (as described in body of paper). *b.* Test-location and loss representation of the measurement shown in Fig. 3a. *c.* Histogram of loss distribution encountered in the measurement in Figs. 3a and b.

HISTOGRAM ADAPTION

One sees from the histogram shown in Fig. 1c that the majority of the measured threshold values show little loss. The region of interest lies roughly in the lower 20 to 30 per cent of the distribution. One can also conceive, though, of meeting with a situation like that shown in Figs. 2a and b. Here, the differential light sensitivity at the *majority* of the test locations is severely diminished and the corresponding region of interest lies in the *upper* 20 to 30 per cent of the distribution.

Thus, it is apparent that if the program is to be truly adaptive to the situation that it finds during a measurement, it would be better if it did not normally operate with fixed loss limits. Rather, it should be able to determine the boundaries where the medium and fine grids become active or cease operation automatically, based on the distribution of loss that is present. This is the notion involved in what we are here calling histogram adaption and this has been incorporated into the SAPRO program design and operation. The ten subprograms mentioned in the preceding section permit the operator to choose between fixed limits (eg. for angioscotoma study) or various loss-histogram percentage levels.

Figures 3a and b show the same visual field as was shown in Fig. 1, but using the loss-histogram adaption. Figure 3a is the gray scale representation and Fig. 3b shows the corresponding test location and loss configuration. One sees that the same scotomous area is equally well resolved. However, the number of stimulus expositions was 919 (a reduction of 930) and the actual examining time was 27 minutes, a time saving of 23 minutes. Figure 3c shows the associated histogram. In this instance, the medium and fine grids were set to be active in the lower 20% of the loss distribution.

CONCLUSION

Some aspects of the SAPRO spatially adaptive program operation have been described, particularly the way it responds to the loss distribution it encounters in any given visual field. By means of an empirical example, we have illustrated the principle of loss-histogram adaption and have shown that it offers distinct advantages over fixed limit response. Thus the SAPRO program becomes not only spatially adaptive, but adaptive to any given loss situation encountered as well. It is hoped that as this versatile and useful program is utilized, it will be further developed and refined into a truly valuable tool in the kit used by those employing automated static perimetry.

REFERENCES

1. Häberlin, H. and Fankhauser, F. Adaptive programs for analysis of the visual field by automatic perimetry — basic problems and solutions, Doc. Ophthalmol. 50: 123 (1980).
2. Häberlin, H., Jenni, A. and Fankhauser, F. Researches on adaptive high resolution programming for automatic perimeter, Int. Ophthalmol. 2: 41 (1980).

3. Fankhauser, F., Häberlin, H. and Jenni, A, Octopus programs SAPRO and F, Albrecht Graefes Arch. Klin. Exp. Ophthalmol. 216: 155 (1981).
4. Häberlin, H., Funkhouser, A. and Fankhauser, F. Angioscotoma: preliminary results using the new spatially adaptive program SAPRO, Doc. Ophthalmol. Proc. 35, Fifth International Visual Field Symposium, Greve, E.L. and Heijl, A., ed., Dr W. Junk, The Hague, 1983.
5. Funkhouser, A. and Fankhauser, F. Erfahrungen mit SAPRO, dem räumlich adaptivem Octopus-Programm (in print).

Authors' address:
University Eye Clinic
Inselspital
3010 Bern
Switzerland

THE AUTOMATED PROGRAM 'GENOA GLAUCOMA SCREENING'

E. GANDOLFO, M. ZINGIRIAN and P. CAPRIS

(*Genoa, Italy*)

ABSTRACT

In a previous paper we have suggested a modification of the Armaly–Drance glaucoma screening strategy suitable for computerized Goldmann perimetry. This so called 'Genoa Glaucoma Screening' program has been applied to a large group of patients affected by ocular hypertension without visual field defect detectable by standard kinetic perimetry. In comparison with traditional screening strategies our program has shown many advantages and few disadvantages.

INTRODUCTION

In a previous paper we have presented a computerized perimetric program for detection of early glaucomatous visual field (v.f.) defects (9). Our strategy consisted of a modification of the Armaly–Drance (A.D.) glaucoma screening technique (1–3, 6). Our aim was to take advantages of the possibilities offered by automation in order to further improve the detection rate of the A.D. program (8).

In comparison with the A.D. strategy the following aspects were modified:

(a) the distribution of the tested points in the paracentral area was rendered more even;

(b) the stimulus adopted for the paracentral static tests was related to the individual threshold at different eccentricities (3, 4);

(c) the number of kinetic trajectories in the nasal v.f. was increased (7);

(d) the sequence of stimuli presentation was randomized (4);

(e) the rate of movement of the kinetic stimuli was related to the eccentricity (5).

MATERIALS AND METHODS

Our glaucoma screening program has been tested in 84 hypertensive eyes without glaucomatous v.f. defects detectable by traditional perimetry (kinetic

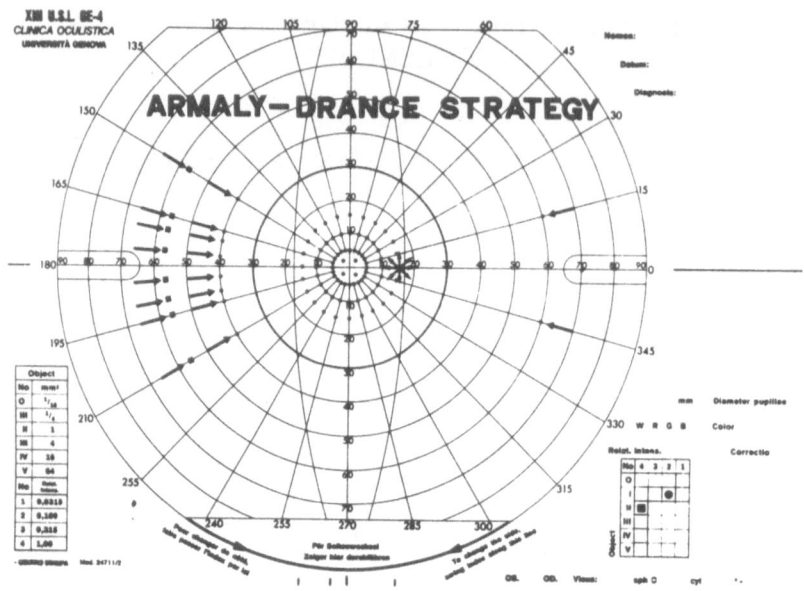

Fig. 1. Armaly–Drance 'Classic' strategy.

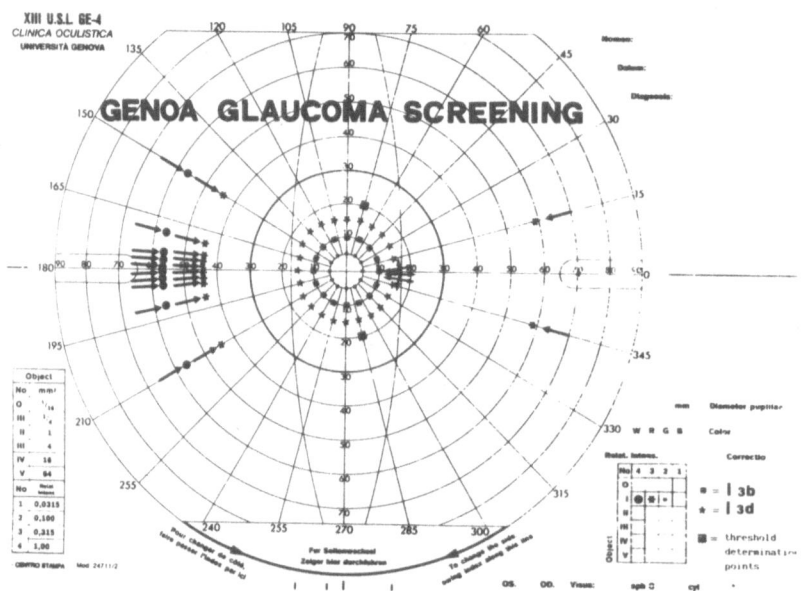

Fig. 2. 'Genoa Glaucoma screening' strategy.

104

Goldmann perimetry with 3 isopters and blind spot determination). All eyes also underwent an original A.D. test and, later, an accurate static-kinetic analysis of the whole v.f. The Automatic Goldmann Perimeter (Perikon) (8) has been the ideal apparatus to carry out this study, since it performs both kinetic and static perimetry and it can be used also as a normal manual Goldmann perimeter.

The automatic evaluation of the Genoa Glaucoma Screening program results was based on the following criteria:

(1) The v.f. was considered normal when:

(a) The blind spot did not exceed pre-determined limits (R.E. = meridians $20°$ and $325°$, parallels $9°$ and $21°$; L.E. = meridians $170°$ and $215°$, parallels $9°$ and $21°$), and

(b) there were no paracentral scotomata (the maximum loss of 3 isolated points was tolerated), and

(c) there was no nasal step (average difference between above below the horizontal meridian less than $3°$), and

(d) the two nasal and the only temporal isopters were wider than the minimum limits ($25°$, $35°$, $40°$).

(2) The response was considered doubtful when:

(a) there was an enlargement of the blind spot, or

(b) there was a doubtful paracentral scotoma (loss of more than 3 isolated points or of 2 neighbouring points), or

(c) there was a doubtful nasal step ($3°-5°$ average difference between above and below), or

(d) there was isopter's contraction.

(3) The response was pathological when:

(a) there was a definite paracentral scotoma (3 or more missed neighbouring points or 2 or more couples of 2 missed points), or

(b) there was a definite nasal step (more than $5°$ of average difference between above and below), or

(c) there were 2 or more doubtful responses.

RESULTS

Among the 84 eyes apparently without glaucomatous damage, the execution of the A.D. screening strategy has discovered 25 anomalies: 12 cases of paracentral scotomata, 7 cases of nasal steps, and 6 cases of combined abnormalities.

Among the 25 eyes classified as pathological by A.D. test, the accurate v.f. analysis performed later showed 24 glaucomatous defects (1 false positive response).

Among the 59 eyes classified as normal by A.D. test, the more complex controls showed 3 cases of v.f. defects (3 false negative responses). The Genoa Glaucoma Screening strategy has almost always confirmed the presence or the suspected existence of a glaucomatous defect. In only one patient, in which the A.D. test had shown a paracentral scotoma, our program did not discover any defect. In this eye, a more accurate v.f. analysis

Table 1. Comparative results.

	TOTAL NUMBER OF EYES	NORMAL VISUAL FIELDS	GLAUCOMATOUS VISUAL FIELDS	FALSE NEGATIVE RESPONSES	FALSE POSITIVE RESPONSES
ARMALY-DRANCE STRATEGY	84	59	25	3	1
GENOA GLAUCOMA SCREENING	84	53	31	1	5
DETAILED VISUAL FIELDS ANALYSIS	84	57	27	0	0

confirmed the presence of glaucomatous damage. On the other hand, in 7 cases classified as normal after A.D. program, our screening strategy has shown the suspected presence of a defect, which was later confirmed in 3 patients by an accurate static-kinetic v.f. study. The defect was, in 2 cases, a paracentral scotoma and, in one, a nasal step.

Among the 31 eyes classified as glaucomatous or suspected by our program, 26 had their abnormality confirmed (5 false positive responses).

Among the 53 eyes considered normal, only one showed glaucomatous alterations (1 false negative response).

COMMENT

In conclusion, our computerized glaucoma perimetric screening program has shown many advantages and few disadvantages compared with more traditional strategies.

The advantages are:
— the test is automatically performed by a computerized perimeter; thanks to this fact the conditions at examination are more constant and standardized;
— the individual threshold determination allows us to carry out a slightly supraliminal test, which increases the probability of detecting a paracentral defect;
— the increased number of kinetic trajectories improves nasal step detection;
— the standardized criteria of results evaluation permit an immediate and automatic classification of the v.f. detected defects.

The disadvantages are:

- there is a higher percentage of false positive responses;
- the cooperation required by the patients is slightly higher in comparison with A.D. strategy;
- a Perikon unit is required.

REFERENCES

1. Armaly, M.F. Ocular pressure and visual field − a ten years follow-up study. Arch. Ophthalmol. 81: 25−40 (1969).
2. Armaly, M.F. Visual field defects in early open angle glaucoma. Trans. Am. Ophthalmol. Soc. 69: 147−159 (1971).
3. Bedwell, C.H. Visual fields. A basis for efficient investigation. Butterworth, London, 1982, pp. 14−15.
4. Fankhauser, F. Problems related to the design of automatic perimeters. Doc. Ophthalmol. 47: 89−138 (1979).
5. Gandolfo, E. Contributo allo studio della soglia retinica differenziale in rapporto a stimoli cinetici. Boll. Oculist. 55: 385−396 (1976).
6. Rock, W.J., Drance, S.M. and Morgan, R.W. Modification of the Armaly visual field screening technique for glaucoma. Can. J. Ophthalmol. 6: 283−292 (1971).
7. Zingirian, M., Calabria, G. and Gandolfo, E. The nasal step: an early glaucomatous defects? Doc. Ophthalmol. Proc. 19: 273−278 (1979).
8. Zingirian, M., Gandolfo, E. and Orciuolo, M. Automation of the Goldmann perimeter. Doc. Ophthalmol. Proc. (1983).
9. Gandolfo, E., Zingirian, M. and Capris, P. Computerized perimetric program for detection of early glaucomatous defects. in press (Doc. Ophthalmol. Proc.).

Authors' address:
Dott. E. Gandolfo
Department of Ophthalmology
University of Genova
Viale Benedetto XV, n° 5
16132 Genova, Italy

PROGRAM SARGON OF THE COMPUTERPERIMETER OCTOPUS IN GLAUCOMA PATIENTS

CHR. FASCHINGER

(*Graz, Austria*)

ABSTRACT

Using the frequency distribution of early visual field defects in glaucoma derived from the results of Octopus perimetry, we developed a special Sargon program (user-defined program). The aim was to create a detection pattern with high resolution in areas with a high frequency of defects and to abandon the targets in areas with a low frequency, in order to shorten the test time.

INTRODUCTION

The aim of every investigator must be to recognize glaucomatous visual field defects as early as possible. The early detection of these small, circumscribed and at first flat scotomas depends not only on the method of examination, that is to say on whether it is kinetic or static, or on whether the instrument used is automatic or manually operated, but also on the number, arrangement and position of the targets. The aim should be the development of a goal-oriented program for the discovery of glaucomatous early field defects which does not last too long and which involves the advantages of the automated perimetry.

MATERIAL AND METHODS

The software of the computerized perimeter Octopus, the so-called program Sargon, allows programs of choice to be developed and continually employed. For any one place a maximum of 66 points can be plotted on a grid using x/y co-ordinates and fed into a computer for storage there.

The determination of the threshold of these 66 points lasts about 9 minutes in the repetitive bracketing process. Possible results are a scheme of figures in decibels ($1 \, dB = 0.1 \log U$) or a comparison between the actual result and the average corresponding to age. A divergence of 5 or more decibels from the norm was considered to be a defect (Fig. 1).

The 66 points were stored according to the scheme of frequency distribution

Heijl, A. and Greve, E.L. (eds.), Proceedings of the 6th Int. Visual Field Symposium.
© *1985, Dr W. Junk Publishers, Dordrecht, The Netherlands. ISBN 978-94-010-8932-6*

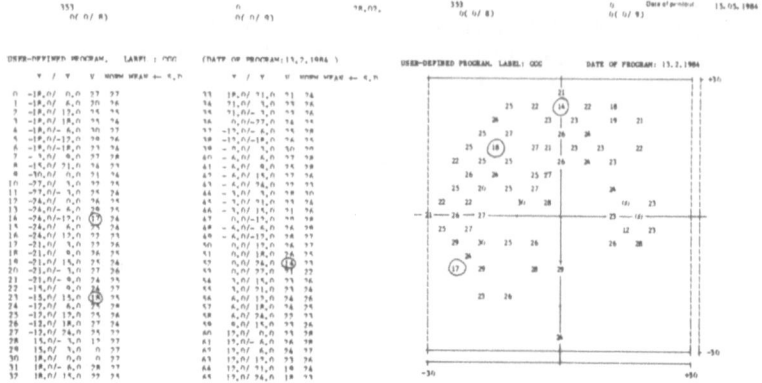

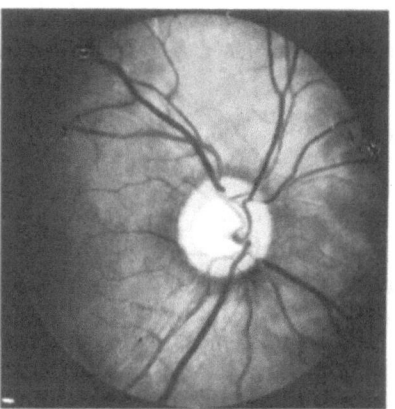

Fig. 1. New pattern of the user-defined program of the computerized perimeter Octopus: The list of the values, the pattern with the results in decibel and the papilla with a glaucomatous excavation. Targets with 5 or more decibel difference to the norm are defects and surrounded.

suggested by Gramer et al. (2) for relative and absolute early field defects, following Aulhorn and Karmeyer's (1) stage II. In areas with high frequency of defects the points were arranged very densely, whereas in zones where early field defects were rare, the points were left out.

DISCUSSION

The distribution scheme of Gramer et al. (2) was obtained by the results of investigations using the Octopus, whereby the program combination 31 and 32 was employed. The zone of eccentricity from 0 to 30 degrees was examined on a 4.2 degree grid. The duration was about 30 minutes. It could be shown, that these early field defects increasingly appear in certain areas,

110

namely nasal and in the upper half, and within a certain level of eccentricity, namely in the upper half near the fixation point and in the nasal upper quadrant from 6 to 30 degrees. This specific frequency distribution, together with the circumstance that the concentration of the mainly elderly glaucoma patients diminished because of an over-lengthy examination, caused us to put our targets only in those areas with a high probability that defects will be discovered. In order to gain valuable time they were omitted temporally and paracentrally in the below half.

We use this search program, which lasts about 9 minutes, along with tonometry, tonography and stereo-papilla-photography, particularly for out-patients. The exact determination of the threshold value in decibels makes possible a check on progress and also on the effectiveness of the therapy.

REFERENCES

1. Aulhorn, E. and Karmeyer, H. Frequency Distribution in Early Glaucomatous Visual Field Defects. Doc. Ophthalmol. Proc. Series, Vol. 14, 75 (1977).
2. Gramer, E., Gerlach, R., Krieglstein, G.K. and Leydhecker, W. Zur Topographie füher glaukomatöser Gesichtsfeldausfälle bei der Computerperimetrie, Mbl. Augenheilk. 180, 515 (1982).

Author's address:
Dr. Chr. Faschinger
Dept. of Ophthalmology
University of Graz
A-8036 Graz, Austria

CARTOGRAPHIC DEFORMATIONS IN AN ORTHOGONAL
PERIMETRIC MAP

LARS FRISÉN

(*Göteborg, Sweden*)

ABSTRACT

Some modern perimeters have replaced the meridians and the parallel circles of the classical perimetric map with an orthogonal grid. Analysis of cartographic deformations in the two maps disclosed practically negligible differences within the central visual field. The intermediary and peripheral parts of the field are depicted differently, however. This may cause difficulties in comparing some types of field defects, particularly those located in octants neighboring the vertical meridian, or in the temporal crescent. Both maps are inappropriate for measuring visual field areas.

INTRODUCTION

Although visual fields primarily are defined in spherical coordinates, practical circumstances force the use of plane field maps. The polar azimuthal equidistant projection has long reigned nearly uncontested. However, some modern perimeters, notably the Octopus, have replaced this familiar map with an orthogonal grid, where horizontal and altitudinal eccentricities are plotted on linear scales. This novel map, which belongs to the family of so-called cylindrical respresentations (6), does not solve the dilemma of faultless representation of spherical coordinates in a plane: like all other types of plane maps, it has its own set of cartographic peculiarities. The differences between the new and old maps may be of diagnostic importance, and merit analysis.

Two ways of illuminating the differences were used here. First, the meridians and parallel circles of the traditional map were transferred into the new map, to show how these familiar references change in appearance. Second, mathematically defined normal isopters were compared with respect to shape and enclosed area. While it is recognized that modern perimeters generally do not use isopters for result representation, it is likely that the user continues to depend on the recognition of broad outlines akin to isopters for the evaluation of results. Therefore, isopters remain useful objects for the analysis of cartographic deformations.

METHODS AND RESULTS

The relationship between coordinates in the two maps is derived in Fig. 1. Application of these formulas to the meridians and parallel circles of the

Heijl, A. and Greve, E.L. (eds.), Proceedings of the 6th Int. Visual Field Symposium.
© *1985, Dr W. Junk Publishers, Dordrecht, The Netherlands. ISBN 978-94-010-8932-6*

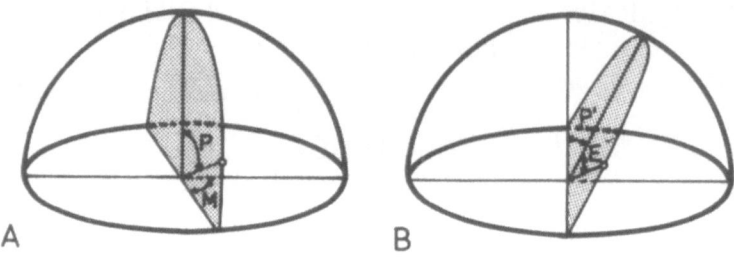

Fig. 1. Relationships between coordinates for a point on the perimeter surface in traditional (A) and novel perimetric maps (B). Polar coordinates are defined with reference to a great circle plane (dotted area) turning around the fixation axis, while the reference plane for the orthogonal map turns around the vertical axis through the eye.

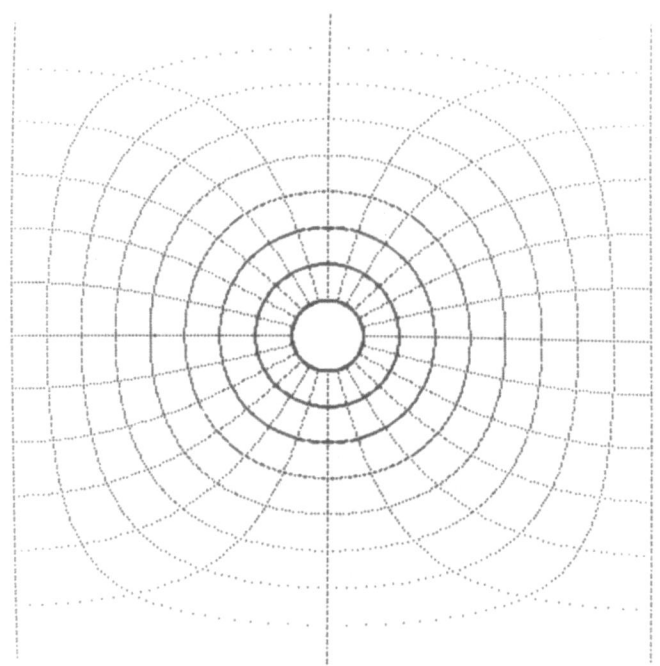

Fig. 2. Transfer of meridians (every 15th degree of polar angle) and parallel circles (every 10th degree of eccentricity) into the orthogonal grid. Dot separation corresponds to 1 degree in polar projection.

classical projection resulted in the orthogonal map given in Fig. 2. Only the centralmost parallel circles retain nearly circular shapes, while more peripheral parallel circles acquire increasingly prominent mid-quadratic bulges. The 90 degree parallel circle is transformed into two vertical lines. There is also distortion along the circumferences of the parallel circles, as shown by the bending of meridians (Fig. 2). This bending increases in prominence both with increasing distances from the center, and with increasing angles relative to the horizontal axis. Meridians running close to the vertical axis acquire bends approaching 90 degrees.

The analysis of isopter transformations is facilitated by the use of an appropriate mathematical model (4). The model used here builds on the observation that the geometrical cones defined by the entrance pupil of the eye and the outlines of normal isopters in the perimetric cupola, approximate right elliptical cones with a 1 : 1.5 axis ratio. With increasing cone diameter, the point of intersection between the cone's axis and the hemisphere moves more peripherally along the 350 degree meridian: the long ellipse axis coincides with this meridian. The model parameters are not critical as the continuous nature of the projection functions causes curves of similar appearances to be deformed similarly.

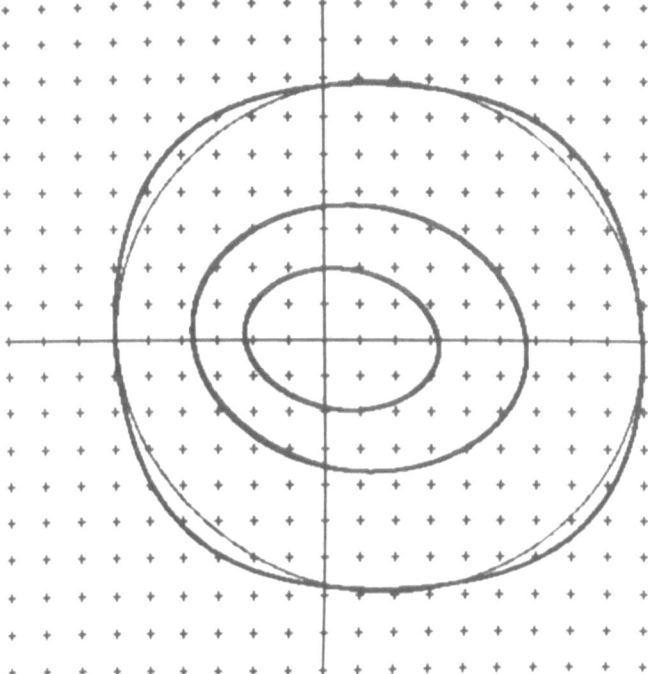

Fig. 3. Appearance of model normal isopters (bold curves) in orthogonal map. The isopters were generated from right elliptical cones (cf. text). The same isopters in conventional projection have been superposed. Differences between the two sets of curves are largely concealed by the limited resolution of the computer screen (512 × 512 pixels). Marked differences occur only for the peripheral isopter (outer curve generated by novel transformation, inner curve by classical projection). Distance between marks represents 10 degrees.

Coordinates were calculated for three different sizes of normal isopters for both maps, and the two plots were superposed in Fig. 3 to show the differences in isopter appearances (the computer program, written in Fortran, can be obtained from the author). There is little difference in the appearance of central and intermediary isopters, while more peripheral isopters acquire outward, mid-quadrantic bulges in the new map. The horizontal and vertical diameters remain unchanged. The transformation involves more than a change in shape, however: once again, there is a considerable and highly variable distortion along the isopter outlines in the orthogonal map, as evidenced by the bending of meridians (Fig. 2). This may have pronounced effects on the shapes of abnormal isopters, particularly if the abnormality affects the peripheral field. Actual computations for abnormal isopters have not been performed because of the lack of suitable mathematical models.

The surface areas enclosed by isopters are sometimes used for analytical purposes. This is valid only if the area measured in the map is proportional to the area enclosed in the perimetric hemisphere. Such proportionality applies only in so-called equivalent maps. Comparison of planimetry results from Lambert's equivalent projection (4) with those obtained in the two maps analysed here demonstrates both their lack of equivalence and their mutual discord (Table 1).

DISCUSSION

Many arguments have been raised against the polar azimuthal equidistant projection (1–3, 6). Its dominance can be attributed to the ease of mechanical implementation of this projection (or an approximation, as in the Goldmann perimeter) (4). Computer-based perimeters are not subjected to these mechanical limitations but allow an unlimited variety of projections and transformations. However, prior to pondering these possibilities, it is sound to examine the user's needs. In the case of clinical perimetry, I firmly believe that tradition needs to be respected. After all, most of the collected clinical knowledge of visual field defects is tied to the traditional projection. For this single reason any novel projections should not deviate to such a degree from accustomed representations that the existing body of knowledge may be difficult to apply. Whether this is the case is often difficult to decide without formal analysis.

Some of the properties of the classical map can be understood intuitively as it can be viewed as a perspective projection, with the projecting center

Table 1. Areal representations (per cent of correct value).

Isopter size*	Conventional map	Orthogonal map
Small	87	89
Medium	100	101
Large	111	118

*See Fig. 3 for definition.

located 2.7 radius units above the tangenting chart plane (6). It can also be viewed as obtained by cutting up the hemisphere along the meridians, and flattening it out in a plane. Meridional distances from the pole are correctly represented to scale, but all other distances are erroneously represented. The projection is neither conformal nor equivalent, i.e., it represents neither angular nor areal relationships correctly (3). The orthogonal grid is more difficult to grasp intuitively as it is defined as trigonometrical transformation. It cannot be thought of as a cutting-and-flattening procedure or a perspective projection. This makes mental comparison with other types of maps difficult. The new map is equidistant solely along the vertical and horizontal axes through the pole. It is neither conformal nor equivalent.

It is worthwhile to consider what may happen during mapping to any properties of symmetry because such properties are very useful in statistical analyses (5). Normal central isopters are symmetrical to a point in the hemisphere, i.e. they will coincide with their original outlines if rotated less than 360 degrees around the center of symmetry. Part of this symmetry is lost during projection to the conventional map, where only symmetry to the long isopter axis is retained (4). The novel map is still more destructive, retaining no symmetry features at all.

The differences between the two maps analysed here may be negligible for most practical purposes within the central visual field. However, problems may occur when dealing with intermediary and peripheral field defects, particularly if they are localized in the octants neighboring the vertical meridian, or if they engage the temporal crescent. Problems may also arise when comparing performances of perimeters employing different maps. Furthermore, areal or angular measurements must not be compared directly: both maps produce inaccurate results in these regards. Kirkham and Meyer (7) have presented a procedure for approximate correction of areal deviations in the conventional projection, but this does not seem to offer any advantages over the exact procedure of planimetry in Lambert's projection (3). Programs for exact determinations of area can easily be provided in computer-based perimeters.

Some other types of maps have been proposed recently, e.g. parabolic projections (1, 2). These novel projections retain meridians and parallel circles, but expand the representation of the central visual field at the expense of the peripheral field. Their cartographic peculiarities remain to be analysed.

REFERENCES

1. Crick, R.P., Crick, J.C.P. and Ripley, L. The representation of the visual field. Doc. Ophthalmol. Proc. Ser. 35: 193–203 (1983).
2. Dannheim, F. Non-linear projection in visual field charting. Doc. Ophthalmol. Proc. Ser. 35: 217–220 (1983).
3. Doesschate, J. ten. Perimetric charts in equivalent projection allowing a planimetric determination of the extension of the visual field. Ophthalmologica 113: 257–270 (1947).
4. Frisén, L. The cartographic deformations of the visual field. Ophthalmologica 161: 38–54 (1970).

5. Frisén, L. and Frisén, M. Objective recognition of abnormal isopters. Acta Ophthalmol. 53: 378—392 (1975).
6. Heissler, V. Kartographie, pp. 73—74. de Gruyter, Berlin (1968).
7. Kirkham, T.H. and Meyer, E. Visual field area on the Goldmann perimeter surface. Correction of cartographic errors inherent in perimetry. Current Eye Res. 1: 93—99 (1981).

Author's address:
Dr. Lars Frisén
Dept. Ophthalmology
Sahlgren's Hospital
S-413 45 Göteborg
Sweden

DEVELOPMENT AND USE OF GRADIENT ISOPTERS IN COMPUTERIZED PERIMETRY

M. MERTZ and U. ZIRKEL

(München, W. Germany)

ABSTRACT

Usually, the presentation of visual field results is done by print-outs of the original data or by greyscale charts obtained by interpolation algorithms. Less often, data are used to calculate the three-dimensional 'hill of vision'. A new method is presented to create isopters of a new kind, based on the evaluation of original Octopus data by image analysis. These 'gradient isopters' contain more information than those generally used, being of different width according to the actual slope of the retinal sensitivity in the area tested. Thus, gradient isopters may be mixed electronically with the corresponding fundus picture, the results giving quantitative information of a 'two step fundus perimetry' based on the use of both optimal fundus photography and perimetry. Problems still arise from the different kind of the concerned projections.

INTRODUCTION

A paper on isopters seems to be not very up to date. In computerized perimetry, we are now used to look at tables of the measured values, or, less accurate but more convenient, at greyscale charts based on the same data but in advance affording any interpolation procedure. The most likely impression and the least accurate one we get looking at three dimensional reconstructions of the concerned visual field. In 1979, in the Zürich Octopus symposium we demonstrated computer procedures to get both of these two forms of visual field representations, 3-dimensional pictures and isopters, already based on the original Octopus data sets (1). Last autumn, in Munich, we showed continuous grey shaded pictures derived from material of the same kind (2). In fact, all these different graphic representations, no matter whether they are 3-dimensional, isopters, profiles or greyscales of any kind, can be converted into each other, all based on an initial calculation of the whole 'hill of vision' (whether shown 3-dimensionally or not), the complete data set of which (containing both measured and interpolated values) can be used to feed any output system, like a printer or a television screen. If an advanced image analysis system (like IBAS/IPS; Kontron) is used for calculations and imaging,

Heijl, A. and Greve, E.L. (eds.), Proceedings of the 6th Int. Visual Field Symposium.
© 1985, Dr W. Junk Publishers, Dordrecht, The Netherlands. ISBN 978-94-010-8932-6

the pictures can be manipulated very easily and can be converted from continuous shading to any defined greyscale.

Alternately, profiles can be cut out of them in any direction. Figures 1 and 2 show a 5-dB-greyscale picture from a 30 degree visual field of myself, and a profile taken out of it along the horizontal marking line.

APPARATUS AND BASIC METHODS

Visual field investigations were performed with the Octopus 201 system, using program numbers 21, 23, 31, and 32. The date gained ('values') were fed into the image analysing computer system IBAS/IPS (Kontron, Eching near Munich) using an automatic figure reading program produced by ourselves. Inside the computer, our non linear spline interpolation was done already published elsewhere (1) in order to create (but not visualize!) the invididual 'hill of vision'. Subsequently, this 'hill' has been 'cut' into horizontal segments, the margins of which can be made visible as isopters.

THE GRADIENT ISOPTER METHOD

In Octopus greyscale pictures, the site of 5-dB-isopters can easily be recognized subjectively merely by looking at it, being the borderlines of the different grey areas. Just as easily they can be located in the profile: isopters have to consist of the total sum of all picture points at which the profile crosses a defined dB step. This threshold observation can also be imaged by the computer. If the crossing of profiles and grey step is defined by the smallest point achievable, this leads to very thin and equally shaped isopter lines. As told in earlier publications we were used to doing so for a long time (1, 2). But as shown in Fig. 3, we now define a certain *range* of this crossing. In this case, the range is 1 dB. The points concerned are marked in the visual field picture (Fig. 4), giving isopters which always contain picture points within the range of one dB. The space between is always representing the rest of the scale, which, is our example, is 4 dB. Thus, these kind of isopters give information not only on the location, but also on the actual slope of the sensitivity distribution in the concerned regions of the visual field. Therefore, we have called them 'gradient isopters'.

THE CLINICAL ATTEMPT: 'TWO STEP FUNDUS PERIMETRY'

We are still at the beginning of these very tedious mathematical experiments. Nevertheless, I would like to give an example of the present state of our research. The fundus picture composed electronically from several photographs (Fig. 5) shows the posterior pole of the left eye of a 35 year old diabetic, who had undergone laser treatment several times. He had deep scotomas in the central 30 degree visual field. We tried to combine these two pictures electronically in order to locate the loss of retinal function in the

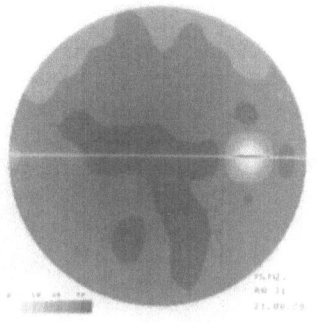

1

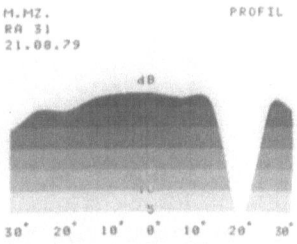

2

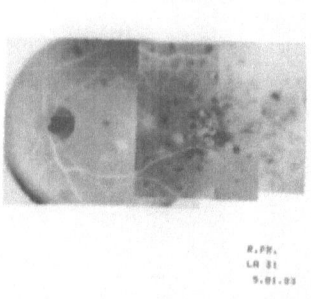

5

Fig. 1. Television imaged, normal central 30 degree visual field (of the author's right eye), based on Octopus program 31 data, non linear rational spline interpolation (4) and cutting into 5 dB-steps.

Fig. 2. Profile including grey scale, extracted from Fig. 1 at the indicated horizontal line.

Fig. 5. Fundus picture of a diabetic young patient treated by laser photocoagulation (see text).

121

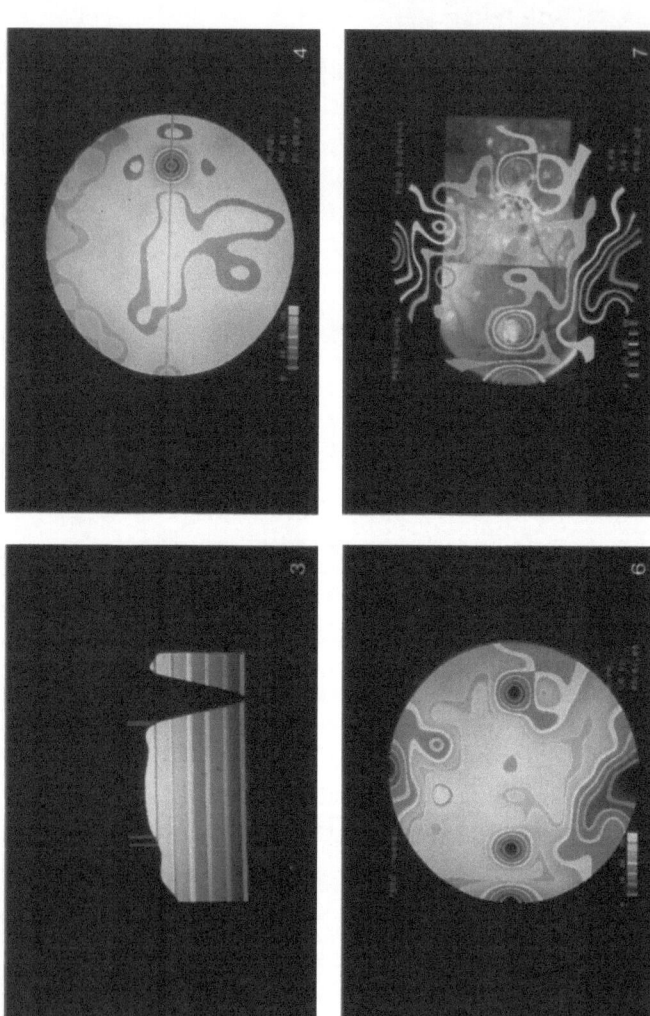

Fig. 3. Introduction of colours marking the different sensitivity levels, the border of which is given by a 1 dB range. At the spots of their intersection with the 3-dimensional profiles system isopters are created, the different width of which is depending on the local slope of the sensitivity curve.

Fig. 4. Visual field displayed in continuous shading with superimposed gradient isopters. Note the flat curve in the paracentral region causing broad isopters, in contrast to the rapid slope around the blind spot, marked by very thin isopters. The colours are introduced to provide a loss of information when these isopters are extracted from the greyscale field to be added to any other related picture, e.g. a fundus photograph.

Fig. 6. Central 30 degree visual field of the same eye (Octopus program 31 + 32, imaging technique see Fig. 1), recalculated upside-down, the gradient isopters added.

Fig. 7. Combined picture of the fundus and the related visual field, shown as coloured gradient isopters. (Projection problems see text.)

122

corresponding areas of the fundus picture. The visual field first had to be turned upside down without changing left and right! (See Fig. 6). Then, the isopters were calculated, extracted and added to the fundus picture, the size relation being taken from the designs of both instruments, the Octopus perimeter and the Zeiss fundus camera. As can easily be revealed, this leads to a first promising result (Fig. 7). Note the blind spot and papilla relation, and the rising scotomas at the vessel arcs (outside the fundus photograph, where massive coagulations could be seen clinically). On the other hand, these seem not to coincide sufficiently. We expected e.g. the paracentral scotoma to lie on the laser scar. Likewise, the point of maximal sensitivity seems to have shifted a little bit from the macula, as does the small laser scotoma from the corresponding scar at the upper arcade.

DISCUSSION

The isopter method had first been developed to compare the results of Octopus and Goldmann perimetry geographically (1). Now, we are using isopters when the original perimetric information should be added to other kinds of 'geographical' information display such as local variations in follow-up examinations (4) or traffic pictures in ergoperimetry (3), or the related fundus picture in our 'two step fundus perimetry'. As concerns the problems of the different projections we have started to improve our calculation system, meanwhile, increasing the accuracy of the projections by using reference points. In this way, the picture can be transformed mathematically as done in satellite photography. This causes a reasonable amount of work still to be done, but will, as we hope, minimize these kind of errors.

CONCLUSION

Coloured gradient isopters can easily be derived from interpolated visual field charts by television image analysis. They contain both sensitivity and local slope information. Extracted from the total visual field concerned, they may be of use in follow-up investigations of functional variability, in ergoperimetry, and in a special kind of fundus perimetry.

REFERENCES

1. Mertz, M. and Schultes, N. Greyscale and isopters. First Internat. Meeting on Automated Perimetry System Octopus. Zürich, 6.–7.4.1979.
2. Mertz, M. Retinale Ortsbestimmung rasterperimetrisch nachgewiesener Skotome. Neuere Entwicklungen in der Ophthalmologie. München, 28.–31.10.1983. Bücherei des Augenarztes, Stuttgart: Enke (in press).
3. Mertz, M. and Zirkel, U. Das binokulare Gesichtsfeld bei intracerebralen Prozessen, untersucht mittels statischer Perimetrie und Bildanalyse. 68. Tagung d. Württemberg. Augenärztlichen Vereinigung, 7.–8.4.1984.
4. Mertz, M. and Zirkel, U. Computerized location of fluctuation and changes in

glaucomatous visual fields. Proc. 2nd Symposium European Glaucoma Society, Hyvinkää/Finnland 18.–20.5.1984 (in press).
5. Weber, B. and Spahr, J. Zur Automatisierung der Perimetrie; Darstellungs-methoden perimetrischer Untersuchungsergebnisse. Acta Ophthalmol. 54, 349 (1976).

Authors' address:
Prof. Dr. M. Mertz
Dipl.-Phys. U. Zirkel
Augenklinik rechts der Isar
der Technischen Universität München
Ismaninger Str. 22
D-8000 München 80
Bundesrepublik Deutschland

THE ROLE OF RETINAL GANGLION CELL DENSITY AND RECEPTIVE-FIELD SIZE IN PHOTOPIC PERIMETRY

JYRKI ROVAMO, ANTTI RANINEN and VEIJO VIRSU

(Helsinki, Finland)

ABSTRACT

The invariance of visibility across the visual field, obtained by magnifying the stimulus (in inverse proportion to the human cortical magnification factor) and reducing its luminance (in inverse proportion to the Ricco's area) with increasing eccentricity, provides a novel method for clinical investigation of visual fields. In this optimal perimetry normal thresholds as a function of visual field location are horizontal lines called perimetrograms. Consequently, visual field defects are readily recognized, as pits in an audiogram.

INTRODUCTION

In photopic vision the number of visual cells analysing one solid degree of visual field decreases with increasing eccentricity. This inhomogeneity of visual sampling is principally determined (6) by the retinal ganglion cells.

To study visual information processing in retinotopically different parts of the central nervous system we have developed a method, called M-scaling (5, 9), that is designed to bypass the effect of ganglion cell sampling. This paper reviews our recent results (3–11) concerning the information transfer from various parts of the human visual field.

METHOD

Contrast sensitivity (10). Sinusoidal gratings were generated under computer control on a white cathode-ray screen. Contrast sensitivity (the inverse of contrast threshold) was determined in a detection task using a computer controlled, two-alternative forced-choice method that indicated the contrast required for a probability of 0.84 of correct choices.

Critical flicker frequency (5). Sinusoidal flicker with a modulation of 30% at 20–70 Hz was generated on a green cathode-ray screen with a linearized luminance response. Critical flicker frequency was determined by means of

Heijl, A. and Greve, E.L. (eds.), Proceedings of the 6th Int. Visual Field Symposium.
© 1985, Dr W. Junk Publishers, Dordrecht, The Netherlands. ISBN 978-94-010-8932-6

the method of adjustment: six, alternatingly ascending and descending trials
were averaged.

The human cortical magnification factor (6). The visual field is represented
topographically in the striate cortex but the central parts have a much larger
representation than peripheral regions. The scale of the map, called cortical
magnification factor (M), indicates the length, in millimetres along the cortical
surface, that corresponds to one degree of arc in the visual field. In monkeys,
the cortical magnification factor squared is directly proportional to the
retinal ganglion cell density corrected for the foveal displacement. Using this
relationship and previously published data on human ganglion-cell and cone
density we have estimated the values of the human cortical magnification
factor along the principal meridians of the visual field.

RESULTS

Contrast sensitivity and grating acuity (cut-off frequency at 100% contrast)
decreased rapidly with increasing eccentricity (Fig. 1A) when the test gratings
had a constant retinal area at different eccentricities.

In Fig. 1B grating acuity became independent of visual field location
when the contrast sensitivity functions of Fig. 1A were replotted (4) as a

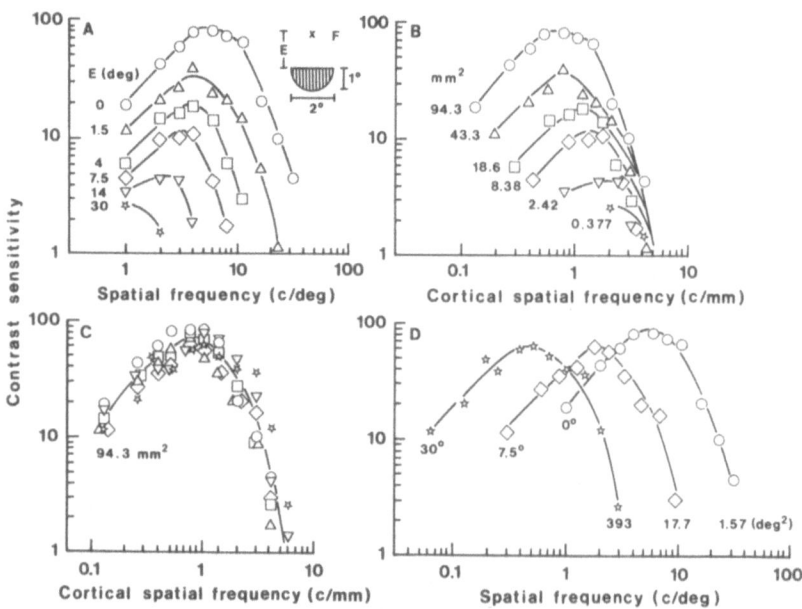

Fig. 1. Spatial contrast sensitivity functions at various eccentricities (E). The inset
depicts the stimulus geometry; F is the fixation point. Modified from (9).

126

function of cortical spatial frequency calculated as F/M where F is the retinal spatial frequency in c/deg of the visual field (11). This means that grating acuity is directly proportional to the human cortical magnification factor. Our recent results suggest that even the local anisotropy of monocular M within ocular dominance columns (7) is reflected in the resolution of gratings oriented along the across meridians in peripheral vision (8).

Despite replotting, contrast sensitivity did not become independent of eccentricity but was found in Fig. 1B to increase with cortical projection area (10) calculated as M^2A where A is the retinal grating area in deg^2 of the visual field (11). This indicates that, although replotting compensates for the variation of cortical spatial frequency with eccentricity, this partial M-scaling, as such, is insufficient for equalizing contrast sensitivity.

However, as Fig. 1C shows, contrast sensitivity functions became almost identical at different eccentricities when the test gratings were M-scaled (9) to produce similar spatial representations in cortical projections originating from different retinal locations: with increasing eccentricity, grating area was increased in inverse proportion to the cortical magnification squared and consequently, the range of test frequencies was extended towards lower spatial frequencies.

Fig. 1C also illustrates the superiority of complete over partial (cf. Fig. 1B) spatial M-scaling by showing that, in addition to spatial frequency, stimulus area must be scaled too. Similarly, if two stimuli, moving at different visual field locations, are to be compared, their cortical translation velocities must also be the same (11).

In Fig. 1D part of the contrast sensitivity functions of Fig. 1C are replotted as a function of retinal spatial frequency (10); the retinal grating areas used in the experiment of Fig. 1C are also indicated.

In comparison with Fig. 1A, contrast sensitivity in Fig. 1D increased markedly at low retinal spatial frequencies and maximal sensitivity reached almost the foveal peak level in the periphery. Also, the shapes and spatial band-widths of the contrast sensitivity functions were similar at all visual field loca-tions tested, indicating a corresponding amount of low-frequency attenuation, but the functions as a whole were shifted on the spatial frequency axis towards lower spatial frequencies at larger eccentricities because resolution was not much affected by M-scaling.

In addition (rev. 5), spatial M-scaling has been found to apply to luminance-modulated, chromatic gratings, to colour contrast, to pattern-reversal evoked potentials, to temporal integration, to fine-grain movement illusion, to detection of coherent movement in random-dot patterns, to differential motion detection and velocity discrimination, and to the slowest velocity needed for perceiving movement.

Critical flicker frequency (CFF) was not independent of eccentricity but first increased and then decreased with increasing eccentricity (Fig. 2A) when the stimulus field had a constant retinal illuminance (3, 5) and area at different eccentricities.

In Fig. 2B, the stimulus area was M-scaled (6): when eccentricity increased

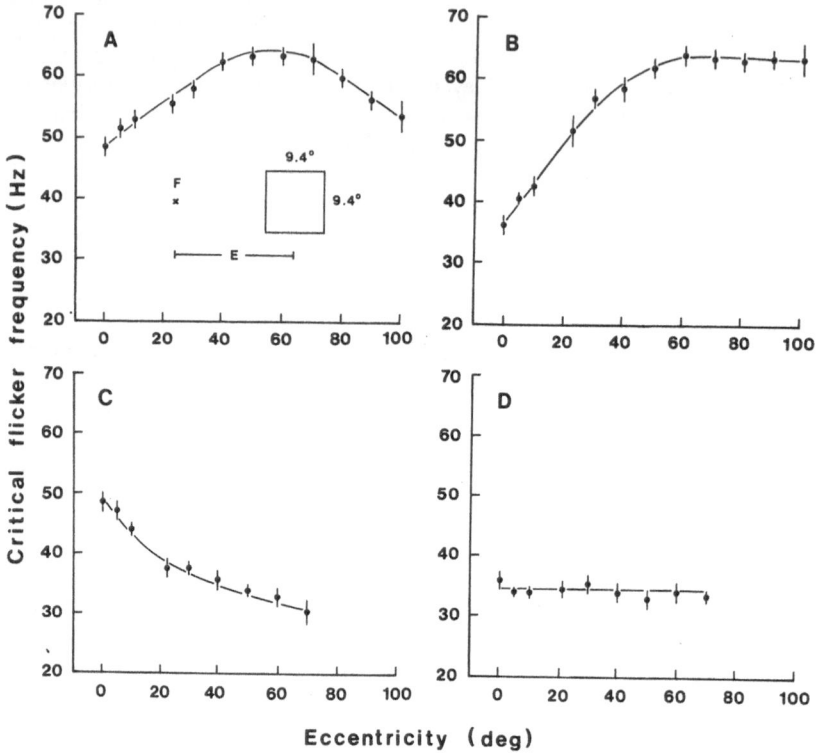

Fig. 2. Critical flicker frequency (Mean ± SD) as a function of eccentricity (E). The inset depicts the stimulus geometry; F is the fixation point. Modified from (5).

from 0 to 100 deg, the stimulus area increased from 0.209 to 369 deg^2 of the visual field. Despite of spatial M-scaling, CCF increased monotonically with eccentricity. The result means that CFF cannot be made independent of visual field location by M-scaling the spatial stimulus parameters. There are (rev. 4) also other measures (e.g. vernier acuity, orientation discrimination, stereoacuity, fusional vergence response, and temporal order detection) that evidently cannot be made independent of visual field location by spatial M-scaling. In agreement with (10), these complications indicate that spatial M-scaling as such is incomplete.

The human cortical magnification factor has been estimated (6) by assuming that magnification is directly proportional to the square-root of retinal ganglion-cell receptive-field density. Hence, M-scaling of spatial stimulus parameters compensates only for the decrease of sampling density of ganglion cells with increasing eccentricity. On the other hand, CFF of single feline ganglion cells increases with flux (1) defined as retinal illuminance multiplied by the area of receptive field centre. This suggests that the monotonical increase of CFF with eccentricity in Fig. 2B results from the

128

increase of receptive field size towards the retinal periphery because retinal illuminance and the number of ganglion cells stimulated were constant.

Ricco's area provides an estimate for the area of receptive field centre in man: by pooling together the results of (2, 12) we found, in agreement with (10), that the radius R of Ricco's area, in degrees, is linearly related to the inverse of cortical magnification: $R = 0.0263 (1 + 3.15/M)$. This suggests that, when expressed in cortical millimetres, the size and overlap of receptive fields are largest in foveal vision and decrease with increasing eccentricity. Our previous results (e.g. 3, 11) indicate, however, that the spatial frequency producing the maximal contrast sensitivity is at all eccentricities directly proportional to the human cortical magnification factor.

In Fig. 2C the area of the stimulus field was constant at all eccentricities but retinal illuminance was M-scaled: stimulus luminance was reduced with increasing eccentricity in inverse proportion to Ricco's area. Thus, when eccentricity increased from 0 to 70 deg, retinal illuminance decreased from 2510 to 40.2 photopic td. CFF decreased now monotonically with increasing eccentricity. The decrease evidently results from the decrease of cortical projection area and retinal ganglion cell density with increasing eccentricity, because retinal illuminance was M-scaled.

In Fig. 2D both the stimulus area and retinal illuminance were M-scaled. Now, CFF became independent of visual field location.

DISCUSSION

Our results support the view that spatiotemporal information processing is qualitatively similar for stimuli presented at different locations of the visual field and that quantitative differences result from retinotopical differences in the density, size and overlap of sampling apertures i.e. ganglion-cell receptive-fields. Also, eye movements and ocular optics evidently contribute to quantitative differences. For example, during steady fixation peripheral stimuli are more stabilized than foveal stimuli because receptive field size grows with increasing eccentricity. On the other hand, peripheral image quality exceeds the requirements of neural sampling which may result in aliasing distortions.

The invariance of visibility across the visual field, obtained by magnifying the stimulus and reducing its luminance with increasing eccentricity, provides a novel method for clinical investigation of visual fields. In this optimal perimetry normal thresholds as a function of visual field location are horizontal lines called perimetrograms. Consequently, visual field defects are readily recognized, as pits in an audiogram.

REFERENCES

1. Enroth-Cugell, C. and Shapley, R.M. Flux, not retinal illumination, is what cat retinal ganglion cells really care about. J. Physiol. 233: 311–326 (1973).
2. Inui, T., Mimura, O. and Kani, K. Retinal sensitivity and spatial summation in the foveal and parafoveal regions. J. Opt. Soc. Am. 71: 151–154 (1981).

3. Rovamo, J. Cortical magnification factor and contrast sensitivity to luminance-modulated chromatic gratings. Acta Physiol. Scand. 119: 365–371 (1983).
4. Rovamo, J., Leinonen, L., Laurinen P. and Virsu, V. Temporal integration and contrast sensitivity in foveal and peripheral vision. Perception, in press.
5. Rovamo, J. and Raninen, A. Critical flicker frequency and M-scaling of stimulus size and retinal illuminance. Vision Res., in press.
6. Rovamo, J. and Virsu, V. An estimation and application of the human cortical magnification factor. Expl. Brain Res. 37: 495–510 (1979).
7. Rovamo, J. and Virsu, V. Isotropy of cortical magnification and topography of striate cortex. Vision Res. 24: 283–286 (1984).
8. Rovamo, J., Virsu, V., Laurinen, P. and Hyvärinen, L. Resolution of gratings oriented along the cross meridians in peripheral vision. Invest. Ophthalmol. Vis. Sci. 23: 666–670 (1982).
9. Rovamo, J., Virsu, V. and Näsänen, R. Cortical magnification factor predicts the photopic contrast sensitivity of peripheral vision. Nature 271: 54–56 (1978).
10. Virsu, V. and Rovamo, J. Visual resolution, contrast sensitivity, and the cortical magnification factor. Expl. Brain Res. 37: 475–494 (1979).
11. Virsu, V., Rovamo, J., Laurinen, P. and Näsänen, R. Temporal contrast sensitivity and cortical magnification. Vision Res. 22: 1211–1217 (1982).
12. Wilson, M.E. Invariant features of spatial summation with changing locus in the visual field. J. Physiol. 207: 611–622 (1970).

Authors' addresses:
Jyrki Rovamo & Antti Raninen
Department of Physiology
University of Helsinki
Siltavuorenpenger 20 J
SF-00170 Helsinki 17
Finland
Veijo Virsu
Department of Psychology
University of Helsinki

A NEW NUMERICAL REPRESENTATION OF THE VISUAL FIELD IN REGARD TO THE RETINAL GANGLION CELL DENSITY

RYUGO HARUTA, KAZUTAKA KANI and TOSHIO INUI

(*Nishinomiya, Japan*)

ABSTRACT

Scales in visual fields are not based on the spread of cortical visual cells. Changes in the density of the retinal ganglion cells with eccentricity linearly correlate with those of cortical visual cells.

We developed a new perimetric chart whose area corresponds to the retinal cell count. The isopters were drawn using a computer system, and a three-dimensional display of the visual islands were made. The volume of the visual island represents the value of the whole visual field. The unit is retinal cell count × sensitivity ($3 - \log\Delta I$ asb).

With this method, we can represent a visual system not only at the retinal, but also at the cortical level.

INTRODUCTION

In clinical use we evaluate the visual function of the patient on the basis of the configuration of the visual field. Classical perimetry, however, is not always suitable for a quantitative estimation of a visual field change with the passage of time. Therefore, various numerical representations of the visual field have been recently devised.

In this study, we present a new numerical representation of the visual field on the basis of the density of receptive fields of retinal ganglion cells.

METHODS

We devised a new perimetric chart, in which the area represents the count of receptive field of the retinal ganglion cells (Fig. 1). This chart is based on Drasdo's formula (1) concerning the relationship of retinal ganglion cell density to the eccentricity from the fovea.

Drasdo's formula is

$$V = 0.005 [1 + 0.59\theta (1 + 3\theta^2 \times 10^{-5} + 8(0.59\theta)^{5.5} \times 10^{-10})]$$

Heijl, A. and Greve, E.L. (eds.), Proceedings of the 6th Int. Visual Field Symposium.
© 1985, Dr W. Junk Publishers, Dordrecht, The Netherlands. ISBN 978-94-010-8932-6

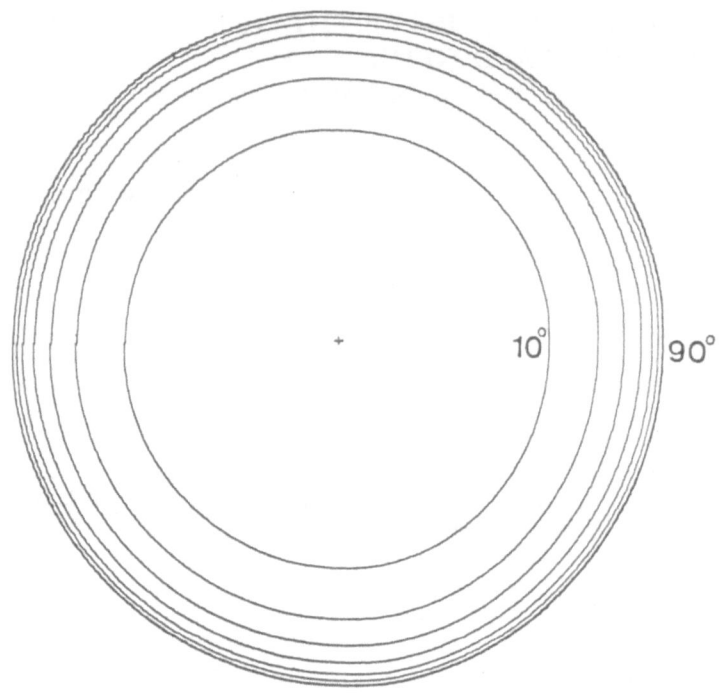

Fig. 1.

Here V is the reciprocal of a square root of the receptive field number per unit of a square root of the receptive field number per unit of a solid angle, and θ is the eccentricity in degree from the fovea.

Prior to the calculation, the visual fields were measured by the Goldmann's kinetic perimeter. The isopter was determined using size-I stimulus (the stimulus area was 0.25 mm^2).

The isopters on the visual field examined by Goldmann's kinetic perimeter were transformed to our new isopters using a SORD M-343 computer and digitizer (Bit Pad One). Furthermore, three dimensional representation of our new method was done for a better understanding of the visual function. The numerical value of visual field was calculated from the visual island in both Goldmann's scale (solid angle on XY plane, retinal sensitivity Z axis) and our new scale (receptive field counts XY plane). The units of our number are steradian × log $(3 - \Delta I)$ and receptive field count × log $(3 - \Delta I)$.

RESULTS

Figure 2 shows a normal visual field. Two dimensional and three dimensional representations of a visual field by Goldmann's scale are demonstrated in the

132

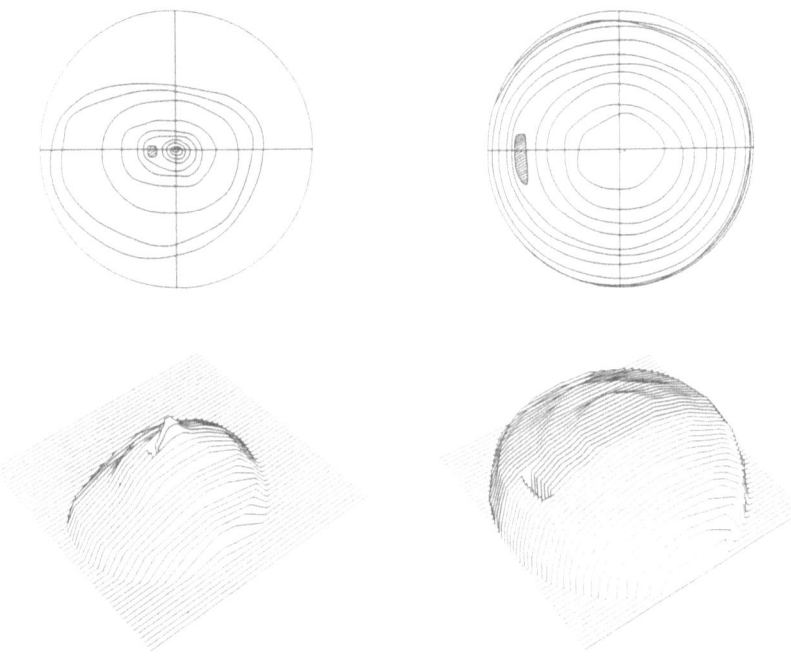

Fig. 2.

left side of Fig. 2. Similar representations of our scale are demonstrated on the right side. In contrast to Goldmann's scale, the central visual field was enhanced in our scale. The numerical value of the ordinary scale is 1.24 and our scale is 2.41×10^6.

Figures 3, 4 and 5 show the temporal changes of the visual field in a case of optic neuritis. Figure 3 indicates the visual field in the first examination plotted on Goldmann's scale (A and B) and on our new scale (C and D), respectively. On our new scale the deterioration of central vision was markedly stressed. The numerical value of the ordinary scale is 0.28 and our scale is 0.16×10^6. Figure 4 is after one week. They show a clear visual field change. The numerical value of the ordinary scale is 0.94 and our scale is 0.16×10^6. Figure 5 shows the visual field ten days after the first examination. The numerical value of the ordinary scale is 0.89 and our scale is 1.69×10^6. Making a comparison between Fig. 4B and 5B the improvement of the visual field is not easily detected. However, Figs. 3D and 4D show a marked trend towards improvement in the central visual field.

The numerical value from our scale shows increasement, on the contrary, the numerical value in ordinary scale shows decreasement in spite of the clinical improvement.

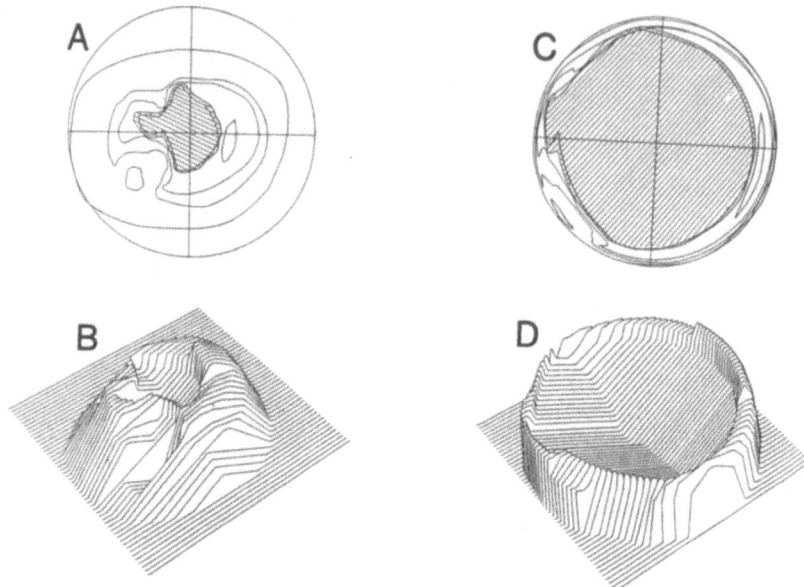

Fig. 3.

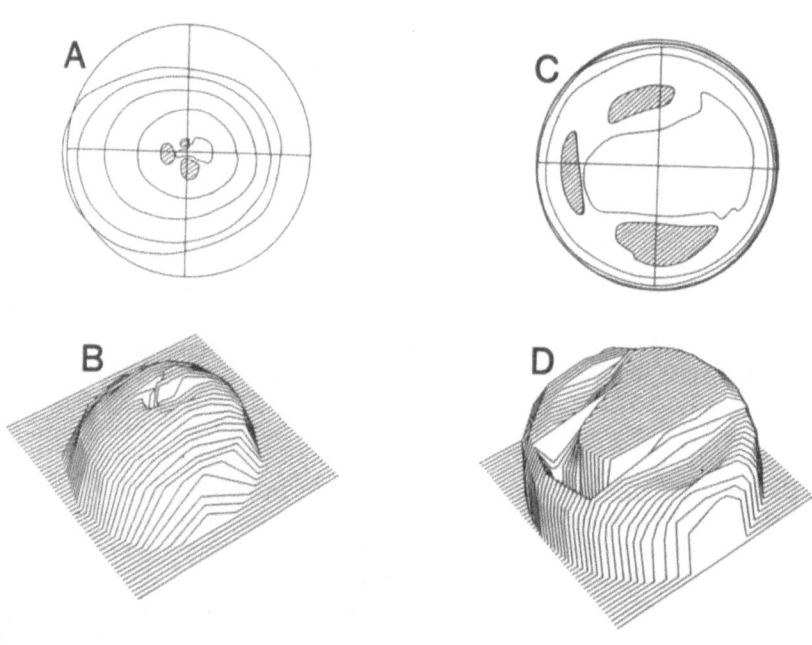

Fig. 4.

134

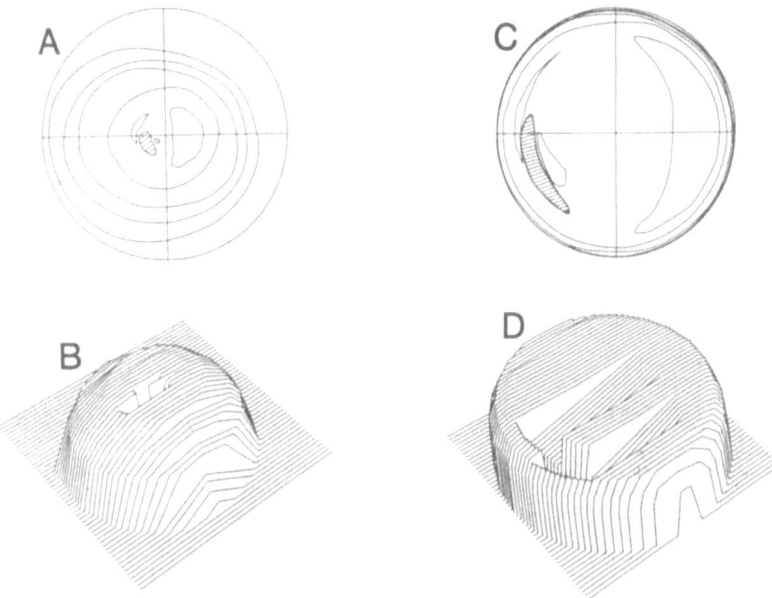

Fig. 5.

DISCUSSION

Several studies on numerical representation of the visual field have been investigated. For example, the area of the representation of the visual field by solid angle units corresponds to the actual visual space (2). However, this does not reflect the well-known fact that central vision is the most important part of the human visual system. Hence a practical, visual field projection method using a parabolic projection (3) and a grid-method for scoring visual fields (4) has recently been devised. In this method is stress on the central visual field.

But these methods have neither an anatomical nor a physiological ground. Our new method was based on both the anatomical and physiological construction of the human retina. It is only in the anatomical structure of the retina that the density of the retinal ganglion cell bodies suddenly become 0 in the fovea. From the physiological findings concerning the retina, the density of the receptive field of the retinal ganglion cells is highest in the fovea. From these facts Drasdo (1) originated his equation concerning the relationship between the eccentricity from the fovea and the receptive field density of the retinal ganglion cells.

Further, Drasdo studied the relationship between the receptive field density of retinal ganglion cells and the cortical magnification factor. This represents the cortical length corresponding to a degree of arc in visual space.

Our new method estimate the visual field by studying the density of retinal ganglion cells based on Drasdo's formula. That is, our scale on the chart represents the number of retinal ganglion cells. Furthermore, in our scale we represent the whole visual field by integrating the retinal ganglion cell counts from Drasdo's formula (X, Y scale) with retinal sensitivity (Z scale). With this method, we can easily estimate the total visual function. The examiner can briefly transform the isopters measured by Goldmann's perimeter to our nre isopters using a personal computer and digitizer.

In all likelihood, this value may furnish us with much information on measuring the VEP and pupillography.

REFERENCES

1. Crick, R.P., Crick, J.C.P. and Repley, L. The representation of the visual field. Doc. Ophthalmol. Proc. Series, 35: 193–203 (1983).
2. Doesschate, J. ten. Perimetric charts projection allowing a planimetric determination of the extension of the visual field. Ophthalmologica, 113: 257–270 (1947).
3. Drasdo, N. The neural representation of visual space. Nature, 266: 554–556 (1977).
4. Esterman, B. Grid for scoring visual fields II. Perimeter, Arch. Ophthalmol. 79: 400–406 (1968).

Authors' address:
Ryugo Haruta, M.D.
Department of Ophthalmology,
Hyogo College of Medicine,
1-1, Mukogawa-cho, Nishinomiya,
Japan, 663

PSYCHOLOGICAL FACTORS IN COMPUTER ASSISTED PERIMETRY; AUTOMATIC AND SEMI-AUTOMATIC PERIMETRY

D.G.M.M. DE JONG., E.L. GREVE., D. BAKKER and
T.J.T.P. VAN DEN BERG
(*Amsterdam, The Netherlands*)

ABSTRACT

The effect of psychological factors on the results of computer assisted perimetry have been underestimated. In order to quantify this effect a group of glaucoma patients was examined twice with a completely automated procedure and twice with a semi-automated procedure on the same instrument, the Peritest. All parameters were similar in both procedures. The examination strategy was also similar. The only difference was the active presence of the examiner during the semi-automated procedure. The examiner judged alertness, fatigue, fixation of the patient and according to his impression determined the speed of examination and provided psychological support.

A psychological score was made during and after the examinations. Defect volumes were calculated for all examinations. In 10 out of 19 cases a significant difference was found between automated and semi-automated procedures. *Intra*-semi-automated defect volumes differences were usually larger than *intra*-automated defect volume differences. Ergo, variation was less in the semi-automated procedure. The somewhat inferior results of the automated procedure were thought to be mainly caused by reaction and judgement problems of the patients. Other factors involved were fatigue, nervousness and fixation problems.

On the basis of these results and on the general experience with computer assisted visual field examination it is advised to offer the option of a semi-automated procedure in every computer assisted perimeter.

INTRODUCTION

Psychological factors in computer assisted perimetry (CAP) have received surprisingly little attention.

It is evident that the interaction between a computer and a human being is not comparable to the interaction between two human beings. In the past it has been emphasized that the human factor – the examiner influence – should be eliminated as much as possible. The human factor – so it is

Heijl, A. and Greve, E.L. (eds.), Proceedings of the 6th Int. Visual Field Symposium.
© *1985, Dr W. Junk Publishers, Dordrecht, The Netherlands. ISBN 978-94-010-8932-6*

137

believed – is a source of considerable variation. It is often overlooked that the human factor may also be a source of psychological support and flexibility. Both statements are correct.

The examiner in manual perimetry has been a source of variation because he was the *brain* behind the examination strategy. The computer has done a better job. The examiner was also the one who set the patients mind at ease, comforted him, encouraged him, corrected and stimulated him. The cool impersonal computer does a worse job here. Would it not be wise to use the computer where it performs best and use the human being where it can not be replaced? A revival of the human factor in computer assisted perimetry.

How do we know whether the human factor has any influence at all? To answer this question we have examined a number of glaucoma patients with an automated procedure and with a semi-automated procedure.

Until now all comparisons between CAP and manual perimetry concerned different instruments and different strategies. Such comparative studies do not tell us anything about the influence of the human factor perse.

We have therefore used the same instrument and the same strategy for this investigation. The only difference was that in the semi-automated procedure the examiner conducted the examination *together* with the computer while in the automated procedure the computer was without human support.

The questions we asked were:
- is there a difference between the results of automated perimetry and the results of semi-automated perimetry as such and in the variability of these results.
- what is the difference between two automated (intra-automatic) and between two semi-automated (intra-automatic) procedures?
- is there a difference between the intra-automatic differences and the intra-semi-automatic differences?
- is there a psychological explanation for these differences?

METHOD AND PATIENTS

With the Peritest (2) 19 patients with visual field defects due to glaucoma were examined.

Each patient had two automated procedures and two semi-automated procedures. Between each procedure a 5 minutes intermission was given. The investigation started with two automated procedures and ended with two semi-automated procedures. This sequence was chosen in order to avoid an effect of the human factor in the semi-automated procedures on the automated procedures. The phases IA and periphery of the Peritest were used (126 locations). The examination was taped, pulse-rate recorded and extensive notes were made on patients behavior. The patient was asked about his impressions at the end of each examination. The major difference between automatic and semi-automatic procedures was the presence of the examiner during the whole semi-automatic procedure.

The examiner did all things he usually does in a manual examination *except* determining the strategy. The examiner determined the speed of the
138

examination, judged patient-response, controled fixation, corrected or encouraged the patient if necessary.

The strategy was kept almost identical to the automated procedure. It was expected that differences between the two procedures would be mainly due to psychological factors. We aimed at a comparison between the *computer* on the one hand and *computer plus examiner* on the other hand.

The patients all had glaucomatous visual field defects with a stage 2 or 3 defect in one or two horizontal visual field halfs or a stage 4 or 5 defect in one visual field half (1).

At the end of each group of examinations the defect volumes (DV) for each procedure were calculated. The DV is the sum of the defect intensities at the individual locations. The defect intensities were measured in steps of 0.6 log. unit, resulting in intensities of 1.2, 1.8 and 2.4 log. units respectively.

The standard deviations of the four measurements per location were calculated and the overall standard deviation was determined, assuming identical uncertainty behavior at all locations.

The psychological factors were quantified in a psychological score: general condition of the patient; did the patient comprehend the first instruction, the second instruction, did the patient have any judgement problems; patient alertness and speed of reaction; patients fatigue; reaction to pseudo-presentations; nervousness; restlessness. The patient was questioned about degree of difficulty of the examination, fatigue, disturbing sounds or silence, speed of examination, judgement problems and a general impression of the examination.

A fluctuation analysis was made. The psychological factors were quantifield in a psychological score.

RESULTS

Some of the results are presented in Table 1. The second column gives a measure for the overall fluctuation, which determines whether the difference between the sum of the defect volume of the two automatic procedures and the sum of the defect volume of the two semi-automatic procedures is significant at the 1% level. In 10 out to 19 cases there was a significant difference between the automated and semi-automated procedures. In 8 of these 10 cases the defect volume was smaller in the automated procedure (third column). In 5 of the 10 cases with a significant difference, this difference was larger than the intra-automated procedure or intra-semi-automated procedure difference (fifth and sixth column).

An example of a result with and without a significant defect volume is shown in Fig. 1.

In Fig. 2. a *histogram* is presented with intra-automated and intra-semi-automatic defect volume differences. From this figure it is clear that there are more semi-automatic defect volume differences among the lower values.

The mean intra-automatic defect volume differences was almost twice as large as the mean intra-semi-automatic difference. However this difference was not statistically significant. The psychological score was low in 4 out of 5 cases where the *inter* defect volume difference was larger than the *intra*

Table 1. Data on defect volume differences and fluctuation.
Column 1: patient number.
Column 2: standard deviation for 4 examinations multiplied by $\sqrt{4.n}$ and 2.5. n = number of positions examined.
Column 3: Δ_1 = difference $(DV\,A_1 + DV\,A_2) - (DV\,SA_1 + DV\,SA_2)$.
Column 4: difference in DV A and DV SA $<$ means DV A smaller than DV SA.
Column 5: Δ_2 = difference $(DV\,A_1 - DV\,A_2)$.
Column 6: Δ_3 = difference $(DV\,SA_1 - DV\,SA_2)$.

Pat #	$2.5^{\Gamma}\sigma$	Δ_1^F	size DVA/NA	Δ_2	Δ_3
1	263	714	$<$	210	24
2	243	1022	$>$	368	48
3	208	162	—	12	18
4	263	156	—	498	138
5	235	18	—	90	376
6	233	170	—	342	48
7	208	38	—	96	74
8	208	261	—	66	147
9	200	72	—	18	30
10	233	438	$>$	738	84
11	180	456	$<$	138	42
12	188	356	$<$	54	45
13	203	270	$<$	42	12
14	293	402	$<$	120	90
15	253	480	$<$	48	348
16	258	622	$<$	78	360
17	245	20	—	222	154
18	290	320	$<$	232	0
19	213	162	—	422	30

defect volume difference. Fifteen of the 19 patients had INSC values with 0.2 log. unit difference in the four examinations.

Four had INSC values that differed more than 0.2 log. unit. In two of these cases the differences were between the automatic and semi-automatic procedures. In one the difference was intra-automatic and in the last one the difference was intra-semi-automatic. All four patients had low psychological scores. The defect volume values can be corrected for INSC differences.

PSYCHOLOGICAL FACTORS

The somewhat inferior results of the automatic procedure were thought to be mainly caused by reaction and judgement problems. Such problems appear only to a certain extent in the false-positive and false-negative scores. Other factors were fixation problems, fatigue and nervousness during the automatic procedure.

DISCUSSION

It did not come as a surprise that we found differences between automated perimetry and semi-automated perimetry. Many of the glaucoma patients are old and have a level and speed of comprehension which causes difficulty to meet the requirements of automated perimetry.

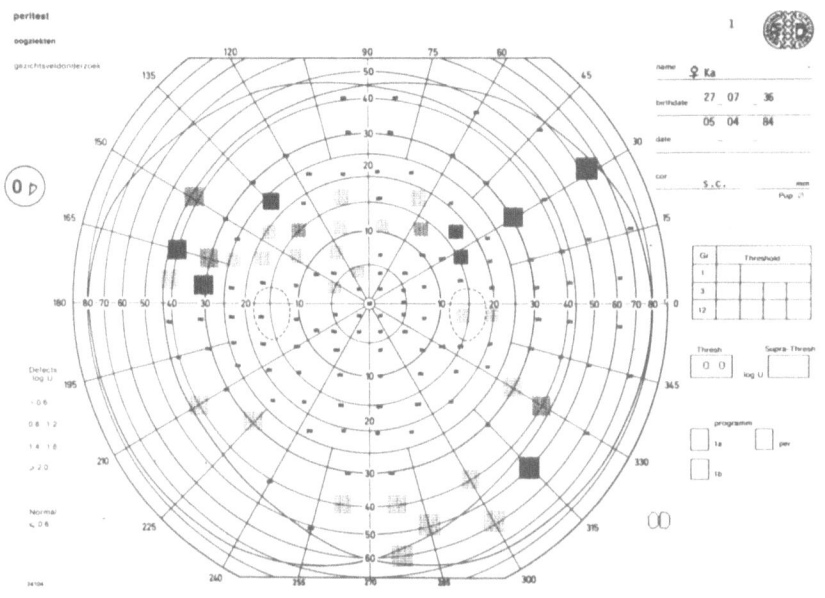

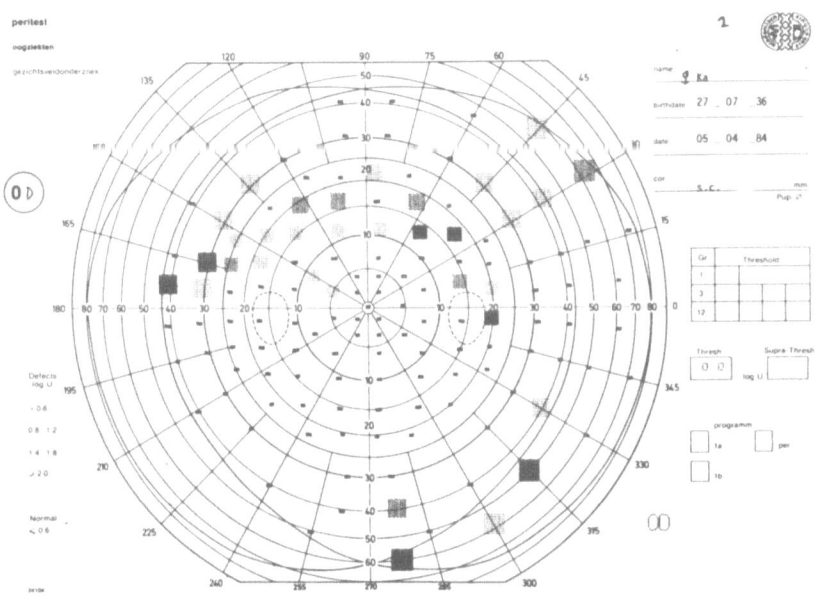

Fig. 1. (a) Four visual fields, without a significant difference of the DV A and DV SA. The two upper fields are automatic. (b) Four visual fields, *with* a significant difference between DV A and DV SA.

141

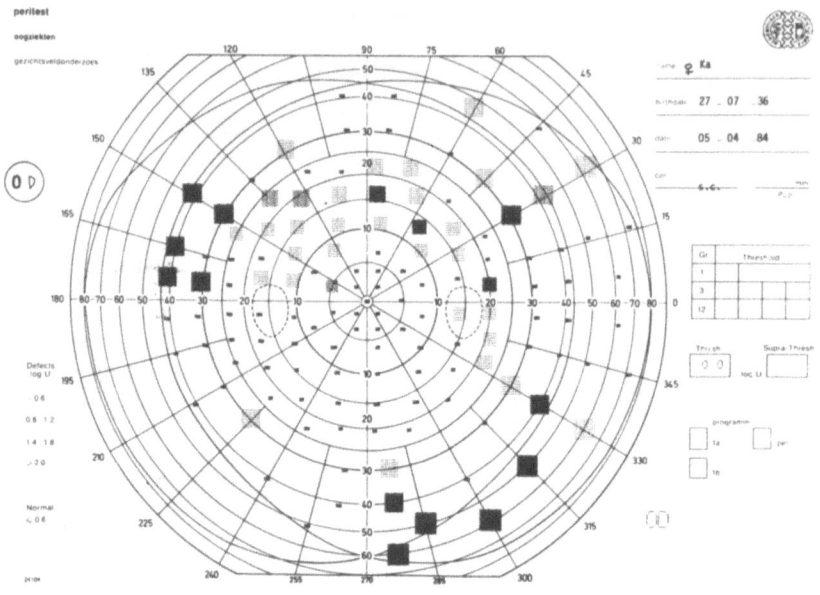

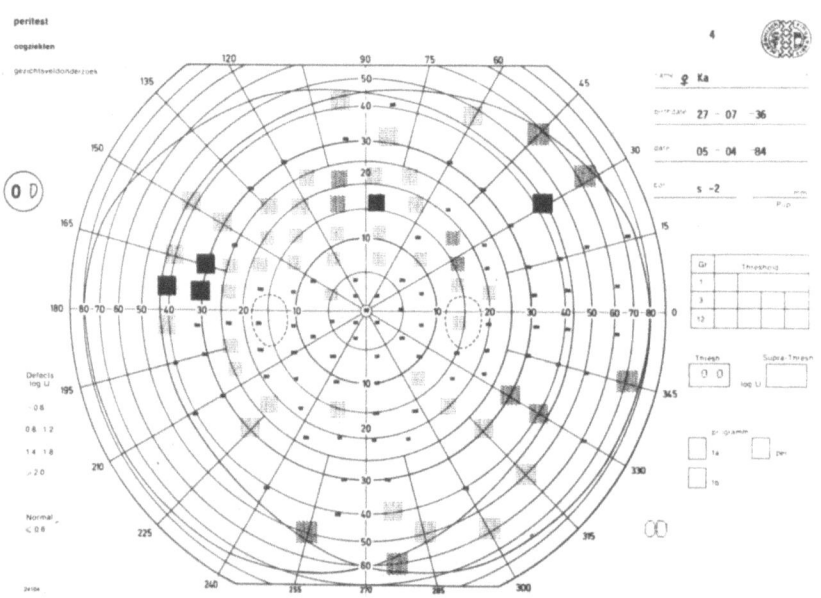

Fig. 1(a). Continued.

142

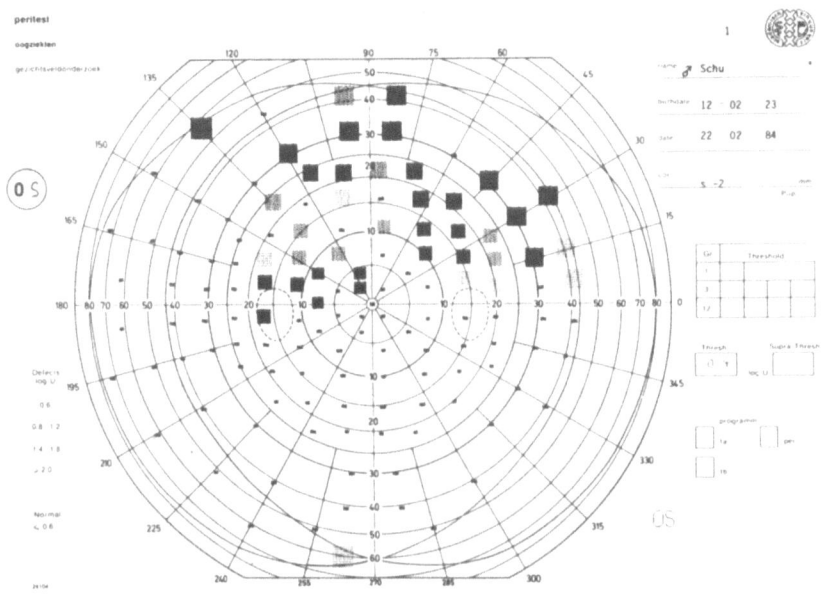

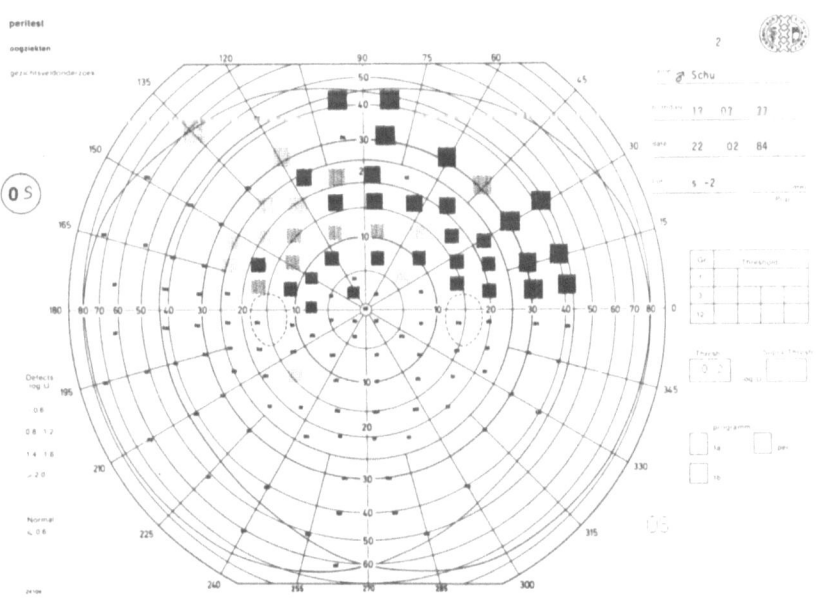

Fig. 1(b). Continued.

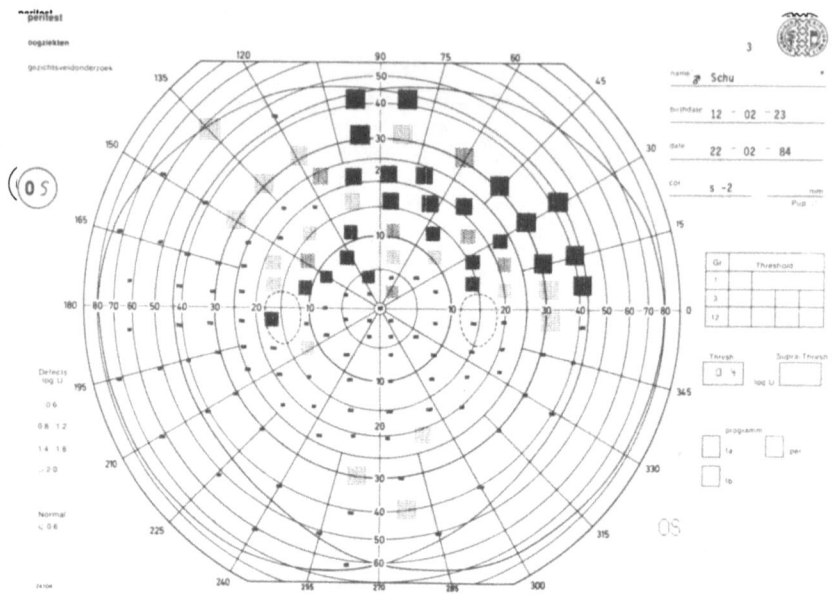

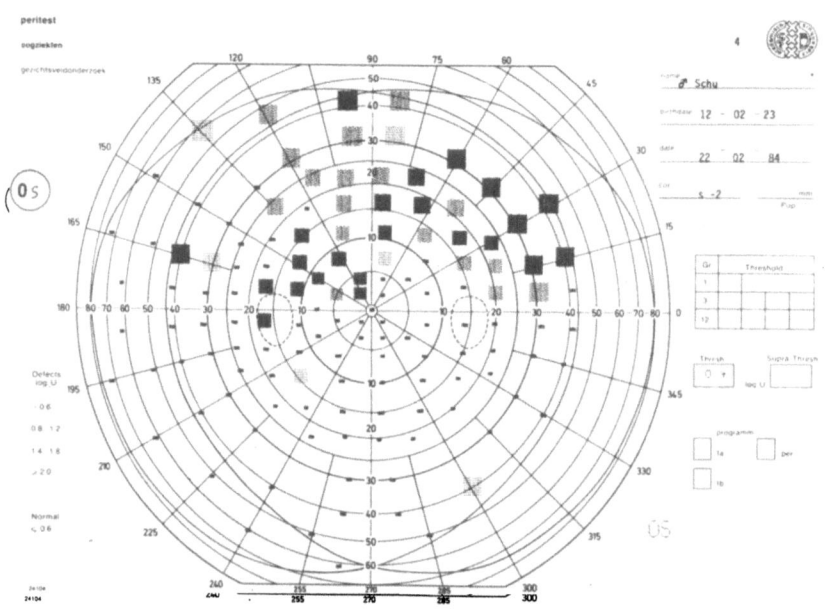

Fig. 1(b). Continued.

144

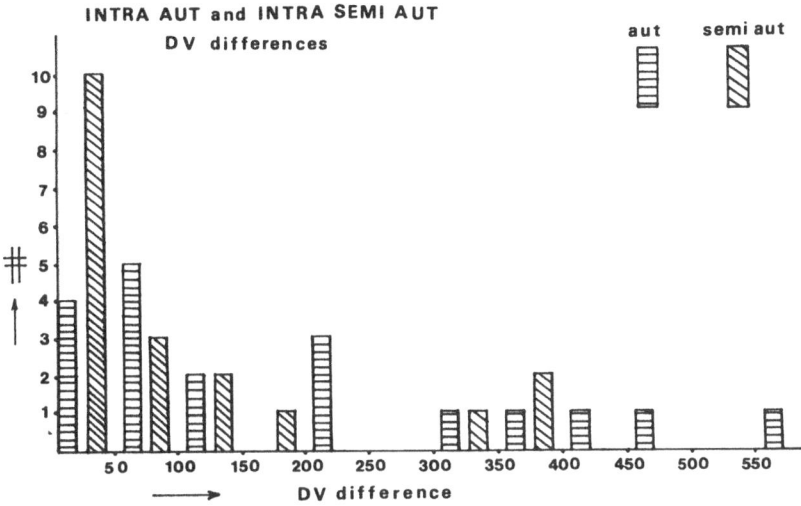

Fig. 2. Histogram indicating the size of the difference between two atuomatic or between two semi-automatic examinations (abscissa). The difference is expressed in dB = 0.1 log. unit. The number of cases that had a certain difference can be found along the ordinate.

We have already reported on the fact that some patients just do not respond well to or do not comprehend automated perimetry (3). It is an almost daily experience of a perimetrist who works with automated perimeters that some patients do very well on full automated perimetry and that others need support.

This investigation shows that there may be differences between automatic and semi-automatic procedures in a substantial number of patients. The results suggest that in these cases the variation between semiautomated examiner-supported procedures is less then in the automated procedures. As expected from clinical experience reaction and judgement were a major cause of the computer-human being interaction problems. Many more details can be extracted out of this study that cannot be discussed here.

It seems reasonable to conclude that in our enthusiasm for the computer guided examination-strategies we have forgotten to pay attention to the human factor.

Psychological support and control may improve the results of automated examination strategies in a number of patients. A semi-automated procedure is necessary in these cases.

REFERENCES

1. Greve, E.L. Performance of computer assisted perimeters. Docum. Ophthal. 53: 343–380 (1982).

2. Greve, E.L., Dannheim, F. and Bakker, D. The Peritest, a new automatic and semi-automatic perimeter. Int. Ophthal. 5: 201–214 (1982).
3. Greve, E.L., Groothuyse, M.T. and Bakker, P. Simulated automatic perimetry. Docum. Ophthal. Proc. Series 14: 23–29 (1977).

Authors' addresses:
Eye Clinic of the University of Amsterdam,
Academic Medical Centre Meibergdreef 9,
1105 AZ Amsterdam,
The Netherlands.
The Netherlands Ophthalmic Research Institute,
P.O. Box 6411, Amsterdam,
The Netherlands.
St. Lucas Hospital,
Dept. of Ophthalmology,
Jan Tooropstraat 164,
1061 AE Amsterdam,
The Netherlands.

PSYCHOPHYSICS OF INTENSITY DISCRIMINATION IN RELATION TO DEFECT VOLUME EXAMINATION ON THE SCOPERIMETER

T.J.T.P. VAN DEN BERG, R. VAN SPRONSEN, W.G. VAN VEENENDAAL
and D. BAKKER

(*Amsterdam, The Netherlands*)

ABSTRACT

For the assessment of changes in the visual fields of patients, parameters have been introduced that relate to the condition of visual field areas as a whole rather than to the behaviour of isolated positions (e.g. the Delta-program from the Fankhauser group). The results of measurements at a number of positions is averaged. The advantage hereof is that changes in the visual field can be determined with a higher degree of accuracy. This accuracy is dependent on the averaging procedure that is performed as well as on the type of the visual field and its defect. In order to optimize the determination of defect volume, basic information is needed on the psychophysics of intensity discrimination in static perimetry with emphasis on the sources of uncertainty involved. Based on the psychophysics involved in normal subjects, we designed a procedure for sensitive assessment of the defect volume.

INTRODUCTION

The concept of the 'Defect Volume' implies the representation of the visual field in a three-dimensional form. The Defect Volume (DV) can be defined as the fall in volume of this three-dimensional form due to defects: Normal Volume minus Actual Volume equals DV. The representation of the visual field and the DV depends on the way the visual field variables are transformed into the three dimensions of the volume. We, for example, use the common way of plotting the visual angles linearly as x and y coordinates which gives the familiar island of vision shape. We plot threshold values in dB, also as usual as z coordinate. However, other choices can be equally justified depending on the application.

Given these choices for the transformations we have studied some points relevant to an accurate derivation of the DV. The study is based on the 'scoperimeter', an experimental, automatized campimeter with a ± 25 degree oscilloscope screen for stimulus and background generation. With the practical limitation that only a limited number of locations can be tested, a correct estimate of the DV can be derived from the sum of threshold values

Heijl, A. and Greve, E.L. (eds.), Proceedings of the 6th Int. Visual Field Symposium.
© *1985, Dr W. Junk Publishers, Dordrecht, The Netherlands. ISBN 978-94-010-8932-6*

in dB's at a number of equidistant locations. For the greater part this was a rectangular grid of 6 degrees (1). Around the blind spot 7 locations of the 6 degree grid have been excluded from the analysis throughout this study.

THE NORMAL VOLUME

We imagine that for each actual, potentially pathological, visual field a 'normal' counterpart can be defined. Each normal field is supposedly a member of the whole population of normal fields for the respective age group (in our case around 70 years of age).

As a control we measured 15 normal fields. The results are examplified in Figs. 1 and 2. Each location was measured twice, the stimulus presentation for the two determinations being randomized. So, the thresholds in series 1 and 2 have no sequential order. The threshold is found after two sign reversals, the first in 4 dB steps, the second in 2 dB steps.

Figure 2 illustrates the general finding that the thresholds scatter increasingly with eccentricity. We have chosen the interpretation that at more eccentricity locations, the lower thresholds represent the true normal sensitivity. Higher thresholds could be due to the location dependent factors and/ or time dependent factors. Time dependent factors can be e.g. blinking or fatigue. On the basis of an Analysis of Variance calculation it proved highly probable that the drop in sensitivity is partly also location dependent (apart from the eccentricity dependence). Inspection of the fields showed that this location dependence is partly concentrated around the blind spot (displaced blind spots, angioscotomata?), partly at the upper margin of the field (glasses, eyelids?) and partly scattered all over the fields in a non-systematic way. Such phenomena pose a restriction on automatic interpretation of pathological visual fields in general. The perimetrist's subjective interpretation takes

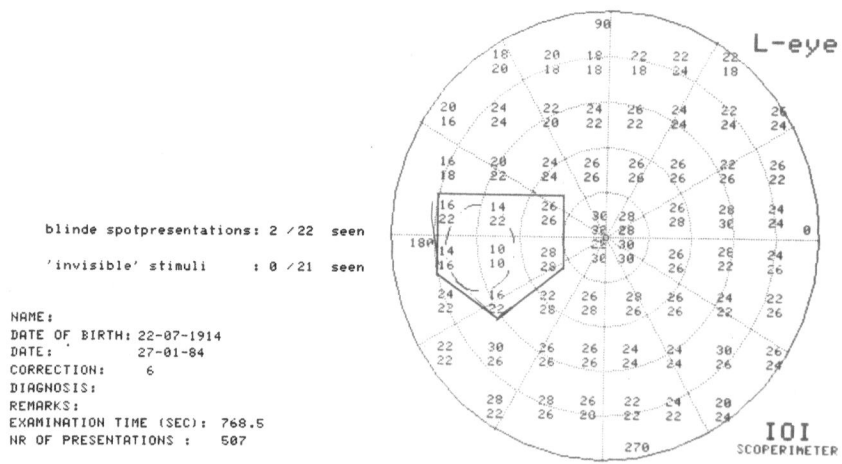

Fig. 1. A printout of the results of the double threshold program for a normal subject.

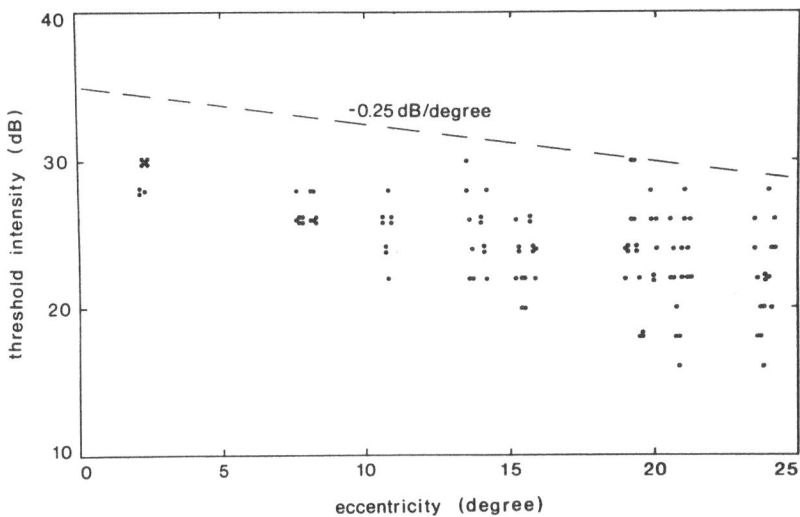

Fig. 2. Data of Fig. 1 plotted against eccentricity (except for the 7 locations around the blind spot).

advantage of more knowledge regarding patient behaviour and the spatial correlation of thresholds and is consequently less bothered by these phenomena. For automatic procedures, we have to keep in mind, that in non-pathological areas low values can be found. Under the assumption of a circular symmetric linear decline of normal sensitivity with eccentricity within the 25° visual field we derived from this group a normal gradient of sensitivity of 0.25 dB/degree (negative sign omitted) and a central sensitivity of 33 dB (observe that 'central sensitivity' is a derived, not directly measured quantity).

According to the above mentioned principle we consider the behaviour of the normal control group to be representative for the normal counterparts of pathological fields. We have to find the patient's linear gradient and normal sensitivity, which should be in the range of the above mentioned values. The gradient is rather constant compared to the central sensitivity, so we initially corrected for this factor (0.25 dB/degree). Accurate assessment of the level of the reconstructed normal field is very important for the calculation of DV measures, since an error in the level is multiplied by the number of locations. The central sensitivity (I_0) is taken as measure for the level, given that the gradient correction is accurate. The normal sensitivity $(I) = I_0 -$ gradient × eccentricity.

I_0 can be estimated as the mean of the thresholds of a number of healthy locations.

For accuracy reasons this number should be as high as possible and the used healthy locations should be an unbiased sample of all healthy locations. However, in general no a priori knowledge about the status of locations is available. One may assume that the highest thresholds indicate healthy points. These threshold values will, however, be biased with respect to the true I_0 because of their statistical behaviour, resulting in an over-estimation of I_0. Therefore we selected healthy points on the basis of series 1 thresholds and averaged the corresponding series 2 thresholds to obtain an unbiased I_0. Recall that the series 1 and 2 thresholds were determined with randomized stimulus presentations. The series 1 thresholds were placed in order of their size. All those series 1 thresholds were selected that were less than 4 dB lower than the third threshold of the order. The third, instead of the first or second was taken to avoid erroneous outlyers. Series 2 thresholds more than 6 dB lower than series 1 were excluded, because of them having a high chance of being pathologic ('pathological spreading').

The so obtained I_0 and the gradient of 0.25 dB/degree are first order estimates of the real values. A better estimate could be obtained by linear regressions analysis of the whole group of healthy locations. Healthy locations can be detected because they will cluster more or less around I_0. The width of the distribution σ around I_0 can be estimated on the basis of the differences between series 1 and series 2 thresholds, assuming that there are no location dependent differences other than the linear gradient. Since pathological points scatter more in the course of one examination than non-pathological points we determined σ on the basis of points that were in the mean not too far below I_0. Regression analysis was performed on all points that were in the mean $> I_0 - k \times \sigma$ (Fig. 3 with k = 2). The factor k should be chosen in such a way that this criterion separates as sharply as possible healthy from

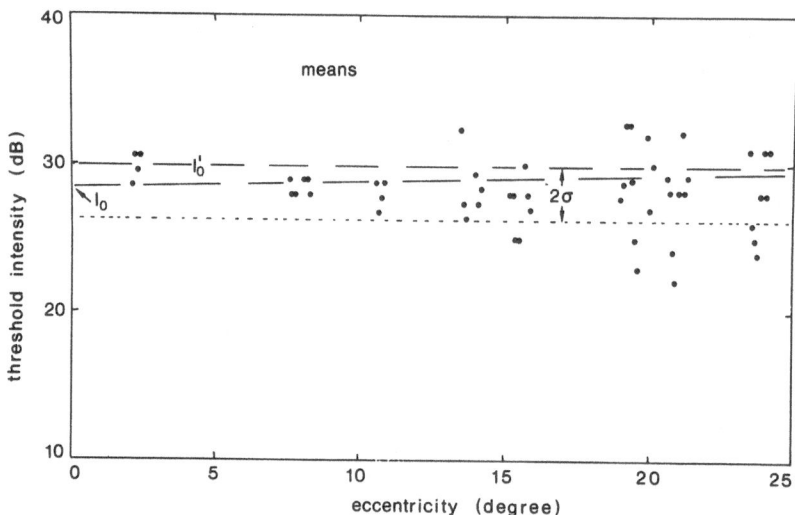

Fig. 3. Same data. Means of the two determinations per location are plotted after correction for a slope of 0.25 dB/degree. Depicted are: The program's first estimate of the central sensitivity (I_0') and the lower 'healthy limit' = $I_0' - 2\sigma$ (chosen k = 2) as well as the regression line, representing the programs best estimate for the subjects' normal sensitivity resulting also in a new estimate of the central sensitivity (I_0).

pathological points. k could be chosen such that the program's opinion on pathological or non-pathological corresponds as well as possible with the perimetrist's opinion for the respective group of patients.

THE DEFECT VOLUME

The regression analysis results in estimated normal values for each eccentricity. The DV is defined as the sum of differences between these normal estimates and the actual values. We also calculate the uncertainty in DV based on the uncertainty in threshold determination during one session. With n and n' the numbers of healthy and pathological locations and σ and σ' the respective standard errors, the standard error in DV can be estimated as the square root of $n'^2\sigma^2/(2n-2) + n'\sigma'^2$. There are, however, other sources of errors as well which we cannot estimate yet. One source related to the described procedure is the separation in normal and pathological points. Much more important, however, might be factors related to patient behaviour such as spontaneous differences between investigations. The results of the DV program to glaucomatous visual function will be described in a separate paper (2).

REFERENCES

1. De Boer, R.W., van den Berg, T.J.T.P., Greve, E.L., and De Waal, B.J. Concepts for automatic perimetry, as applied to the Scoperimeter, an experimental automatic perimeter. Int. Ophthalmol. Clin. 5: 181–191 (1982).
2. Langerhorst, C.T., van den Berg, T.J.T.P., van Spronsen, R. and Greve, E.L. Results of a fluctuation analysis and DVC (Defect Volume Change) program for automated static threshold perimetry with the scoperimeter. Doc. Ophthalmol. Proc. Series, this volume.

Authors' addresses:
T.J.T.P. van den Berg, R. van Spronsen,
W.G. van Veenendaal,
The Netherlands Ophthalmic Research Institute,
P.O. Box 12141, 1100 AC amsterdam.
T.J.T.P. van den Berg,
Laboratory for Medical Physics,
University of Amsterdam.
D. Bakker,
Eye Clinic, University of Amsterdam,
The Netherlands.

COMPARING DIFFERENT AUTOMATED STRATEGIES FOR STATIC THRESHOLD DETERMINATION

E. GANDOLFO, P. CAPRIS, G. CORALLO, and M. ZINGIRIAN

(*Department of Ophthalmology, University of Genova, Italy*)

ABSTRACT

Three different static perimetric strategies in normal and pathological visual fields are clinically compared.

The first strategy is the widely used method of limits, and the second is the repetitive 'up and down' method. The third strategy, the so-called double resolution method of limits, represents a certain modification of the method of limits, by adopting infra-liminal stimuli with two different incremental ratios of target luminance; 0.5 L.U. steps luminance increase for a first threshold approximation and 0.1 L.U. steps increase for the threshold assessment phase were adopted. A computerized Goldmann perimeter was employed.

Our study demonstrated only small differences in the results obtained with the three methods, if a traditional meridian examination is clinically performed.

Practical advantages and disadvantages are discussed.

INTRODUCTION

The study of the optimal static perimetric strategy to obtain the best reliability and reproducibility of measured results with a maximum information gain has been carried out by many Authors (1–8).

In particular Bebié et al. (1, 2) have compared the so-called method of limits with the repetitive up and down strategy by means of computer simulation and the advantages and disadvantages of these two strategies have been noted.

To reduce the disadvantages of the method of limits and create a fast strategy applicable to classical meridian and circular static perimetry according to Goldmann, a modified method of limits was studied. This method, called the double resolution method of limits, was utilized in the computerized Goldmann Perimeter (Perikon-Optikon) (9), and clinically compared with the repetitive up and down method and the manual method of limits.

Heijl, A. and Greve, E.L. (eds.), Proceedings of the 6th Int. Visual Field Symposium.
© *1985, Dr W. Junk Publishers, Dordrecht, The Netherlands. ISBN 978-94-010-8932-6*

(1) The first strategy tested was the repetitive up and down method according to the description of Bebie et al. (1) adopting correction steps of 4, 2, 1. Light intensity of the first stimulus was always chosen at 12.5 asb. which is the middle point of a normal static sensibility curve (3–8).

(2) For the second strategy (manual method of limits) a series of light stimulus steps was used and the first stimulus was chosen about 2–4 dB below the mean threshold of normal subjects. The value corresponding to a series of two perceptions of the same stimulus out of three presentations was considered as the threshold.

(3) The third strategy was the double resolution method of limits. It consists of two interactive methods that occurs alternatively according to the behaviour of the tested point.

Method a: Starting from infraliminal values put at 2 dB below the normal light sensitivity for that point, single presentations were made with a luminance increase of 5 dB till perception was achieved. At this point a series of 4 presentations of 1 dB step increase were made starting from the last non-seen light value. The lower light intensity perceived was considered as the threshold.

Method b: This method was carried out when a series of retinal points was studied according to a meridional or parallel static procedure. It consists of sequential presentations on the points selected by the program. The light intensity was chosen 2 dB lower than the sensitivity of the preceding point. If the target is perceived the threshold is determined by readopting the method a. On the contrary, if no perception was noticed the luminance was increased by 2 dB steps for three presentations and then by 5 dB steps till a response was obtained. A positive response was verified with an other series of presentations with a 1 dB light intensity increase, starting from the last negative response.

MATERIALS AND METHODS

Comparison of the three strategies for static perimetry in our study was carried out by an automated Goldmann perimeter (Perikon-Optikon). For the traditional normal method of limits the same device was utilized but the choice of the stimulus light intensity was made by an expert perimetrist. In such a way the same conditions of stimulus presentation time, background and target light intensity were always maintained.

Eight normal and eight pathological eyes in different subjects underwent perimetric static examination along the temporal horizontal hemimeridian at the following eccentricities: $0°, 3°, 6°, 9°, 12°, 15°, 18°, 21°$.

Every examination was carried out three times adopting the three different strategies previously described. The examination was repeated four times for every subject on different days. A meridional centrifugal sequential presentation was always adopted with random order of the strategies. Patients were not informed about the differences in the three procedures.

Optic correction for near-sightedness was adopted and eye fixation control was guaranteed by the automatic telescopic system of the Perikon.

RESULTS

The mean value profiles obtained by the three methods do not differ significantly.

The average threshold values obtained with the manual method was almost always (76% of the tested points) lower than that obtained by the double resolution method of limits.

The average threshold values obtained with the up and down method are frequently (64% of the tested points) at an intermediate level between the other two methods.

Figure 1 shows the average threshold values and standard deviation of all the normal subjects obtained by the three strategies.

The difference between the highest and the lowest average threshold value with the three strategies in the same point is not significant (maximal value = 3 dB; average = 1.39 ± 0.73 dB) in both normal and pathological subjects. The average σ (SD) for the three methods for all the points tested are the following:

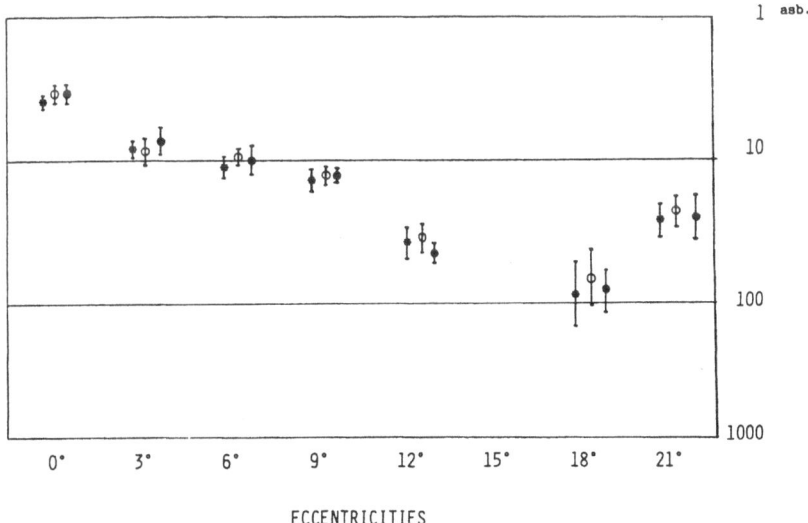

ECCENTRICITIES

Fig. 1. Average static threshold values of four examinations for each strategy: vertical bars represent the standard deviation. * = double resolution method of limits, ○ = manual method of limits and ● = up and down method.

155

	Normal subjects	*Pathological subjects*
Manual method of limits	0.84 ∓ 0.60	0.92 ∓ 1.13
Double resol. M. limits	1.02 ∓ 0.98	1.04 ∓ 0.73
Up and down method	1.03 ∓ 0.97	1.10 ∓ 0.93

An accuracy comparison of the three methods was performed by means of the variance ratio (F) of all the normal and pathological subjects. The variance ratios (F) of the three methods in the various eccentricities are represented in Table 1.

Table 1. The average number of stimuli presentations to obtain total profiles for the three methods are comparable in the three methods: manual = 28.3; double = 37.8; U/D = 36.2

Eccentricities. Methods	0°	3°	6°	9°	12°	15°	18°	21°
Double res.m.limits vs. up-down method	1.21	1.26	1.06	0.76	1.05	1	1.45	1.25
Manual m.limits vs. double res.m.limits	1.14	1.10	1.04	1.34	1.04	1	1.45	1.41
Up-down method vs. manual m.limits	1.39	1.14	1.11	1.03	1.10	1	1.42	1.11
$F = 1.54 \quad p < 0.01$								

COMMENT

Clinical comparison of the three strategies reliability in our study has not shown significant differences.

The accuracy difference, evaluated by means of the variance ratio, is not significant and the number of presentations to obtain a total profile is comparable in the three methods. The disadvantages of the manual method of limits, constituted by time consumption and dependence of the threshold on target luminance for initial presentation (as pointed out by Bebie et al. (1)) is therefore overcome by the adoption of the double resolution strategy. This later method, therefore, is fairly accurate and maintain the small number of supraliminal stimuli of the manual method of limits.

This method represents a computerized version of classical static perimetry according to Goldmann with the advantages of automation represented by a gain in time and reliability.

ACKNOWLEDGEMENTS

This study was supported from a grant of the Consiglio Nazionale delle Ricerche, Progetto Finalizzato Medicina Preventiva e Riabilitativa, Sottoprogetto Malattie Degenerative, Obiettivo n.47a, Rome, Italy.

REFERENCES

1. Bebie, H., Fankhauser, F. and Spahr, J. Static perimetry: strategies. Acta Ophthalmol. 54: 325–338 (1976).
2. Bebie, H., Fankhauser, F. and Spahr, J. Static Perimetry: accuracy and fluctuations. Acta Ophthalmol. 54: 339–348 (1976).
3. Boer, T.J.T.P. (de), Berg, E.L. (van den), Greve, E.L. and Waal, B.J. (de) Concepts for automatic perimetry, as applied to the Scoperimeter, an experimental automatic perimeter. Int. Ophthalmol. 5: 181–191 (1982).
4. Capris, P., Spinelli, G. and Zingirian, M. Comparing continuous and stepwise luminance variation in static campimetry using the Grignolo-Tagliasco-Zingirian projection campimeter. International Ophthalmology (in press).
5. Fankhauser, F. and Bebie, H. Threshold fluctuations, interpolations and spatial resolution in perimetry. Doc. Ophthalmol. Proc. 19: 295–309 (1979).
6. Fankhauser, F., Koch, P. and Roulier, A. On automation of perimetry. A.v. Graefes Arch. klin. exp. Ophthalmol. 184: 126–150 (1972).
7. Gauger, E. Computer simulation of examination procedures for the automatic 'Tubinger perimeter'. Doc. Ophthalmol. Proc. 14: 31–36 (1977).
8. Greve, E.L. Single and multiple stimulus static perimetry in glaucoma: the two phases of perimetry. Doc. Ophthalmol. 36: 1–347 (1973).
9. Zingirian, M., Gandolfo, E. and Orciuolo, M. Automation of the Goldmann perimeter. Doc. Ophthalmol. Proc. 35: 365–369 (1983).

Authors' address:
University Eye Clinic
Viale Benedetto XV, 5
16132-Genova
Italy

PRELIMINARY CLINICAL TRIALS WITH THE HUMPHREY FIELD ANALYZER

RICHARD A. LEWIS, JOHN L. KELTNER, and CHRIS A. JOHNSON

(*Davis, CA, USA*)

ABSTRACT

The Humphrey Field Analyzer is a new automated perimeter that performs static threshold testing and suprathreshold static testing. The static threshold test procedures use a target presentation pattern and staircase testing strategy that is similar to those employed on the Octopus and Squid automated perimeters. This paper describes our preliminary clinical evaluations of the central visual field threshold test procedure of the Humphrey Visual Field Analyzer. Manual kinetic testing on the Goldmann perimeter and Humphrey visual field tests were performed on 50 eyes with glaucoma or neuro-ophthalmologic disorders. The Humphrey static threshold test times ranged from 8.3 to 19.2 minutes per eye, with an average time of 15 ± 2.6 minutes. We found fair to excellent correlation of the field results in 94% of the cases.

A variety of automated perimeters have been shown to be reliable in the detection and monitoring of visual field defects (1–5). As new perimeters are introduced clinically, validation studies are necessary to evaluate their usefulness when compared to established techniques. The Humphrey Field Analyzer is a new automated perimeter that performs static threshold and suprathreshold testing. In this study we conducted a preliminary comparison of results obtained with the central 30 degree static threshold test of the Humphrey Field Analyzer to manual kinetic perimetry using the Goldmann perimeter.

METHODS

A total of 50 eyes were evaluated: thirteen eyes with glaucoma and thirty-seven eyes with other retinal, optic nerve or neurologic disorders. Each underwent manual visual field testing with the Goldmann and Humphrey Field Analyzer. Most tests were performed on separate days within a four week time span. Pupils were dilated whenever possible to 3 mm or greater for all visual field tests.

Goldmann kinetic fields were performed by highly skilled perimetrists,

Heijl, A. and Greve, E.L. (eds.), Proceedings of the 6th Int. Visual Field Symposium.
© *1985, Dr W. Junk Publishers, Dordrecht, The Netherlands. ISBN 978-94-010-8932-6*

according to our standard protocol described previously (4, 5). This consisted of two isopters beyond 30 degrees from fixation and three isopters within 30 degrees. Extensive spot checks were performed within the central 30 degrees. An appropriate refractive correction was used for examining the central 30 degrees. The standard background luminance of 31.5 asb was used.

Visual field testing with the Humphrey Field Analyzer utilized the screening strategy of the threshold test, central 30-2. This procedure included a background luminance of 31.5 asb, a stimulus duration of 0.2 seconds, and an average interval of 1−1.5 seconds between stimuli. A Goldmann equivalent size II target and appropriate refractive correction was used. Targets were presented in a random sequence. Each field was printed with a gray scale and numeric value representation.

Three examiners evaluated each pair of fields. These were correlated according to the detection and general similarity of the field abnormality. For this preliminary evaluation, the degree of correlation was rated on a 1 to 4 scale with 4 the most similar and 1 the least. In addition, the amount of time to complete field testing with the Humphrey instrument was determined.

RESULTS

Fifty eyes of 27 patients were included in the study. The average age was 47.9 ± 13.2 years. The most common diagnosis was glaucoma (13 eyes). Other diagnoses included retinal or optic nerve disease (26 eyes) and neurologic tumors or infarcts (11 eyes).

We found good to excellent correlation (rated 3 or 4) between the Humphrey and Goldmann visual fields in 37 (74%) eyes (12 eyes were rated excellent while 25 were rated good). In 10 of the eyes (20%) there was a fair correlation (rated 2) but outstanding differences between the two fields were noted. In 3 eyes from two patients (6%) the correlation was poor with the pair of fields appearing almost unrelated.

The average time for the Humphrey test was 15 ± 2.6 minutes with a range from 8.3 minutes to 19.2 minutes. There was no correlation between the duration of testing and any specific diagnosis. Generally, the more advanced the defect, the less time necessary to complete the test.

REPORT OF CASES

(1) A 67-year-old man had a history of glaucoma, visual field loss, and cupping. Examination showed a visual acuity of 20/20 in each eye and a tension of 14 mm Hg in the right eye and 16 mm Hg in the left eye while taking Timolol in each eye. Fundus examination showed extension of each cup inferiorly. Kinetic perimetry on the Goldmann perimeter and Humphrey static fields are shown in Fig. 1.

The Goldmann kinetic field in the right eye showed a dense superior arcuate scotoma to the V/4e target. In a test that required 13:17 minutes the Humphrey also showed superior field loss. Correspondence between the Humphrey and kinetic perimeter was judged to be excellent.

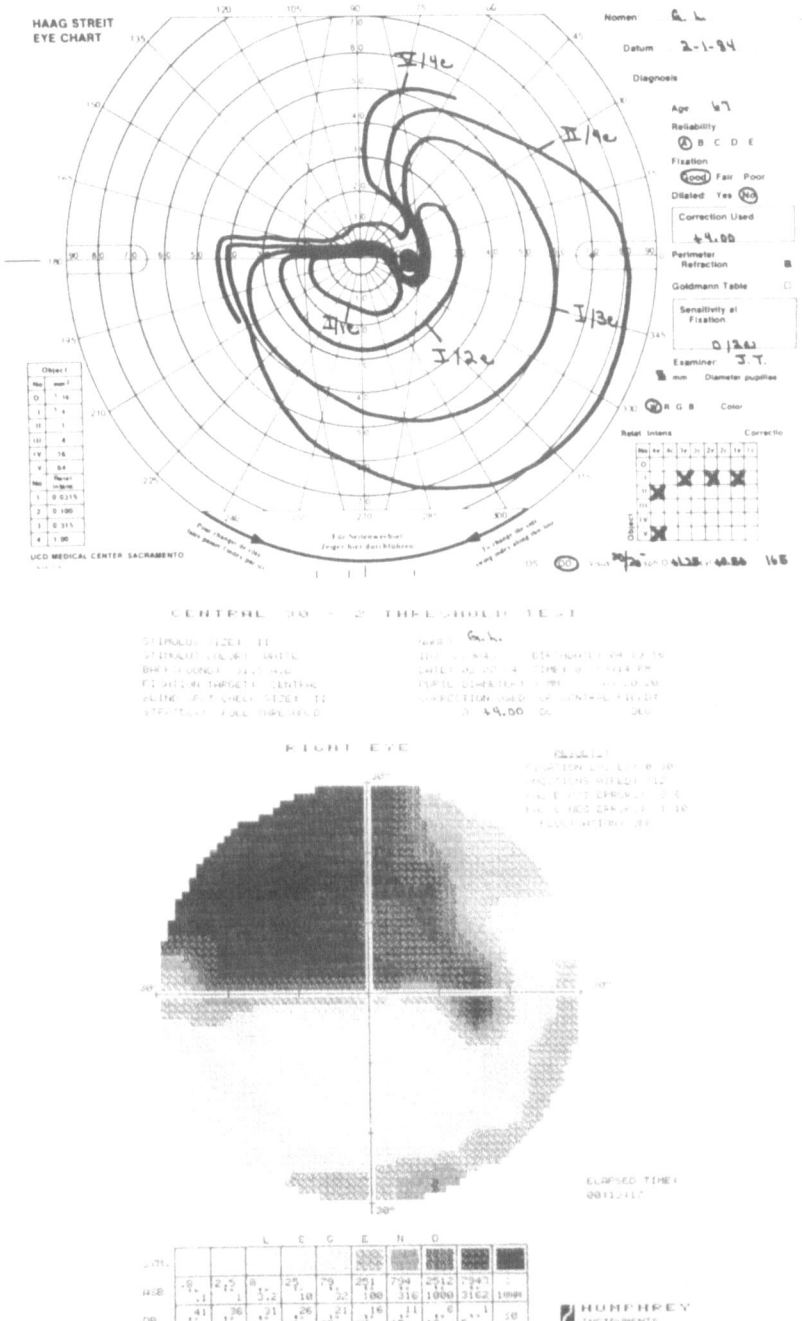

Fig. 1. Goldmann kinetic field (A) and Humphrey static field (B) demonstrate a dense superior arcuate scotoma.

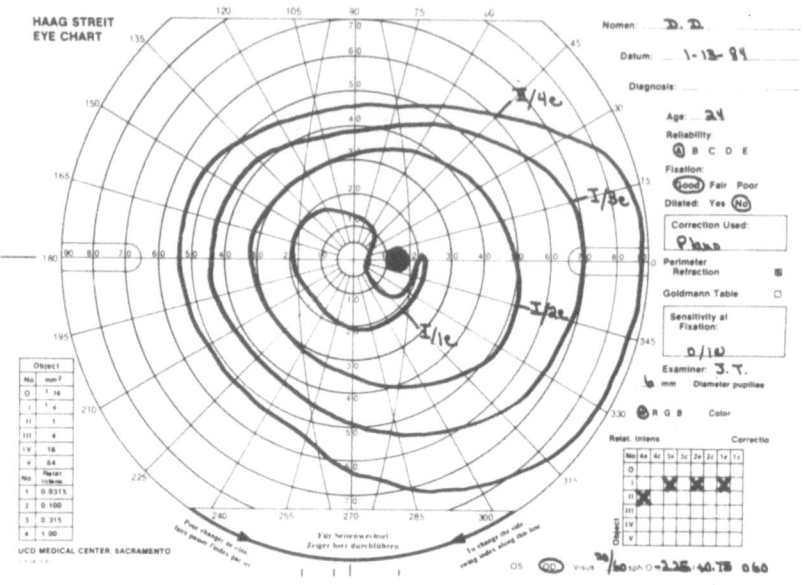

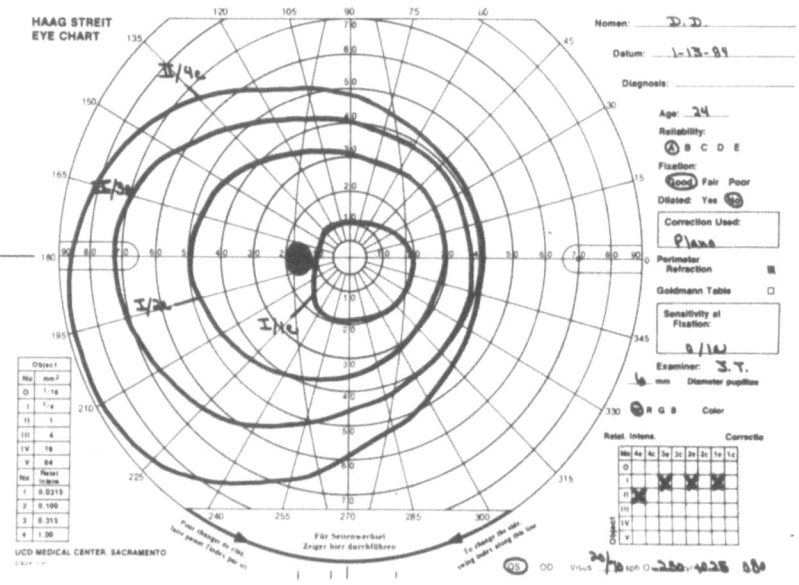

Fig. 2. Goldmann kinetic field – right eye (A) and left eye (B). Humphrey static field – right eye (C) and left eye (D). Note the poor correlation between fields probably because of statokinetic dissociation.

162

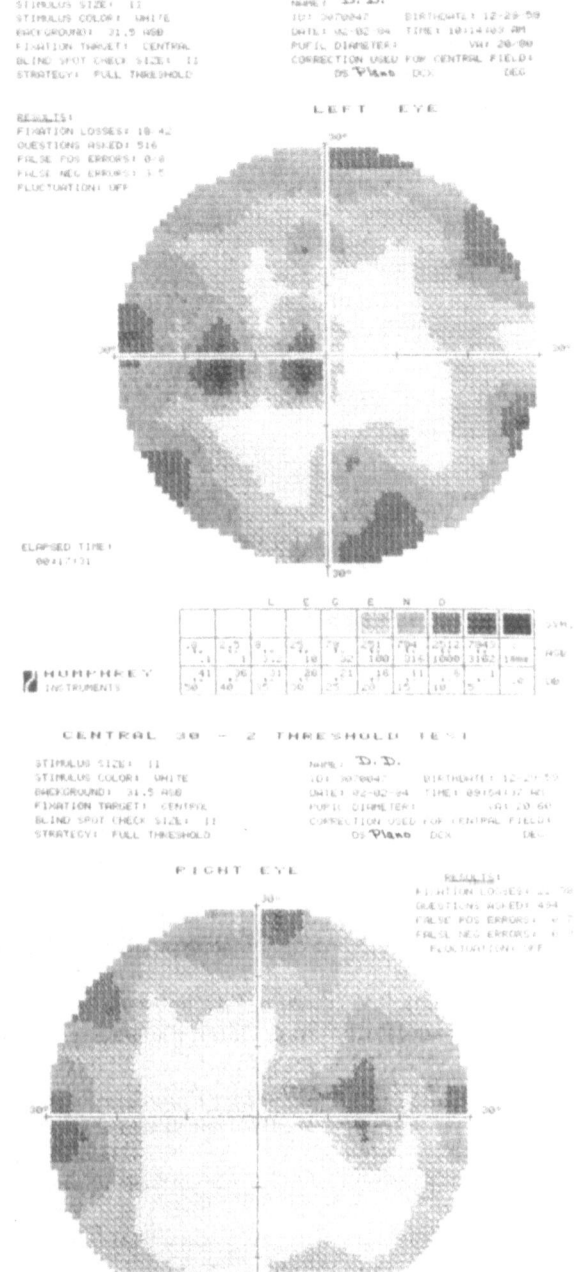

Fig. 2. Continued.

(2) A 23-year-old man had a history of demylinating disease. Examination showed a visual acuity of 20/60 OD and 20/70 OS, no afferent pupillary defect and bilateral temporal pallor. Goldmann kinetic perimetry and the Humphrey static field are shown in Fig. 2.

The kinetic field showed missed spot checks around the pericentral area in both eyes but no definite central scotoma. The Humphrey field showed decreased sensitivity in both eyes especially superiorly. The Humphrey field required 16:52 minutes OD and 17:31 OS. Correspondence was judged to be poor, probably because of statokinetic dissociation (6).

DISCUSSION

Our preliminary study suggests that the Humphrey Field Analyzer showed fair to excellent correlation with standard Goldmann kinetic perimetry in 94% of the cases. However, in 3 eyes the correlation between the two tests was so poor as to suggest unrelated problems. Two of these eyes appeared to demonstrate statokinetic dissociation and, thus, the lack of correlation can be attributed to a difference in the use of static versus kinetic testing (6, 7). The third case could also be attributed to a failure of our kinetic test procedure. In all three cases, repeat testing and evaluation with other automated perimeters confirmed the findings of the Humphrey Field Analyzer.

As with other automated perimeters, the Humphrey static threshold test has definite advantages and disadvantages over kinetic perimetry. Both forms of perimetry require good patient reliability and cooperation. The Humphrey Field Analyzer required an average of 15 minutes per test which compares favorably with kinetic perimetry, with the exception that kinetic perimetric testing evaluated both the central and peripheral visual fields. Although static testing of the periphery can be accomplished with the Humphrey, we feel that it is too time consuming to be widely used clinically. Also, many patients prefer field testing with the Goldmann perimeter because of the human interaction with the perimetrist.

Dense visual field defects appear to be detected with equal frequency for each form of testing. Humphrey static perimetry is probably more sensitive in the detection of early field defects than Goldmann kinetic perimetry. In neuro-ophthalmologic disorders this is due to statokinetic dissociation (6, 7). This also may account for the poor correlation of the fields in some patients during our study.

Although the indirect method of monitoring fixation (Heijl–Krakau blind spot technique) and the noise associated with stimulus movement make the Humphrey Field Analyzer potentially more susceptible to spurious results, we noted no significant effects on the quality of information obtained in this study.

In summary, perliminary evaluation of automated static threshold testing with the Humphrey Field Analyzer offers a sensitive means of detecting visual field loss that correlates well with standard kinetic perimetry. Further study is necessary to compare the various programs of the Humphrey with other automated static threshold perimeters.

REFERENCES

1. Fankhauser, F., Spahr, J. and Bebie, H. Three years of experience with the Octopus automatic perimeter. Doc. Ophthalmol. Proc. Series 14: 7–15 (1977).
2. Heijl, A. and Drance, S.M. The value of an automatic perimeter (Competer) in detecting early glaucomatous field defects. Arch Ophthalmol. 98: 1560–1563 (1980).
3. Dannheim, F. Clinical experiences with a new automated perimeter 'Peritest'. Documenta Ophth. 35: 309–312 (1983).
4. Keltner, J.L., Johnson, C.A. and Balestrery, F.G. Suprathreshold static perimetry: Initial clinical trials with the Fieldmaster automated perimeter. Arch. Ophthalmol. 97: 260–272 (1979).
5. Johnson, C.A. and Keltner, J.L. Automated suprathreshold static perimetry. Am. J. Ophthalmol. 89: 731–741 (1980).
6. Safran, A.B. and Glaser, J.S. Statokinetic dissociation in lesions of the anterior visual pathways; a reappraisal of the Riddoch phenomenon. Arch. Ophthalmol. 98: 291–295 (1980).
7. Keltner, J.L. and Johnson, C.A. Automated and manual perimetry – a 6 year overview. Ophthalmol. 91: 68–85 (1984).

Authors' address:
Department of Ophthalmology,
University of California,
Davis, California, U.S.A.

TWO YEARS OF EXPERIENCE WITH THE PERIMETRON AUTOMATIC PERIMETER IN GLAUCOMATOUS PATIENTS.

PAOLO BRUSINI and CLAUDIA TOSONI

(*Udine, Italy*)

ABSTRACT

A computerized automatic perimeter (Perimetron) was used for visual field examination of 122 patients affected by open-angle glaucoma in various stages of development.

Static-kinetic programs were found to be suitable in the screening and with some reservations in the assessment phase. The examination is often too long and tiring if perimetric defects are severe and complex also because the software is sometimes inadequate. Long-term follow-ups (up to two years) have demonstrated the usefulness of this instrument in sequential visual field evaluation of glaucomatous patients. The reliability of the results, nevertheless, is very dependent on the level of collaboration of the patient and the type of program used.

INTRODUCTION

Automatic perimetry, in spite of some limitations, represents today a real progress in the management of patients with chronic open-angle glaucoma. Several studies have already confirmed the validity of various types of automatic perimeters for the detection of glaucomatous field defects (e.g. 1, 2, 5, 6, 8, 10, 11). The correct assessment of the detected defects, however, is still a problem and can only be reliably done with the most sophisticated of the automatic instruments which can determine the threshold in a fixed number of points.

The benefits of automatic perimetry in the follow-up of glaucomatous patients with sequential visual field evaluations have been studied little and have not yet been clearly shown (3, 4, 7, 9).

We report here more than two years experience with the Perimetron automatic perimeter used for detection, assessment and follow-up of the visual field in a group of patients with glaucoma.

MATERIALS AND METHODS

231 eyes from 122 pateints in various stages of chronic open-angle glaucoma were examined. The ages ranged from 32 to 84 (average 63.3). The ocular

Heijl, A. and Greve, E.L. (eds.), Proceedings of the 6th Int. Visual Field Symposium.
© *1985, Dr W. Junk Publishers, Dordrecht, The Netherlands. ISBN 978-94-010-8932-6*

media were clear and there were no other associated eye diseases. Visual acuity ranged from 20/30 to 20/20 with optical correction. A control group of 43 normal subjects (82 eyes) were selected, aged between 17 and 63 (average 34.4).

The Perimetron (Coherent Medical Division) was used for the automatic visual field tests. It is a computerized projection perimeter which employs both kinetic and static techniques, using stimuli of the same size and intensity as that of the Goldmann perimeter. The fixation can be checked automatically by an infra-red monitor or manually through a telescope.

The following programs have been used in this study (the two numbers in brackets directly after the program number indicate the number of normal and glaucomatous eyes tested respectively):

— program 6 (33 and 32): 2 isopters kinetic perimetry (I/4/e and I/2/e) and blind spot delimitation (I/4/e);

— program 8 (52 and 14): 1 isopter kinetic perimetry (I/2/e), scan of the peripheral nasal step (I/4/e), blind spot delimitation (I/4/e) and static testing of 74 points within 25° (I/2/e, if missed I/4e);

— program 10 (146 and 36): 3–5 isopters kinetic perimetry (stimuli selected by the computer based on individual sensitivity), blind spot delimitation (I/4/e) plus static testing of 129 points is the central 25° area (the stimulus used in that for the surrounding isopter, if missed, increases in intensity in steps of 0.5 log. units).

All the patients were also tested manually with the Goldmann perimeter using kinetic perimetry, and suprathreshold static testing between isopters.

Criteria for interpreting automatic tests. Nasal steps equal to or greater than 7° were considered abnormal as were isopteric irregularities of more than 10° at more than one point. In program 8, missed stimuli at the maximum intensity (1000 asb) and groups of 3 or more missed stimuli at 100 asb were considered abnormal. In program 10 isolated static missed points were disregarded if their intensity was less than 0.4 log. units above that of the surrounding isopter, or if their intensity was less than or equal to 32 asb. Finally, missed stimuli within 5° from the blind spot and at 25° from fixation between the 60° and 120° meridians when a corrective lens was used, were not considered.

Follow-up. 37 patients (67 eyes) underwent a total of 94 automatic control tests over a period of 27 months. Program 6 was used 24 times; program 8, 23 times and; program 10, 47 times. 26 patients (47 eyes) were tested twice; 7 patients (13 eyes), 3 times and; 4 patients (7 eyes), 4 times.

RESULTS

Sensitivity. Program 6: 21 out of 33 abnormal visual fields were correctly classified giving a sensitivity of 63.6%. Program 8: 43 out of 52 cases were reliably identified (sensitivity 82.7%). Program 10: 123 out of 146 visual fields were correctly classified as abnormal (sensitivity 84.2%).

Specificity. Program 6: 2 out of 32 normal visual fields were falsely classified as pathological, giving a specificity of 93.8%. Program 8: only one result out of 14 was a false-positive, a specificity of 92.9%. Program 10: 5 out of 36 visual fields were falsely classified as abnormal, a specificity of 86.1%.

Test time. The test time required by the different programs was calculated, excluding the time taken for the patients to rest or to add corrective lenses. The test time with program 6 ranged from 6 to 12 minutes for glaucomatous patients (average 9.2 minutes) and from 6 to 9 minutes for normals (average 7.4 minutes). For program 8 the test time ranged from 7 to 16 minutes for glaucomatous patients (average 11.3 minutes) and between 6 and 13 minutes for normals (average 9.6 minutes). Program 10's test time ranged from 16 to 45 minutes for the glaucomatous (average 24.7 minutes) and between 14 and 31 minutes for normals (average 19.8 minutes).

Follow-up. Program 6 gave results useful for long-term follow-up, such that an accurate judgement was possible on the progression or non-progression of visual field loss, in 15 out of 24 cases (62.5%). Program 8 was useful in 16 out of 21 cases (76.2%) and program 10 in 42 out of 47 (89.4%).

DISCUSSION

The Perimetron is substantially different to other automatic perimeters, which are based on the presentation of static stimuli. It on the other hand has been designed with the aim of completely automating those conventional techniques, above all kinetic, that can be used by an expert perimetrist on a Goldmann perimeter. This created difficult strategic problems, which have in part been satisfactorily resolved. The huge range of available programs (more than 20) ensures great flexibility, but also requires a clear understanding of the problems of perimetry to get the best results in the shortest time. Program 6 proved to be useful for developed isopteric defects, such as those which appear in some neuro-ophthalmological diseases or in advanced glaucoma. However, generally, it is not sensitive enough to detect early glaucoma defects. The static-kinetic programs were found to be more reliable, even though they had certain limitations. Program 8 allows for a rough analysis of the visual field, differentiating absolute from relative defects. It is a short test and can be used for glaucoma screening. Program 10, specifically designed for glaucoma, allows for an extensive exploration of the whole visual field, including the extreme periphery. The depth of the paracentral defects is measured in steps of 0.5 log. units. However, the shape and margins are not always particularly clear. The sensitivity is good, but could be even better if the static stimuli were presented in a randomized sequence as for example in the suprathreshold static programs 2, 3 and 4. Program 10 is sometimes limited, when there are complex perimetric alterations, by inadequate software. Kinetic examination, for instance, contracts concentrically when there is a central remnant of the visual field, ignoring any possible islands of vision in the peripheral field. Where the central visual field defects are numerous and

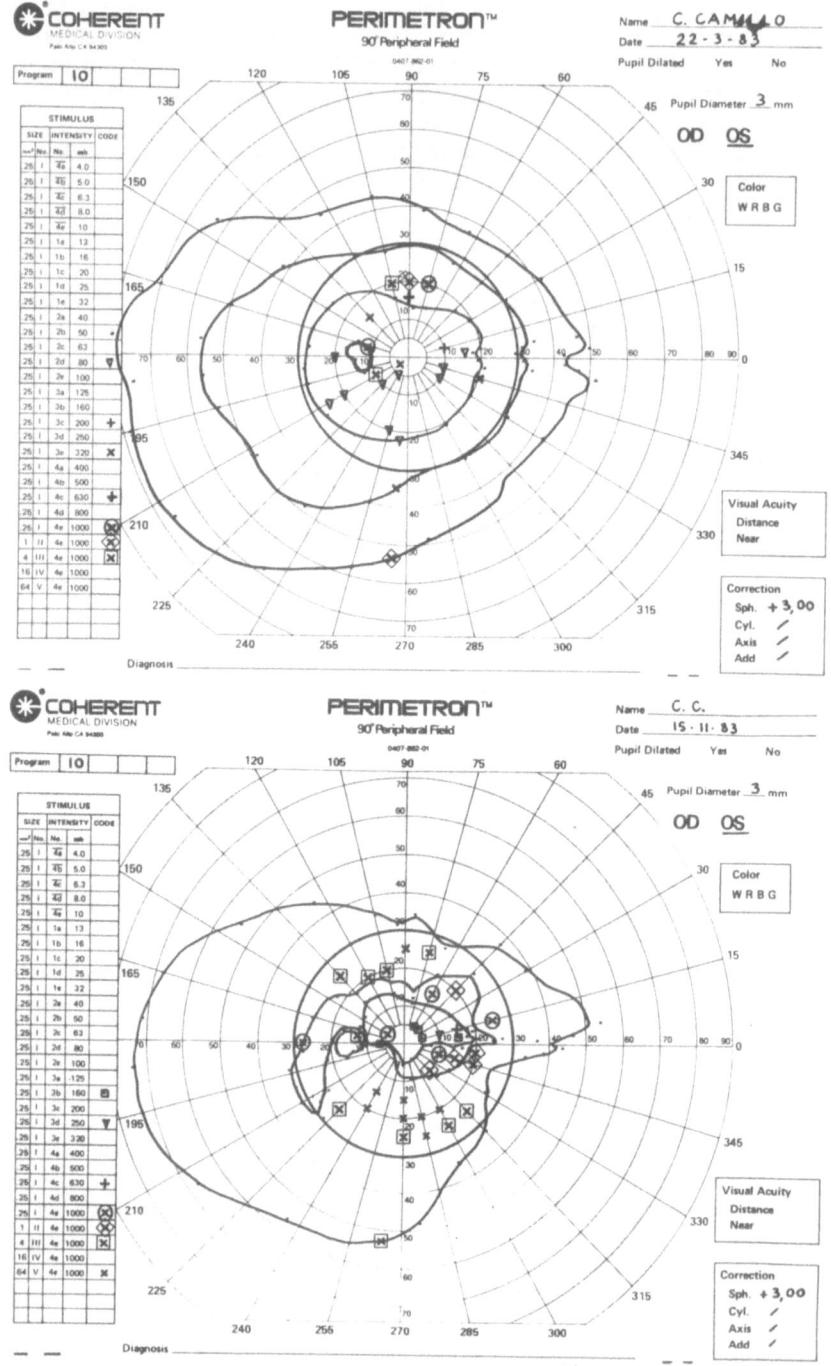

Fig. 1. Important visual field deterioration in 8 months, clearly illustrated by program 10.

170

extensive, static testing proceeds very slowly, making the test excessively long and laborious. Another problem with this program is the interpretation of results which is often confused by variously shaped and coloured symbols indicating the intensity of missed static stimuli. In many cases, however, the intensities of missed stimuli are very low and the defects should be disregarded according to the criteria already mentioned. Such obstacles could be eliminated by modifying the data output system, for example, by using non-interpolated grey scales.

An important point, often forgotten in many studies of automatic perimeters, is the ability of an instrument to follow the progression or regression of a visual field defect over time. The Perimetron is not designed for automatic comparisons between tests carried out at different times (only possible with some of the latest generation automatic perimeters furnished with specific statistical programs). However it gives equally good results in the follow-up phase. Program 10, in particular, gave roughly a 90% correct appraisal of the control tests (Fig. 1). Other programs used were not so good at following the course of a perimetric defect, mainly due to their low sensitivity in the presence of initial glaucomatous defects, e.g. small paracentral scotomas.

In general the reproducibility is good, but in some cases the results can be affected by threshold fluctuations, which can reach high values if the subject does not collaborate well or if there are serious visual field defects.

Comparison with manual tests, done by the Goldmann perimeter, is generally fairly easy, thanks to analagous charts and standards used by the two instruments. However, with the same stimuli, the isopters are larger and the blind spot smaller with the Perimetron, which is partly due to the elimination of operator reaction time.

The Perimetron has a positive role, especially for patients without advanced visual field defects. The automatic testing is too time-consuming and laborious for patients with serious or complex defects. These cases are more suited for manual testing.

In conclusion we think that the Perimetron, correctly used (patients and programs carefully selected, appropriate criteria for interpreting automatic tests, etc.), could lead to a significant improvement in the quality of perimetric screening and follow-up of patients with chronic glaucoma.

REFERENCES

1. Brusini, P. Perimetria automatica nel glaucoma: prime esperienze cliniche con un perimetro computerizzato (Perimetron). Atti VII Congr. S.O.Si. 54–60 (1982).
2. Dannheim, F. Clinical experiences with a new automated perimeter 'Peritest'. Doc. Ophthalmol. Proc. Series 35: 309–312 (1983).
3. Gloor, B. and Schmied, U. Erfahrungen bei Verlaufsuntersuchungen von Glaukomatoesen Gesichtsfeldern mit dem automatischen Perimeter Octopus. Klin. Mbl. Augenheilk. 176: 545–546 (1980).
4. Gloor, B., Schmied, U. and Fässler, A. Changes of glaucomatous field defects. Analysis of Octopus fields with programme Delta. Doc. Ophthalmol. Proc. Series 26: 11–15 (1981).

5. Heijl, A. and Drance, S.M. A clinical comparison of three computerized automatic perimeters in the detection of glaucoma defects. Arch. Ophthalmol. 99: 832–836 (1981).
6. Heijl, A., Drance, S.M., and Douglas, G.R. Automatic perimeter (Competer): Ability to detect early glaucomatous defects. Arch. Ophthalmol. 98: 1560–1563 (1980).
7. Holmin, C. and Krakau, C.E.T. Automatic perimetry in the control of glaucoma. Glaucoma 3: 154–159 (1981).
8. Johnson, C.A., Keltner, J.L. and Balestrery, F.G. Suprathreshold static perimetry in glaucoma and optic nerve disease. Ophthalmology 86: 1278–1286 (1979).
9. Keltner, J.L. and Johnson, C.A. Effectiveness of automated perimetry in following glaucomatous visual field progression. Ophthalmology 89: 247–254 (1982).
10. Krieglstein, G.K., Schrems, W., Gramer, E. and Leydhecker, W. Detectability of early glaucomatous field defects. A controlled comparison of Goldmann versus Octopus perimetry. Doc. Ophthalmol. Proc. Series 26: 19–25 (1981).
11. Li, S.G., Spaeth, G.L., Scimeca, H.A., Shatz, N.J. and Savino, P.J. Clinical experiences with the use of an automated perimeter (Octopus) in the diagnosis and management of patients with glaucoma and neurologic disease. Ophthalmology 86: 1302–1312 (1979).

Authors' address:
Dr. Paolo Brusini
Divisione Oculistica
Ospedale Civile
33100 Udine
Italy

AUTOMATIC PERIMETRY IN GLAUCOMA: A CLINICAL COMPARISON OF TWO COMPUTER-ASSISTED PERIMETERS (PERIMETRON AND OCTOPUS 2000)

PAOLO BRUSINI and CLAUDIA TOSONI

(*Udine, Italy*)

ABSTRACT

Two automatic computerized perimeters (Perimetron and Octopus 2000) were used to test the visual fields of 43 patients (78 eyes) with open-angle glaucoma in various stages of development. A control group of 14 normal subjects (27 eyes) was also taken into consideration.

The sensitivity of the two instruments was good, with high rates of detection of visual field defects. In the test of normal patients, both instruments demonstrated a good specificity, with a low number of false-positive results.

The automatic perimetry results are very closely connected to the type of program used, the criteria adopted for the classification of test results, the gravity of visual field defects and the level of collaboration of the subject examined.

The most important advantages of the Perimetron and Octopus 2000 over manual perimetry are the objectivity and standardization of the test parameters. An improved fixation control device, and some modification of the software would make the two instruments even more reliable.

INTRODUCTION

The importance of visual field examination in the management of glaucomatous patients does not have to be underlined. Such research, normally carried out by tangent screens or hemispheric perimeters by varyingly trained technicians, can now be achieved with the use of automatic instruments that can run this test totally without (or with minimum) intervention by the operator.

Only the threshold static perimeters can offer a detailed and precise analysis of the visual field, being capable of determining the depth and morphology of a defect.

The first and most noted amongst the perimeters of this type is the Octopus from Interzeag, introduced in 1976 (1, 4, 6). More recently, a cheaper model has been built: the Octopus 2000 which retains most of the characteristics of its older brother (3).

The Perimetron (Coherent Medical Division), however, has been designed

Heijl, A. and Greve, E.L. (eds.), Proceedings of the 6th Int. Visual Field Symposium.
© 1985, Dr W. Junk Publishers, Dordrecht, The Netherlands. ISBN 978-94-010-8932-6

with completely different criteria: in practice it is the first attempt to automatize the Goldmann classic perimeter, and to carry out all the manual kinetic and static techniques.

Below, we report our personal experience based on the use of the Perimetron for nearly two years and the Octopus 2000 for about 6 months. During this period. a few hundred patients with varying optic diseases were examined. The only results which have been taken into consideration here are those of a controlled study of patients with glaucoma, to test the reliability of the two instruments and to check carefully any deficiencies.

MATERIALS AND METHODS

Patient Population. 43 patients (26 male and 17 female) affected by chronic open-angle glaucoma at various stages were considered (a total of 78 eyes). In particular 37 eyes had incipient glaucoma; 28 established; and 13, terminal stage. The ages varied between 34 and 84 (average 65.4).

Also a control group of 14 normal subjects (average age 39.6) were examined (a total of 27 eyes).

Instruments. The Perimetron is an automatic projection perimeter allowing kinetic perimetry with tests selected by the computer or operator, suprathreshold static examination and finally, meridional and circular static perimetry. The stimuli are identical in sizes and intensities to those of the Goldmann perimeter; all the test parameters could be modified by the operator at any time. The fixation could be checked automatically by an infra-red monitor regulated according to two sensitivity levels, or, alternatively, manually through a telescope. At the end of the examination a plotter traces the graph of the visual field on Goldmann type charts.

The Octopus 2000 is a computer-assisted projection perimeter using static stimuli and is furnished with a series of scanning and basic programs, memorized on floppy disk. The tests are shown for 0.1 second in a randomized sequence. The background is at 4 asb and is unchangeable. The fixation is monitored by an infra-red camera connected to a TV monitor and the sensitivity of such a test is adjustable. The patients' replies are recorded and printed-out using a printer with a variety of print modes (grey scale mode, value table mode, symbol mode). A comparison can be made between the examined patients and their age-corrected normal values.

Research on the Perimetron was run using program '10', which is designed for glaucoma: this program kinetically plots 3–5 isopters with tests selected by the computer based on individual sensitivity and performs static examination of 129 paracentral points at the threshold level of the enveloping isopter with a threshold increment in the missed points. As regards the classification of results we have not considered pathological the following distortions: 1) nasal steps less than 7°; 2) non specified irregularities of the nasal isopter segment which crosses the horizontal meridian; 3) isopteric irregularities relative to only one point; 4) isolated static missed tests, if their intensity is less than 0.4 log. units above that of the surrounding isopter or if their intensity is equal to or less than 32 asb; 5) missed points within 5° from the blind spot; 6) missed points at 25° from the fixation, between 60° and 120°, in which case a corrective lens is used. 3 or more close missed points at an intensity of more than 32 asb was considered as abnormal.

Program '31' was used with the Octopus 2000: the threshold is measured in 73 points with 30° from fixation, with a 6° interstimulus distance. Ten independent test points are determined twice to evaluate the threshold fluctuation. The stimulus size was 3 mm.

According to Heijl and Drance (2), the following have been treated as abnormal: 1) the points with a threshold of at least 1.5 log. units above that of the highest registered threshold sensitivity; 2) a discrepancy greater than 1 log. unit between the upper and lower emifield with adjacent points having a threshold either equal to or greater than 0.5 log. units. The most peripheral test points were disregarded to avoid lens rim artefacts as were the 6 points situated in the blind spot area (2 points on the horizontal meridian at 12° and 18°, and their 2 closest points above and below).

Procedure. All the subjects were examined with both of the automatic perimeters and manually with the Goldmann perimeter. A 3–5 isopters kinetic perimetry, and a static suprathreshold examination between the isopters were used for the manual test. The test sequence with the various instruments was random, in many cases the three tests were all performed the same day or within a few days. Whereever there was a discrepancy between the results of the various instruments, the patients were re-examined with the Goldmann perimeter, concentrating the research on the suspected area. In cases of poor patient collaboration where the test was unreliable, the subject was eliminated from the research.

RESULTS

In order to appraise the sensitivity of the two automatic perimeters we have separately considered the three groups of patients examined (incipient, established and terminal glaucoma).

The Perimetron correctly identified 33 of the 37 early field defects with a sensitivity rate of 89.2%; while the Octopus 2000 gave 29 correct results, with a sensitivity rate of 78.4%.

In the group of patients with established glaucoma, out of 28 abnormal fields, the Perimetron correctly identified 26 and the Octopus 2000, 27 with a respective sensitivity rate of 92.9% and 96.4%.

All the 13 cases with terminal glaucoma defects were identified by both instruments with a sensitivity rate of 100%, in both cases.

In the control group the Perimetron falsely classified 3 of the 27 fields as abnormal, with a specificity rate of 88.9%, while the Octopus 2000 gave only one false-positive result, with a specificity rate of 96.3%.

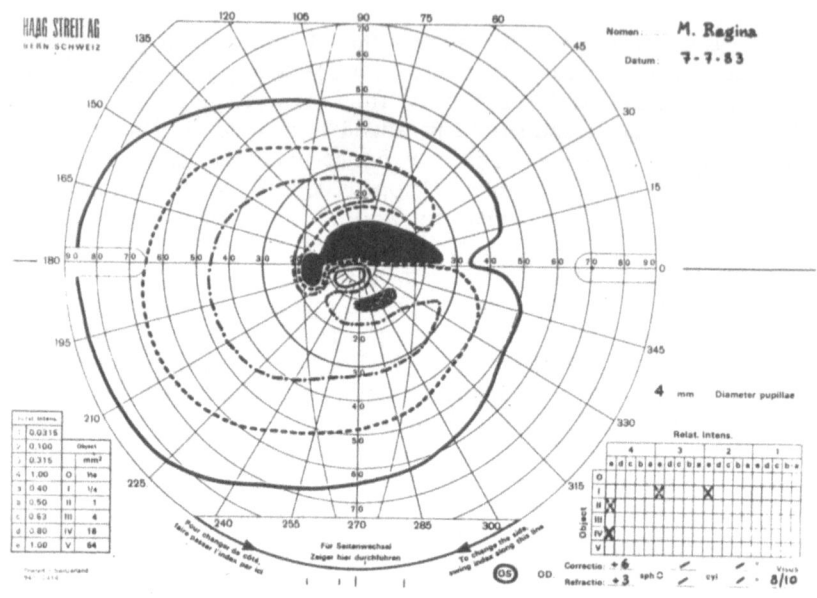

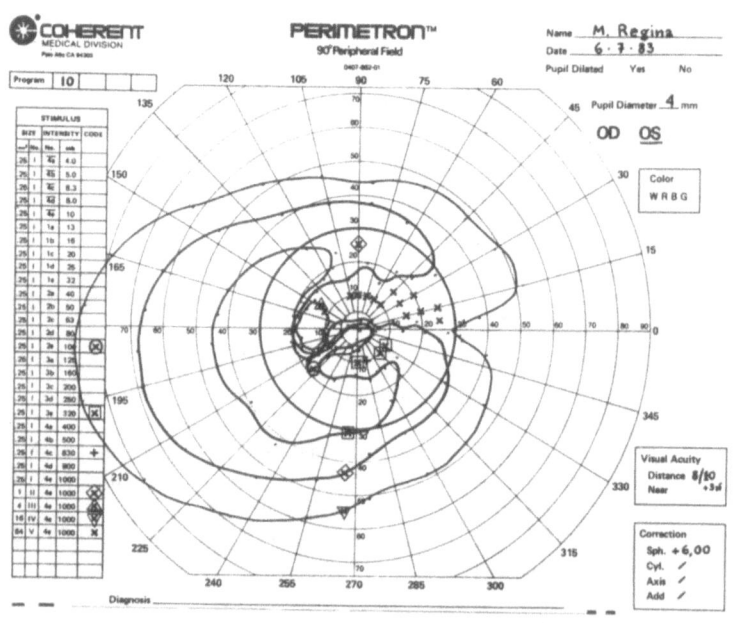

176

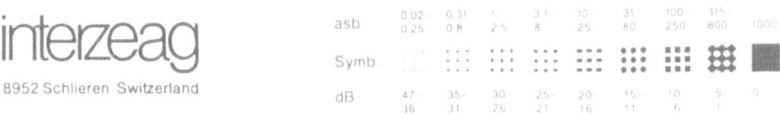

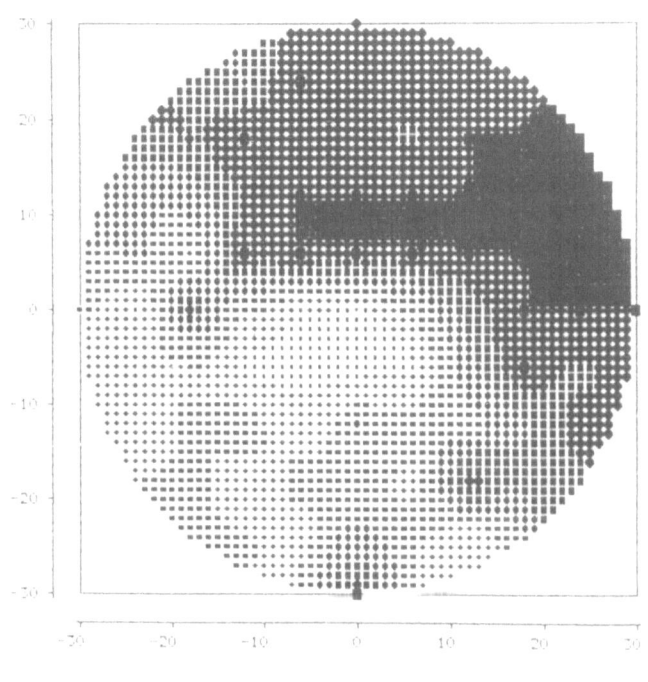

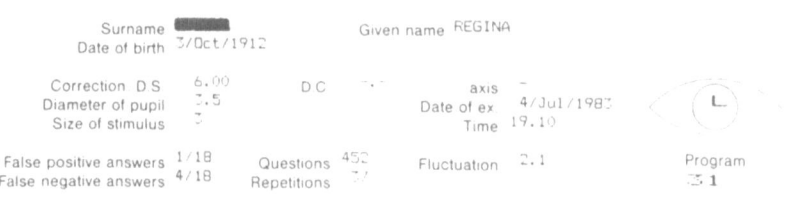

Fig. 1. Severe arcuate scotoma proceeding away from the blind spot and initial inferior nerve fibres bundle defect in a 70-year-old patient with established glaucoma. Manual reference perimetry corresponds very closely to output from both of the automatic perimeters.

177

DISCUSSION

The automatic perimetry results are closely correlated to the following factors: 1) type of program used; 2) criteria selected for the classification of the automatic test results; 3) type and severity of field defects; 4) quality of reference perimetry; 5) degree of collaboration of subject examined.

The program used clearly influences the quantity, quality, and reliability of the results obtained. The more complex programs provide more information but significantly increase the time necessary, augmenting the probability of error due to lack of attention or tiredness.

The program '10' of the Perimetron, specifically designed for glaucoma, explores the whole visual field, but unfortunately for defects of a certain complexity the time needed (more than 30 minutes) is too long. Moreover, the nonrandomized presentation of the static stimuli can be criticized, because it makes correct fixation more difficult thus facilitating false-negative results.

Program '31' of the Octopus 2000 is a good compromise between time and precision, rarely going above 20 minutes. The exploration, however, is limited to 30° from fixation and the resolution (6°) is not very high. It is, though, possible to combine: program '32', which then doubles the number of points examined and increases the resolution; and program '43' (and/or '44'), that examines the annular band between 30° and 60° from the centre.

Another important point, when judging an automatic perimeter, are the criteria used to classify the results. The sensitivity and specificity rate of an instrument in fact varies enormously depending on the strictness of these criteria. For the Octopus 2000 we have based ourselves on the standards suggested by Heijl and Drance (2), but which nevertheless seem to us rather broad, even accepting as normal, quite evident defects (enlargement of the blind spot, paracentral scotomas, etc.). However we agree with the above mentioned authors that; using more restrictive criteria such as those suggested by Schmied (5), the number of false-positive results becomes excessive therefore reducing the specificity rate to an unacceptable level.

As regard the Perimetron we have modified the criteria used by Heijl and Drance on the basis of our experience, to obtain the greatest sensitivity rate without lowering excessively the specificity rate.

The severity of defects should be taken well into consideration when evaluating the sensitivity of an automatic perimeter. Both instruments gave good results with terminal glaucoma defects, but often the test-time was shorter and the graphic interpretation simpler with the Octopus 2000. As regards the patients with developed perimetrical defects the results were good with both the Octopus 2000 and the Perimetron (Fig. 1): more than 9 out of 10 cases were correctly identified by both. The results were interesting also with initial glaucomatous defects; the sensibility rate of the Perimetron was 89.2% as against 78.4% with the Octopus 2000. It should be stated that we are talking of very subtle defects, that, in some cases, where identified by both of the automatic instruments, but not considered as abnormal according to the criteria previously mentioned.

In this type of study the quality of the manual perimetry used as a reference is very important: the more accurate the manual test, the lower the sensitivity of the automatic will appear to be and vice-versa.

Lastly, we consider a factor which comes to the foreground in a research based on subjective replies: the degree of collaboration of the examined subject. Without good collaboration, it is impossible to be sure of the reliability of the results and the test has to be rejected. With the Perimetron the only indication of poor collaboration is when the automatic fixation control interrupts the test. This occurs each time the examined eye fails to look correctly in the direction of the central target. Even though the device is equipped with two tolerance levels, it often proves to be too sensitive to disturbances, forcing the operator (from time to time) to revert to manual control. The Octopus 2000, on the other hand, is equipped with a variety of systems to estimate the patient reliability: 1) presentation of zero intensity stimuli; 2) presentation of stimuli at maximum intensity (1000 asb) at locations in which sufficient sensitivity has already been ascertained during the test; 3) recording of the number of repetitions; 4) double determination of the threshold in ten independent points (only with program '31' and '32'); and 5) calculation of the threshold fluctuation.

In conclusion, the most important advantages of the two instruments are the objectivity and satandardization of the test parameters. The reproducibility, generally satisfactory, depends, to a large extent, on the degree of collaboration of the subject examined.

Problems with the instruments, apart from their elevated cost, should be easily sorted out: for the Perimetron we should remember the excessive sensitivity of the automatic control of fixation, and the sometimes inadequate software (nonrandomized presentation of static stimuli and strategy of kinetic exploration, which is not always up to the complex perimetric defects).

Among the short comings of the Octopus 2000 should be mentioned; the automatic control of fixation, sometimes barely sensitive to even large shifts of the examined eye; the impossibility of following the course of events on the monitor during the test, and the lack of a selective program to concentrate the analysis on a suspected zone (like program '61' for the big Octopus).

We feel, however, that the results obtainable with the two automatic instruments are superior to those from routine manual perimetry. They could with a little modification become even more reliable, greatly benefitting both the ophthalmologist and his patients.

REFERENCES

1. Fankhauser, F.. Spahr, J. and Bebie, H. Three years of experience with the Octopus automatic perimeter. Doc. Ophthalmol. Proc. Series 14: 7–15 (1977).
2. Heijl, A. and Drance, S.M. A clinical comparison of three computerized automatic perimeters in the detection of glaucoma defects. Arch. Ophthalmol. 99: 832–836 (1981).
3. Leuenberger, A.E. Erfahrungen mit dem Praxisperimeter Octopus 2000. Klin. Mbl. Augenheilk 182: 510–511 (1983).
4. Li, S.G., Spaeth, G.L., Scimeca, H.A., Schatz, N.J. and Savino, P.J. Clinical

experiences with the use of an automated perimeter (Octopus) in the diagnosis and management of patients with glaucoma and neurologic diseases. Ophthalmology 86: 1302–1312 (1979).
5. Schmied, U. Automatic (Octopus) and manual (Goldmann) perimetry in glaucoma. Proc. 1st Int. Meeting on Automated Perimetry System Octopus. Schlieren, Switzerland, Interzeag Publishers, 53 (1979).
6. Spahr, J. Zur Automatisierung der Perimetrie: I. Die Anwendung eines computer-gesteuerten Perimeters. Albrecht von Graefes Arch. klin. exp. Ophthalmol. 188: 323–338 (1973).

Authors' address:
Dr. Paolo Brusini
Divisione Oculistica
Ospedale Civile
33100 Udine
Italy

REAL TIME PATTERN RECOGNITION AND FEATURE ANALYSIS FROM VIDEO SIGNALS APPLIED TO EYE MOVEMENT AND PUPILLARY REFLEX MONITORING

JACQUES R. CHARLIER[1,2], JEAN-LUC BARISEAU[1], VINCENT CHUFFART[3], FRANÇOISE MARSY[3] and JEAN-CLAUDE HACHE[4]

(*Lille, France*)

ABSTRACT

Original techniques for real time pattern recognition and feature analysis from standard video signals have been applied to the monitoring of eye movements and pupillary size during visual field examinations in routine ophthalmological practice.

INTRODUCTION

The evaluations of eye orientation and pupil size are of great interest in ophthalmology as eye movements and pupil contractions provide relevant informations on the proper operation of the visual sensory-motor system. The accuracy of fixation and the pupil size also play an important part in many visual function tests (3) including the visual field examination, since they determine the position and intensity of the retinal stimulus.

A desirable method for monitoring eye fixation, eye movements or pupil size during routine clinical examinations should require minimal subject training, co-operation, discomfort and set-up time. It should allow relatively free natural head movements and measure the rotation of the eye independently of its position. Furthermore, an eye-monitoring device should be positioned in such a way that it does not interfere with the visual examination.

Conventional intruments used for monitoring eye fixation exhibit a high sensitivity to head motion, and require frequent readjustment and reinstruction of the patient (7, 9). Some of these instruments compare the light reflection from the iris and cornea to a reference level set during proper alignment. Other instruments are tracking the position of the iris or the corneal reflection. Both types of instruments do not separate lateral and rotary motions of the eye. An eye rotation of 1° can be shown to be equivalent to a head transverse motion of only 0.17 mm (4). Maintenance of the head fixed within such limits is difficult, uncomfortable and not suitable for clinical examinations lasting for more than 10 minutes.

In a previous work (2), we described a new instrument for monitoring eye fixation and pupil size during visual field examinations. The major

Heijl, A. and Greve, E.L. (eds.), Proceedings of the 6th Int. Visual Field Symposium.
© *1985, Dr W. Junk Publishers, Dordrecht, The Netherlands. ISBN 978-94-010-8932-6*

features of this instrument will be reviewed in the background section. The eye orientation was determined from the position of the corneal reflection relative to the bright pupil. Standard video equipment and LSI circuitry were used.

Intensive clinical evaluation for 3 years and over more than 6000 eyes indicated satisfactory performance in about 60% cases. The remaining 40% of cases resulted from severe perturbations of the ocular video image including partial occlusions of the pupil with eye lids and eye lashes, amplitude fluctuations of the video signal and parasite light reflections. In order to increase the performance of the instrument to an acceptable range, new developments were undertaken which will be presented in this paper.

BACKGROUND

The optics of the instrument have been described previously (2, 8, 10). The eye of the patient is illuminated with near i.r. radiation obtained from a tungsten filament lamp filtered to the 800–900 nm band, which is sufficiently far into the i.r. region to be almost invisible.

Part of the incident light beam is reflected by the front of the cornea and produces the so-called corneal reflection. The boundary between the pupil and the iris, which normally exhibits very low contrast, is enhanced with the bright pupil effect: the illumination and collection apertures of the optical systems are made coincident (Fig. 1) so that incident light rays are refracted

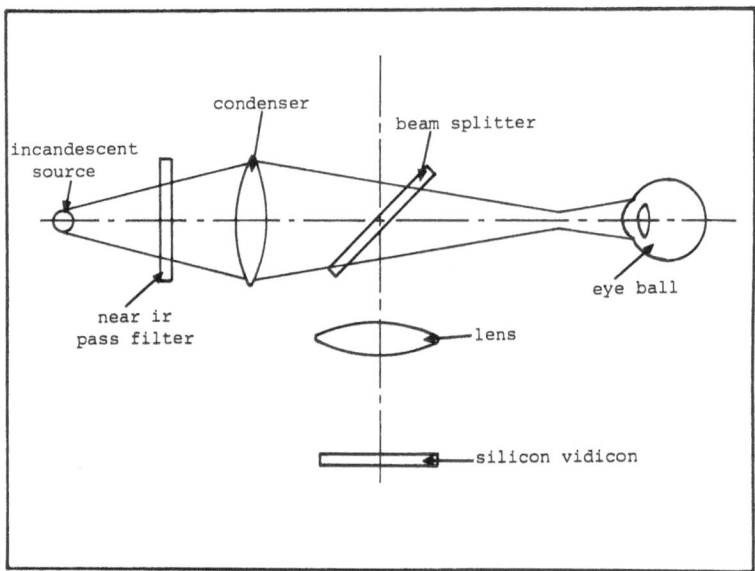

Fig. 1. Schematic of the optical system.

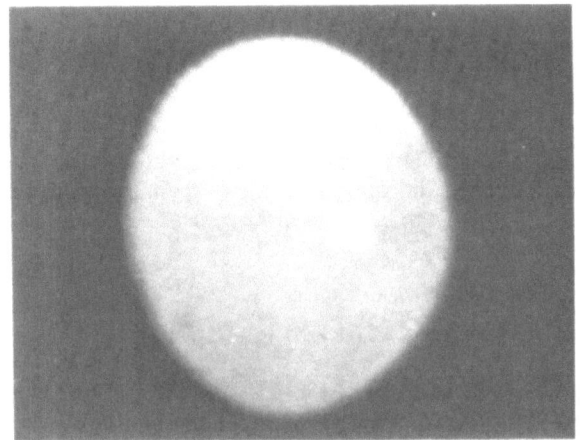

Fig. 2. Video image of the eye.

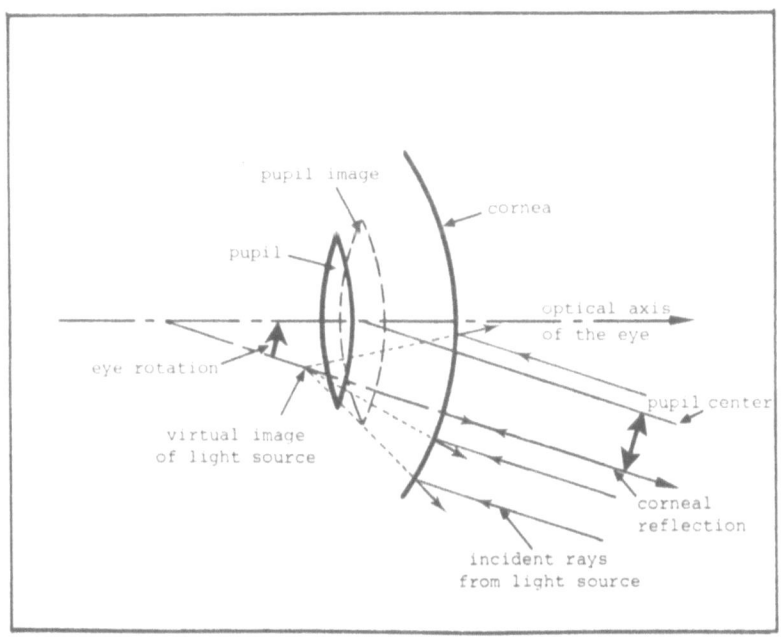

Fig. 3. The origin of the bright pupil and corneal reflection.

back from the retina and back light the pupil. The resulting image of the eye
(Fig. 2) shows the pupil as a bright disk against a dark background superimposed upon the corneal reflection. The corneal reflection and the bright

pupil images are located in two different optical planes. Their relative position is not affected by translation movements of the eye and is only related to its rotations (8) (Fig. 3). A standard 625 interlaced scanning lines, 50 frames per second, television camera is used as an image transducer. The resolution of 312 lines per frame allows for a precision of one degree of eye angular motion with an approximative 2 cm by 2 cm image area at the eye.

Eye orientation and pupil size are extracted from the camera video signal. Eye orientation is evaluated from the displacement of the corneal reflection relative to the pupil center.

FEATURE SELECTION

Previous design. In a first design (2), processing of the video signals involved two major steps. A preprocessing interface determined over each scanning line the co-ordinates of the beginning and end of the bright pupil as well as of the corneal reflection. Further calculations were carried out by a Motorola 6802 microprocessor.

The processing interface included amplitude threshold detectors which triggered a 5 MHz clock counter at the leading and trailing edges of the bright pupil and corneal reflection. The pupil center was calculated as the barycenter of the detected points which were likely to belong to the pupil perimeter.

This first design has been in the Lille ophthalmologic clinic for three years. More than 6000 examinations including visual fields and pupillary reflex evaluations have been performed. The instrument is found to be very convenient for routine clinical examinations in about 60% of the subjects. In these cases, it does not require any training, co-operation of discomfort. The error in measurement of eye orientation is typically less than ± 1 degree. Head movements within 10 mm amplitude do not affect the results significantly. The examination can be interrupted at any time and still no initiation of the eye monitor is needed when the examination is resumed. Pupil surface area is measured with satisfactory accuracy and recordings of pupillary contractions have been used for the clinical investigation of the pupillary light reflex (6).

Ocular video image perturbations. The remaining 40% of cases result from severe perturbations of the ocular video image involving several types of problems.

Pupil contour detection. The bright pupil intensity depends upon the pupil aperture and the opacity of ocular media. The contour of the pupil can hardly be detected when the contrast of the bright pupil is low. This situation is found when the pupil is less than 2.5 mm in diameter, as in glaucomatous patients treated with pilocarpine (Fig. 4) or when the ocular media are opaque, as in patients with cataracts. In some patients wide fluctuations of the pupil diameter require periodic readjustment of the amplitude detection threshold.

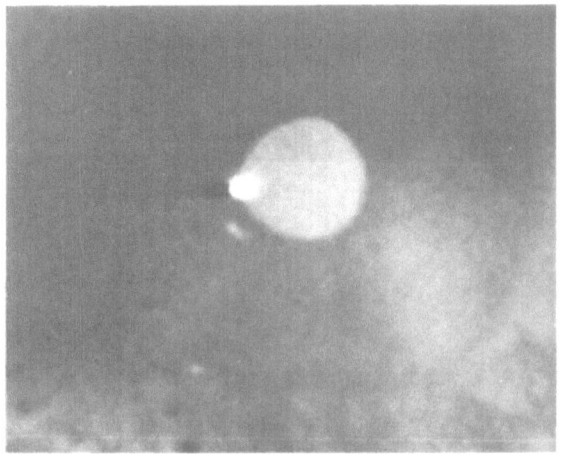

Fig. 4. Low contrast pupil.

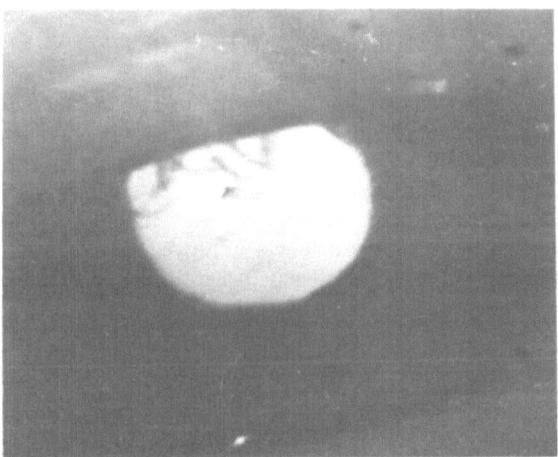

Fig. 5. Obstruction of the pupil with eye lashes.

Obstruction of the bright pupil. A large part of the pupil is often obstructed by the eyelids of eyelashes (Fig. 5). In these cases, the calculation of the barycenter leads to false determinations of the pupil center.

Corneal reflection detection. In a number of cases, parasite reflections occur on the sclera, on the skin or on optical glasses which are often needed for the evaluation of central vision (Fig. 6). These situations result in false identification of the corneal reflection.

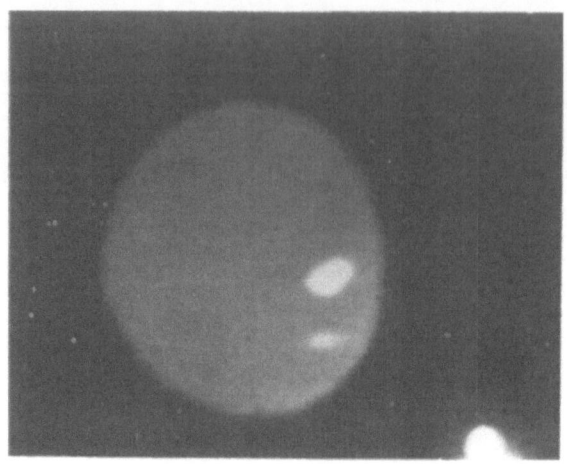

Fig. 6. Parasite reflections.

FEATURE DETECTION, IDENTIFICATION AND ANALYSIS

New solutions have been developed in order to incease the performance of the instrument to an acceptable range. The basic scheme involving, in a first step, the extraction of pupil boundary and corneal reflection from each individual scanning line and, in a second step, the determination of pupil center and the calculation of relative corneal reflection displacement and pupil surface area, has been kept. It was improved significantly by the introduction for more specific ('intelligent') algorithms for feature detection, feature identification and reduction as well as feature analysis.

Feature detection. A shape detector circuitry was developed for the detection of the leading and trailing edges of the pupil and of the corneal reflection within the video signal. Figures 7 and 8 illustrate the results obtained from a sample video image. Using shape detection instead of amplitude level or amplitude variation detection improves performance significantly with low contrast images. It eliminates the problems associated with variations of the detection thresholds with pupil size fluctuations. A better discrimination is also obtained of the corneal reflection which is usually sharper than parasite reflections.

Feature identification and reduction. Further processing is carried out on a Z80 microprocessor after direct memory access of the data. Considerable thought has been given to minimizing calculation time to permit real time operation of the system, i.e., the complete analysis of each image within 20 ms. Specific, fast operating algorithms have been developed and implemented in assembly language. The present algorithms can process about

186

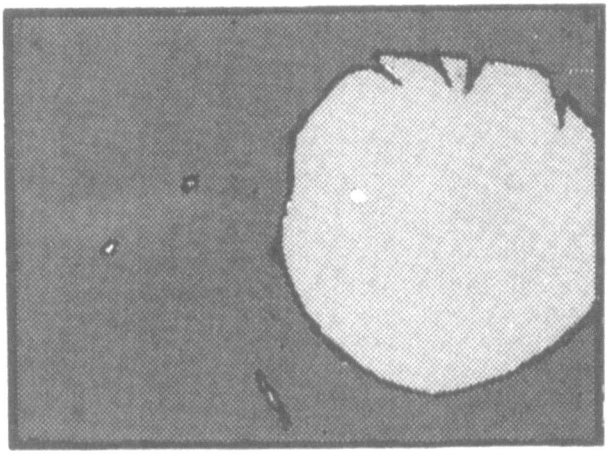

Fig. 7. Sample video image with eye lashes and parasite reflections.

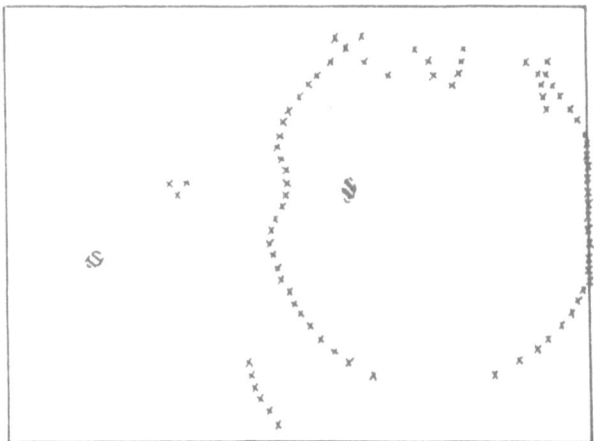

Fig. 8. Pupil boundary and corneal reflection detection.

100 detected leading and trailing edges within 20 ms. These data are clustered in data chains using algorithms based on contour continuity (Fig. 9) and curvature consistency (Fig. 10) of the pupil boundary. The data chains are scored according to these two criteria. The two data chains which obtained the highest scores are selected for further processing. This processing eliminates data chains resulting from parasite reflections and eye lashes.

Feature analysis. The purpose of feature analysis is to calculate the pupil center and diameter from the selected data chains. A fast algorithm

187

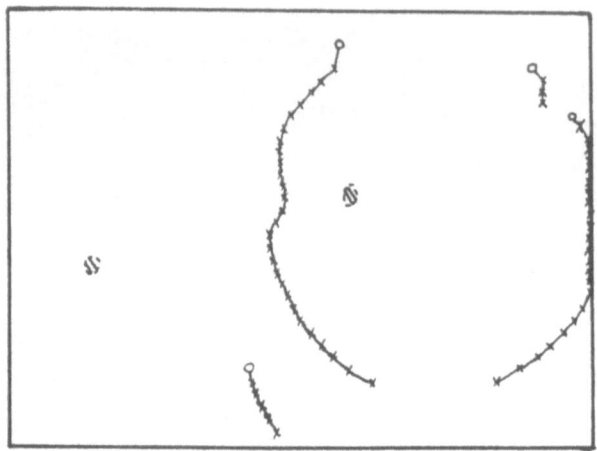

Fig. 9. Data chain extraction based on contour continuity.

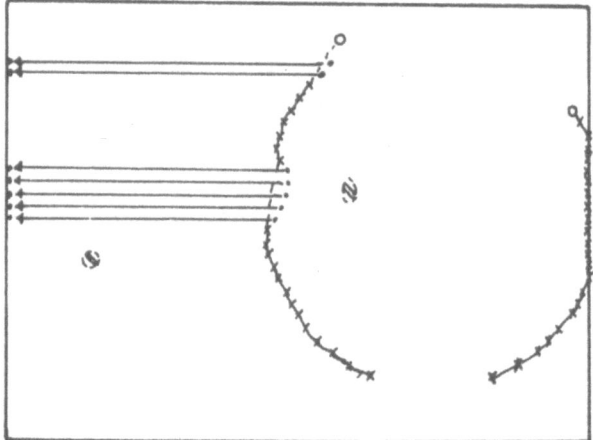

Fig. 10. Data chain extraction based on curvate consistence.

determines the center of the circle which fits the two data chains with a minimum distance error. The circle radius is computed as the average distance between the circle center and 8 data points chosen at regular intervals along the selected data chains. Finally, the corneal reflection is selected from the detected data according to its location within a perimeter centered on the pupil.

CONCLUSION

This work demonstrates the possibility of implementing fast, 'intelligent' image analysis systems providing an answer to the difficult problem of fixation and pupil size monitoring under clinical conditions.

The basic features of the resulting instrument are:

(1) The use of low-cost hardware, i.e. standard video equipment and LSI circuitry.

(2) The measurement eye orientation from the position of the bright pupil relative to the corneal reflection.

(3) 'Real time' processing and high data throughout of 50 samples per second, allowing pupillary and oculomotor reflex analysis.

(4) Specialized hardware and software permitting an adjustment free feature identification and analysis directly from video signals. Severe perturbations of the ocular video images can be handled by the system, including partial occlusions of the pupil with eye lids or eye lashes, fluctuations of amplitude levels and parasite light reflections.

Further clinical evaluation is needed in order to evaluate the improvement provided by this new design.

REFERENCES

1. Baseville, M. 'Détection de contours: méthodes et études comparatives', Ann. Telecom. 34: 559–579 (1979).
2. Charlier, J. and Hach, J.C. 'New instrument for monitoring eye fixation and pupil size during the visual field examination', Med. Biol. Eng. Comput. 20: 21–28 (1982).
3. Charlier, J. and Hache, J.C. 'Optimization of computer assisted visual field examination', Fifth International Visual Field Symposium, Junk Pub. 359–364 (1983).
4. Ditchburn, R.W. and Ginsborg, B.L. 'Involontary eye movements during fixation', J. Physiol., 119: 1–9 (1953).
5. Gale, A.G. 'A note on the remote oculometer technique for recording eye movements', Vision Research 22: 201–202 (1982).
6. Hugeux, J.P., Bariseau, J.L., Charlier, J., Hache, J.C. and Moschetto, Y. 'Acquisition, traitement et analyse d'image de l'oeil pur l'étude du réflexe pupillaire', Innovation et Technologie en Biologie et Médecine 4: 159–168 (1982).
7. Keltner, J.L., Johnson, C.A. and Balestrery, F.G. 'Suprathreshold static perimetry: Initial clinical trials with the Fieldmaster automated perimeter', Arch. Ophthalmol. 77: 260–272 (1979).
8. Merchant, J. and Morrissette, R. 'Remote measurement of eye direction allowing subject motion over one cubic foot of space', IEEE Trans. BME 21: 309–317 (1974).
9. Portney, G.L. and Krohn, M.A. 'Automatic perimetry: background, instruments and methods', Surv. Ophthalmol. 22, 271–278 (1978).
10. Young, L.R. and Sheena, D. 'Survey of eye movement recording methods', Behavior Research Methods Instrumentation 7: 397–429 (1975).

Authors' addresses:
[1] C.T.B. Inserm, 13–17, rue Camille Guérin 59800 Lille, France
[2] Essilor International, 6, rue Pastourelle 75003 Paris, France
[3] I.S.E.N., 3, rue François Baes, 59056 Lille, France
[4] Centre Hospitalier, Place de Verdun, 59000 Lille, France

THE EARLIEST VISUAL FIELD DEFECTS IN MID-CHIASMAL COMPRESSION

LARS FRISÉN

(*Göteborg, Sweden*)

ABSTRACT

Analysis of visual field records from 254 personally examined pituitary adenoma patients allowed identification of the earliest visual field defect attributable to mid-chiasmal compression. This took the form of a bitemporal foreshortening of central isopters, not extending beyond 15 degrees of eccentricity, usually somewhat more pronounced above, often lacking a clear vertical step, and often asymmetrical between the eyes. These defects seemed to be more difficult to detect in static profiles.

INTRODUCTION

Detailed knowledge of the different stages of chiasmal compression and their associated perimetric signs dates back to the systematic studies of Cushing and Walker (1), reported in 1915. Their findings have been amply corroborate by a long list of later investigators. The very earliest visual field defects in mid-chiasmal compression seem to have escaped definition, however. Very subtle field defects have certainly been encountered by many examiners (e.g., Dannheim (2)), but still subtler defects might be revealed by systematic search. This possibility has important implications for the design of maximally efficient screening procedures.

Identification of the earliest stage of a field defect is always a difficult task as the defect by definition will deviate only marginally from the normal visual field with all its individual variations. Extrapolation from knowledge of the more advanced stages of disease may be misleading. The same objection applies to studies of minimal defects remaining after treatment. There are at least two better approaches. One is to keep watch for the appearance of field defects in individuals with known pituitary tumors who were found to be normal in careful baseline examinations, and where treatment was deferred or postponed. Another useful approach is to compare pre- and post-treatment visual field records from individuals lacking obvious field defects in the first examination, to see if there were any changes after treatment. Both approaches were used here. The study was limited to patients with pituitary

Heijl, A. and Greve, E.L. (eds.), Proceedings of the 6th Int. Visual Field Symposium.
© *1985, Dr W. Junk Publishers, Dordrecht, The Netherlands.. ISBN 978-94-010-8932-6*

adenomas as adenomas are the only types of sellar tumors that frequently are diagnosed prior to the stage of gross chiasmal dysfunction.

PATIENTS AND METHODS

Selection of cases was made among 254 personally examined patients with endocrinological, radiographical, and/or surgical evidence of a pituitary adenoma. First, all cases with easily discernible visual field defects were excluded, as were those with complicating conditions or anomalies: only those who had *normal or questionably normal visual field examinations prior to treatment* were retained for further selection. Their pre-treatment and post-treatment visual field records were compared, and those cases who had identical results in the two examinations were excluded. There remained 3 cases showing a visual field expansion after treatment: these were thought to represent the very earliest stage of chiasmal compression in the present series. Additional observations were obtained from 1 patient, who was followed for a period of time during the evolution of early chiasmal dysfunction. These 4 cases constituted 1.6% of the population under study. None had any visual complaints.

Visual field examinations were made with a Haag-Streit 940 ST perimeter. As the tests were run in a busy practice it was not possible to adhere to a blind, standardized multi-isopter, multi-profile strategy. Instead, a screening strategy crystallized from many years of experience was used. This involves the charting of two isopters at about 10 and 15 degrees of nasal eccentricity, using appropriately dimmed targets of the I series. This is complemented by checking for subjective symmetry of perception across the vertical meridian for the fainter target. In many instances, the limits for target 14e are also charted. The full test usually requires 10 to 15 minutes, including instructions. Static sections are obtained only in cases where there is some doubt whether the kinetic results are normal or not. Any profiles bisect the area of suspicion, using target II at two-degree intervals. This usually requires an additional 10 minutes, including the time for perimeter modification. Finally, a check is made of subjective symmetry across the vertical meridian of the saturation of a supra-liminal red reflecting target. This is presented against a black tangent screen illuminated by 30 1x. Apparent color saturation is also compared in central vision between the two eyes, using alternate cover.

RESULTS AND DISCUSSION

The visual field defects observed in the selected 4 cases were strictly limited to the central part of the temporal visual field and became undetectable outside some 15 degrees of eccentricity. Only depressions were encountered: there was no instance of a scotomatous defect. The depressions were always most clearly seen in the inner of the two central isopters, and they gradually tapered out with increasing eccentricity. Typical examples of these early defects are shown in Figs. 1 and 2.

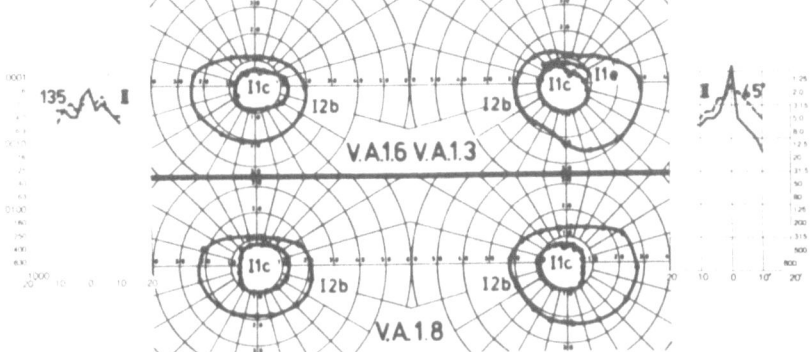

Fig. 1. Case of moderate acromegaly, operated transsphenoidally. Computed tomography showed 4 mm of suprasellar extension of tumor. The subtle temporal depressions in the pre-operative visual fields (top kinetic charts and solid lines in static profiles) were combined with bitemporal desaturation of color: this regressed after surgery. Note improvement also in visual acuity.

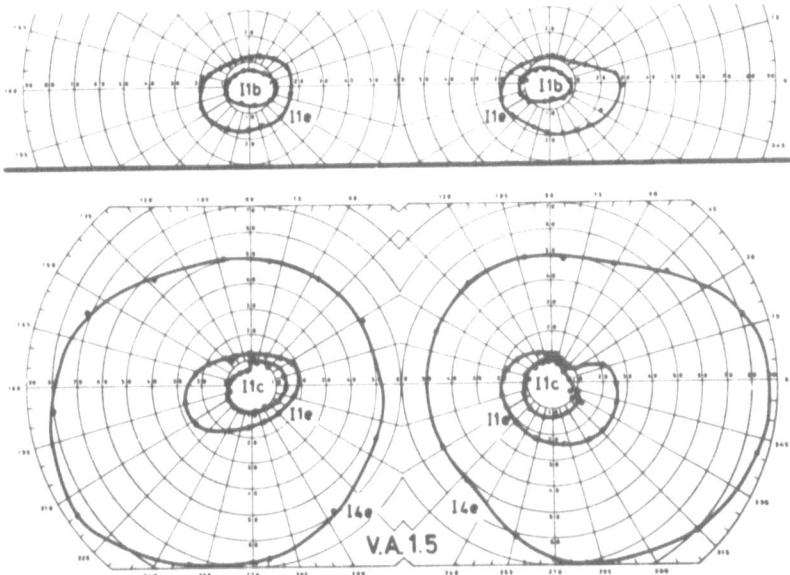

Fig. 2. Case of pituitary adenoma followed without treatment for 1 year. Top chart represents one of several visual field examinations thought to be normal, with later progression (bottom chart). At surgery, chiasm was found to be prefixed, and elevated by tumor. After surgery, the isopters assumed the same appearance as in the top chart.

Curiously, these early defects seemed not to respect the vertical meridian very clearly, as might be expected from extrapolation from cases with more advanced stages of chiasmal compression (1). Their most conspicuous

193

characteristic was a smooth foreshortening of the temporal halves of the central isopters. The typical failure to find a vertical step might be artificial, however, and related to the technical difficulties of manual perimetry in the cramped central area in the Goldmann perimeter. Support for this notion came from the observations of subjective desaturation of supraliminal color stimuli: there seemed to be a relatively abrupt change in saturation when the target crossed the vertical meridian. At the same time, the color test supported the impression that temporal foreshortening was the major isopter abnormality because desaturation usually appeared to be nearly equally pronounced above and below the horizontal meridian. Incidentally, no case with an isolated abnormality of color saturation was encountered in the present series.

Another factor contributing to the failure of identifying vertical steps is the fact that the highest point on the circumference of *normal* central isopters usually is situated somewhat nasally (5), meaning that for equal elevations in the central visual field, temporal thresholds usually are somewhat higher than nasal thresholds. This normal state of affairs is in opposition to the classical emphasis on vertical steps as early indicators of chiasmal conduction failure. This does not hinder that vertical steps remain reliable signs of somewhat later stages of chiasmal (and retro-chiasmal) visual pathway failure. Foreshortening remains a major component of the field defect also in later stages.

These early defects were generally easier to detect in isopters than in static profiles, presumably due to the difficulty of detecting the shallow slope of the distal defect area. Hence, kinetic perimetry seems preferable for screening for early chiasmal defects. Incidentally, at least some of the defects analysed here might have escaped detection by the screening procedure recently proposed by Trobe and coworkers (6), which heavily emphasizes vertical cuts.

Visual acuity was found to be affected in all cases where it was determined carefully enough (cf Fig. 1). This attests to the notion that also non-crossing nerve fibers are affected at an early stage of chiasmal compression, long before the appearance of nasal perimetric defects (4).

As stated in the introduction, the definition of the very earliest type of field defect is a difficult task, not the least because of the rarity of opportunities to study cases with very early lesions. Furthermore, progression may occur within days once the first defects have appeared (7). Although the number of early cases reported here is small, I feel confident in concluding that perimetric screening for early mid-chiasmal compression can be limited to careful charting of one single kinetic isopter of small radius (say, 8—12 degrees in the nasal field), complemented with a check for symmetry of apparent color saturation both across the vertical meridian and between the eyes, and a careful test of visual acuity. Application of an objective isopter shape test (5) might increase sensitivity additionally. There is no point in adding more peripheral isopters if this critical isopter is normal: this will not enhance the diagnostic yield.

REFERENCES

1. Cushing, H. and Walker, C.B. Distortions of the visual fields in cases of brain tumour. Chiasmal lesions with especial reference to bitemporal hemianopsia. Brain

37: 341–400 (1915).

2. Dannheim, F. Perimetrie beim Chiasmasyndrom, schwellennahe und überschwellige Reize. Klin. Mbl. Augenheildk. 171: 468–477 (1977).

3. Frisén, L. A versatile color confrontation test for the central visual field. A comparison with quantitative perimetry. Arch. Ophthalmol. 89: 3–9 (1973).

4. Frisén, L. The neurology of visual acuity. Brain 103: 639–670 (1980).

5. Frisén, L. and Frisén, M. Objective recognition of abnormal isopters. Acta Ophthalmol. 53: 378–392 (1975).

6. Trobe, J.D., Acosta, P.C. and Krischer, J.P. A screening method for chiasmal visual-field defects. Arch. Ophthalmol. 99: 264–271 (1981).

7. Van Dalen, J.T.W. and Greve, E.J.. Rapid deterioration of visual fields during bromocriptine-induced pregnancy in a patient with a pituitary adenoma. Br. J. Ophthalmol. 61: 729–733 (1977).

Author's address:
Dr. Lars Frisén
Dept. Ophthalmology
Sahlgren's Hospital
S-413 45 Göteborg
Sweden

A STUDY OF THE DEPTH OF HEMIANOPIC FIELD DEFECTS FOR OPTIMIZING COMPUTERIZED PERIMETRY

H. BYNKE

(Lund, Sweden)

ABSTRACT*

Although the test point pattern of the computerized perimeter 'Competer' has been enlarged, focal diagnosis is in many cases difficult since the area outside 35° of eccentricity cannot be examined. Further improvements of the instrument requires knowledge about the depth at various eccentricities of common neurological field defects. This was calculated in bitemporal and suprageniculate homonymous defects. Forty-one eyes with chiasmal defects and 36 eyes with suprageniculate defects were compared with 26 normal fields. Generally, the central area was more or less intact in relative hemianopias, probably because of the large proportion of macular fibres in the visual pathways, and the depth was found to increase towards the mid-periphery. The results indicate that with a simplified test strategy for the mid-peripheral area, few hemianopic defects would be missed by the 'Competer'. In this way, the examination of the mid-peripheral area could be shortened. Without prolonging the total test session, which is already 15–20 min per eye, focal diagnosis could be facilitated by adding and testing a number of points in the area outside 35° of eccentricity. Such modifications are in progress.

Author's address:
H. Bynke, M.D., Ph.D.
University Eye Clinic
S-221 85 Lund
Sweden

---

*The paper will be published in full in Neuro-Ophthalmology (Amsterdam).

Heijl, A. and Greve, E.L. (eds.), Proceedings of the 6th Int. Visual Field Symposium.
© *1985, Dr W. Junk Publishers, Dordrecht, The Netherlands. ISBN 978-94-010-8932-6*

EVALUATING THE USEFULNESS IN NEURO-OPHTHALMOLOGY OF VISUAL FIELD EXAMINATIONS PERIPHERAL TO 30 DEGREES*

ANNA-LENA HÅRD-BOBERG and JONATHAN D. WIRTSCHAFTER

(*Minneapolis, USA*)

ABSTRACT

The value of the information obtained from Goldmann manual kinetic perimetry beyond 30° was examined. Of 229 randomly selected patients in a University eye clinic who had visual fields performed for reasons other than glaucoma or ocular hypertension, only three patients had abnormalities confined to the peripheral visual field (PVF) of one or both eyes. In none of these three patients was the PVF necessary to detect disease (Graves' disease, two cases; retinoschisis, one case). The PVF was useful in determining the localization of the disorder and/or the therapeutic management in 14 patients of whom four had retinitis pigmentosa, and five had other retinal disorders where the PVF showed the extent of the retinal damage. For ergo-ophthalmologic purposes the PVF was useful in 45 patients; most frequently because the extent of abnormality provided a basis for warning the patient. In some cases the PVF was considered to be useful for economic disability determination or to exclude significant PVF defects in a patient with only one visually useful eye. In 77 patients the PVF of each eye was abnormal, but not of ergo-ophthalmologic significance.

If these data can be extrapolated to automated static perimetry, there will be a very great incremental cost for any clinically useful information obtained from the examination of the PVF. Because the cost-effectiveness of the examination must be compared with competing methods of obtaining information, it is proposed that the PVF be examined (1) whenever indicated for ergo-ophthalmologic reasons, or (2) when the central visual field (CVF) examination does not resolve a clinical problem for which there is a reasonably high probability that (a) additional clinically useful information will be obtained by examination of the PVF *after* the results of the CVF examination have been analyzed, or (b) the eye is likely to have a condition that can be detected or followed best by PVF examination.

*Note: An expanded version of this paper was presented at the American Ophthalmological Society, 1984.

Heijl, A. and Greve, E.L. (eds.), Proceedings of the 6th Int. Visual Field Symposium.
© *1985, Dr W. Junk Publishers, Dordrecht, The Netherlands. ISBN 978-94-010-8932-6*

INTRODUCTION

The increasing use of automated perimetry has made it imperative to determine the cost-effectiveness of examining the peripheral visual field (PVF), because this region is not examined in passing as was the case with Goldmann manual kinetic perimetry. We must know when the PVF must be examined because only perimetry can provide the needed information, and when it may be examined because there is a reasonable prior probability that perimetry can provide information of better quality than would be obtained by using alternative and competing techniques.

Prior studies of the usefulness of the PVF may not be applicable to the present problem because (1) some studies were performed prior to the introduction of the Goldmann perimeter, (2) varying definitions of 'peripheral' as defined by varying degrees of eccentricity, (3) 'peripheral' defined by the size and intensity of the stimulus rather than by degrees of eccentricity, (4) the studies were related to specific disorders, or they, (5) do not integrate both clinical and ergo-ophthalmologic considerations in a single study.

In 1958, Blum et al (1) had reviewed 3078 'paired fields' from 1892 patients. In only 25 fields of 22 patients (1.16%), did they demonstrate defects in the PVF when the central visual field (CVF) was normal, and in none of these did the PVF yield information that was important for the diagnosis or management of the case. The routine use of PVF testing was questioned.

Ogawa and Suzuki (9) in 1978 reported the results of kinetic perimetry by the Goldmann perimeter in 1296 eyes, PVF defects were defined as focal defects within V/4 or constriction of V/4 to less than the V/4 standard boundary isopter. Only six eyes in six patients showed isolated PVF changes, but at least two of these had CVF defects in the other eye. Five eyes had ophthalmoscopically detectable retinal degenerations. The remaining eye had a CVF defect before a pituitary tumor operation. The conclusion was that CVF examination is fully sufficient for the detection phase, and that PVF examinations should be performed in the assessment phase, if necessary.

On the other hand, there are several conditions in which the earliest VF defects almost always occur exclusively in the periphery. Deutman (4) describes the VF defects of retinitis pigmentosa (RP) as an annular scotoma extending from 30° to 50° from fixation, later spreading centrally and peripherally. Constriction of the PVF may be caused by drugs toxic to retinal ganglion cells including quinine, salicylates, thioridazine, hydrochloride and carbon monoxide (6). Whether these changes appear with totally normal CVF is not known to us.

Constriction of the PVF may also be caused by 'classical' neuro-ophthalmologic disorders such as optic disc drusen. In idiopathic intracranial hypertension (pseudotumor cerebri) constriction of the PVF is the most important indicator of failing vision. In *Chamlin's* (2) study of 100 patients with optic neuritis, one case was reported to have an isolated peripheral defect. In this case, however, 'peripheral' meant that the defect was not connected to the blindspot. There was involvement of the entire periphery extending centrally as close as 12° from fixation. In 1938, Sloan and Woods

(11) examined 56 patients with syphilitic primary atrophy of the optic nerve. The fields were charted with the Ferree-Rand perimeter and the tangent screen. Seven patients had concentric peripheral contraction of the fields and in early stages the defect was limited to the far periphery. Walsh (13) described peripheral constriction as the characteristic VF defect in syphilitic optic atrophy of the primary type.

In 1957, *Chamlin* (3) studied 33 eyes in 23 patients with mass lesion compression of the optic nerve well in front of the chiasm. In 4 cases the secondarily involved eyes showed PVF defects only, with normal central fields and in no case was there a central scotoma with normal periphery. He concluded that such a compression first causes PVF defects, with central involvement as an extension of the PVF defect. In none of the cases, however, was there PVF defect with normal central fields in both eyes.

In retrochiasmal neuro-ophthalmologic problems the PVF may be characteristic. For example, in disorders of the anterior tip of the calcarine fissure there may be a unilateral temporal crescent. In this condition the visual field defect is seen only in the periphery. Abnormalities of the temporal lobe and lateral geniculate body may also be more pronounced in the PVF than the CVF.

In open angle glaucoma (OAG) a peripheral nasal defect has been found to be the first VF defect in a number of investigations. LeBlanc and *Becker* (8) reported the occurrence of an isolated peripheral nasal step in 11% of 81 eyes with glaucomatous field defects. However, there were localized depressions within 30° in the two cases whose fields are shown in the paper. Phelps, Hayreh, and Montague (10) compared the VF defects in low tension glaucoma (LTG), primary open angle glaucoma (OAG), and anterior ischemic optic neuropathy (AION). In about 4% of eyes with each disorder, they found a peripheral nasal step not extending to within 30° from fixation as the only evidence of visual field damage. Drance (5) examined 35 eyes of 30 patients who developed VF defects due to glaucoma. In two eyes (6%) with normal central fields he found a nasal step only in the periphery. Hart *et al.* (7) studied the visual fields of patients with ocular hypertension. They found that reduction in the peripheral isopter area was associated with impending field loss.

METHODS

A computer search was made covering all patient visits to the University of Minnesota Ophthalmology Service and Clinics in the year 1983. In that period, a total of 1972 visual fields were recorded as having been performed, some of which represent multiple examinations on a given patient. Five hundred and ten hospital charts were obtained without any known systematic bias. These were reviewed and 61 were excluded from this study, because they did not contain Goldmann manual kinetic visual fields. Patients whose visual fields were performed only for glaucoma or ocular hypertension were also excluded. Two hundred and twenty-nine hospital charts with non-glaucoma visual fields have been analyzed to date.

Although the performance of a visual field examination in 1983 was the first criterion for entrance into the study, the VF examinations we evaluated were the initial ones for each patient. Some of these were recorded as early as 1960. The examinations had been performed by a number of perimetrists with obvious variations in technique.

Two persons reviewed each chart and the initial visual fields were evaluated. The patients' complete medical records were available in the charts. Each central and peripheral visual field was classified as normal or abnormal, and the VF defects present were described. The additional value of the information from the PVF examination over the information from the CVF was assessed as it related to the detection of the existence of VF defects, topographic localization of the lesion, management of the patient, and ergo-ophthalmologic purposes.

The criteria for abnormality were relatively subjective. They depended largely on the performance of the patient and the original examiner. Examinations thought to be unsatisfactory by the original examiner or the evaluator were excluded. The criteria for generalized constriction of isopters were approximate. The evaluators were more certain when generalized depression was present in one eye than in both. More certainty was present in the description of localized field defects such as localized depressions and scotomas. The patients were classified into eight diagnostic categories at the time results were analyzed.

Even with the availability of the clinical record it proved difficult to determine the contribution of the PVF to the many factors that led to clinical decision-making. The PVF was considered of value for detection if there were VF defects outside 30° with normal CVF. The major reason to consider a PVF valuable for determining topographic localization and/or management of the patient was demonstration of VF defects typical for a certain disorder only in the periphery, e.g. ring scotoma in retinitis pigmentosa (RP), or that it showed the extent of retinal or optic nerve involvement, or that the PVF was the site of the only remaining function in the eye. A peripheral field was evaluated as able to alter the ergo-ophthalmologic assessment (1) if it was done for the purpose of evaluation of an injury (whether the field was abnormal or normal), (2) when the evaluator thought that the patient or the patient's family would have been warned about an occupational hazard or mobility limitation on the basis of the PVF examination or (3) when the patient had only one visually useful eye.

RESULTS

Diagnostic classification of each case was done on the basis of the stated problem for which the visual field was performed, unless subsequent events proved that the visual field better correlated with the subsequent diagnosis than the initial problem.

The largest group of patients (91) were in the group designated as having neuro-ophthalmic symptoms. These patients had complaints of fluctuating

Table 1. Distribution of results of visual field abnormalities of all patients whose initial visual field examinations were not performed to follow glaucoma or ocular hypertension. The result code is central field right eye, peripheral field right eye, central field left eye, peripheral field left where N = normal, A = abnormal, X = not examined. Note that abnormalities of the peripheral visual field are not predicted by the central field of that eye in the middle grouping. Detailed descriptions of the diagnostic categories are given in the text.

Diagnosis	N-Ophth symptoms	Optic neuritis	Vascular N'pathy	Orbital	Pituitary adenomas	Retinitis pigmentosa	Other Retina	Cornea, lens, etc.	Total
Result									
NNNN	26	2		1	11		1	4	45
XXNN + NNXX								1	1
NANA									
NANN + NNNA				1			1		2
NAXX + XXNA				1					1
AANA + NAAA									
ANNA + NAAN	1			1					2
AAAA	38	4	13	1	11	7	16	10	100
AANN + NNAA	10	5	2				1	1	19
AAAN + ANAA	5		1		1	2	2	1	12
ANAN	3	2	1		4		2		12
ANNN + NNAN	4	2		1	2		3	4	16
XXAA + AAXX	4	2	2		2		4	4	18
XXAN + ANXX					1				1
Totals	91	17	19	6	32	9	30	25	229

vision, migrainous scotomas, headaches, diplopia, cloudy vision and other symptoms and/or known intracranial tumors other than pituitary adenoma. Hereditary and unclassified optic atrophies were also in this group (Table 1). Twenty-six of these patients had completely normal fields. One patient had only peripheral abnormalities in one eye and central in the other. This patient was thought to be a false positive as the patient was diagnosed as having psychogenic complaints. Of the remaining (64) patients, no eye had PVF defects with an entirely normal central field. Abnormalities of both central and peripheral fields occurred in both eyes in 38 patients. In no case, would the presence of field defects have been missed, had the PVF not been performed. The PVF was considered important for topographic localization and/or management in two cases. One was a child with optic atrophy secondary to malnutrition, where a temporal island of vision was found in an eye without vision within the 30° CVF. In a patient with falx-meningioma and occipital lobe involvement, the sparing of a temporal crescent helped localize the lesion to the posterior portion of the calcarine fissure. In 16 cases the PVF was useful for ergo-ophthalmologic purposes, while in 27 cases where the PVF was abnormal it was not useful.

The patients characterized as having optic neuritis included those who were diagnosed as having multiple sclerosis. Seventeen patients were in this group and only two had normal fields (Table 1). None of the patients had abnormalities confined to the PVF, and in none of the cases was the PVF required for localization or management. In two cases the information from the PVF was considered useful for ergo-ophthalmologic purposes. In four cases, the PVF of both eyes was abnormal, but did not provide a basis for an ergo-ophthalmologic warning.

The category of vascular optic neuropathy includes cases of anterior ischemic optic neuropathy (AION) of both the arteritic and non-arteritic type as well as patients examined for low tension glaucoma (Table 1). There were 19 patients in this category of whom only two were judged on review to have peripheral visual fields which aided in the diagnosis of therapeutic management. In one case the CVF had only a small remaining island of vision and the PVF had a similar remaining island, indicating that the entire optic nerve was affected. The other case had a localized area of constriction in the temporal periphery not continuous with existing CVF defects which were nasal. In both cases the PVF showed the extent of damage. Four of these patients had positive and useful ergo-ophthalmologic examinations, while the PVF of 11 patients were abnormal which did not aid in the ergo-ophthalmologic evaluation.

There were six patients with orbital tumors, pseudotumors and proptosis (Table 1). Half of these patients had abnormal PVF results not predicted by an abnormal CVF in the affected eye. While the PVF detected a VF abnormality it did not detect the presence of disease, contribute to the localization or therapeutic management, nor contribute positive and useful ergo-ophthalmologic information.

There were 32 cases of pituitary adenomas (Table 1). Eleven patients had normal VF and 21 had at least one abnormal CVF with or without additional abnormality of the PVF. The PVF did not provide localizing or therapeutic information greater than that available from the CVF alone. In five cases useful and positive ergo-ophthalmologic data was obtained while in 8 cases the PVFs were abnormal, but not of ergo-ophthalmologic importance.

There were nine patients with retinitis pigmentosa (Table 1). In no case was the PVF critical for detection. In four cases the PVF gave useful topographic information. Three cases had unspecific CVF defects and a ring scotoma could be identified in the periphery only. In one case the PVF was useful in completing the demonstration of a ring scotoma that was partially demonstrated in the central field. In five cases where the PVF was abnormal it gave positive and useful ergo-ophthalmologic information whereas, in two cases an abnormal PVF did not provide a basis for warning the patient. Thus the PVF examination proved to be particularly useful in determining the extent of the lesion and the ergo-ophthalmologic status of patients with retinitis pigmentosa, and the PVF examination competes favourably with funduscopy and electroretinography in the evaluation of such patients.

Retinal disorders, other than retinitis pigmentosa and other related degenerations were present in 30 cases (Table 1). The presence of field defects could be detected only in the PVFs of a patient with ophthalmoscopically diagnosed retinoschisis. In one of this patient's eyes the PVF defect served as a basis for photocoagulation therapy and therefore influenced the management of the patient. Altogether, in five cases of the 30, PVF was useful for localization or management. One patient of these five had venous stasis retinopathy secondary to vasculitis and was initially thought to have disc shunt vessels of meningioma. Normal PVF helped rule out compressive neuropathy. In three of the five cases with diabetic retinopathy the PVF was useful in showing the extent of damage. The reasons for considering a PVF not useful was that it added nothing to the information obtained by ophthalmoscopy or that the changes found were nonspecific. In six of the 30 cases the PVF was judged useful in the ergo-ophthalmologic evaluation of the patients, whereas in 15 cases abnormal PVF were not of ergo-ophthalmologic significance.

In 25 patients there were miscellaneous ocular disorders, most of which involved the anterior segment (cornea and lens) with questions relating to the coexistence of neuro-ophthalmologic problems such as optic nerve disease, secondary glaucomas, or macular disorders (Table 1). In none of these patients was there a PVF abnormality in the absence of a CVF abnormality. In one patient with traumatic cataract the PVF was reviewed as useful in determining the topographic localization and therapeutic management because the only remaining vision was in the peripheral field. In seven cases the PVF was useful for ergo-ophthalmologic purposes whereas, in 8 cases an abnormal PVF was not of ergo-ophthalmologic significance.

Altogether, 29% of all eyes examined in this study had normal visual fields, 57% had abnormalities of both central and peripheral fields, 13% had normal peripheral fields with abnormal central, and in 1.6% of eyes there were field defects exclusively in the periphery. However, two patients in the last group had a central field abnormality in the opposite eye, and one of those two was thought to be a flase positive. For the other three patients (two cases of proptosis, one of retinoschisis – 1.3% of patients in the study), the PVF was useful in detecting the presence of visual field defects, but the presence of disease had already been detected by other means. For about 6% of patients the PVF was useful for localizing the lesion and/or changing the management of the case. Two-thirds of these cases had retinal problems. In 20% of all the patients in the study the PVF provided useful ergo-ophthalmologic information.

DISCUSSION

Weinstein and Fineberg (14) in their book, *Clinical Decision Analysis*, point out that a diagnostic test is introduced to resolve diagnostic, prognostic and therapeutic uncertainties to help in reaching a specified goal, such as the preservation of sight.

If there is a small probability that a given test e.g. PVF testing, in a given population will positively influence the outcome of management of the patient, and the PVFs are performed on all patients in that population — the incremental cost of the outcome (the cost of all PVFs performed divided by the number of valuable PVFs) will be very high.

With static threshold automated perimetry the PVF testing is time consuming and tiring for the patient. The number of examinations that can be performed is limited by the number of automated perimeters available, or the examining hours a day. Approximately twice as many patients could share the benefits of automated perimetry if only or mostly CVF examinations were done.

In this study we have reviewed a number of Goldmann manual kinetic fields in order to assess the circumstances under which information gained by examination of the visual field peripheral to 30° will be useful subsequent to the performance of central automated static perimetry. Prospective studies on a large number of patients are needed to determine the probabilities of obtaining useful PVFs in population with specific disorders. Our results confirm those of others (Blum, Suzuki), that the PVF is of little importance in detecting the presence of field defects. It is remarkable that two of three patients with exclusively PVF defects had orbital disease. It would be interesting to further investigate the probabilities of finding peripheral changes with a normal central field in conditions such as retinitis pigmentosa, drug toxicity, AION including normotensive glaucoma and mass compression of the optic nerve anterior to the chiasm and at the optic nerve-chiasmal junction.

For localization of the lesion and for management of the case, our results indicate that the value of PVF is limited. The usefulness in most cases was to show the extent of damage in retinal or optic nerve disease. In no case could we prove that the information from the peripheral field helped change the visual outcome.

The examination of the PVF appeared to be particularly relevant to the assessment of visual disability. We are aware that conventional visual fields do not provide the best information for evaluating the patient's visual ability to function in daily life (12). Nevertheless, decisions concerning, for example,

204

the patient's ability to drive a car often have to be based on that information. In those paitents with complete homonymous hemianopia of the CVF we automatically evaluated the PVF as useful for ergo-ophthalmologic purposes, but it would be interesting to discover how often the contralateral peripheral hemifields are abnormal or the ipsilateral peripheral hemifields retain some function.

Weinstein and Fineberg note that a test can be considered valuable even if it does not improve the clinical outcome. Improvement of disability assessment and/or resource utilization are other favourable effects of the additional information it provides. Even if the test results do not perform these functions, the physician may elect to perform the test anyway because it provides improved detection of disease, localization of the lesion, prognostic information and/or research information. The information might be satisfying to the physician in terms of the clinical reasoning or the ability to communicate with the patient concerning the condition.

If the data in this study can be extrapolated to automated static perimetry there will be a very great incremental cost for any clinically useful information obtained from the examination of the PVF. It is therefore proposed that the PVF be examined (1) whenever indicated for ergo-ophthalmologic reasons, or (2) when the CVF examination does not resolve a clinical problem for which there is a reasonably high probability that (a) additional clinically useful information will be obtained by examination of the PVF after the results of the CVF examination have been analyzed, or (b) the eye is likely to have a condition that can be detected or followed best by PVF examination.

REFERENCES

1. Blum, F.G., Jr., Gates, K. and James, B.R. How important are peripheral fields? Arch. Ophthalmol. 61: 1–8 (1959).
2. Chamlin, M. Visual field changes in optic neuritis. Arch. Ophthalmol. 50: 699–713 (1953).
3. Chamlin, M. Visual field defects due to optic nerve compression by mass lesions. Arch. Ophthalmol. 58: 37–58 (1957).
4. Deutman, A.F. Rod-cone dystrophy: Primary, hereditary, pigmentary retinopathy, retinitis pigmentosa. In: Archer D (ed.): Krill's Hereditary Retinal and Choroidal Diseases. Vol 2. Clinical Characteristics. Hagerstown, Harper & Row (1977), pp. 511–512.
5. Drance, S.M. Earliest visual field disturbances in glaucoma. In: Krieglstein GK, Leydhecker, W. (ed). Glaucoma Update: International Glaucoma Symposium, 1978. Berlin, Springer-Verlag (1979), pp. 61–64.
6. Harrington, D.O. The visual fields: A textbook and atlas of clinical perimetry. 4th ed. St. Louis, Mosby (1976), pp. 225–230.
7. Hart, W.M. Yablonski, M., Kass, M.A. and Becker, B. Quantitative visual field and optic disc correlates early in glaucoma. Arch. Ophthalmol. 96: 2209–2211 (1978).
8. LeBlanc, R.P. and Becker, B. Peripheral nasal field defects. Am. J. Ophthalmol. 72: 415–419 (1971).
9. Ogawa, T. and Suzuki, R. Relation between central and peripheral visual field changes with kinetic perimetry. Doc. Ophthalmol. Proc. Ser. 19: 469–474 (1979).
10. Phelps, C.D., Hayreh, S.S. and Montague, P.R. Visual fields in low-tension glaucoma, primary open angle glaucoma, and anterior ischemic optic neuropathy. Doc. Ophthalmol. Proc. Ser. 35: 113–124 (1983).

11. Sloan, L.L. and Woods, A.C. Perimetric studies in syphilitic optic neuropathies. Arch. Ophthalmol. 20: 201–253 (1938).
12. Verriest, G., Barca, L., Dubois-Poulsen, A., Houtmans, M.J.M., Inditsky, B., Johnson, C., Overington, I., Ronchi, L. and Villani, S. The occupational visual field: I. Theoretical aspects: The normal functional visual field. Doc. Ophthalmol. Proc. Ser. 35: 165–185 (1983).
13. Walsh, F.B. Syphilis of the optic nerve. Trans. Am. Acad. Ophthalmol. Otlaryngol 60: 39–42 (1956).
14. Weinstein, M.C. and Fineberg, H.V. Clinical Decision Analysis. Philadelphia, Saunders (1980), pp. 298–303.

Authors address:
Department of Ophthalmology,
University of Minnesota,
Minneapolis, MN,
USA.

USEFULNESS OF PERIPHERAL TESTING IN AUTOMATED SCREENING PERIMETRY

RICHARD P. MILLS, M.D.

(*Seattle, Washington, U.S.A.*)

ABSTRACT

Peripheral field exploration consumed 40% of testing time during a study involving the Fieldmaster 200 and Dicon AP2000 perimeters used in a screening mode. In 3% of eyes found abnormal by reference quantitative Goldmann perimetry, the peripheral field detected an abnormality which the central field had missed. In 10% of cases, a diagnostic characterization was made possible or improved in quality by the peripheral visual field. In an additional 52% of cases, the peripheral field confirmed an abnormality detected on central field testing, and enhanced confidence of the validity of the central field data. Strategies for screening fields should thus de-emphasize, but not ignore, the peripheral visual field.

INTRODUCTION

I recently reported the results of a study comparing the Dicon AP2000, Fieldmaster 200, and Goldmann perimeters used in a screening mode (4). There were no significant differences in the abilities of these devices to fulfill reasonable objectives of screening: detection of abnormal fields at rates over 90% and false alarms in normal fields at rates below 10%.

Peripheral field testing consumed 40% of the testing time at the two automated perimeters using the screening strategy to be described. Whether peripheral testing generated sufficient useful information to warrant this large time expenditure was investigated and forms the basis for this report.

METHODS

The simple test strategy used at the three screening perimeters was selected because it was available as standard equipment on the automated devices, and a similar manual method had been previously validated (5, 6). On each device, a single intensity stimulus was used for testing the central field and a second stimulus one log unit stronger was used for the peripheral field. At the

Heijl, A. and Greve, E.L. (eds.), Proceedings of the 6th Int. Visual Field Symposium.
© *1985, Dr W. Junk Publishers, Dordrecht, The Netherlands. ISBN 978-94-010-8932-6*

Fieldmaster 200, 82 central and 57 peripheral spots were tested (total 139), while at the Dicon 2000, 70 central and 74 peripheral locations were tested (total 144).

The central stimulus was chosen related to a single point threshold determination at 25 degrees eccentricity temporal to the blind spot. If the threshold seemed unusually high, an alternate point was selected at the same eccentricity inferiorly. The threshold determinations were made independently at each perimeter, and the central testing was done with a stimulus no stronger than 0.5 log units above the threshold determination. The screening fields were compared to a multiple isopter quantitative field done at the Goldmann perimeter.

Criteria for classification of a field as 'normal' or 'abnormal' were those used by Kelter and Johnson (2, 3): (1) marked contraction of a major portion of the visual field, (2) two or more adjacent locations missed with a single stimulus intensity, surrounded by locations which were detected, and (3) a single location missed at both intensity levels tested (in this study only the 30 degree eccentricity was tested at two intensities). All fields on each patient were completed in a single test session of about one hour. An appropriate corrective lens was provided for testing in the central 30 degrees and all missed stimuli were retested before recording a 'miss'.

RESULTS

Patients were selected from a general eye clinic population on the sole basis that the examining ophthalmologist felt a field defect was likely to be present. 123 eyes of 122 patients were enrolled in the study. Only 4 patients could not complete testing due to fatigue or language barrier. Ages ranged from 8 to 84 years with a median of 45 years. 33 eyes were classified as normal and 86 eyes abnormal on the basis of the reference quantitative field. Approximately 1/3 (28) of the abnormal fields were due to glaucoma, 1/3 (28) to other optic neuropathy, and 1/3 (30) were caused by either intracranial or retinal disease. Similarly, 1/3 (27) of the field defects were subtle, with only small, shallow scotomas. 1/3 (32) were classified as mild, with denser scotomas appearing in only one quadrant of the field, or involving generalized nonspecific constriction. 1/3 (27) were severe, with dense scotomas involving more than one visual field quadrant.

Among the normal fields, 7% were incorrectly classified as abnormal on the basis of the automated screening charts. Of these 5 false alarms, 4 occurred because of abnormality in central field testing, but only one occurred because of peripheral field results. In that case two adjacent missed spots at 30 and 40 degrees eccentricity were surrounded by locations which were seen. Neither Fieldmaster nor Goldmann fields on this patient confirmed this aberrant finding.

Among the 86 abnormal eyes, 92% were detected using this simple screening strategy at the automated perimeters (172 fields). In only 3% of these eyes, the peripheral field was *solely* responsible for detecting the abnormality. That is, since the screening central field was normal, the abnormal peripheral field was the reason the field was classified as abnormal. This occurred in 2 cases of optic atrophy, 1 case of retinal disease, and one case of glaucoma with a temporal wedge defect. Thus, from the limited standpoint of screening alone, the peripheral field data was necessary only 3% of the time.

However, considerable information is contained on screening visual field charts beyond that required to determine normality or abnormality. Physicians use that additional information to make a diagnostic characterization of the defect found by screening. Because those characterizations are subjective, they are difficult to quantify. Accordingly, the automated fields from this study were divided into broad categories, as follows:

Group I.   Field charts with good defect characterization allowing diagnosis without further visual field testing.

Group II. Field charts with fair defect characterization indicating a probable diagnosis, but further visual field testing was necessary to be sure.

Group III. Field charts were uncertain defect characterization, requiring further testing for diagnosis.

Group IV. Field charts on which the defect was missed entirely.

Analysis was then made of the frequency with which peripheral test data improved the defect characterization which had been made with the central field data alone. In 10% of the automated fields, an improvement of at least one classification was achieved by peripheral field test results. Predictably, this improvement in classification occurred less frequently among defects which were subtle and among defects caused by optic neuropathies other than glaucoma, which often spared the peripheral field.

Finally, analysis was made of the frequency with which peripheral test data confirmed the defect characterization suggested by the central field data. Such confirmation tends to make the physician more confident of his diagnostic interpretation, since the defect has been demonstrated twice. This occurred in 52% of the automated fields, though much less frequently in the subtle defects. Stated differently, in 35% of the cases, the peripheral field was normal, and was of no assistance whatever in diagnostic characterization (Table 1).

DISCUSSION

The capability of testing the central and peripheral visual field separately at different intensity levels is available on most inexpensive automated perimeters as standard equipment. With the addition of a manually determined threshold at one or two points, a simple and rapid threshold-related screening is easily performed.

Used on a population of patients thought to represent a typical mixture of

Table 1. Proportion of peripheral visual field charts (n = 172) fulfilling various criteria of usefulness.

Criterion of usefulness	Percent of peripheral fields
Detection of abnormality missed on central test	3%
Improvement of diagnostic characterization made by central test	10%
Confirmation of central field diagnostic characterization	52%
No value in screening or diagnostic characterization	35%

field defects likely to be discovered in a general ophthalmic practice, the strategy detected over 90% of defects while suffering a false-positive rate of under 10%.

A multiple-isopter quantitative field done at the Goldmann perimeter was selected as a standard against which to measure the automated screening fields. Because of the known difficulties of judging static visual fields against a kinetic standard (1), no attempt was made to correlate scotoma size or depth discovered with the various instruments. Some of the 'false positives' discovered by the automated units may well have been truly abnormal, had manual threshold static perimetry been done on all patients. However, the performance of the automated perimeters relative to each other and the usefulness of central vs. peripheral field data should not have been materially affected by the use of a kinetic standard.

40% of the time in visual field screening with the automated perimeters was spent exploring the peripheral field. Yet in only 3% of cases was the peripheral field information crucial in determining that a field was in fact, abnormal. In the remainder, central field information alone was sufficient to make this determination. One might conclude on that basis that peripheral testing is not necessary for screening.

The theoretical division of visual field tasks into screening, diagnosis, and quantitation is useful to understand how visual field strategies should be designed. However, users of perimeters are not willing to accept a device which provides no information beyond assignment of a field into a normal or abnormal category. Diagnostically useful data, at least, and preferably some quantitative information on abnormal fields should be available upon completion of any visual field examination. To accomplishing this requires that a device be sufficiently interactive in its software to make the transitions in tasks from screening to diagnostic characterization to quantitative exploration (as good perimetrists always do).

Even with simple, non-interactive strategies such as the one selected for this study, some diagnostically useful information can be recovered. The peripheral visual field improved the diagnostic characterizations provided by the central field in 10% of cases, and confirmed central field characterizations in 52%. In only 35% was the peripheral field information of no measurable value.

Exploration of the peripheral field as part of enhanced screening strategies is therefore viewed as important because of its utility in enhancing or confirming diagnostic suspicions generated by central field data. The optimal ratio of central to peripheral test loci is not known. It is probably excessive to commit 40% of testing time to the peripheral field, as was the case for the automated strategies in this study, and fewer points could have been tested without significantly affecting the diagnostic assistance provided by the peripheral field. Designers of strategies for automated screening perimetry should thus de-emphasize, but not ignore, the peripheral field.

REFERENCES

1. Heijl, A. and Drance, S.M. A clinical comparison of three computerized automatic perimeters in the detection of glaucoma defects. Arch. Ophthalmol. 99: 832–6 (1981).
2. Johnson, C.A. and Keltner, J.L. Automated suprathreshold static perimetry. Am. J. Ophthalmol. 89: 731–741 (1980).
3. Keltner, J.L., Johnson, C.A., and Balestrery, F.G. Suprathreshold static perimetry – initial clinical trials with the Fieldmaster automated perimeter. Arch. Ophthalmol. 97: 260–72 (1979).
4. Mills, R.P. A comparison of Goldmann, Fieldmaster 200, and Dicon AP2000 perimeters used in a screening mode. Ophthalmology 91 (in press) (1984).
5. Rock, W.J., Drance, S.M., and Morgan, R.W. A modification of the Armaly visual field screening technique for glaucoma. Can. J. Ophthalmol. 6: 283–92 (1971).
6. Trobe, J.D., Acosta, P.C., Shuster, J.J., and Krischer, J.P. An evaluation of the accuracy of community-based perimetry. Am. J. Ophthalmol. 90: 654–60 (1980).

Author's address:
Richard P. Mills, M.D.
Department of Ophthalmology,
University of Washington RJ-10,
Seattle, Washington 98195, U.S.A.

VER-ANALYSIS WITH SIMULTANEOUS HEMIFIELD STIMULATION OF TRANSIENT POTENTIALS

F. DANNHEIM and W. WESEMANN

(*Hamburg, W. Germany*)

ABSTRACT

Simultaneous stimulation of transient cortical potentials by checkerboard reversal of both hemifields is comparable to successive stimulation. Even mild hemiopic visual field impairment by lesions of the central visual pathways correspond to significant deformations of potentials for the affected hemifield. Advantages are a real comparability of the two hemifields, since both are equally affected by the noise in the EEG, and a reduction in the duration of the test by a factor of about two.

INTRODUCTION

Cortical responses for the temporal or nasal half of the visual field in neuro-ophthalmology are usually recorded by successive stimulation of each hemifield (2). A disadvantage is the long duration of the test. The response of each hemifield might furthermore be differently affected by interfering factors in the EEG. A simultaneous stimulation of steady state potentials in the four quadrants of the visual field applying a Fast Fourier Analysis (1) showed some improvement in this respect. The temporal characteristics of the cortical response, however, appeared more valuable than just the amplitude.

The following describes a new method for the simultaneous hemifield stimulation of transient cortical responses.

METHOD

A television checkerboard pattern is computer generated using an Imaging Technology picture processing system IP-512 controlled by a Z80 micro-computer (Fig. 1). The right and left hemifield of the pattern can be inverted independently. A vertical, 0.5° wide black bar separates the two fields and excludes interfering effects from small eye movements. Cortical responses are recorded bipolar median.

Heijl, A. and Greve, E.L. (eds.), Proceedings of the 6th Int. Visual Field Symposium.
© *1985, Dr W. Junk Publishers, Dordrecht, The Netherlands. ISBN 978-94-010-8932-6*

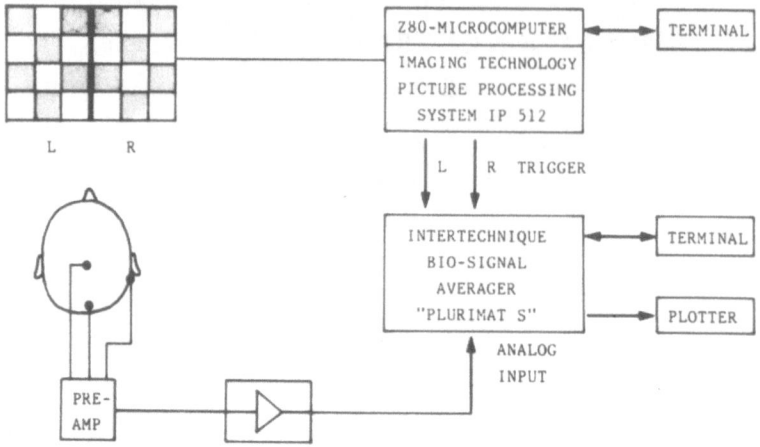

Fig. 1. Experimental setup.

The sequence of the VER measurement is shown in Fig. 2. After the start the microprocessor
- changes the pattern in the right hemifield,
- sends a trigger pulse to the signal averager 'plurimat S' to indicate that the first sweep in the right field has started and
- sets an internal counter-timer to 250 ms followed by a random time delay of 250 to 350 ms.

The signal averager samples the VER response for the right hemifield in a 500 ms sweep. When the total delay has passed, the picture processor inverts the pattern in the left field and triggers the averager to start sampling the response for the left field. A 30 Hz digital filter is applied to the accumulated 100 responses, providing smooth, reproducible curves.

The main feature of this recording technique is the pattern reversal taking place in one hemifield, while the rhythmic after-discharge from the other hemifield is still going on. Thus the overall pattern reversal frequency lies close to 4 Hz, even though the frequency in each hemifield is 2 Hz, as in conventional set-ups. This allows simultaneous separate measurements in both hemifields in the time necessary for a single field. A random time delay prevents interference of signal correlated responses in the after-discharge of

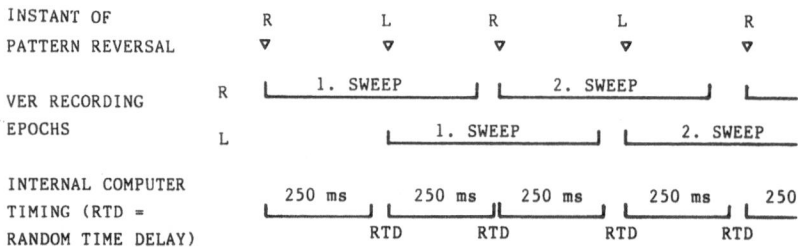

Fig. 2. Timing diagram.

214

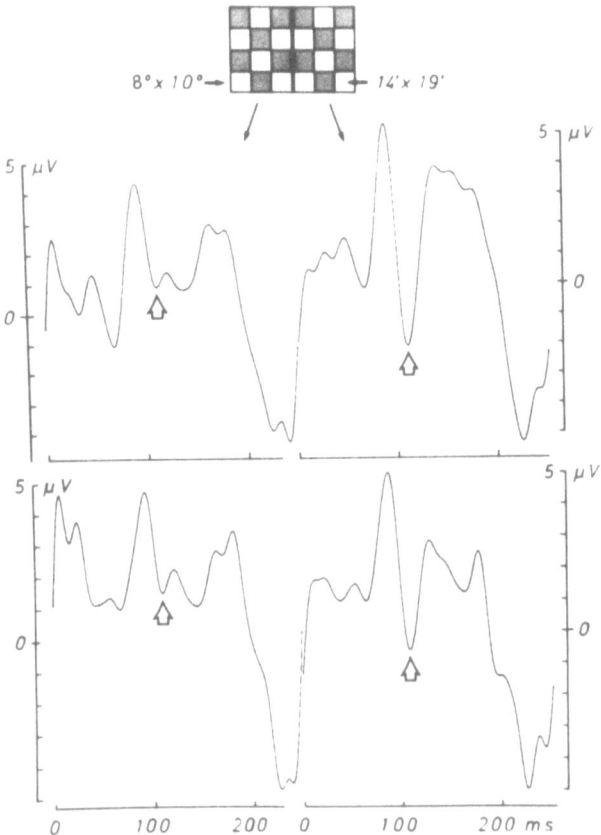

Fig. 3. Two consecutive VER records in a health subject, both hemifields simultaneously stimulated. P 100 latency in the normal range (arrow).

one hemifield with the response of the other hemifield within the first, most important, 200 ms. These after-discharges are added up in random phase and are thus extinguished by the averaging process.

CLINICAL RESULTS

The described method has been applied to a group of healthy subjects and to patients suffering from lesions of the central visual pathways. The average normal response resembles the one found with the usual successive stimulation (Fig. 3).

If the television screen shows the alternating pattern only in one hemifield, potentials are obtained for this hemifield alone, whereas the other hemifield produces no proper response (Fig. 4). This illustrates the independency of

215

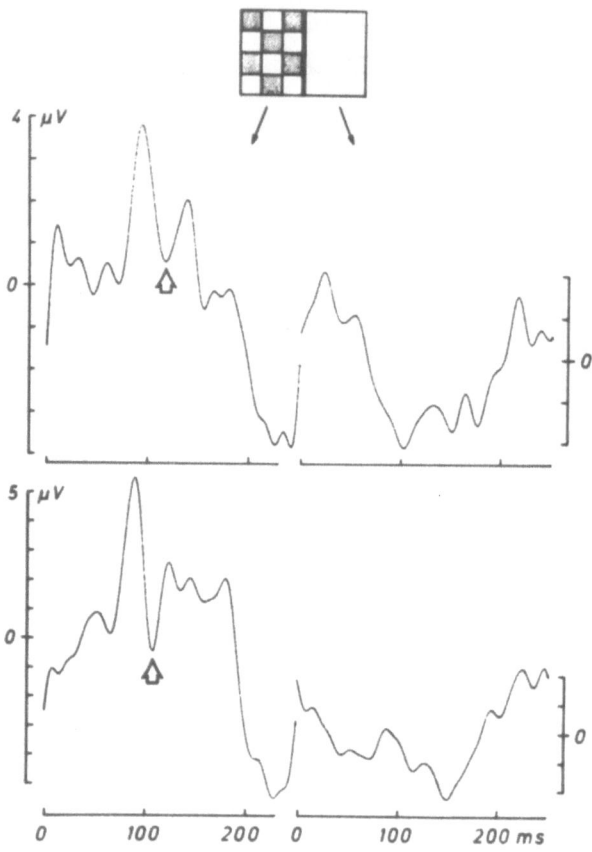

Fig. 4. Same eye as in Fig. 3, stimulation of left hemifield only. No proper response in record of unstimulated hemifield.

the two hemifields. In cases with chiasmal compression the mild hemiopic reduction of sensitivity corresponds well with a marked deformation of potentials only for the affected hemifield (Fig. 5).

The limitations of the described method, especially in elderly, less cooperative patients, are obviously similar to those of the classical successive VER technique. The shorter test duration, however, is valuable in this respect.

ACKNOWLEDGEMENTS

We are indebted to Mrs. K. Bieganowski who carried out the experiments for this study in preparation of her thesis. The technical setup was supported in part by a Grant of the DFG.

216

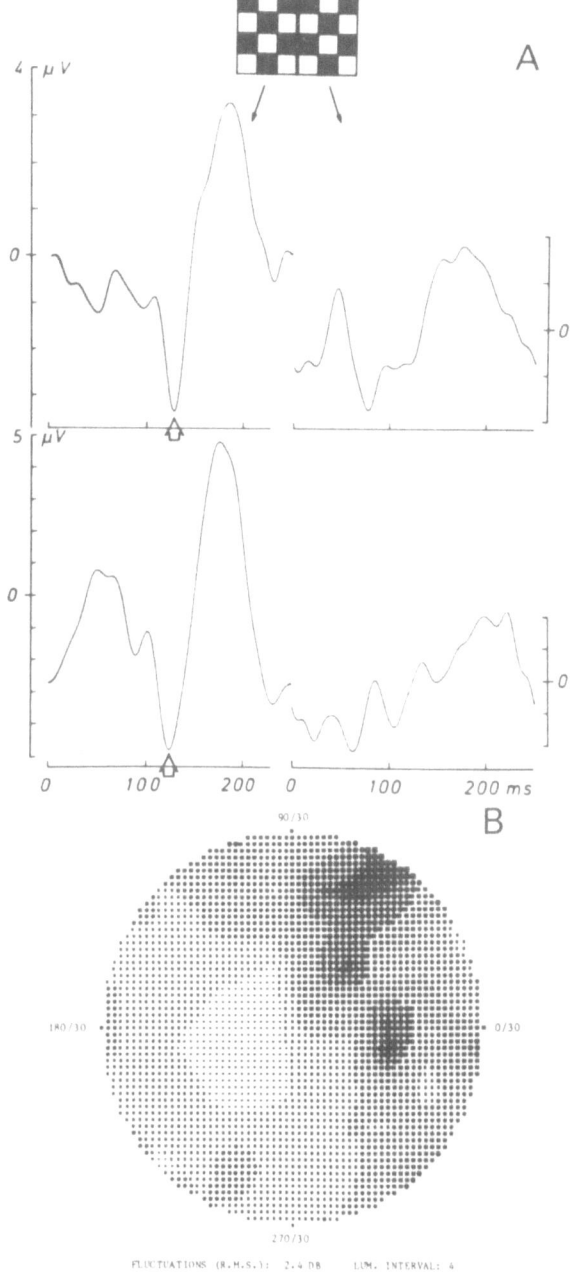

Fig. 5. 40 year old male with chiasmal lesion and bitemporal field defects, right eye demonstrated. A) 2 VER records, simultaneous hemifield stimulation: Marked deformation for temporal hemifield corresponds to depression of sensitivity in the temporal visual field in the Octopus program 32 printout.

217

REFERENCES

1. Dannheim, F. and Wesemann, W. Visuell evozierte Potentiale in der perimetrischen Diagnostik chiasmanaher Sehbahnläsionen. Bücherei des Augenarztes, Enke Verlag (in print).
2. Wildberger, H.G.H., Van Lith, G.H.M., Wijngaarde, R. and Mak, G.T.M. Visually evoked cortical potentials in the evaluation of homonymous and bitemporal visual field defects. Brit. J. Ophthal. 60: 273–278 (1976).

Authors address:
Priv.-Doz. Dr. F. Dannheim,
Universitäts-Augenklinik,
Martinistrasse 52,
2000 Hamburg 20,
West Germany

VISION CHANGES IN PARKINSON'S DISEASE: ELECTROPHYSIOLOGICAL AND PERIMETRIC FINDINGS

G. CALABRIA, E. GANDOLFO, C. BURTOLO, A. ONETO and N. PIZIO

(*Genoa, Italy*)

ABSTRACT

It has been demonstrated that in Parkinson's disease VEP latency is frequently abnormal. The aim of this paper is to evaluate the possible existence of visual correlate to VEP changes in Parkinsonians. Therefore in the same group of patients VEP have been compared with the results of automated perimetry (Perikon and Peritest) and chromatic sense analysis (Farnsworth 100 Hue Test). Preliminary results indicate that the considered parameters are correlated. To establish if the visual changes are specific, the results obtained in the Parkinsonians are compared to those of a matched control group.

INTRODUCTION

It has been recently demonstrated that in Parkinson's disease visual evoked potential (VEPs) are frequently characterized by a pathological increase in the latency of their main positive peak (1, 6).

However, data are lacking on whether such a pathological change is correlated to clinically detectable visual impairment. The aim of this paper is to evaluate the possible existence of visual correlate to VEP changes in Parkinson's disease. Specifically, visual field (V.F.) abnormalities and chromatic sense alterations have been searched for, since it was shown that careful examination of such parameters may be as useful as the assessment of VEPs in identifying the presence of damage in the visual system, at least in multiple sclerosis (2).

MATERIALS AND METHODS

24 paitents, 14 men and 10 women, ranging in age from 42 to 72 (mean: 59.4; S.D. = 8.9) were studied. Duration of illness ranged from 6 months to 24 years (mean: 7.9; S.D. = 7.0). All patients were on medication with variable combination of L.DOPA, DOPA decarboxylase inhibitors, anticholinergic drugs and bromocriptine; none of them presented on-off

Heijl, A. and Greve, E.L. (eds.), Proceedings of the 6th Int. Visual Field Symposium.
© *1985, Dr W. Junk Publishers, Dordrecht, The Netherlands. ISBN 978-94-010-8932-6*

phenomena. The symptom severity rated from Score 1 to 3 of the Hoehn and Yahr scale (5). The control group consisted of 22 subjects, 13 men and 9 women, ranging in age from 49 to 72 years (mean: 60.8; S.D. = 7.7) suffering from neurological illness not involving the visual system. Both Parkinsonians and control subjects had no evident ocular disorders and only the eyes with visual acuity of not less than 0.8 were examined.

Patterns were generated by a standard system (MPS LACE 01) on a TV screen. We employed 2 different stimuli: (a) a checkerboard subtending $10°$ of visual angle with simple checks of $55'$ aperture at a distance of 171 cm from the eye; (b) a grating with sinusoidal luminance profile subtending $4°$ of visual angle at the same distance and with spatial frequency of $2 c/°$. In both cases the dark elements presented a luminance of 0.6 cd/mq and the light ones 30 cd/mq. VEPs were evoked by pattern reversal at a temporal frequency of 2 reversals per sec. The latency of the evoked potentials was measured as the time from the onset of the pattern reversal to the peak of the major positive component at the occipital electrode (4).

The ophthalmological examination consisted of a complete check-up followed by perimetric and colour tests.

1. Perimetry

The patients underwent standard kinetic perimetry and static perimetry along the horizontal meridian carried out by means of the Automatic Goldmann Perimeter Perikon (7); the V.F. examination was concluded by an automatic supraliminar test performed by Peritest (3).

2. Chromatic sense

All subjects were examined with the Farnsworth 100 Hue Test. The following criteria of results evaluation were adopted:

VEP: the evoked responses underwent a statistical analysis in order to be classified as normal or pathological. Following the 'one-tailed' criterium, the latency values significantly pathological were:

checkerboard: p 0.05 = latency = 118 msec.
checkerboard: p 0.01 = latency = 123 msec.
grating   : p 0.05 = latency = 121 msec.
grating   : p 0.01 = latency = 126 msec.

Perikon Perimetry: the kinetic results were evaluated by means of a clinical criterium based on the isopters' width; the static results were considered normal when the threshold luminance at the fixation point was less than 10 asb for the stimulus I ($1/4$ mm^2), and the sensitivity profile had the characteristic gradient.

Peritest Perimetry: and individual threshold of 0.4 L.U. or less was considered normal. The absence of scotomata in the whole V.F. was necessary to classify the results as normal.

Chromatic Sense: the Farnsworth 100 Hue Test results were classified as normal or pathological on the basis of normal clinical criteria.

Table 1. Obtained results in Parkinson's group and in control group.

SUBJECTS	TYPE OF THE RESPONSE	VISUAL EVOKED POTENTIALS (latency)		VISUAL FIELD (PERIKON)		VISUAL FIELD (PERITEST)		CHROMATIC SENSE (Farnsworth 100 hue test)
		checkerboard	grating	static perimetry	kinetic perimetry	individual threshold	static perimetry	
PARKINSON GROUP (24 pts, 46 eyes)	eyes with normal responses	40 (87%)	22 (48%)	22 (48%)	25 (54%)	26 (57%)	18 (39%)	10 (22%)
	eyes with pathological responses	6 (13%)	24 (52%)	24 (52%)	21 (46%)	20 (43%)	28 (61%)	36 (78%)
CONTROL GROUP (22 pts, 44 eyes)	eyes with normal responses	41 (93%)	35 (80%)	28 (64%)	32 (73%)	34 (77%)	32 (73%)	28 (64%)
	eyes with pathological responses	3 (7%)	9 (20%)	16 (36%)	12 (27%)	10 (23%)	12 (27%)	16 (36%)

Table 2. Statistical analysis performed on visual evoked responses.

	PARKINSON GROUP	CONTROL GROUP
CHECKERBOARD $p < 0.05$ = latency $\geq$ 118 msec $p < 0.01$ = latency $\geq$ 123 msec	112.15 ± 6.86 msec	107.97 ± 6.05 msec
GRATING $p < 0.05$ = latency $\geq$ 121 msec $p < 0.01$ = latency $\geq$ 126 msec	123.22 ± 11.44 msec	110.40 ± 6.63 msec

RESULTS

Table 1 shows the obtained results.

VEP

The VEP latency was pathologically increased in the 52% of the Parkinsonians, but the statistical analysis of the data demonstrated that only responses evoked by grating stimuli were significantly altered (see Table 2).

Visual field

The tests performed by Perikon unit showed a high percentage of pathological results both in static (52%) and kinetic (46%) perimetry. In the first case the alterations were characterized by an elevation of central threshold values (mean = 12.5 asb) and by a certain flattening of the senstivity profile in the paracentral V.F. In kinetic results we often noted an irregular concentrical isopteric constriction.

The Peritest results indicated a frequent (43%) threshold alteration

221

(mean = 0.6 L.U.) and the presence of paracentral scotomata of different width and depth (61%).

Chromatic sense

The Farnsworth 100 Hue Test showed almost always (78%) pathological results in Parkinsonians. The alteration was often relevant and of a global type, without preferential axis.

COMMENT

The results of our study have confirmed the increase in VEP latency already demonstrated by several researchers in Parkinsonians. The accurate V.F. and chromatic sense examinations performed indicated that the electro-physiological findings correlated to well defined visual disturbances. The frequence of V.F. defects or colour discrimination abnormalities still seemed higher than VEP alteration. The comparison with a control group has shown that the detected pathological alterations were really present and not due to normal visual function decay linked to age. The large number of examined cases and the consistency of results were other factors in favour of our conclusions. To establish the origin of such visual disorders appeared more difficult, even if a complex alteration involving both photoreceptors and optic nerve fibers seemed to be present. Ulterior studies will be necessary in order to acquire more complete knowledge about visual system disorders connected to Parkinson's disease.

REFERENCES

1. Bodis-Wollner, I. and Yahr, M.D. Measurements of visual evoked potentials in Parkinson's disease. Brain. 101: 661–671 (1978).
2. Dalen, J.T.W. and Spekreijse, H. Comparison of visual field examination and visual evoked potentials in multiple sclerosis patients. Doc. Ophthalmol. Proc. 27: 139–147 (1981).
3. Greve, E.L. and Dannheim, F. The Peritest, a new automatic and semi-automatic perimeter. Int. Ophthalmol. 5: 201 (1982).
4. Halliday, A.M., McDonald, W.I. and Mushin, J. Visual evoked responses in the diagnosis of multiple sclerosis. Br. Med. J. 4: 661–664 (1973).
5. Hoehn, M.M. and Yahr, M.D. Parkinsonism: onset, progression and mortality. Neurology (Minneapolis) 17: 427–442 (1967).
6. Tartaglione, A., Pizio, N., Bino, G., Spadavecchia, L. and Favale, E. VEP changes in Parkinson's disease are stimulus dependent. J. Neurol. Neurosurg. Psychiatry 47: 305–307 (1984).
7. Zingirian, M., Gandolfo, E. and Orciuolo, M. Automation of the Goldmann perimeter. Doc. Ophthalmol. Proc. 35: 381–385 (1983).

Author's address:
Prof. G. Calabria,
Department of Ophthalmology,
University of Genova,
Viale Benedetto XV,
no 5, 16132 Genova,
Italy.

PUPILLARY SIGNS IN RETINAL AND OPTIC NERVE DISEASE

H. STANLEY THOMPSON
(Iowa City, USA)

ABSTRACT

Pupillary signs can be fit into the diagnostic puzzle of retinal and optic nerve disease if the relative afferent pupillary defect (RAPD) is first quantified. This can be done with neutral density filters (6). Using this technique, certain clinical rules of thumb have emerged.

Optic neuritis. More than 90% of patients with an optic neuritis (past or present) — have a RAPD. If a patient with a 'unilateral' optic neuritis does *not* have a RAPD, then bilateral disease should be suspected. A *fresh* optic neuritis may have a RAPD of almost any size — from 0.3 to 3 whole log units — it just depends on how much damage has been done to the nerve, and how many fibers have stopped conducting. The mean RAPD in fresh cases of optic neuritis is 1.7 log units, but the variance is large (2). On the other hand, the mean RAPD in an old 'recovered' optic neuritis is 1.0 log units, and very few have a RAPD greater than 1.5 log units or smaller than 0.5 log units (Cox, ibid.).

Amblyopia. You should *expect* a small RAPD in an amblyopic eye. It is not always there, but, if you look carefully, you will see a RAPD in more than half of the cases. The pupil defect in the amblyopic eye is generally less than 0.5 log units. If, in an amblyopic eye, you see a RAPD between 0.5 and 1.0 log units, this should be considered suspiciously large, and only reluctantly accepted as due to the amblyopia. If the RAPD is more than 1.0 log unit, don't blame it on the amblyopia. Look for some other cause. The size of the RAPD does not correlate well with the acuity of the amblyopic eye (5).

Macular disease. In pure macular disease (e.g., disciform) there *is* a rough correlation between the RAPD and the visual acuity. This is because — in the macula — both of these functions (pupil and acuity) are related to the size of the macular lesion and the size of the central scotoma. The one relationship in all of this that seems to hold good for any part of the retina is that the pupil loss is proportional to the size of the field loss (7). If the visual acuity

Heijl, A. and Greve, E.L. (eds.), Proceedings of the 6th Int. Visual Field Symposium.
© *1985, Dr W. Junk Publishers, Dordrecht, The Netherlands. ISBN 978-94-010-8932-6*

is no worse than 20/200 don't expect a RAPD any bigger than 0.5 log units. It is hard to get a RAPD larger than 1.0 log unit with a lesion confined to the macula. When unilateral macular disease causes a RAPD of 1.2 log units, the central scotoma is generally large enough to include the blind spot.

Central serous retinopathy. The RAPD is very small in CSR – as would be expected in a macular disease producing very little field loss. Initially there may be as much as 0.3 log units of RAPD, but when the subretinal fluid disappears, so usually does the pupil defect (4).

Retinal detachment. One quadrant of fresh retinal detachment (with the macula on) produces approximately 0.3 log units of RAPD, and 2 quadrants produces 0.6, etc. (3). As you might expect, when the macula comes off, the RAPD jumps up by about 0.9 log units (1). Thus a fresh, complete retinal detachment would be expected to have a RAPD of more than 2.0 log units.

Cataracts. If an eye with a cataract has a RAPD, don't blame the RAPD on the cataract – no matter how brunescent the lens. There seems to be something about a cataract which boosts the overall sensitivity of the retina – or, at least, the light responsiveness of the pupils. In unilateral cataract this may produce a small RAPD in the *other* eye. The prognosis for aphakic acuity is not *necessarily* poor in the presence of a pre-operative RAPD – an AION or glaucoma may cause loss of field and a RAPD, but spare the central acuity.

Anisocoria. More light gets through the bigger pupil producing a real RAPD in the eye with the smaller pupil. Generally this is not clinically significant until the anisocoria in bright light is greater than 2.0 mm. When one pupil is fixed, then figure on 0.1 log unit of RAPD in the eye with the smaller pupil for every millimeter of anisocoria in bright light.

Functional visual loss. Functional visual loss does *not* produce a RAPD. If an eye with functional visual loss shows a RAPD, then something else is going on in addition to the function visual loss.

REFERENCES

1. Bovino, J.A. and Burton, T.C. Measurement of the RAPD in retinal detachment. Am. J. Ophthalmol. 90: 19–21 (1980).
2. Cox, T.A., Thompson, H.S. and Corbett, J.J. Relative afferent pupillary defects in optic neuritis. Am. J. Ophthalmol. 92: 685–690 (1981).
3. Fineberg, E. and Thompson, H.S. Quantitation of the Afferent Pupillary Defect. N-0 Update, Smith, J.L. (Ed.), Masson and Cie, N.Y., pp. 25–29 (1980).
4. Folk, J.C., Thompson, H.S., Han, D. and Brown, C.K. Central serous retinopathy. Arch. Ophthalmol., in press (1984).
5. Portnoy, J.Z., Thompson, H.S., Lennarson, L. and Corbett, J.J. Pupillary defects in amblyopia. Am. J. Ophthalmol. 96: 609–614 (1983).
6. Thompson, H.S., Corbett, J.J. and Cox, T.A. How to measure the relative afferent pupillary defect. Surv. Ophthalmol. 26: 39–42 (1981).

7. Thompson, H.S., Montague, P., Cox, T.A. and Corbett, J.J. The relationship between visual acuity, pupillary defect, and visual field loss. Am. J. Ophthalmol. 93: 681–688 (1982).

Author's address:
H. Stanley Thompson, M.D.
Department of Ophthalmology
University of Iowa
Iowa City, Iowa
52242, U.S.A.

IMPORTANCE OF VISUAL FIELD TESTS OF PATIENTS WITH PITUITARY ADENOMA DURING PREGNANCY AND POST-PARTUM LACTATION

YOSHIHITO HONDA and AKIRA TAKAHASHI

(*Kyoto, Japan*)

ABSTRACT

Visual fields of 20 patients with radiological evidence of pituitary adenoma were measured monthly or bimonthly by Goldmann perimeter during pregnancy and post-pregnancy lactation period. Amonorrhoea was treated with administration of bromocriptine and/or Hardy's operation (4 patients). The appearance and enlargement of the visual field defects during the period were found to occur more frequently (8/20 cases: 40%, including minor changes) than in previous reports. Visual acuity was not affected. The visual field test is safer than radiological tests for the pregnant patients and more sensitive to adenoma growth. Pregnancy-associated visual field defects induced in patients with pituitary adenoma subsided when bromocriptine was administrated or following delivery. In some cases, post-delivery lactation delayed recovery of visual field defects.

INTRODUCTION

Prolactin (PRL)-producing pituitary adenoma usually induces amenorrhoea and sterility (Badawy, Nusbaum and Omar 1980). Recently advanced treatment using bromocriptine or clomiphene has made it possible for women suffering from PRL-producing adenoma to become pregnant. However, in these women the adenoma increases in size during pregnancy, resulting in compression of chiasma with enlargement or the appearance of visual field defects (3, 5, 9, 13). In this study, visual fields of 20 patients with PRL-producing adenoma were evaluated during pregnancy and the post-pregnancy lactation period.

PATIENTS AND METHODS

The Kyoto University Hospital sterility clinic succeeded in achieving 21 pregnancies in 20 patients with PRL-producing pituitary adenoma employing Hardy's operation and/or oral administration of bromocriptine (5–10 mg

Heijl, A. and Greve, E.L. (eds.), Proceedings of the 6th Int. Visual Field Symposium.
© *1985, Dr W. Junk Publishers, Dordrecht, The Netherlands. ISBN 978-94-010-8932-6*

Table 1. Status of patients before treatments, kinds of treatment (Br. indicates bromocriptine) and results of pregnancy.

case No	adenoma	history of pregnancy	grade of amenorrhoea	PRL level before (ng ml)	therapy	visual disturbance	delivery	baby sex	weight (gr)
1	macro	none	Am II	223 7	Hardy+Br	–	normal (40w)	female	3260
2	macro	none	Am I	220 0	Hardy	+	suction (41w)	male	3060
3	macro	none	Am I	281 3	Hardy	–	twin (38w)	female female	2350 2400
4	macro	abortion 1	Am I	766 6	Hardy+Br	–	twin (37w)	male male	2750 1800
5	micro	abortion 2	Am I	230 1	Br	+	suction (36w)	male	2520
6 - 1	micro	none	Am I	528 0	Br.	+	normal (37w)	male	3065
6 - 2	micro	delivery 1	Am I	211 0	Br.	+	normal (38w)	male	3260
7	micro	delivery 1	Am I	186 8	Br.	–	normal (39w)	female	3690
8	micro	delivery 1	Am II	173 0	Br.	+	normal (40w)	male	3090
9	micro	delivery 1	Am I	84 6	Br.	–	normal (38w)	female	
10	micro	none	Am II	772 0	Br.	–	normal (41w)	female	2740
11	micro	abortion 1	Am II	212 7	Br.	–	normal (40w)	female	3240
12	micro	none	Am I	195 0	Br.	+	normal (40w)	female	3280
13	micro	none	Am II	123 5	Br.	+	normal (39w)	male	2510
14	micro	delivery 1	Am II	396 1	Br.	+	normal (40w)	female	3170
15	micro	none	Am I	63 4	Br.	–	normal (40w)	female	2850
16	micro	delivery 1	Am I	155 1	Br.	–	spontaneous abortion (13w)		
17	micro	none	Am I	340 0	Br.	–	normal (39w)	female	3220
18	micro	none	Am I	173 5	Br.	?	normal (37w)	female	2570
19	micro	none	Am I	154 0	Br.	–	normal (34w)	male	2560
20	micro	delivery 1	Am I	51 0	Br.	–	normal (38w)	male	2980

daily) (Table 1). Pituitary adenomas were classified into macroadenoma and microadenoma before pregnancy by Hardy's criteria (6). Amenorrhoea was classified into grade I or II, according to ovulation difficulty. PRL-level in blood was measured by radioimmunoassay, and the values before and during pregnancy are shown in the table. Visual fields were measured by Goldmann perimeter monthly or bimonthly during pregnancy and the post-pregnancy lactation period. Isopters of V/4, I/4, I/3, I/2 and I/1 were routinely employed. Field tests of patient 18 were not performed during the last 4 months of pregnancy (no change until this time) which was therefore excluded from statistical analsysis of field changes.

RESULTS

Plus marks in the column of visual disturbances of the table indicate that a field defect appeared for the first time (patients 2, 5, 12 and 13) or defects were enlarged (patients 6, 8 and 14) during the period. A minor change of inner isopters was counted as a positive sign of field change even if the patient did not complain of the defect. The frequency of abnormality was 40% (8/20 pregnancies, excluding patient 18). The first change usually appeared on the temporal side and progressed to the center.

Figure 1 shows a typical change of fields of patient 8. Selected fields at five time points are shown. Defects on the temporal field of the right eye became indistinct after delivery. Enlarged or newly appearing defects during

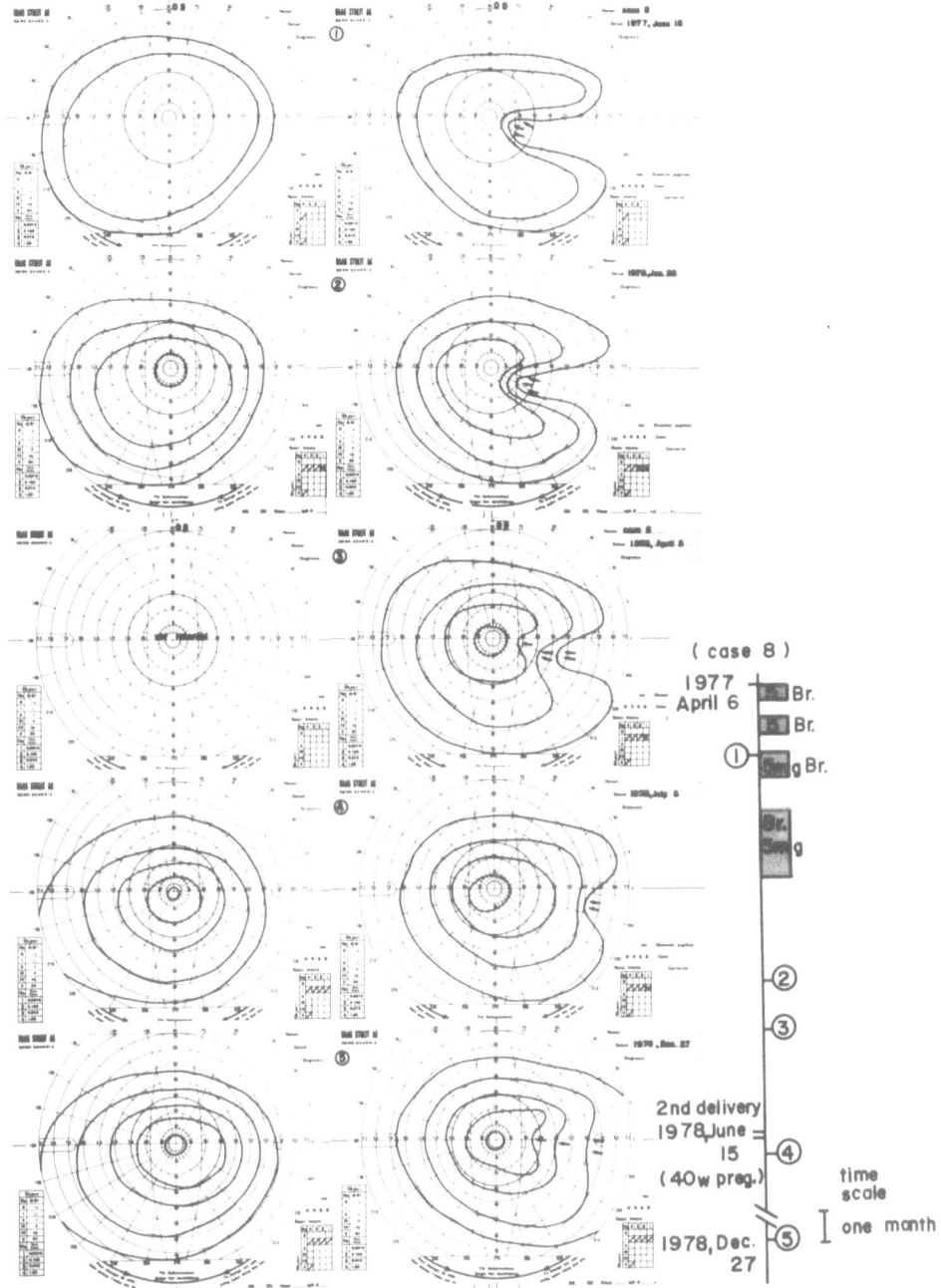

Fig. 1. Representative findings of visual fields of patient 8. Time course of administration of bromocriptine is shown on the right side with numbers indicating the times when these fields were tested.

229

pregnancy were reversible in these patients when bromocriptine was administered or following delivery. In some cases, post-delivery lactation delayed recovery of field defects. Central visual acuity was not affected in any of the patients throughout pregnancy.

DISCUSSION

Recent advances in immunoradioassay have made it possible to detect pituitary adenoma in an early stage. This is due to the fact that a group of pituitary adenomas induce hyperprolactinemia. This diagnostic technique is sometimes superior to conventional radiological examinations in detecting micro-adenoma.

Adenomas increase in size during pregnancy. Under such circumstances a microadenoma has a possibility of increasing in size, thus compressing the chiasma and resulting in field defects. Until now the frequency of visual field defects in PRL-producing adenoma has been studied by several investigators (4, 7, 10, 12). Reviewing these reports we found that the rates of abnormalities varied widely and that previous field tests employed in these papers were inadequate and incomplete. The 40% rate of visual field defects observed in the present study by employing many isopters is higher than the rates reported previously in patients with PRL-producing pituitary adenoma during pregnancy and the post-pregnancy lactation period. Furthermore, our findings show that defects are reversible when discovered and treated in an early stage.

Bromocriptine diminished adenoma size, resulting in normalization of visual fields (8, 11, 16), reported that in 5 of 6 cases defects disappeared when bromocriptine was administrated. Bromocriptine therapy rather than Hardy's operation seems to be preferable for treating this disease.

The timing for commencement of therapy can be accurately deduced through field tests. If progress of defects is slow it is safe to wait until normal delivery. Since delivery also results in a cessation of defects. However, once the mother has started lactating, special attention should be paid to defect progressing and delaying recovery.

REFERENCES

1. Badawy, S.Z.A., Nusbaum, M.L. and Omar, M. Hypothalamic-pituitary evaluation in patients with galactorrhea-amenorrhea and hyperprolactinemia. Obsterics & Gynecol. 55: 1–7 (1980).
2. Bergh, T., Nillius, S.J. and Wide, L. Clinical course and outcome of pregnancies in amenorrhoeic women with hyperprolactinaemia and pituitary tumours. Brit. Med. J. I: 875–880 (1978).
3. Child, D.F., Gordon, H. and Mashiter, K. et al. Pregnancy, prolactin, and pituitary tumours. Brit. Med. J. II: 87–89 (1975).
4. Corenblum, B. Successful outcome of ergocryptine-induced pregnancies in twenty-one women with prolactin-secreting pituitary adenomas. Fertility and Sterility 32: 183–186 (1979).
5. Gemzell, C. Induction of ovulation in infertile women with pituitary tumors. Am.

J. Gynecol. 121: 311–315 (1975).

6. Hardy, J. Transsphenoidal surgery of hypersecreting pituitary tumors, in Kohler, P.O. and Ross, G.T. eds.: Diagnosis and treatment of pituitary tumors. International Congress Series 303. 179–194, Excepta Medica, Amsterdam (1973).

7. Jewelewicz, R. and Vande Wiele, R.L. Clinical course and outcome of pregnancy in twenty-five patients with pituitary microadenomas. Am. J. Obstet. Gynecol. 136: 339–343 (1980).

8. Lamberts, S.W.J., Seldenrath, H.J., Kwa, H.G. et al. Transient bitemporal hemianopsia during pregnancy after treatment of galactorrhea-amenorrhea syndrome with bromocriptine. J. Clin. Endocrinol. and Metab. 44: 180–184 (1977).

9. Magyer, D.M. & Marshall, J.R. Pituitary tumors and pregnancy. Am. J. Obstet. Gynecol. 132: 739–751 (1978).

10. March, C.M., Kletzky, O.A. and Davajan, V. et al. Longitudinal evaluation of patients with untreated prolactin-secreting pituitary adenomas. Am. J. Obstet. Gynecol. 139: 835–844 (1981).

11. Spark, R.F., Baker, R. and Bienfang, D.C. et al. Bromocriptine reduces pituitary tumor size and hypersecretion. JAMA 247: 311–316 (1982).

12. Speroff, L., Levin, R.M. and Haning, Jr. R.V. et al. A practical approach for the evaluation of women with abnormal polytomography of elevated prolactin levels. Am. J. Obstet. Gynecol. 135: 896–906 (1979).

13. Swyer, G.I.M., Little, V. and Harries, B.J. Visual disturbance in pregnancy after induction of avulation. Brit. Med. J. 4: 90–91 (1971).

14. Thorner, M.O., Edwards, C.R.W. and Charlesworth, M. et al. Pregnancy in patients presenting with hyperprolactinaemia. Brit, Med. J. II: 771–774 (1979).

15. Van Roon, E., Van der Vijver, J.C.M. and Gerretsen, G. et al. Rapid regression of suprasellar extending prolactinoma after bromocriptine treatment during pregnancy. Fertility and Sterility 36: 173–177 (1981).

16. Was, J.A., Williams, J. and Charlesworth, M. et al. Bromocriptine in management of large pituitary tumors. Brit. Med. J. 284: 1908–1911 (1982).

Author's address:
Department of Ophthalmology (Y.H.) and Gynecology (A.T.),
Kyoto University Faculty of Medicine, Sakyo-ku,
Kyoto 606, Japan

QUANTITATIVE VERSUS SEMIQUANTITATIVE PERIMETRY IN NEUROLOGICAL DISORDERS

O. MEIENBERG, H. MATTLE, A. JENNI and J. FLAMMER

(*Bern, Switzerland*)

ABSTRACT

72 patients (135 eyes) with visual field defects from various neurological disorders were examined on the Octopus automated perimeter using both a quantitative and a semi-quantitative procedure. The semiquantitative strategy tests only whether the sensitivity is normal, relatively or absolutely disturbed. When it was used, normal values and absolute defects agreed in about 90% of the test locations with the quantitative measurements. Relative defects, however, were falsely negative (i.e. 'normal') or positive (i.e. 'absolute defect') in more than 50% of the test locations with the semi-quantitative procedure. Since in optic nerve and chiasmal lesions a frequent occurrence of relative defects must be expected, quantitative measurements should be performed in these disorders. In suprageniculate lesions, on the other hand, absolute defects often predominate. In most of these cases semiquantitative examinations, which are much more time saving, deliver sufficient information to the clinician.

INTRODUCTION

The Octopus automated perimeter has two types of programs, quantitative and semiquantitative. In the quantitative programs the actual threshold of the differential light sensitivity is determined with a bracketing strategy. The semiquantitative screening programs test only whether the sensitivity is normal, relatively or absolutely disturbed. While a quantitative examination gives more information, but is time consuming, a semiquantitative examination gives less information, but is time saving. Since in neurological patients the ability to cooperate sometimes is limited by psychic alteration or fatigue, the results of time consuming quantitative measurements could be less reliable than those of a simpler and shorter semiquantitative procedure. The aim of this investigation, therefore, was to determine in which neurological conditions semiquantitative examinations deliver sufficient information, and in which conditions quantitative measurements provide significant additional information.

Heijl, A. and Greve, E.L. (eds.), Proceedings of the 6th Int. Visual Field Symposium.
© *1985, Dr W. Junk Publishers, Dordrecht, The Netherlands. ISBN 978-94-010-8932-6*

PATIENTS AND METHOD

72 patients (135 eyes) with visual field defects due to various neurological disorders were examined on the Octopus automated perimeter with both a semiquantitative and a quantitative procedure. The semiquantitative screening program used – hereafter referred to as program 09 – had been adjusted geometrically so that the test locations coincided with the combined quantitative standard Octopus programs 32 and 42. This allowed direct comparisons between the semiquantitative and quantitative measurements for each test location. The strategy in program 09 is identical to that used in the Octopus programs 03 and 07 (see Octopus system 201 operators manual, or Funkhouser *et al.*, 1983).

All 135 eyes were first examined with the semiquantitative program 09, and then additionally with the quantitative programs 32 and/or 42 (86 eyes with 32; 63 eyes with 42; 23 eyes with 32 and 42). In order to keep fatigue effects at a minimum, patients often were examined in two separate sessions on the same day or within a few days.

RESULTS

The number of patients and eyes examined in each of the four diagnostic groups of clinically manifest optic nerve lesions, subclinical optic nerve lesions in multiple sclerosis, chiasmal lesions, and suprageniculate lesions are given in Table 1. Furthermore, the duration of the examinations with programs 09, 32 and 42 is indicated. It is evident that semiquantitative examinations save time for all kinds of lesions when compared with quantitative. A screening of almost the whole visual field of both eyes with program 09 took about a quarter of an hour, while a quantitative examination of the same areas with the combined programs 32 and 42 took about one hour for both eyes.

Figure 1 shows a comparison between the results obtained with quantitative and semiquantitative procedures. For quantitatively determined normal test locations, the semiquantitative procedure was correct in about 90% in all four diagnostic groups. Absolute defects were correctly indicated by the screening method in about 90% of the test locations in the clinically manifest optic nerve lesions and in the suprageniculate lesions, while in the chiasmal lesions the results were correct in 80%, and in the subclinical optic nerve lesions in 50% only. The relative defects were either false negative (i.e. missed) or false positive (i.e. indicated as absolute defects) in over 50% of the test locations with the semiquantitative method in all four groups.

Figure 2 illustrates the distribution of the relative and absolute defects found with the quantitative measurements in the four groups of neurological disorders. In the first three groups, relative defects markedly predominate. In the suprageniculate lesions, on the other hand, about 60% of the defects are absolute. In addition, these defects generally were large, i.e. hemianopias or quadrantanopias, and in 26 of the 29 patients (90%) the clinically relevant information could be drawn also from the semiquantitative data.

234

Table 1. Number of patients in the different diagnostic groups, and duration of the examinations with semiquantitative (program 09) and quantitative (programs 32 and 42) procedures.

	Number of patients	Number of eyes	Mean duration of examination (minutes)		
			09	32	42
Group 1 Clinically manifest optic nerve lesions	14	24	6.5 (5–7.5)	13.6 (11–22)	14.6 (12–18)
Group 2 Subclinical optic nerve lesions (MS)	14	26	6.2 (4.5–8)	12.3 (8–15)	14.5 (10–20)
Group 3 Chiasmal lesions	15	27	6.5 (4–8)	14.4 (10–19)	12.0 (11–13)
Group 4 Suprageniculate lesions	29	58	6.5 (5–9)	13.1 (11–20)	12.7 (10–21)
Total	72	135	6.4 (4–9)	13.4 (10–22)	13.4 (10–21)

DISCUSSION

Two questions are essential for the choice of programs for automated examination of the visual fields: (1) Which area of the visual field is of particular interest? and (2) How can the most reliable results be obtained?

In most ophthalmological disorders optimal information will result from examinations of more or less circumscribed areas with relatively high spatial resolution and quantitative threshold determinations. In neurological disorders often an overview of the whole visual fields of both eyes is of interest. This area is tested with Octopus program 21. The spatial resolution of this program, however, is low and the borders of visual field defects, therefore, are usually ill-defined. An improved spatial resolution could be obtained by combinations of program 21 with other quantitative programs. However, a long duration of the examination can markedly reduce the reliability of the results, especially in neurological patients, whose ability to cooperate not infrequently is limited by mental alteration and fatigue. In such situations semiquantitative examinations could even give more reliable information.

As our results have shown, in those neurological disorders in which relative defects predominate or in which follow up examinations are important, such as in optic nerve and chiasmal lesions, quantitative examinations should be performed when possible. In suprageniculate lesions, where absolute defects often predominate, the defects usually are extended and the patients' ability to cooperate is often limited, semiquantitative examinations generally deliver the clinically relevant information.

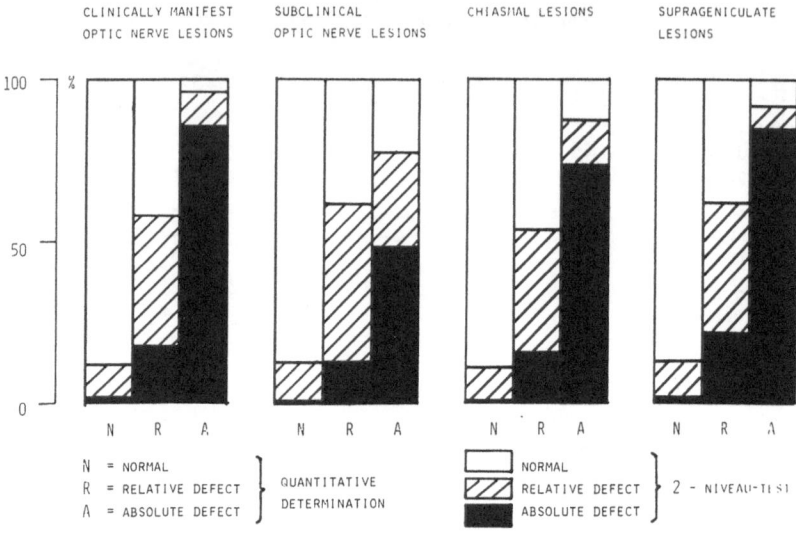

Fig. 1.

DISTRIBUTION OF RELATIVE AND ABSOLUTE VISUAL FIELD DEFECTS IN THE DIFFERENT
GROUPS OF NEUROLOGICAL DISORDERS (QUANTITATIVE DETERMINATIONS)

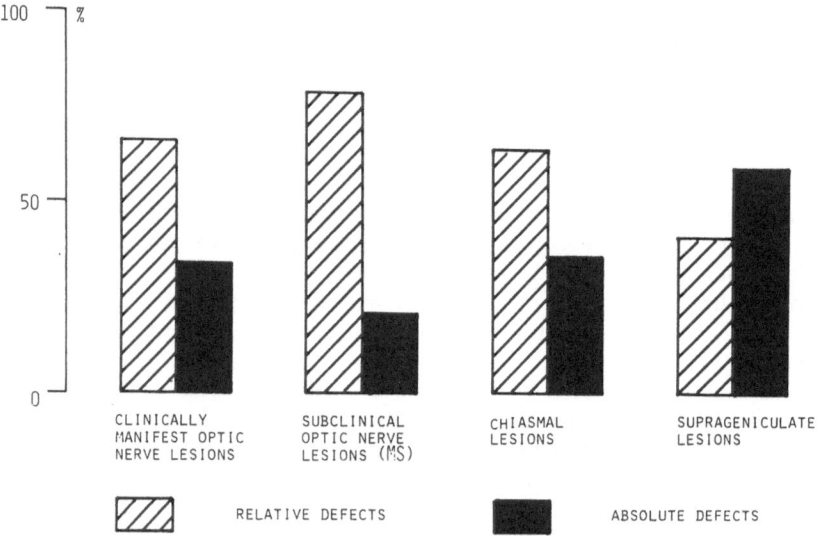

Fig. 2.

REFERENCES

Funkhouser, A., Wetterwald, N. and Fankhauser, F. The accuracy of screening programs. A preliminary report on an ongoing longitudinal investigation to ascertain the quantitativeness of qualitative 2-niveau-test procedures. In: Greve, E.L., Heijl, A. (eds.) Fifth International Visual Field Symposium. 1983. Dr. W. Junk Publishers, The Hague.

Author's address:
O. Meienberg, M.D.
Department of Neurology
University of Basel
Kantonsspital
CH-4031 Basel/Switzerland

COLOR PERIMETRY OF CENTRAL SCOTOMAS IN DISEASES OF THE MACULA AND OPTIC NERVE

WILLIAM M. HART, Jr., GREGORY KOSMORSKY and RONALD M. BURDE

(*St. Louis, U.S.A.*)

ABSTRACT

We have used a microcomputer controlled color video tangent screen to examine 23 patients with isolated central visual field defects that have resulted from either optic nerve or macular disease. Colored test objects were used for kinetic perimetry. Test object luminance was matched to the luminance of a white surround at 10 ft lamberts by using flicker photometry. Central scotomas that were present by conventional kinetic perimetry (luminance increment sensitivity) were also present for color modulated test objects (color saturation increment sensitivity). In no case were defects found in the visual field for colored test objects that could not also be demonstrated by conventional luminance increment techniques. Qualitative shape characteristics of central visual field defects were of more value in distinguishing optic nerve and macular diseases, than was any difference between luminance and color perimetry.

INTRODUCTION

Acquired dyschromatopsias have been thought by some investigators to differ when produced by optic nerve disorders as opposed to macular diseases (1–3). Since acquired dyschromatopsias are such a prominent feature of these disorders, it has commonly been felt that the use of color as a distinguishing feature of perimetric test objects should produce a more sensitive test of the central visual field. We have developed a perimetric test system, using a color video tangent screen as the test instrument, so that the luminance of test objects and their surrounds can be independently controlled. Matching of luminance of colored test objects to a colorless surround by means of flicker photometry allows for the generation of colored test objects whose luminance has been empirically matched to the surround. The degree of color within the test object (saturation) can then be varied while maintaining a constant luminance. This permits testing of the visual field by means of an isolated color detection function, allowing differentiation of visual field defects for color perception from defects of luminance increment detection.

METHODS

The theoretical design and construction of the color video tangent screen system has been previously reported (4, 5). The system uses a 19 inch triphosphor color video instrument which is controlled by a microcomputer through an electronic interface that allows independent manipulation of the red, green and blue phosphors of the video screen. A white background of 10 ft lamberts is maintained by driving all 3 phosphors simultaneously to appropriate levels of luminance. Prior to each visual field test the color of test object to be used is matched in luminance to the 10 ft lambert white surround by means of flicker photometry. Test objects are then presented in kinetic fashion within the white surround. For this study test object sizes were between 1 and 3 degrees in angular subtense, test object color saturations varied between 0 and 25% of maximum, and only red and blue test objects were used. Twenty three patients were examined. All had central visual field defects. Prior to color perimetry, all defects were fully characterized by a combination of conventional manual kinetic and static perimetry. In 5 cases manual static perimetry was augmented by use of the Octopus 2000 perimeter system.

RESULTS

Of 23 patients examined, 11 had optic nerve diseases, while 12 had retinal disorders. Of those with optic nerve disease 4 had retrobulbar optic neuritis, one had dominant optic atrophy, one had a glioma of the optic nerve, and 5 had extrinsic compression of the optic nerve by either orbital neoplasms or intracranial aneurysm or neoplasm. Of the 12 patients with retinal disease, 3 had had branch artery occlusions, 2 had primary macular dystrophies, 3 had epiretinal macular membranes, and 4 had senile macular degeneration with subretinal neovascular membranes.

In all cases central scotomas that were plotted by luminance increment perimetry were detected with the use of color modulated test objects. The most striking finding was that the boundaries of visual field defects mapped with color increment test objects followed very closely the boundaries of the same defects when plotted with luminance increment techniques. The primary difference found between the two techniques was that generalized depression of sensitivity in the central visual field was often more profound when mapped with colored test objects than by luminance increment techniques. In patients with partially recovered optic neuritis color isopters were markedly constricted so that the most brightly colored test objects were required to demonstrate the boundaries of the central visual field defects.

Colored test objects did not appear to be any more sensitive in the detection or characterization of these central visual field defects when

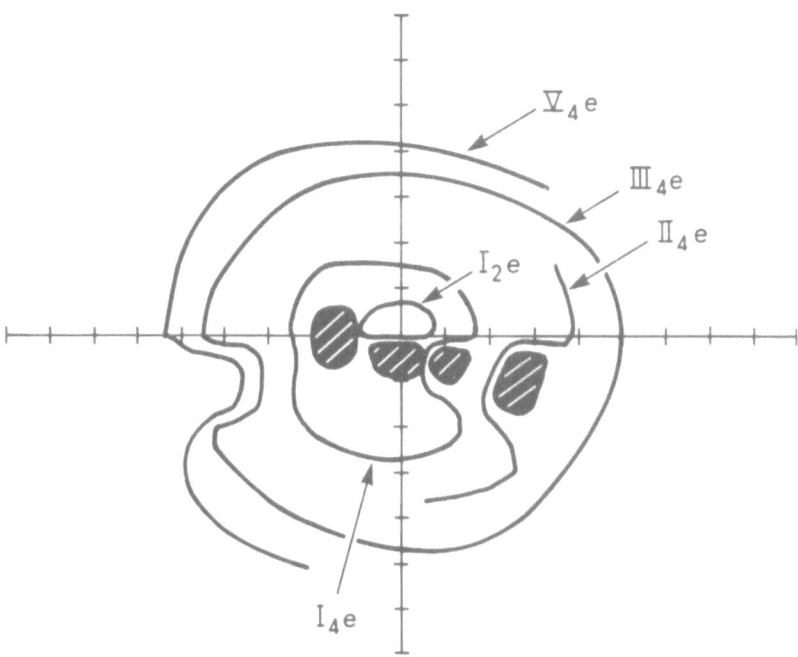

Fig. 1. Goldmann visual field. Case 1, demonstrating dense, narrow, inferior nerve fiber bundle defect splitting fixation.

compared to luminance increment techniques. Differentiation of optic nerve from macular disorders was likewise not improved by the use of the color techniques. Rather, such distinctions were more reliably made on the basis of the morphology of central visual field defects. Defects arising from optic nerve diseases more frequently produced cecocentral scotomas with borders obeying the distribution of nerve fiber fascicles within the papillo-macular bundle, while primary diseases of the macula more frequently produced isolated central scotomas that could be plotted separate from the physiologic blind spot.

Two cases will be described. The first patient was a 66 year old man with sudden onset of optic nerve compression caused by a small intracranial aneurysm arising at the origin of the left ophthalmic artery. This diagnosis was confirmed by a combination of C-T scanning and selective arteriography. Goldmann visual fields (Fig. 1) demonstrated the presence of a dense nerve fiber bundle defect containing a series of dense scotomas abutting the nasal horizontal meridian. Color perimetry with blue test objects (Fig. 2) showed a dense nerve fiber bundle defect in the same distribution. Although the defect was apparently denser when plotted with colored test objects, its boundaries precisely matched those mapped by Goldmann perimetry. Indentical results were obtained with the use of red test objects.

The second patient was a 31 year old man with dominantly inherited optic atrophy. Visual acuity was 20/60 in the right eye and 20/200 in the left.

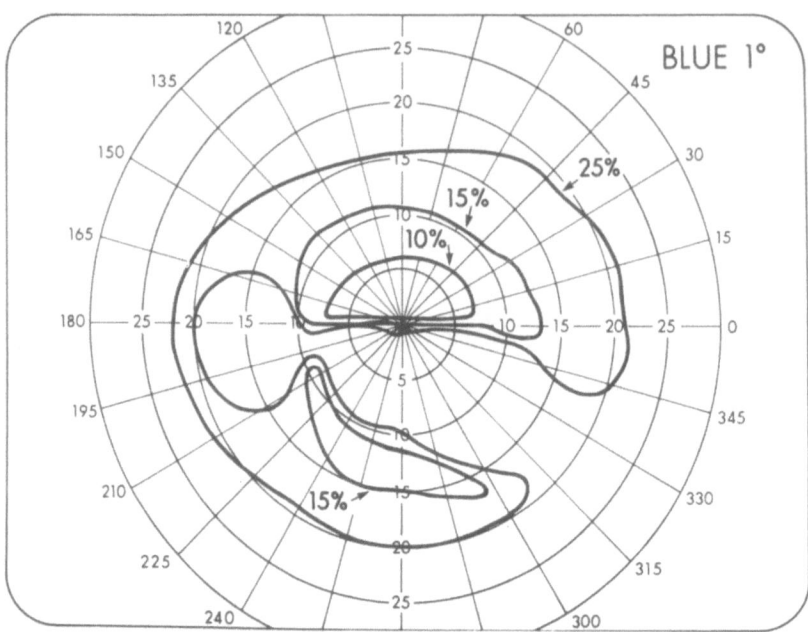

Fig. 2. Color perimetry of left eye of Case 1 with inferior nerve fiber bundle defect. Note that the defect plotted with blue test objects is dense, but has identical peripheral boundaries to that obtained by the Goldmann perimetric technique. Percentage figures indicate percentage of maximum test object color saturation. Angular size of all test objects was 1 degree.

There were bilateral ceocentral scotomas. Static perimetry with the Octopus 2000 system (Fig. 3) demonstrated a dense cecocentral scotoma in the right eye. Fundus examination revealed only mild atrophy of the temporal portions of the optic discs. Color perimetry using red test objects in the right eye likewise demonstrated the presence of a dense cecocentral scotoma with boundaries that fell along the horizontal meridian between the physiologic blind spot and the point of fixation. The boundaries of the scotoma when plotted with the red test objects did not extend beyond those that had been mapped by luminance increment testing.

DISCUSSION

That the use of colored perimetric test objects might be a more sensitive or specific means of differentiating and detecting central visual field defects from retinal and optic nerve disorders has been suggested by two classes of information. Acquired dyschromatopsias in these diseases are subjectively marked and are frequently the first symptom to be noted by the patient. In addition, there is an apparent dissociation of luminance and color defects in such disorders as recovered optic neuritis. Visual acuity may return to normal levels while defects in hue discrimination remain profound (6). A

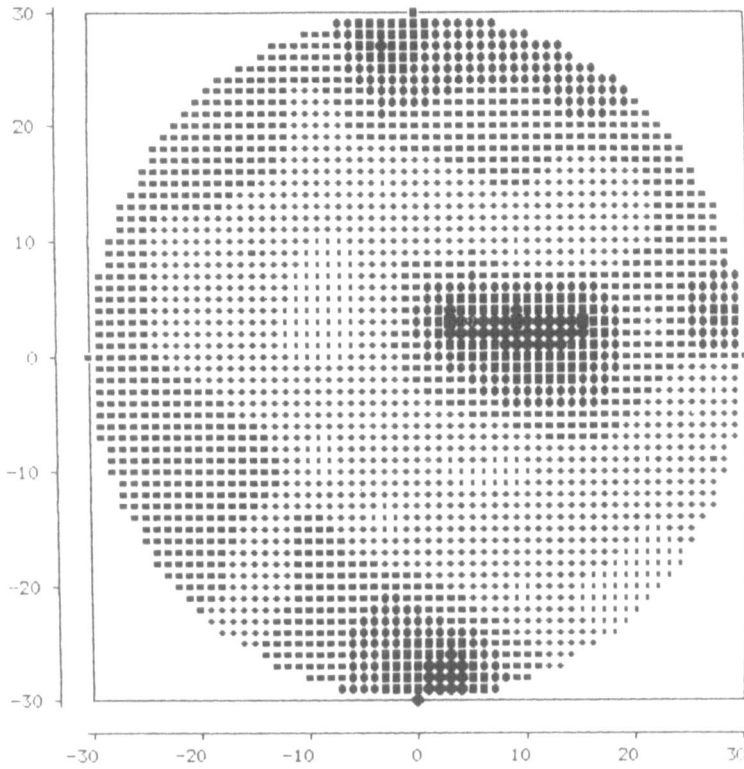

Fig. 3. Case 2. Perimetry of right eye with Octopus 2000-R system, program 34. Note pattern of dense cecocentral scotoma extending from physiological blind spot into superior half of macular field.

second class of information is that which is based on studies of luminance and color coding in the afferent visual system. Ganglion cells, optic nerve fibers and lateral geniculate cells having receptive field properties that show color opponency with a center-surround organization are known to conduct their information at the level of the optic nerve by way of neurons that are anatomically smaller than those with phasic firing properties, thought to be predominantly mediators of luminance information (7). There is a partial functional and anatomic segregation of luminance and color information encoded in the afferent visual system, suggesting that there might be differential sensitivity of these two broad classes of information to pathologic insult at the level of the optic nerve (8). However, this feature may be limited to color discriminations along the blue—yellow axis, since only the blue-on/yellow-off cells of the primate visual system are known to detect color contrast independent from luminance differences (9).

In the limited series of central visual field defects resulting from optic nerve and macular disorders that we have studied, we have not been able to demonstrate any qualitative difference between the distribution (shape or

243

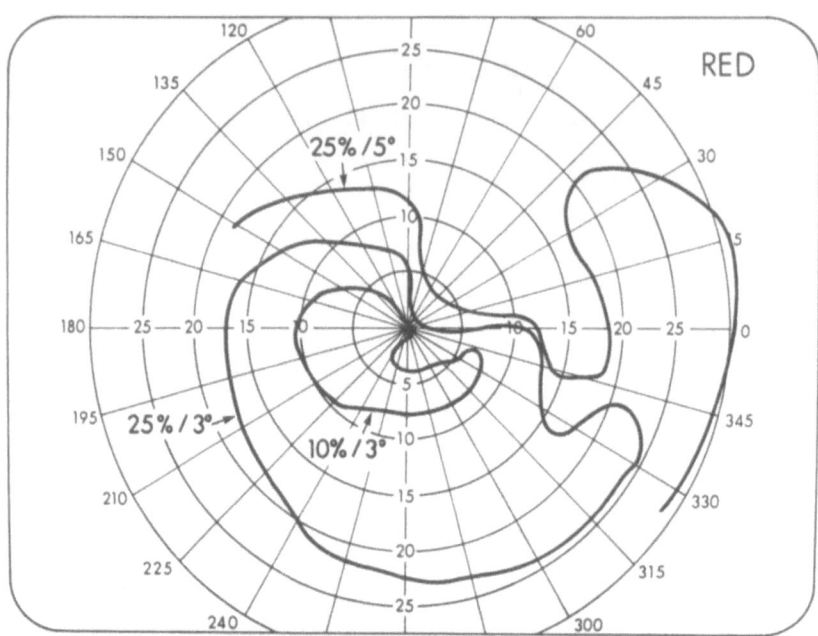

Fig. 4. Case 2. Color perimetry of central field of right eye using red test objects. Percentage marks indicate percentage of maximal color saturation of red test objects; degree marks indicate angular size of test objects. Note the dense cecocentral scotoma for color saturation detection, having boundary along horizontal meridian between physiological blind spot and point of fixation, and marked depression of isopters for red saturation sensitivity.

size) of visual field defects mapped with color increment as opposed to luminance increment testing techniques. Two qualifications should be noted. The first is that color increment testing cannot be directly compared to luminance increment testing on a quantitative basis, since sensitivity to color saturation is an entirely different visual function than is brightness sensitivity. The second problem is that we have studied only those patients in whom visual field defects have already been demonstrated by the luminance increment technique. It remains to be determined whether visual field defects for color increment testing might exist in patients in whom there is no known visual field defect by conventional testing techniques. In spite of the lack of apparent additional sensitivity for the detection or characterization of central visual field defects by the color contrast technique, we would like to encourage other investigators to pursue this same avenue of investigation, especially in those instances where relatively subtle central visual field defects must be analyzed. Such disorders would include suspected early toxic maculopathies and neuropathies, and possibly the detection of earliest glaucomatous visual field defects in the Bjerrum region.

ACKNOWLEDGEMENTS

This work was supported by grant EY-03703 from the National Eye Institute.

REFERENCES

1. Cox, J. Color vision defects acquired in diseases of the eye. Brit. J. Physiol. Opt. 18: 3–32 (1961).
2. Krill, A.E. and Fishman, G.A. Acquired color vision defects. Trans. Am. Acad. Ophth. & Oto. 75: 1095–1111 (1971).
3. Dubois Poulsen, A. Acquired dyschromatopsias. Acquired colour vision deficiencies. Int. Symp., Ghent 1971. In: Mod. Prob. Ophthalmol. 11: 84–93 (1972).
4. Hart, W.M. Jr., Hartz, R.K., Hagen, R.W. and Clark, K.W. Color contrast perimetry. Invest. Ophthalmol. Vis. Sci. 25: 400–413 (1984).
5. Hart, W.M. Jr. and Gordon, M.O. Color perimetry of glaucomatous visual field defects. Ophthalmology 91: 338–346 (1984).
6. Burde, R.M. and Gallin, P.F. Visual parameters associated with recovered retrobulbar optic neuritis. Am. J. Ophthalmol. 79: 1034–1037 (1975).
7. Gouras, P.L. Antidromic responses of orthodromically identified ganglion cells in monkey retina. J. Physiol. (London) 204: 407–419 (1969).
8. DeValois, R.L. Processing of intensity and wavelength information by the visual system. Invest. Ophthalmol. 11: 417–427 (1972).
9. Gouras, P. and Eggers, H. Hering's opponent colour channels do not exist in the primate retinogeniculate pathway. Ophthalmic. Res. 16: 31–35 (1984).

Author's address:
Department of Ophthalmology,
Washington University School of Medicine,
St Louis, MO 63110, U.S.A.

EFFECTS OF COLOUR ON THE CONTRAST SENSITIVITY FUNCTION AS A FUNCTION OF ECCENTRICITY

JEAN-PIERRE MENU

ABSTRACT

Stationary sinusoidal gratings red, green and blue ($40\,\mathrm{cd/m^2}$) were presented to eight subjects using a psychophysical adjustment technique to establish sensitivity functions; 1 — in foveal vision; 2 — in peripheral vision: $10°, 20°, 30°, 40°$, nasal retina on the horizontal meridian.

Result quantification indicates: 1 — that there is no difference among colours in foveal vision; 2 — that perception is greatly and equally reduced for all colours in peripheral vision; 3 — that this phenomenon depends on spatial frequencies.

The least deteriorated frequencies are medium range spatial frequencies (1 cycle/deg.). This method is the basis of the studies presently conducted to quantify decreases in visual function.

1. INTRODUCTION

The contrast sensitivity function has been the object of numerous studies. Green (1968) (4) and Kelly (1974) (5) analyzed the role of the colour parameter in foveal vision. Bourdy et al. (1983) (3), Rovamo (1983) (8) studied this factor in peripheral vision. However these studies used low photopic, even mesopic, light stimulation and the rest of the retina was not excited (scotopic environment). Noorlander et al. (7) used brighter photopic stimuli but as all other authors, conducted these experiments on a very small number of subjects. Aside from this, the evolution of the phenomenon was not really quantified.

The purpose of this experiment was to define objectively, on a larger number of subjects (8), the evolution of contrast sensitivity for red, green and blue at retinal eccentricities of $10°, 20°, 30°, 40°$ (nasal retina).

The stimulus was presented at a high photopic level in an equally bright environment, stimulating all photoreceptors ($40\,\mathrm{cd/m^2}$).

Quantification which allows objective evaluation was based on a gain calculation method (Bonnet, 1982) (2).

Heijl, A. and Greve, E.L. (eds.), Proceedings of the 6th Int. Visual Field Symposium.
© 1985, Dr W. Junk Publishers, Dordrecht, The Netherlands. ISBN 978-94-010-8932-6

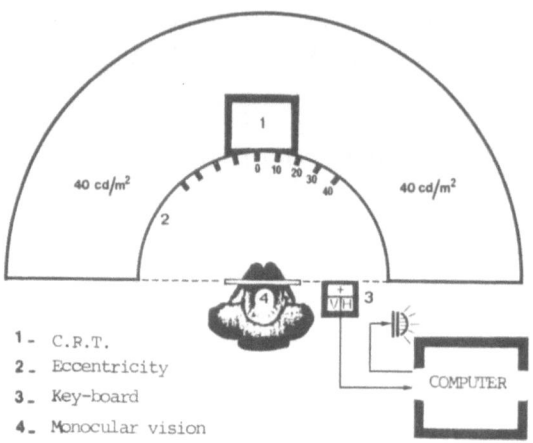

1 - C.R.T.
2 - Eccentricity
3 - Key-board
4 - Monocular vision

Fig. 1.

2. MATERIAL AND METHOD

2.1 Apparatus and stimuli

Stationary sinusoidal gratings were generated by a computer and displayed on a high resolution colour monitor with a frame frequency of 50 Hz. Colour parameters (luminance and trichromatic coordinates) were controlled by a Pritchard 1980B spectro-photometer. Colours were the primaries of the cathode ray tube: red (x = 0.665, y = 0.305), green (x = 0.365, y = 0.557), blue (x = 0.142, y = 0.072). The area of the stimulation field was 8° seen in near vision (1 meter). Controlled light environment provided an homogeneous isoenergetic field on all spectral wavelengths (white light x = 0.37, y = 0.38). Fixation points were positioned on a transparent half dome every 10° on the horizontal meridian up to an eccentricity of 40°. The observer's head was fixed on a bite-board. Thresholds were measured in central monocular vision and in the temporal field at 10°, 20°, 30° and 40° on the eye with natural pupil.

2.2 Experimental procedure

A psychophysical ascending adjustment method determined contrast sensitivity functions for each subject.

Using a button, the observer increased the stimulus contrast until he detected a vertical or an horizontal pattern. Ten horizontal and vertical spatial frequencies from 0.08 cycle/deg to 10 cycles/deg were presented three times in a random order.

Raw data is presented in Log-Log coordinates. Curves are the representation of the cone approximated from raw data, using least squares.

In order to quantify the observed differences, a gain value was calculated for each spatial frequency as a function of the various factors, according to the following formula:

$$G = 10 \, \text{Log} \frac{\text{Eccentricity Contrast}}{\text{Central Contrast}}$$

This gain is expressed in decibels.

The representation of the gain as a function of spatial frequencies evidences three types of frequencies: low, medium and high. In reported results, only the central frequency of each class of frequencies is used, i.e. $0.3 \, c/°$ for low frequencies, $0.7 \, c/°$ for medium frequencies, and $5 \, c/°$ for high spatial frequencies.

A negative gain value expressed an attenuation. For the three considered spatial frequencies, the evolution of attenuation for each subject, each colour and orientation is represented. These values were adjusted by linear regression. Since the coefficient of determination r2, calculated after adjustment by regression, is always greater than 0.8, attenuation as a function of eccentricity may be considered as a monotonous and linear function. Modeling and comparison between straight lines thus become possible.

Rather than comparing slopes, the equation of the median straight line of each family was formulated. The difference between attenuation at the beginning and attenuation at $40°$ of eccentricity gives a value for the three spatial frequencies and by colour.

2.3 Subjects

Eight experienced subjects (6 men and 2 women, age $21-36$) participated in this experiment. All had normal vision. Their foveal colour acuity tested with Ishihara and Farnsworth 100 hue was normal.

3. RESULTS

3.1. Sensitivity curves as a function of eccentricity, per subject, per orientation and per colour

For all subjects, in central vision, the three superimposed curves red, green, and blue, show that there is no difference between colours.

In peripheral vision, sensitivity decreases as eccentricity increases. This is particularly obvious for medium range, and even more so for high spatial frequencies.

3.2. Representation of attenuation for colours and eccentricity

The envelopes of regression lines presented in Figs. 3, 4, 5 for each primary colour as a function of eccentricity show that the evolution of the three groups of spatial frequencies is not similar for all three colours. Result dispersion is greater for red, especially at high frequencies. For blue, dispersion is smaller at all frequencies. Globally, results presented in Fig. 6 show that, under the present experimental conditions, blue is no more attenuated than red or green.

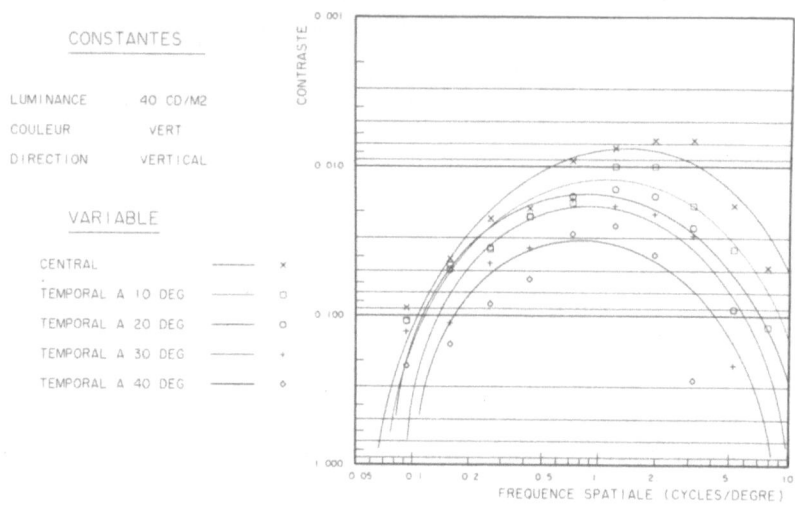

Fig. 2.

4. DISCUSSION

In central vision, contrast values for all three colours are similar to those reported by other authors. Attenuation which exists in the eccentric field shows that although colours are not as well perceived as in central vision, they are still seen (Gordon and Abramov (1), Noorlander et al. (7)). High spatial frequencies are the most altered, which supports the hypothesis of an enlargement of receptor field as a function of eccentricity (Koenderink et al. (6)). The bandpass character of the contrast sensitivity function is reinforced in peripheral vision (Bourdy et al. (3)).

All three colours were equally attenuated, which slightly differs from results obtained by Noorlander et al. (7). The high photopic level and the stimulation of all types of photo-receptors on the entire retina must be partially responsible for this phenomena. The Troxler effect is also involved.

In addition to this overall attenuation, especially pronounced on high spatial frequencies, the general dispersion is another factor to be taken into consideration. This dispersion is actually greater on medium range red frequencies. Subjectively, this result reveals the difficulty encountered by subjects when picking up information in this colour in parafoveal vision. It may be difficult for subjects to perceive fine detail in red in eccentric vision. This concept completes Rovamo's work and indicates that in peripheral vision, the spatial structure of the stimulus has to be taken into consideration.

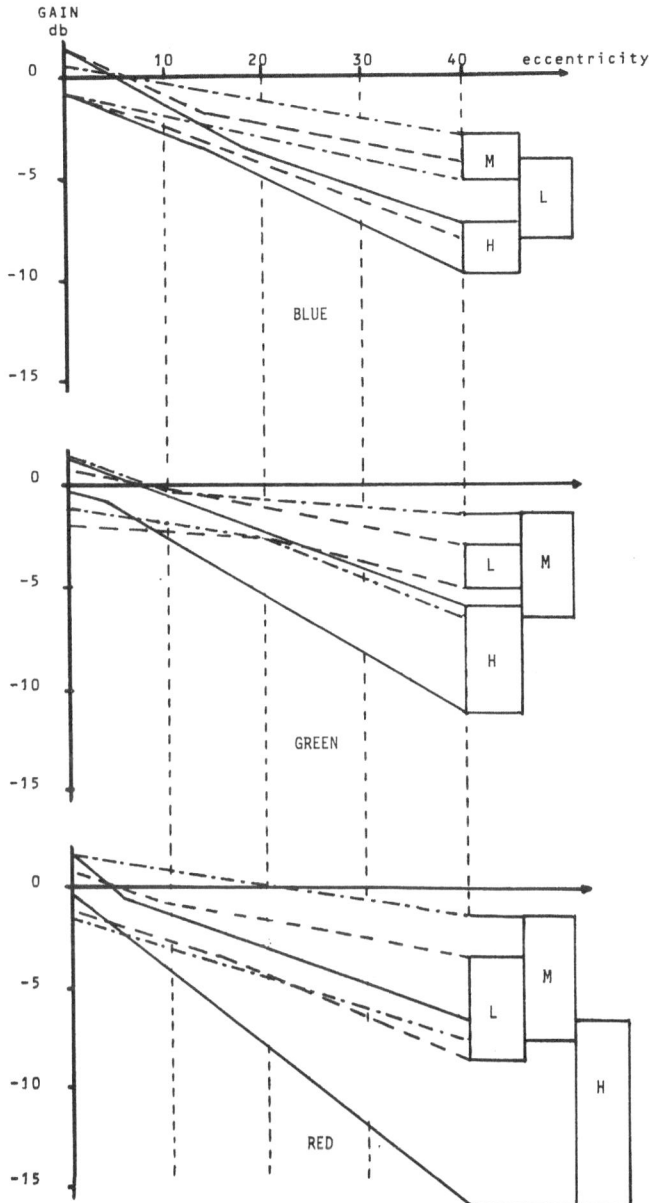

Figs. 3, 4, 5. Evolution of the gain or attenuation expressed in decibels as a function of temporal eccentricity (10°, 20°, 30°, 40°) for blue, green and red. The general envelopes of regression lines for the eight subjects are indicated for a medium range, a low and high frequency. Inter-subject dispersion is minimum at medium range and high spatial frequencies; it is greater at low frequencies. Attenuation is greatest at high frequencies and smallest at medium range frequencies.

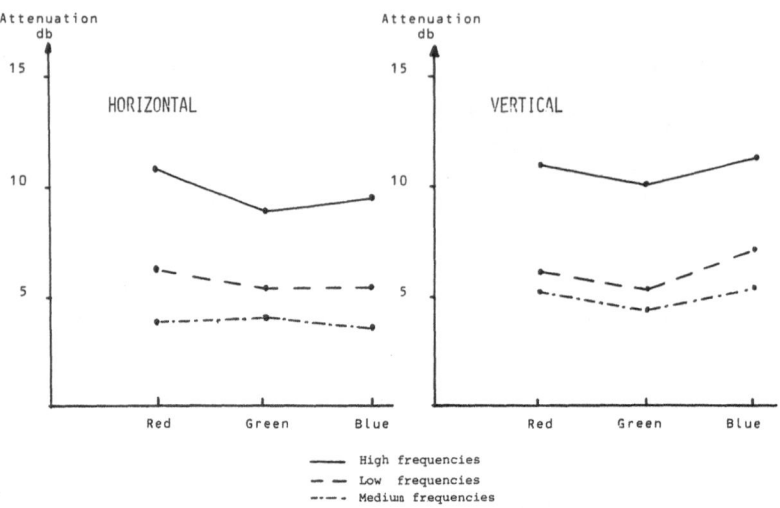

Fig. 6.

This finding is very important for the ergonomics of colour peripheral visual information: medium range spatial frequencies must be more widely used as they are the least attenuated.

ACKNOWLEDGEMENTS

The author is grateful to Dr. Santucci, G., Timball, J. and Miss Batejat, D., Seigneur J-M., Barrault, B. for their technical participation, to D. Freund for her assistance in preparing the English translation of this text, and to the eight subjects for their willingness to participate in this experiment.

REFERENCES

1. Abramov, I. and Gordon, J. Color vision in the peripheral retina: I – spectral sensitivity. J. Opt. Soc. Am., Vol. 67, 2, 195–202.
2. Bonnet, C., Le Gall, M. and Lorenceau, J. L'adaptation neuro-sensorielle au mouvement visuel. L'année psychologique, 82: 7–17 (1982).
3. Bourdy, C., Vienot, F., Monot, A. and Chiron, A. Spatial sensitivity of the human visual system under selective chromatic adaptation: Shape of the contrast sensitivity curves, foveal versus peripheral vision. J. Optics (Paris), Vol. 14, 5: 225–233 (1983).
4. Green, P.G. The contrast sensitivity of the colour mechanisms of the human eye. J. of Physiology (London), 196: 415–429 (1968).
5. Kelly, D.H. Spatio temporal frequency characteristics of color mechanisms. J. Opt. Soc. Am., 64: 983–990 (1974).
6. Koenderink, J.J., Bouman, M.A., Bueno de Mesquita, A.E. and Splappendel, S.

252

Perimetry of contrast detection thresholds of moving spatial sine wave patterns. I – The near peripheral visual field. J. Opt. Soc. Am., Vol. 68, 6: 845–849 (1978).

7. Noorlander, C., Koenderink, J.J., Den Ouden, R.J. and Edens, B.W. Sensitivity to spatio-temporal colour contrast in the peripheral visual field. Vision Res., Vol. 23, 1–11.
8. Rovamo, J. Cortical magnification factor and contrast sensitivity to luminance modulated chromatic gratings. Acta Physiol. Scand., 119: 365–371 (1983).

EXTRAFOVEAL RELATIVE RED-GREEN SENSITIVITY

KENJI KITAHARA, RYUTARO TAMAKI, HIROSHI KITAHARA,
JUN NOJI and ATSUSHI KANDATSU
(*Tokyo, Japan*)

ABSTRACT

In order to investigate opponent color channel damages in optic nerve diseases, the ranges of the red-green hue cancellation were measured for up to 10° from the fovea along the horizontal meridian on two normal observers and on a patient with optic nerve disease. In the normal observers, the red-green hue cancellation ranges widened and higher red-green ratios were obtained with an increase in eccentricity. In the patient with optic nerve disease, the red/green hue cancellation range was wider than that of the normal observers even at the fovea, and in the extrafovea abnormally wide ranges were found.

INTRODUCTION

To study the relative red and green sensitivities, the colour matching method with a model I Nagel anomaloscope is useful in examining color vision deficiencies for retinal diseases. The reason for that is the color matching method is used to detect the properties of visual pigments in general.

In order to investigate the red and green opponent channel damages for optic nerve diseases clinically, a hue cancellation method was applied. In doing this, the mixing complementary color method (1, 2) was applied for up to 10° of the visual field.

METHOD

The apparatus used for this study was a three channel Maxwellian view optical system. These channels provided two 1° diameter circular test fields (500 nm and 680 nm) superimposed in the center of an 8° white circular background field. The light source was a 150 W xenon arc with a suitable stable power supply. Narrow-band (7 nm half-band width) interference filters were used for both test lights. The observers' pupils were dilated with 1%

Heijl, A. and Greve, E.L. (eds.), Proceedings of the 6th Int. Visual Field Symposium.
© *1985, Dr W. Junk Publishers, Dordrecht, The Netherlands. ISBN 978-94-010-8932-6*

tropicamide. Their fixation was controlled by a small red light from an accessary system. The biting board was adjusted at each eccentric position in order to allow the test and the background light to pass directly through the center of the pupil. The intensity of both of the background and the green (500 nm) test light was fixed at the luminance of 1000 photopic trolands. The red (680 nm) test light was super-imposed on this green test light. Then, the discrimination limens were determined by increasing the intensity of the red test light until the observer reported a visible red color and then decreasing the red test light until the observer reported a visible green color. This procedure was repeated at least five times until the results became stable in each retinal position.

RESULTS

The red/green hue cancellation ranges were measured along the horizontal meridian in the temporal retina at every degree out to 10°. The results for the two normal observers (K.K. on the left and J.N. on the right) are shown in Fig. 1. The discrimination limens for both red and green in terms of red/green ratios were plotted as a function of degrees in eccentricity. The upper solid lines for both observers represent the average limens for red (i.e., the point at which red was reported visible), while the lower solid lines show the average limens for green (i.e., the point at which green was reported visible). The error bar limits show the ±1 SD of five measurements. The pattern for both normal observers showed similar trends, that is, the red/green hue cancellation ranges widened and higher red/green ratios were obtained with an increase in eccentricity. Also, the observer K.K. showed wider ranges of error bars with an increase in eccentricity.

The results for the patient are shown in Fig. 2. The patient has optic neuritis in both eyes with the left eye being more affected. The mean values with error bars, connected with solid lines in terms of red/green ratios, were plotted as a function of degrees in eccentricities. The red and green hue cancellation range for observer K.K. was shown by the dotted lines in this figure for comparison. The limens for the right eye (shown on the left) in terms of red/green ratios for both red and green showed similar values up to 4 degrees and began to fall at 5 degrees. Beyond 5° the patient could not perceive the stimulus as green even with the red light removed. The results for the left eye (shown on the right) showed a wide range of hue cancellation even at the fovea, with even higher red/green ratio and wider ranges obtained at 1°. Beyond 1°, the patient could not perceive the stimulus as green even in the complete absence of the red light.

DISCUSSION

The purpose of this experiment was to determine whether or not the hue cancellation method using a background field could be applied to investigate opponent color damages in optic nerve diseases. The patient studied in this

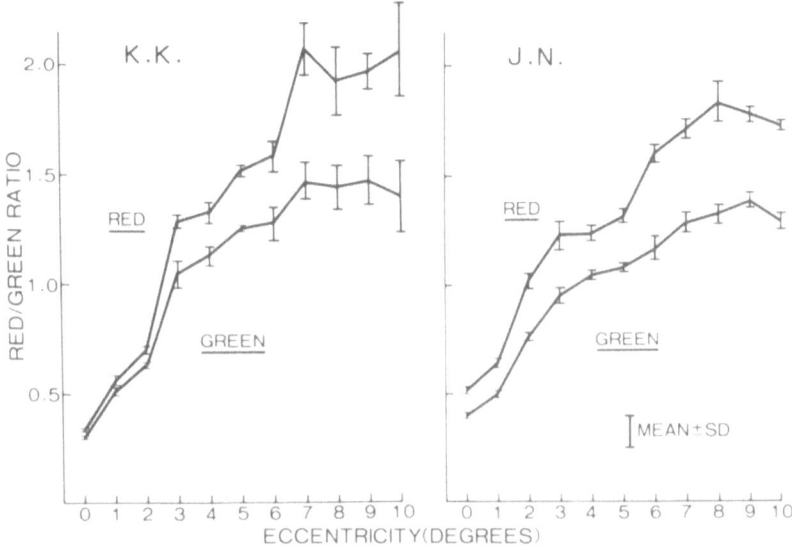

Fig. 1. The red/green hue cancellation ranges for the two normal observers K.K. (on the left) and J.N. (on the right).

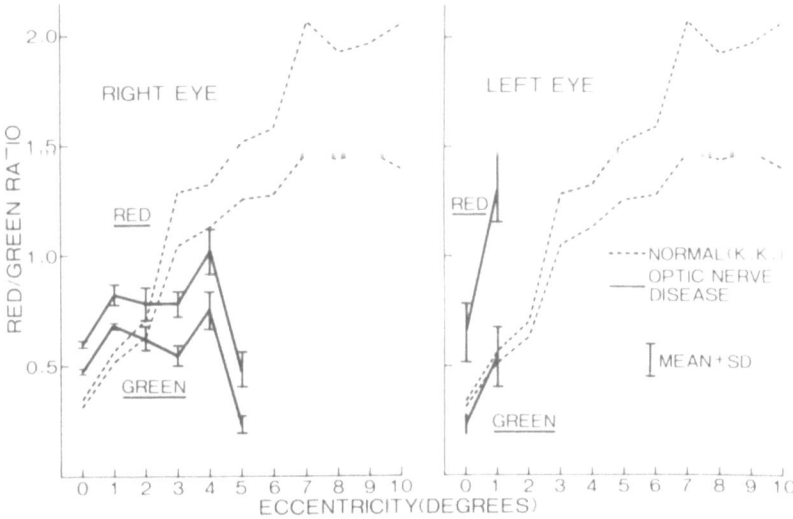

Fig. 2. The red/green hue cancellation ranges for the patient who has optic neuritis in both eyes with the left eye being more affected. The dotted lines indicate the results for one of the normal observers (K.K.).

experiment showed normal Rayleigh equation for both eyes with a Nagel model I anomaloscope. But using the red/green hue cancellation method,

257

abnormal findings were obtained. Therefore, it is felt that this method can be useful in investigating opponent color damages in optic nerve diseases.

REFERENCES

1. Connors, M.M. & Kinney, J.A.S. Relative red-green sensitivity as a function of retinal position. J. Opt. Soc. Am. 52 (1): 81–82 (1962).
2. Stevens, S.S. The relation of saturation to the size of the retinal image. Am. J. Psychol. 46: 70–79 (1934).

Author's address:
Kenji Kitahara
Department of Ophthalmology
19-18 Nishi-Shinbashi 3-chome, Minato-ku, Tokyo,
Japan

INCREMENT THRESHOLD VERSUS INTENSITY CURVES FOR RODS

KENJI KITAHARA, RYUTARO TAMAKI, JUN NOJI, ATSUSHI
KANDATSU and HIROSHI MATSUZAKI

(Tokyo, Japan)

ABSTRACT

The increment threshold versus intensity (t.v.i.) curve for rods was studied using Stiles' two color threshold technique at $10°$ temporal retina on two normal observers. The results show that the t.v.i. curves for rods for both observers were shallower than the t.v.i. curves for rods which Stiles (1939) (1) described. The possibility that the t.v.i. curve for rods may consist of two brances was suggested. In order to examine the results with the Field Additivity Law, the t.v.i. curve for rods for a 430 nm test on a 480 nm background, and bichromatic mixtures of fields of 480 nm and 598 nm were measured at $10°$ temporal retina. In this field mixture experiment, the increment threshold for rods obeyed the Field Additivity Law.

INTRODUCTION

In a previous paper (Kitahara (2), 1982) we studied the increment threshold versus intensity (t.v.i.) curves for cones at retinal eccentricities of up to $10°$ to lay the ground work for theoretically sound color perimetry.

In the present experiments, the t.v.i. curves for rods were studied using Stiles' two color threshold technique.

METHOD

A three channel Maxwellian view optical system was used in this study. The light source was a 150 W xenon arc lamp. A $1°$ diameter circular test light was superimposed in the center of an $8°$ circular main background field. In the mixture experiment, an auxiliary background field was superimposed on the main field. The test light was exposed for 200 msec every two seconds. Narrow band (7 nm half band width) interference filters were used for the test and also for both the main and auxiliary background lights. A small red light served as the fixation point, with the test light $10°$ to its nasal side along the horizontal meridian. The biting board was adjusted in order to

Heijl, A. and Greve, E.L. (eds.), Proceedings of the 6th Int. Visual Field Symposium.
© *1985, Dr W. Junk Publishers, Dordrecht, The Netherlands. ISBN 978-94-010-8932-6*

allow the test flash and the background lights to pass through the center of the pupil.

Measurements were made on the right eye of two normal male trichromats. Their pupils were well dilated with 1% tropicamide. Prior to a series of measurements the observers were dark-adapted for one hour. Then they were adapted to each background light for one min plus whatever additional time was needed for the measured results to become stable. For a measurment, the intensity of the test flash was adjusted by the subjects and the test thresholds were measured at least five times for each background condition using the adjustment method. The radiances of the test flash and the background lights were determined with a calibrated PIN-10 silicon photodiode (United Detector Technology) for each experiment.

RESULTS

The t.v.i. curves were measured for a 478 nm test on a 480 nm background at $10°$ temporal retina. Figure 1 shows the results of the t.v.i. curves for observer K.K. (on the left) and J.N. (on the right). The left ordinate gives the log test intensity at threshold (log photons sec^{-1} deg^{-2}) while the abscissa specifies the background intensity (log photons sec^{-1} deg^{-2}). Each circle represents the mean value of five measurements. The arrows indicate the absolute threshold for cones for each observer. These values were determined by measuring the dark adaptation curve for a 478 nm test flash. The t.v.i. curves obtained for rods both observers showed almost the same pattern. Looking at these results, it could be said that the t.v.i. curves for rods for both observers consist of one branch. But, compared to the t.v.i. curve for rods which Stiles (1939) described, these curves for rod for both observers were shallower than Stiles' t.v.i. curve which is shown by the solid line in this figure. Furthermore, it was found that one of these t.v.i. curves has a very slight kink. Because of these findings, it was felt that there exists the possibility of t.v.i. curves for rods consisting of two branches. Possible upper branches for both observers are shown by the dotted lines. This dotted line also indicates Stiles' (1939) t.v.i. curve for rods.

In order to examine the field-additivity for the π_0 t.v.i. curve, the t.v.i. curves for a 430 nm test on a 480 nm background, and bichromatic mixture of fields of 480 nm and 598 nm were measured at $10°$ temporal retina. The t.v.i. curve obtained for a 430 nm test on a 480 nm background for rods showed almost the same pattern as the t.v.i. curve for a 478 nm test on a 480 nm background. Then, the 480 nm backgrounds were fixed at two different background intensities, one of which was in the lower branch and the other in the upper branch of the π_0 t.v.i. curve. Then a series of 598 nm fields of increasing radiance were superimposed and the threshold was measured for each mixture. Figure 2 shows the results of the field-mixture experiment. The dotted line indicate Stiles' t.v.i. curve for rods. In this field-mixture experiment for the π_0 t.v.i. curve, the increment threshold for rods obeyed the Field Additivity Law.

260

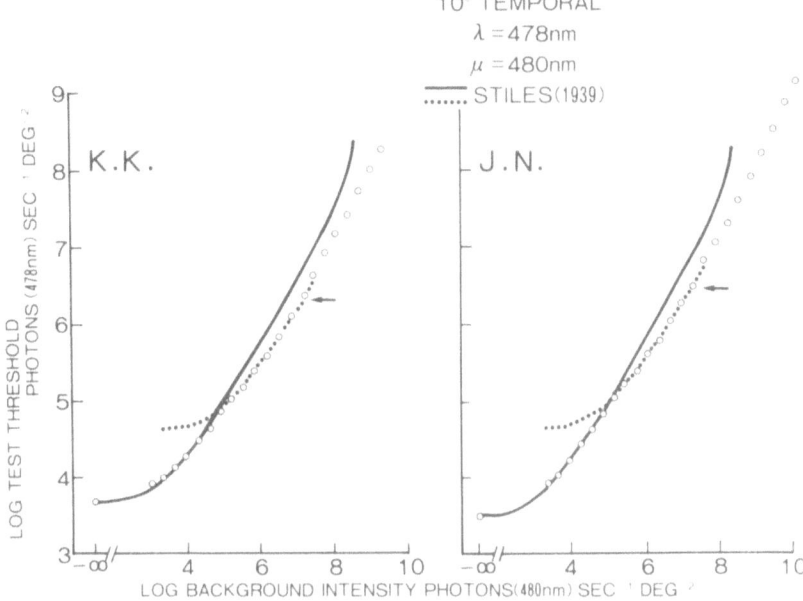

Fig. 1. The t.v.i. curves for a 478 nm test on a 480 nm background at 10° temporal retina for observer K.K. (on the left) and J.N. (on the right). The arrows indicate the absolute threshold for cones for each observer. Both the solid line and the dotted line show the t.v.i. curve for rods of Stiles (1939).

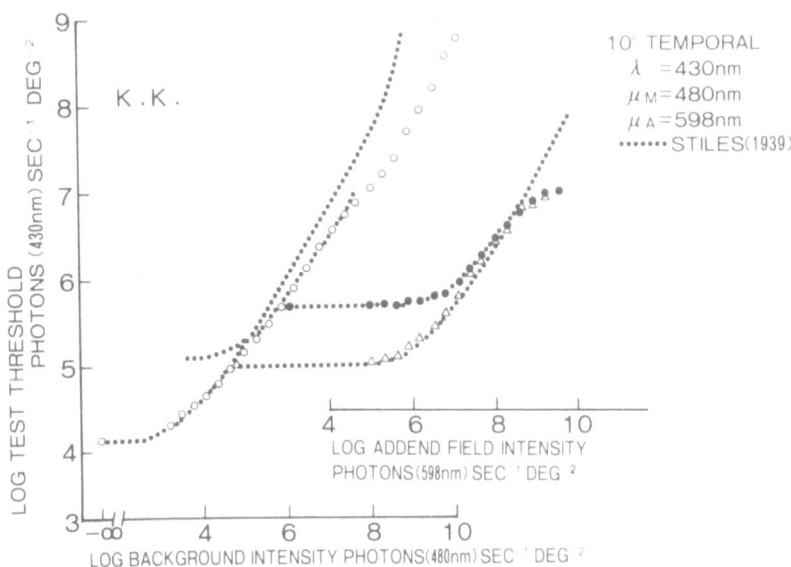

Fig. 2. The results of the field-mixture experiment. The dotted lines indicate Stiles' t.v.i. curve for rods (1939).

DISCUSSION

Stiles (1939) showed the t.v.i. curve for rods as being shallower than the t.v.i. curve for cones. Our results showed the t.v.i. curves for rods even more shallow than the t.v.i. curves which Stiles showed. The reason for this difference may lie in the fact that somewhat different experimental conditions were used. After careful study of these results, it is felt that the possibility that the t.v.i. curve for rods may consist of two branches is one that cannot be discarded. This is a possibility that may need to be investigated further.

In order to investigate the detection properties in this t.v.i. curve, the field mixture experiment was conducted. The wavelengths for the test light and both background fields selected were from one of the combinations that Pugh (1976) (3) used in investigating the field-additivity for the π_1 mechanism. In this field-mixture experiment, the π_0 t.v.i. curve obeyed the Field Additivity Law. This suggests that the t.v.i. curve obtained in this experiment is determined by one class of receptors (rod receptors).

REFERENCES

1. Stiles, W.S. The directional sensitivity of the retina and the spectral sensitivities of the rods and cones, Proc. Roy. Soc. (London), B127, 64 (1939).
2. Kitahara, K., Tamaki, R., Noji, J., Kandatsu, K. and Matsuzaki, M. Extrafoveal Stiles' mechanisms, Doc. Ophthalmol. Proc. Series 35: 397–403 (1982).
3. Pugh, E., The nature of the π_1 mechanism of W.S. Stiles, J. Physiol. 257: 713 (1976).

Author's address:
Kenji Kitahara
Department of Ophthalmology
The Jikei University School of Medicine
19-18 Nishi-Shinbashi 3-chome, Minato-ku, Tokyo,
Japan

SUPRATHRESHOLD RED-GREEN TEMPORAL RESPONSIVENESS ACROSS THE VISUAL FIELD

LUCIA R. RONCHI and VANNA GALASSI PRINCIPE

(*Florence, Italy*)

ABSTRACT

Two pulses of different hues, red and green, are delivered in succession. The task consists in matching their brightnesses, at various eccentricities, and under different degrees of defocus. Although highly skilled, our observers exhibit a 'training' effect, in that the red source appears increasingly brighter than the green one, in subsequent sessions. The dependence on presentation order represents one of the difficulties met in the photometric specification of perimetric tests. The duration of our pulses (800 ms) is probably not long enough to apply a 'steady state' photometry. The implications in perimetric testing with interruped light (e.g. flash-and-recovery-cycle technique) still wait elucidation.

AIM OF THE WORK

The 5th IPS Circular of Research Group of Colour Perimetry (8) tackled, amongst others, the photometric specifications for achromatic increment threshold perimetry on coloured background. In particular, the comparison of two stimuli of different dominant wavelengths was suggested. In supra-threshold perimetry, the problem is further complicated by the brightness-luminance discrepancy. Some technical solutions to overcome this in central vision have been suggested (5). In extrafoveal vision there are difficulties because 'spectral sensitivity is locus specific and changes with . . . recording procedure' (3), the number of colour perimetry parameters is large (2), and the inter- and intra-observer variability is known to be large. Suprathreshold perimetry is of importance in some occupations, because of the role of colour vision in speeding the search process (ref. 1, p. 297), and the quality of colour vision depends critically on stimulus size (ref. 2, p. 384).

The data obtained in the present experiment aim at affording a contribution of possible practical relevance, imbedded in a controversial theoretical substrate (6, 7).

Heijl, A. and Greve, E.L. (eds.), Proceedings of the 6th Int. Visual Field Symposium.
© 1985, Dr W. Junk Publishers, Dordrecht, The Netherlands. ISBN 978-94-010-8932-6

MATERIALS AND METHOD

Source: a square raster, where eight red LEDs (HLMP 0300) and eight green LEDs (HLMP 0500) are intermingled. The chromaticity coordinates are: $x = 0.42$; $y = 0.45$ and $x = 0.72$ and $y = 0.28$, respectively. The intercentre (between adjacent LEDs) distance is 40 min. of arc, the raster diagonal 4.4 degrees (the viewing distance being 33 cm). The background $(1 \text{ cd/m}^2$ luminance) is lit by daylight fluorescent tubes.

Calibration: performed by placing the detector of an EG.G Photometer Radiometer System, Mod. 450, at eye's place. Illuminations are of the order of 10^{-2} lux, when measured for unlimited exposure.

Observers: three normal subjects (ages: 36; 39; 55), highly experienced in matter of visual research, were tested monocularly.

Method: two flashes of equal duration (800 ms) and different hues are delivered in succession (interpulse interval practically zero), the one flash being all the red LEDs, and the other all the green LEDs. Contiguous retinal areas are therefore stimulated by each pulse. In some presentations, the red flash comes first, in others the green one. Green illuminance (E_g) is kept the same throughout the whole experiment (log $E_g = 2.155$). The red illuminance is varied, from trial to trial, in steps less than 0.1 log unit. The task consists in telling whether the red flash is brighter, less bright, the same brightness as the green one. Red illuminance E_r, at the brightness match, is recorded by the use of constant stimulus method and Probit Analysis. When desired, a defocussing lens is placed close to the eye, perpendicularly to the line joining the center of the raster to the center of the pupil.

FINDINGS AND DISCUSSION

(a) The dependence on eccentricity is shown in Fig. 1 (which refers to the red-before-green presentation order): the red illuminance needed to match a given green pulse decreases as the distance from the fovea increases.

(b) The dependence on 'training' (recall that our subjects are highly skilled) leads to need for the red LED to be made dimmer to achieve a brightness match. This is shown, for instance, in Fig. 1 (VP' and VP", data recorded by the same observer, in two sessions one month far apart from one another), and in Fig. 2, where observer LR exhibits a shift of 0.7 log units across a few months. By considering, in addition, the strong inter-individual differences in response level (Fig. 1), one sees how difficult the problem of peripheral photometric specification is. Note, paradoxically, that the standard foveal response seems to hold even at large eccentricities, E_r being very close to E_g. This applies particularly in the preliminary sessions.

(c) The dependence on the presentation order has been investigated by presenting, in alternation, in the same session, a red-before-green and a green-before-red pair, every other parameter being equal. The contribution to brightness of the red still depends on whether it is shown before or after the green. (The dependencies on both eccentricity and degree of blur cannot be described here, for the sake of space.) This fact is probably related to a

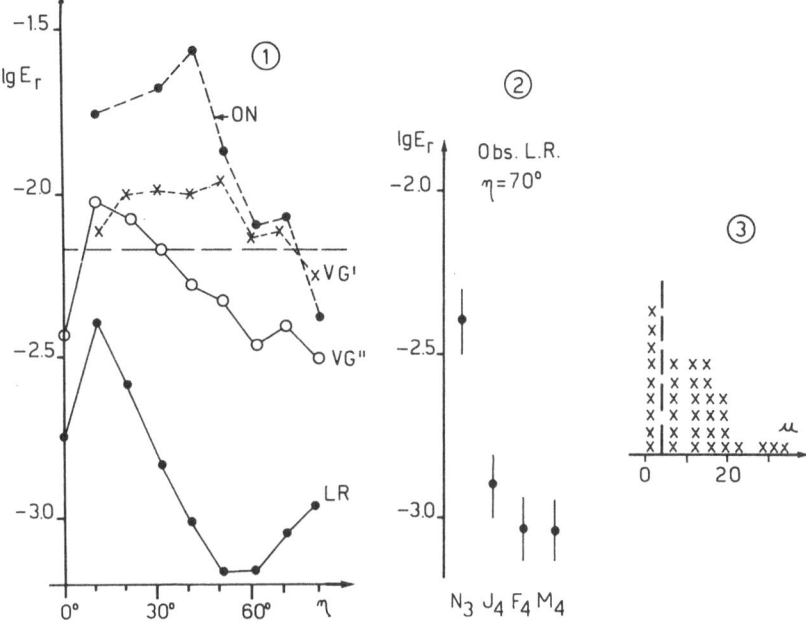

Fig. 1. Abscissae: retinal eccentricity (horizontal meridian, nasal retina). Ordinates: log red illuminance (E_r, in lux), at the brightness match. The illuminance of the (fixed) green pulse is at the level of the (horizontal) broken line. Labels: the observers. Dashes: 1st and 2nd sessions.

Fig. 2. Log red illuminance, at the brightness match, for the same observer, in four successive sessions (capital letter, the month; labels 3, 4, the year, 1983 or 1984).

Fig. 3. Frequency histograms of estimates of u-statistics. The effect of presentation order is significant ($P = 0.05$) for points at the right of the broken line.

difference in pulse response shapes. The rod contribution to the green response (but not to the red one) does not fully explain the effect above, since even in foveal vision the sequential presentation order is a factor of relevance (ref. 1, p. 334). The average difference in liminal log E_r values is found to be 0.21 ± 0.12 l.u. outside 45°. By applying a strengthened chi-square test (4), statistics u is found to lie above the significance level in the majority of cases.

(d) The effect of retinal blur is visualized in Fig. 4: the plot of log E_r versus the dioptric power of the defocussing lens changes in shape, when passing from the fovea to the periphery, being either inverted-U-shaped, or U-shaped or flat, or exhibiting a slowly declining trend. The eccentricities where the transitions from one to another shape occur, depend on the orientation of the tested meridian. The different shaped curves may be due to the enlargement of the image area due to defocus. A bias is due to the intrinsic differences in the sizes of red and green images, being differentially focussed because of eye chromatic aberration. The size of the raster was chosen to ensure adequate peripheral responses covering at least the whole extent on one peripheral receptor unit.

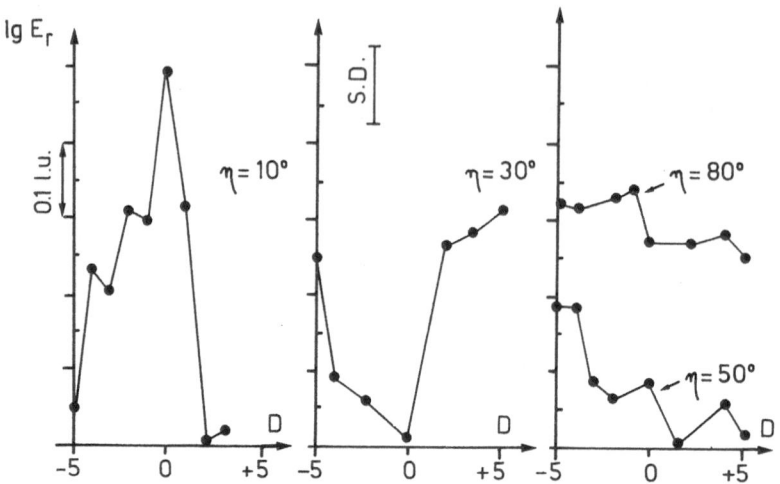

Fig. 4. Abscissae: degree of defocus of extrafoveal image, in dioptres. Ordinates: log red illuminance, at the brightness match. Label denotes eccentricity (horizontal meridian). Observer, L.R.

CONCLUDING REMARKS

The photopic photometry allows, for instance, to regulate two flashes of different hues (red and green), to exhibit the same luminance. If these flashes are now presented to the peripheral retina, the brightness match may not exist. The discrepancy may be even as large as 0.5–0.7 log units. The question arises whether it is legitimate to neglect this deviation, or whether the photometric assessment of peripheral testing requires an evaluation 'ad hoc'. Of interest, from the ergo-ophthalmological stand point, seems the fact that the situation in the plane where the eye is at focus differs from those in other planes, both closer and farther from the observer, in terms of red compared to green. Hence, the photometric assessment is bi- but not tri-dimensional!

REFERENCES

1. Boynton, R.M. Human Color Vision, Holt-Rinehart-Winston, New York (1979).
2. Carlow, T.J., Flynn, J.T. and Shipley, T. Color perimetry parameters, Doc. Ophthal. Proc. Ser. 14: 429–439 (1976).
3. Hedin, A. and Verriest, G. Is color perimetry useful? Doc. Ophthal. Proc. Ser. 26: 161–184 (1981).
4. Kincaid, W.M. The combination of 2 × m contingency tables, Biometrics, 18: 224–228 (1962).
5. Kinney, J.A.S. Brightness of colored self-luminous displays, Color Res. Apll. 8(2): 82–89 (1983).
6. Kuyk, T.K. Spectral sensitivity of the peripheral retina to large and small stimuli, Vision Res. 22: 1293–1297 (1982).

7. Uchikawa, P., Kaiser, P.K. and Uchikawa, K. Color vision deficiency in the peripheral retina, Color Res. Appl. 7(3): 264–269 (1982).
8. Verriest, G. Chairman's Report on the Answers and Comments on the 3rd Questionnaire issued by the IPS Res. Group on 'Colour Perimetry', 5th Circular, June 1st (1978).

Author's address:
Istituto Nazionale di Ottica, ,
6, Largo E. Fermi,
50125 Florence, Italy

267

CONSIDERATION ON STILES π MECHANISMS IN GLAUCOMATOUS BJERUM AREA

J.L. VOLA, P. GASTAUT and B. GONDOIS

(*Marseille, France*)

ABSTRACT

Fundamental colour mechanisms were explored by means of the Stile's two colours threshold method in the Bjerrum area of glaucomatous patients with early perimetric alterations.

To standardise normal curves: 21 normal subjects were tested and 18 patients were examined. In all the cases alterations of π_4 (medium-wavelength-green-mechanism) and sometimes π_1 (short wavelength-blue-mechanism) were detected but the red mechanism: long wavelength mechanism π_5 was always found normal.

This method suggests that in glaucoma peripheral colour mechanisms defects seem to precede field impairments.

The aim of this work which is not really a perimetric problem is to investigate the paracentral colour mechanisms at the intersection of the 15° parallel and the 45° temporal meridian in the Bjerrum area, when early perimetric alterations appear in open angle glaucomas.

The Stile's colour technique that we have used since 1974, seems to be an appropriate method for evidencing the extra-foveal fundamental colour mechanisms (Stiles, Kitahara et al). The long (red π_5), medium (green π_4) and short (blue π_1) wavelength sensitive mechanisms are respectively obtained with 650 nm light adaptation background and are represented by thresholds versus radiance (T.V.R. curves). The fixation point's enlargement up to 11° of Tubingen perimeter was used as adaptation background. A circular test of 11 mm $(1, 59°)$ presented for 500 ms was superimposed on the background. The test thresholds were plotted after 10 mn of dark adaptation starting at the lowest intensity of the background.

On the extrafoveal area as Stiles and Kitahara et al. show it, a new branch at the beginning of the light adaptation appears and represents the rod mechanism called π_0..

To standarise the normal curves, 21 normal subjects were tested: 11 from 30 to 50 years old and 10 from 50 to 65.

Heijl, A. and Greve, E.L. (eds.), Proceedings of the 6th Int. Visual Field Symposium.
© 1985, Dr W. Junk Publishers, Dordrecht, The Netherlands. ISBN 978-94-010-8932-6

18 patients with chronic open angle with slight early alterations of the Bjerrum area were examined. The age of these patients was between 44 and 80.

The observer was asked to fix a red fixation point adjusted on the visual field diagram of the apparatus in order to investigate the chosen area.

RESULTS

(a) Normal subjects: means of 21 curves.

The π_5 T.V.R. curve is a single curve with a high initial threshold with regard to the other T.V.R. curves. The first part of the curves is flat.

The slope rises smoothly and regularly.

The first standard deviation is only 0.2 log units.

(b) The π_4 T.V.R. curve medium wavelength sensitive mechanisms obtained with the combination 525/650 presents two main branches: the lower branch corresponding to rod senstivity (π_0) and a second branch corresponding to π_4. The first standard deviation is between 0.4 and 0.3 log units.

(c) With the 480/650 combination the T.V.R. curve included 3 branches. π_0, π_4 and π_1. The standard deviation varies from 0.4 to 0.3 log units.

The π_1 curve is flat as shown by Kitahara, and short because the apparatus has not enough high radiance to define completely this mechanism.

(d) Pathologic cases.

To approach the pathologic results we have to define a semeiology of the T.V.R. curves: with regard to the first standard deviation.

1. Raising the initial threshold,

2. Raising of the thresholds with a steeper gradient of one or more mechanisms corresponding to the branches of the curve and displacement of the curve upward and on the left of the graph,

3. Shortening of one or several branches of the curves.

The pathologic cases were divided into 3 groups:

(a) exclusion of the blind spot,

(b) Seidel scotoma with blind spot exclusion,

(c) Seidel and pericentral scotomas.

We were unable to find an aggravation of the pathologic curves with the increasing defects of the Bjerrum area.

But in all these pathologic groups we observed:

1) A prominence of π_0 with a shortening of π_4 and π_1, and 2) in some cases the initial threshold of π_0 is increased. The curve the most often impaired is the 480/650 (π_0, π_4 and π_1).

The curves are shifted upward and on the left of the graph by the increasing thresholds. The initial thresholds of π_4 and sometimes π_1 are increased.

The π_4 curve given by the 524/650 combination is less impaired and in our 21 cases the π_5 curve is always normal and in the range of the first standard deviation.

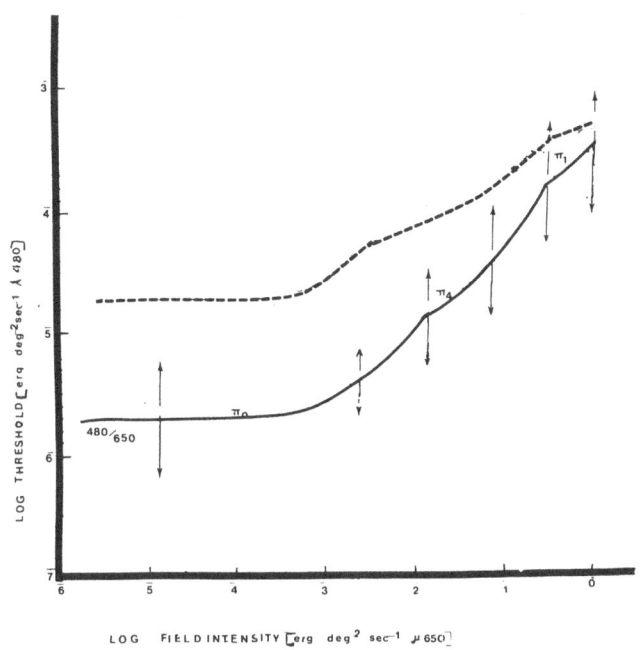

LOG THRESHOLD [erg deg⁻²sec⁻¹ Å 480]

$480/650$

π_0

π_4

π_1

LOG FIELD INTENSITY [erg deg² sec⁻¹ μ 650]

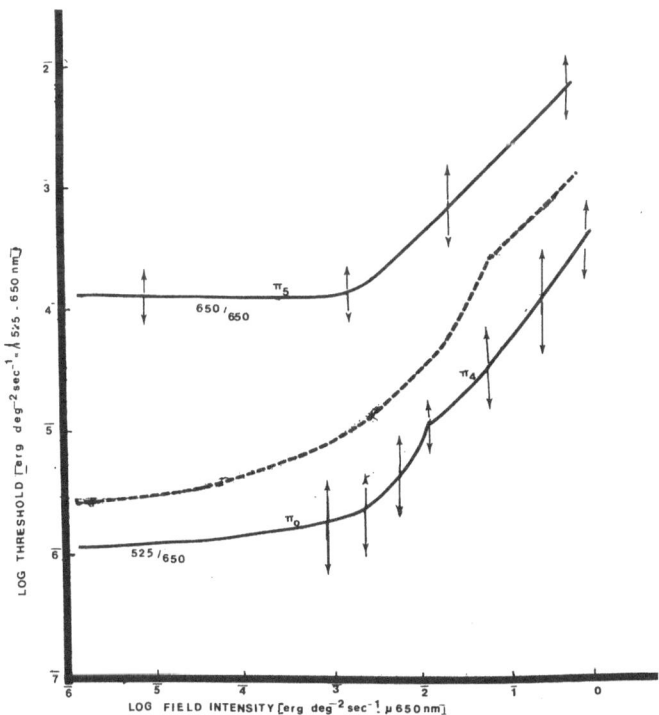

LOG THRESHOLD [erg deg⁻²sec⁻¹ Å 525 - 650 nm]

$650/650$

π_5

$525/650$

π_4

π_0

LOG FIELD INTENSITY [erg deg⁻²sec⁻¹ μ 650 nm]

DISCUSSION

The papers of Kitahara and associates give us a very good opportunity to discuss our results.

In spite of a different method used by the authors the π_0, π_4 and π_1 were identified.

The shapes of the curves plotted by Kitahara are flatter, except for π_1 and the branch of rods is more prominent. But in comparison with the fovea curves recorded, a good agreement was found between the two works. An important discrepancy is the evidence of a rod branch on the π_5 Kitahara curves.

The difference could be perhaps explained by the time of the dark adaptation: 30 mn for Kitahara, 10 mn for us.

Whatever methods are used the colour mechanisms on an extra foveal could be explored.

Concerning the pathologic cases: in this investigation where there are only early and slight alterations of the visual field in the open angle glaucomas it could be said that:

1. The long wavelength mechanism stayed strictly normal, no matter what defect was found.

2. In all the cases, alterations of π_4 and sometimes π_1 mechanisms can be detected and are characterized by an increase of either the initial threshold or by all thresholds with a displacement of the curve upward and on the left of the graph. A steeper slope of the curve can be noticed.

The 480/650 T.V.R. curve is the most often affected.

It can be concluded that the T.V.R. curves are interesting in the diagnosis of early impairments in open angle glaucomas. Conversely it could be suggested that peripheric colour mechanisms defects precede early visual field alterations.

REFERENCES

Kitahara, K., Tamaki, R., Noji, J., Kandatsu, A. and Matsuzaki, H. Extra foveal Stiles' π mechanisms. Doc. Ophthalmol. Proc. Series. 35: 397–403 (1982).

Kitahara, H., Kitahara, K., Irie, J., Shirakawa, A. and Matsuzaki, P. Extra foeveal Stiles' π 5 mechanisms. Doc. Ophthalmol. Proc. Series 26: 185–191 (1980).

Stiles, W.S., Colour vision: The approach throught increment threshold sensitivity. Proc. N.A.S. Vol. 45 (1959).

Vola, J.L., Cornu, L., Chovet, M. and Saracco, J.B. Applications Cliniques de la Technique des Doubles Seuils Colorés de Stiles. Ann. Therap. Clin. Ophthal. 25: 308–312 (1974).

Vola, J.L., Leprince, G., Langle, D., Cornu, L. and Saracco, B. Preliminary results on the clinical interpretation of Stiles two colour thresholds method. Mod. Probl. Ophthal. 19: 266–269 (1978).

Author's address:
Docteur J. Vola
38, rud Jean Mermoz,
13008 – Marseille, France

COLOR PERIMETRY WITH A COLOR NAMING METHOD

M. IKEDA, N. SEKIGUCHI and S. SHIOIRI

(*Yokohama, Japan*)

ABSTRACT

Color visual fields were determined by a quantitative color naming method for test stimuli 450, 510, 570 and 650 nm, approximately representing unique blue, green, yellow and red. When one of the stimuli was presented at a certain retinal location, a subject estimated the amount of achromatic and chromatic components perceived in the stimulus, and estimated further the amount of unique hues. Three normal subjects participated in the experiment and their color visual fields were determined. The fields indicated a good hue perception at the fovea, a rapid decrease till about 20°, and a gradual decrease at a further periphery for blue, green and red unique hues. A gradual decrease from the fovea to the periphery was found for the yellow perception.

INTRODUCTION

In the color perimetry in which a colored stimulus is employed, we can ask various questions to subjects. One is a mere light sensation. Subjects may respond with 'yes' whenever they detect a light. The second is a color sensation. Subjects respond with 'yes' when they notice any color in the stimulus. The third is a hue perception. Subjects respond with 'hue-names' that they perceive in the stimulus. We can further ask them about the amounts of the hues.

Implications of results should differ depending on what response was given by subjects. In the past, the distinction was not necessarily clearly made or at least not shared in reports. Some old reports (1, 2), therefore, are not so much useful as commonly considered. New data with clear distinction are needed, but only few are available at the present to our knowledge (3). In the present paper quantitative color visual fields will be obtained with the color naming method.

EXPERIMENT

On to a hemi-spherical screen of diameter 60 cm, a test spot of diameter 2° arc of visual angle was projected through a small projecting optical unit whose

Heijl, A. and Greve, E.L. (eds.), Proceedings of the 6th Int. Visual Field Symposium.
© *1985, Dr W. Junk Publishers, Dordrecht, The Netherlands. ISBN 978-94-010-8932-6*

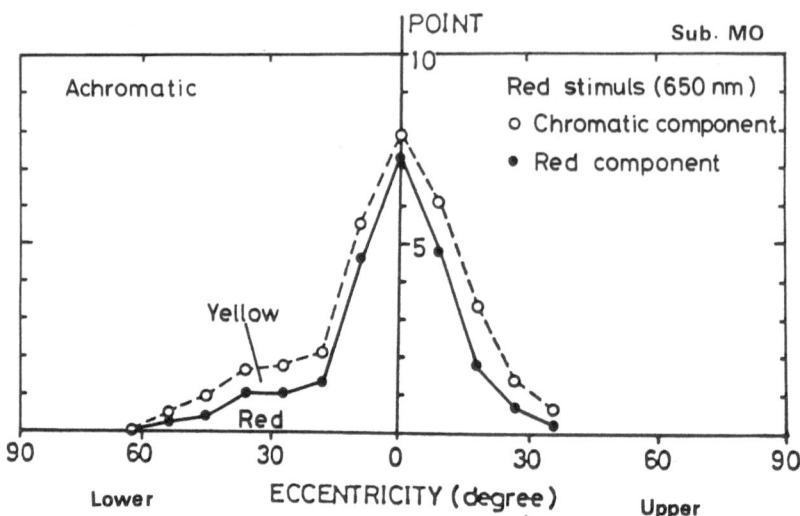

Fig. 1. Profile of the chromatic component for the red stimulus. Vertical direction. Subject, MO.

direction was controlled with a micro-computer. The optical unit was connected to a light guide through which lights of four different colors were supplied. Their wavelengths were 450, 510, 570 and 650 nm obtained through interference filters and corresponded approximately to the unique hues of blue, green, yellow and red, respectively. The test stimulus was presented along the twelve directions and at distances with 9° steps from the fovea. The luminance of the test stimuli was about 3 cd/m² . No background light was used.

The subject used his right eye located at the center of the hemi-spherical screen. He released a shutter by himself to have a test stimulus of 500 msec duration while fixating his eye to the center of the field. He estimated the amounts of achromatic and chromatic components perceived in the stimulus, and gave them points out of 10, such as 2 achromatic and 8 chromatic. He further estimated the amounts of unique hues in the chromatic component such as 3 yellow and 7 red, using also a total of 10 points. This stimulus was thus perceived as 2 achromatic, 8 chromatic with 2.4 yellow and 5.6 red. The subject could observe the stimulus repeatedly until he could reach the responses.

Locations and colors of test stimulus were randomly selected by the computer and the experiment continued until the entire visual field was covered. Three normal experienced subjects participated in the experiment.

RESULTS AND DISCUSSION

Figure 1 shows an example of profile of color naming response along a vertical direction. Each point is the average of 10 determinations. The

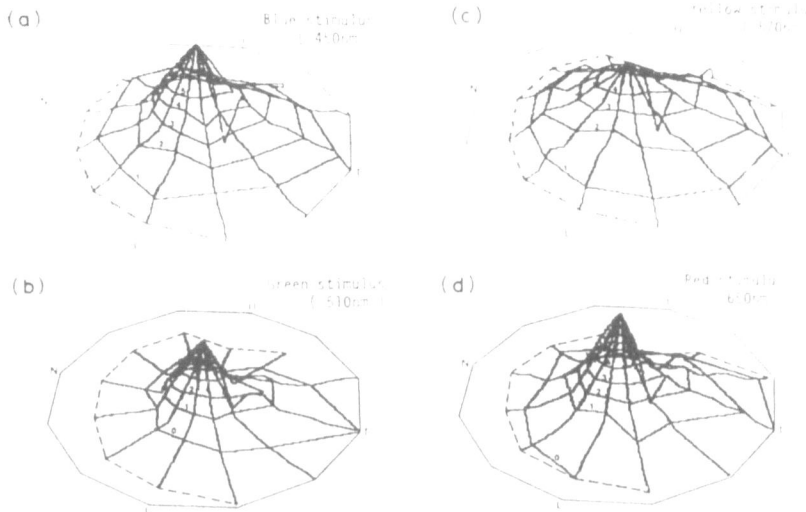

Fig. 2. Three dimensional display of four unique hues points from the subject NS. Dotted lines show the limit of light sensation. The curve of point 0 shows the limit of the unique hue sensation.

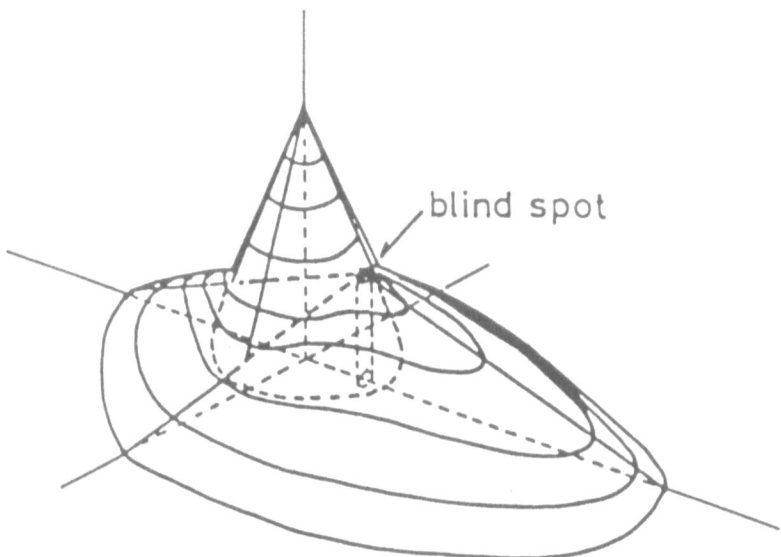

Fig. 3. A scheme of two layers construction of the color field.

achromatic component is represented by the area above the open circles and the chromatic component by the area below them. The chromatic

275

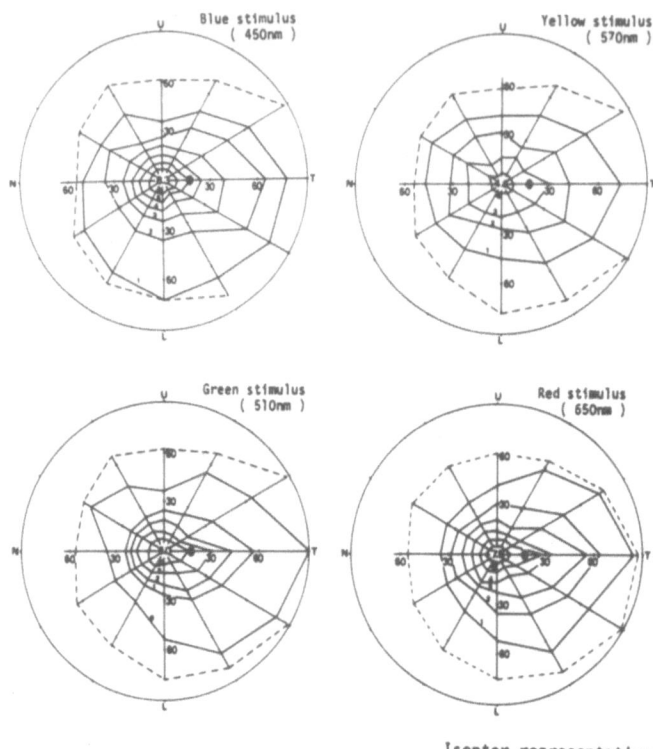

Unique color component

Sub. TF

Blue stimulus
(450nm)

Yellow stimulus
(570nm)

Green stimulus
(510nm)

Red stimulus
(650nm)

Isopter representation

Fig. 4. Isopter display of four unique hues components for the subject TF.

component shows a rapid decrease till about 20° from the fovea and a gradual decrease further out.

The filled circles represent quantities of the dominant unique hue. Therefore, the interval between the filled and open circles shows the amount of the secondary unique hue perceived in the chromatic component. It must be recalled, however, that the size of this interval depends upon the wavelengths chosen as the stimulus. If a stimulus were chosen such that its color exactly coincided with the unique red of this subject, the interval would have been zero.

Figure 2 is the three dimensional display of the four unique hues constructed from the profiles such as shown in Fig. 1. Numbers along contours indicate the points given to the unique hue. The property of the rapid-and-then-gradual decrease of amount of unique hue is quite evident, though the decrease of yellow hue is dominated by the gradual change and that of green hue by the rapid change, particularly at the nasal side.

The shape of these three dimensional representations suggests us two

276

underlying pyramids as schematically shown in Fig. 3. One sharp pyramid has its peak at the central fovea, while the other shallow pyramid has its peak at the papilla. This two layers composition might be explained along the embryological view point.

Figure 4 is the isopter display in which numbers indicate the points as in Fig. 2. If we compare the isopters for the point 1 among the unique hues, the yellow is the largest and the green is the smallest, but for the point 4 the red is the largest and the yellow the smallest. It is almost meaningless, therefore, to represent the color field by only one isopter for one unique hue such as done by OSA (2).

REFERENCES

1. Ferree, C.E. and Rand, G. Effect of size of stimulus on size and shape of color fields. Am. Jr. Ophthal. 10: 399–411 (1927).
2. Committee on Colorimetry, Optical Soc. of Amer. The science of color. 101–105, Crowel (1953).
3. Uchikawa, H., Kaiser, P.K. and Uchikawa, K. Color-discrimination perimetry. Color Res. and Appl. 7: 264–272 (1982).

Author's address:
Tokyo Institute of Technology,
Dept. of Information Processing,
Nagatsuta, Midori-ku,
Yokohama 227, Japan

A MODIFICATION OF THE GOLDMANN PERIMETER
DESIGNED FOR COLOUR PERIMETRY

EGILL HANSEN, BORGAR TØRRE OLSEN, THORSTEIN SEIM
and DONALD WORMALD
(*Oslo, Norway*)

With an increasing interest for quantitative colour perimetry it is felt desirable to obtain a better light transmission, especially in the short wave range. There is also a need for an accurate regulation of the exposure times used for the adapting field as well as for the presentation of coloured lights of the stimulus. This is necessary for studying the temporal effect during selective chromatic adaptation in the visual field. We have taken advantage of the regulation of the stimulus lights by the grey filter battery used in the Goldmann perimeter,

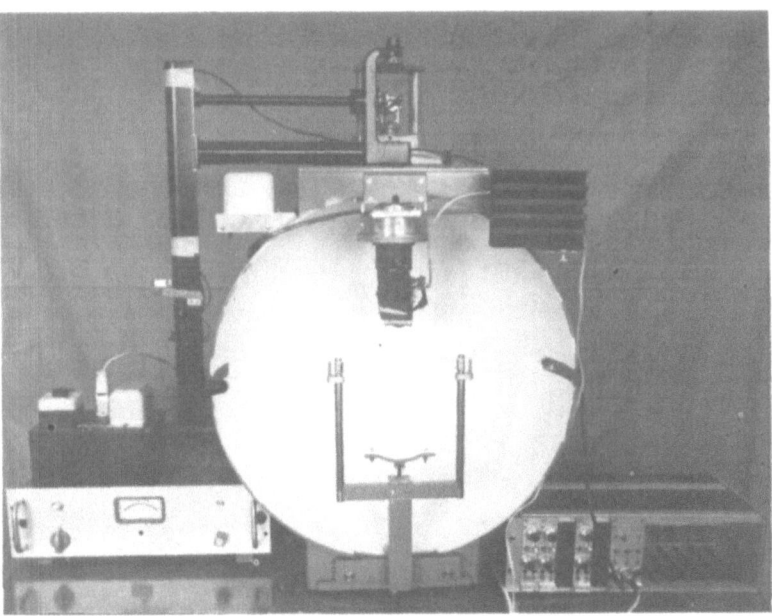

Fig. 1. A: Lamp house B: Cooling rib C: Inserted interference filter D: Electromagnetic shutter E: Regulated power supply and high voltage starting device F: Programmable timers.

Heijl, A. and Greve, E.L. (eds.), Proceedings of the 6th Int. Visual Field Symposium.
© 1985, Dr W. Junk Publishers, Dordrecht, The Netherlands. ISBN 978-94-010-8932-6

279

which has earlier been calibrated (Hansen and Seim 1978) and which has been essentially unchanged in later models of the apparatus.

In this modification of the perimeter the lamp has been changed with a Xenon arc lamp of 75 W giving a near ideal light source of great intensity. There is possibilities for accurate adjustments of the position of the lamp in relation to the optic system. A cooling rib is attached to the perimeter and connected to the lamp house by a heat pipe. At the same time a limited but highly intensive background field is obtained from the same light source by means of an optical system built into the lamp house. The field which measures 6–10 cm in diameter, can be set at any perimetric angle along the horizontal diameter. The maximum intensity of the adapting field (measured for white light) is approximately $5,000 \, cd/m^2$ and that of the stimulus light approximately $6,500 \, cd/m^2$. Presentation of the central stimulus field and the surround fields are regulated by means of two electro-magnetic shutters. Programmable timers control the duration and timing of the light stimuli. Interchangable interference filters are inserted in a slit in the projection arm of the apparatus. Spectral sensitivity measurements can be done in this way with a series of interference filters. The modified perimeter has been used for registration of Stiles' functions in the visual field. Experiments are being carried out with transient tritanopia phenomenon in normals as well as in patients with ocular pathology.

REFERENCE

Hansen, E. and Seim, T. Calibration of the Goldmann perimeter and accessories used in specific quantitative perimetry. Acta Ophthal 56: 241–51 (1978).

THE OCCUPATIONAL VISUAL FIELD: II. PRACTICAL ASPECTS: THE FUNCTIONAL VISUAL FIELD IN ABNORMAL CONDITIONS AND ITS RELATIONSHIP TO VISUAL ERGONOMICS, VISUAL IMPAIRMENT AND JOB FITNESS

GUY VERRIEST (EDITOR), IAN L. BAILEY, GIOVANNI CALABRIA,
EMILIO CAMPOS, RONALD P. CRICK, JAY M. ENOCH, BEN
ESTERMAN, ALAN C. FRIEDMANN, ADRIAN R. HILL,
MITSUO IKEDA, CHRIS A. JOHNSON, IAN OVERINGTON,
LUCIA RONCHI, SHINYA SAIDA, ANTONINA SERRA, SERGIO
VILLANI, ROBERT A. WEALE, MYRON L. WOLBARSHT and
MARIO ZINGIRIAN

ABSTRACT

This second portion of the official report from the IPS Task Committee on the Functional Visual Field describes the effects of age, refractive error and its correction, ocular and neuro-ophthalmic disease, hypoxia, drugs, physical exercise, environmental lighting and noise on the functional visual field. Relationships between the functional visual field and ergonomics are also discussed, particularly with regard to driving, piloting an airplane, control tasks, illumination engineering, optical instruments, visual display units, and the design of spectacles and other devices that partially obstruct or interfere with peripheral vision. A third section examines visual field loss as a form of visual impairment, especially with regard to the definitions of visual disability, low vision and blindness, the prediction of functional capabilities, and the design of treatment regimens. Relationships between visual field properties and job fitness are discussed in a fourth section, with an emphasis on existing regulations and how they might be improved for driving, aviation and other areas. The last report section consists of technical notes pertaining to testing distance, measurement of eye and head movements, assessment of the dynamic functional visual field, and detection of visual field defects within the context of industrial medicine and automobile driver licensing requirements.

The report was intended only as a review of the present knowledge about an interdisciplinary topic. It suggests lines along which progress may be directed, but does not include actual practical recommendations.

THE FUNCTIONAL VISUAL FIELD IN ABNORMAL CONDITIONS

This section will discuss abnormalities of both the observer and the environmental conditions of the observer's surroundings.

Heijl, A. and Greve, E.L. (eds.), Proceedings of the 6th Int. Visual Field Symposium.
© 1985, Dr W. Junk Publishers, Dordrecht, The Netherlands. ISBN 978-94-010-8932-6

In ergonomics and illumination engineering, younger and older *age* groups have to be considered as 'abnormalities' when reference is made to data obtained from young adult populations.

Under the conditions of clinical perimetry, teenagers have higher peripheral sensitivity and lower central sensitivity than adults, whereas elderly individuals have lower sensitivity throughout the visual field, but especially in the periphery (Verriest and Uvijls, 1977: see Fig. 1). This sensitivity loss is secondary to the large changes in crystalline lens transmittance properties (Weale, 1981) and to the reduced number of receptors (Marshall, 1984). It has already been reported in Part I of this report that extraction of information in the periphery is poorer for children than for adults, particularly in the presence of a foveal load or a competing non-visual task. Information about the functional visual field in the elderly is lacking, although it is known that the latency of saccadic eye movements is increased (Abel, Troost and dell'Osso, 1983). Also, longer reaction times (Surwillo, 1961) may be one of the main factors responsible for the deterioration of decision-making behavior.

With regard to visual anomalies, we will first consider the influence of *refractive error* on the functional visual field.

For static and dynamic orientation properties of visual behavior, peripheral vision is largely independent of refractive error, provided that stimulation is well above threshold (Leibowitz, Post and Ginsburg, 1980). However, for threshold detection conditions, all perimetrists are aware that retinal image blue due to uncorrected refractive error lowers visual resolution and increment threshold sensitivity, especially for smaller targets and more central visual field locations (Sloan, 1961; Fankhauser and Enoch, 1962; Serra, 1983; see Fig. 2). Refractive errors and their effects on vision remain consistent (less than 0.5 diopters of change) from the fovea out to about 30 degrees eccentricity. Beyond 30 degrees, there are significant 'off-axis' refractive errors, the correction of which does not improve visual resolution and increment thresholds, but does improve some specific visual functions such as sensitivity for movements of short duration (Post and Leibowitz, 1981). There is an interaction between the effects of practice and correction of refractive error in peripheral movement sensitivity, practice being more effective without correction (Johnson and Leibowitz, 1974). This suggests that such practice effects may be related to blur interpretation.

Correction of refractive error can be more harmful to the functional visual field than refractive error per se.

Indeed, because of their prismatic effect, plus lenses minify while minus lenses magnify the field of gaze corresponding to specific angular movements of the eye. By the same principle, the transition from the visual field seen through the lens to the visual field outside of the lens creates an 'annular scotoma' at the edge of a plus lens (not a true physiological scotoma since there is no gap in the retinal response to illumination, but a missing region of visual space pronounced by the

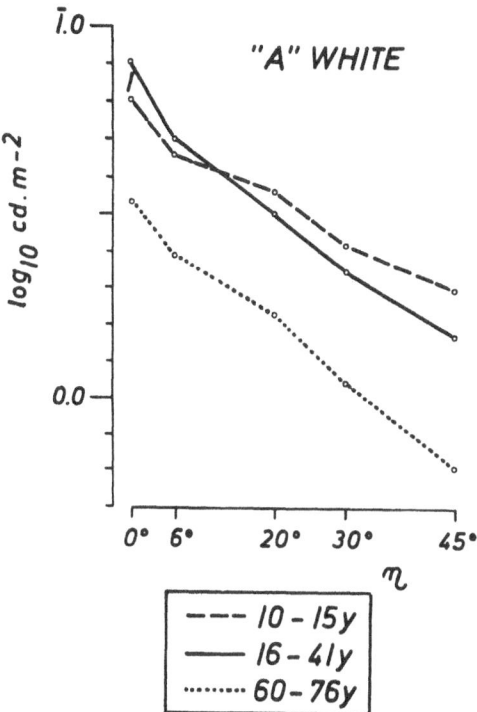

Fig. 1. Mean macular static increment threshold vs. eccentricity in three age groups of normal subjects. Tübingen perimeter, round target of 116′, background luminance of 10 cd.m⁻². From Verriest and Uvijls (1977).

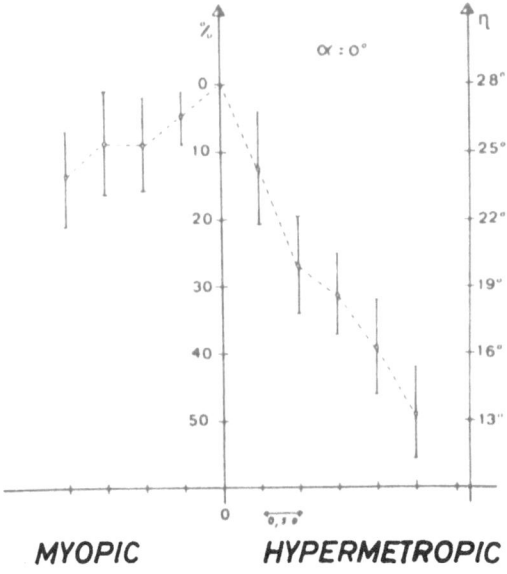

Fig. 2. Procentual and absolute change in mean radius of the Goldmann II/2 isopter on the horizontal meridian when changing refraction by means of glasses. From Serra (1983).

magnification of the scene through the lens). In the case of a minus lens, there is an annular zone of diplopia produced by the minification effect of the lens. The magnitude of this effect depends on the power of the lens and the vertex distance; the annular zone can reach an extent of 15 degrees. Spectacle frames create another blurred outline of an annular scotoma, which can achieve a size of 7.4 degrees in the case of a 4 mm rim.[*] The width of the spectacle frame scotoma must be added to the lens scotoma for a plus lens, and must be deducted from the diplopia ring associated with a minus correction (Hager, 1961a; see Fig. 3).

The wearer of high plus lenses is hampered by the reduction of visual fields and gaze fields, particularly when he has to clearly see objects away from the primary point of regard such as the steps of a descending staircase (see Fig. 4). Moreover, part of the 'annular scotoma' moves toward the fixation point as the eye moves away from the primary point of regard. This can result in the disappearance of the sought object (the 'jack in the box' phenomenon). In addition, vision becomes less distinct in peripheral gaze directions because of the optical abberations of the lens. Vision is distorted even when the subject turns his head without moving his eyes, since the prismatic effect increases towards the periphery of the lens to produce often a changing curvature to vertical contours (Bronner et al., 1983).

Most of the above-mentioned difficulties with the wearing of spectacles can be avoided by using better quality lenses, as the 4-drop lenses for aphakia, or, more effectively, by prescribing contact lenses. Following cataract extraction, an intraocular implant (pseudophakia) can also be used. Both hard and soft contact lenses provide a larger and less distorted visual field, with a more natural viewing environment for the patient with marked ametropia (see Fig. 5). In pseudophakia, peripheral visual acuity is somewhat better than for aphakia corrected by a spectacle lens (Meur, 1983) but the limits of the peripheral visual field can be reduced by about 10 degrees (Binkhorst, 1983).

---

[*]There is a distinction to be made between three kinds of restrictions that can be created by spectacles or other obstacles within the visual field. Let us consider the case of a simple aperture mounted in front of the eye. If one maintains central fixation and also has a pinpoint pupil the field of view will be determined by the angular size the apertures subtend at the center of the pupil. Next there is a field of gaze, the field over which foveal fixation can be achieved. The field of gaze is determined by the angular size of the aperture at the center of rotation of the eye. Clearly it is smaller than the field of view. Next there is what could be called 'the field of visibility' which is larger than the field of view. Should the observer move his eye so that he fixates towards the extreme right hand of the aperture, the eye pupil will translate towards the right hand side thereby enabling more of the left hand visual field to be seen. This means that objects to the left may become detectable only when the eye moves to the right. These three kinds of field become even more complicated when pupil diameter is taken into account (and for occupational visual field pupil size should be considered). The scotoma created by a 4 millimeter rim of a spectacle frame will, in object space, have a triangular cross section with its base at the rim of the spectacle frame and its apex some distance away. The apex of this triangular blind area will depend on the magnitude of the difference between the eye pupil and the width of the obstruction (Bailey).

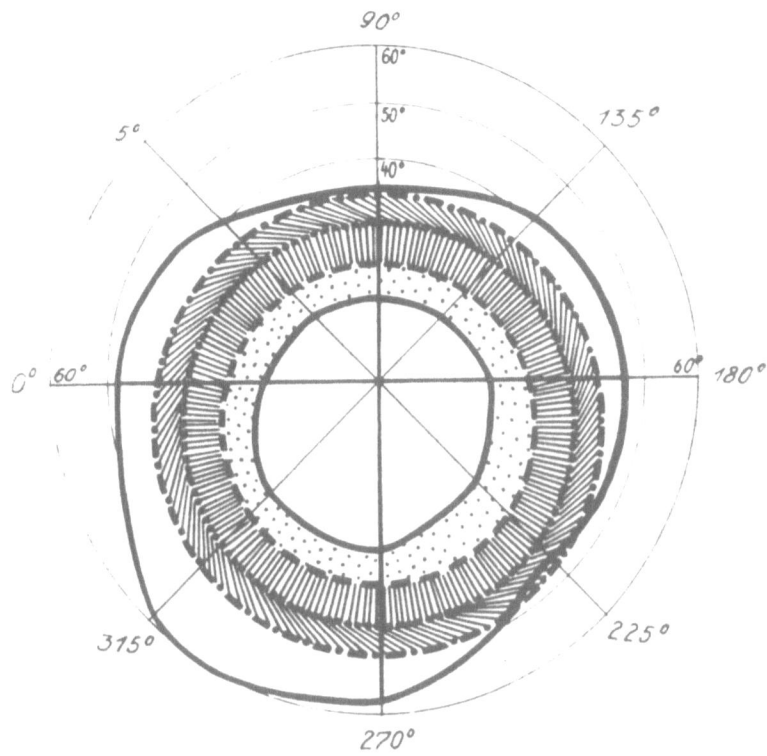

Fig. 3. Limitation of the field of gaze of an aphakic eye by a round glass of 10 dptr. ———— : gaze field without glass. — · — — : external limit of the frame scotoma. . . . . . inner limit of the frame scotoma. — — — : extreme outer limit of the gaze field left by the primatic effect. ———— : limit of the gaze field in a given observed case. From Hager (1961a).

With regard to tinted spectacle lenses, contact lenses and windshields, it should be noted that lighter shades of tint do not appreciably influence photopic vision (Verriest et al., 1981), although sensitivity thresholds can be augmented in mesopic and scotopic vision (Cristiani, 1981; Gloria and Sulli, 1981).

Let us now consider *ocular and neuro-ophthalmic disease.*

Aulhorn (1975) found that when fixation becomes eccentric in *maculopathies*, the macular scotoma generally shifts upward or to the right, with smaller scotomas usually shifting mostly to the right (Fig. 6), thereby not disturbing binocular vision. When the macular scotoma is larger, fixation is unstable and more peripheral.

Measurement of the individual size and shape of the functional visual field used for reading and for professional activities is of paramount importance for determining which retinal area should be photo-coagulated in diseases such as diabetic retinopathy.

Studies of the *binocular visual field* are just beginning, although it is

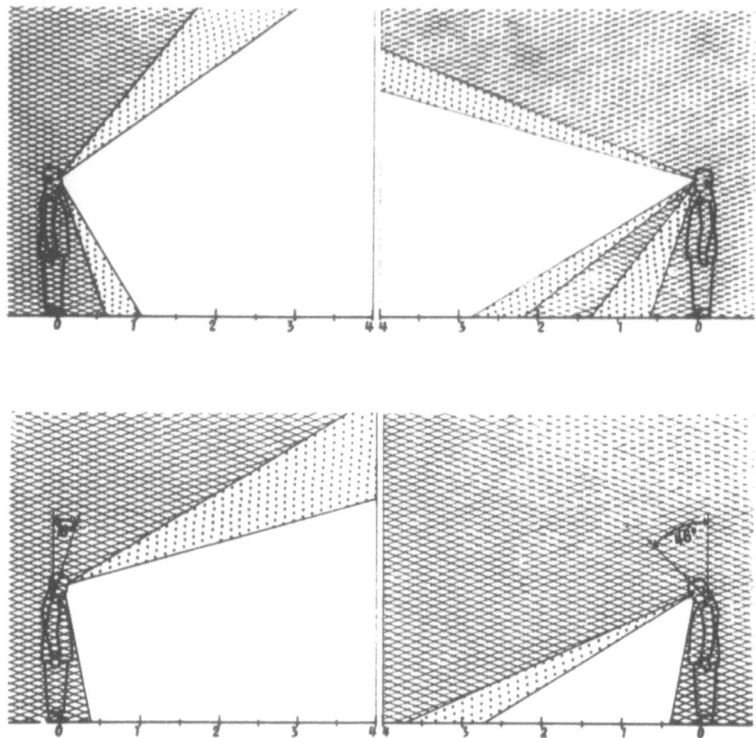

Fig. 4. Above: gaze field (white) and visual field (punctate) of an emmetropic subject (left) and of an aphakic subject corrected by spectacles (right) when looking straight ahead. Below: the same when looking a point 30 cm before the feets (for descending a staircase). From Hager (1961a).

already known that the binocular visual field is often larger than the sum of the two monocular visual fields. This is not only because non-seeing areas in one eye are compensated by an overlapping seeing area in the other eye, but also because of greater sensitivity in the overlapping portions of the visual field with sloping field defects (Esterman, 1982; see Fig. 7). Calabria, Capris and Burtolo (1983) found that deficits in the central visual field of glaucoma patients showed a binocular sensitivity summation that was less efficient than in other forms of visual impairment (e.g., pigmentary retinopathy). This may explain why glaucoma patients with extensive visual field loss display greater difficulties in visually guided behavior than other patients with similar visual field deficits. Moreover, Ross (1983) evidenced a strong positive relationship between (monocularly measured) field loss and visual disability in a glacuoma group, whereas no such relationship was found in a cataract group.

In other *optic nerve lesions* facilitation and summation effects associated with binocularity also appear to be reduced or absent. In

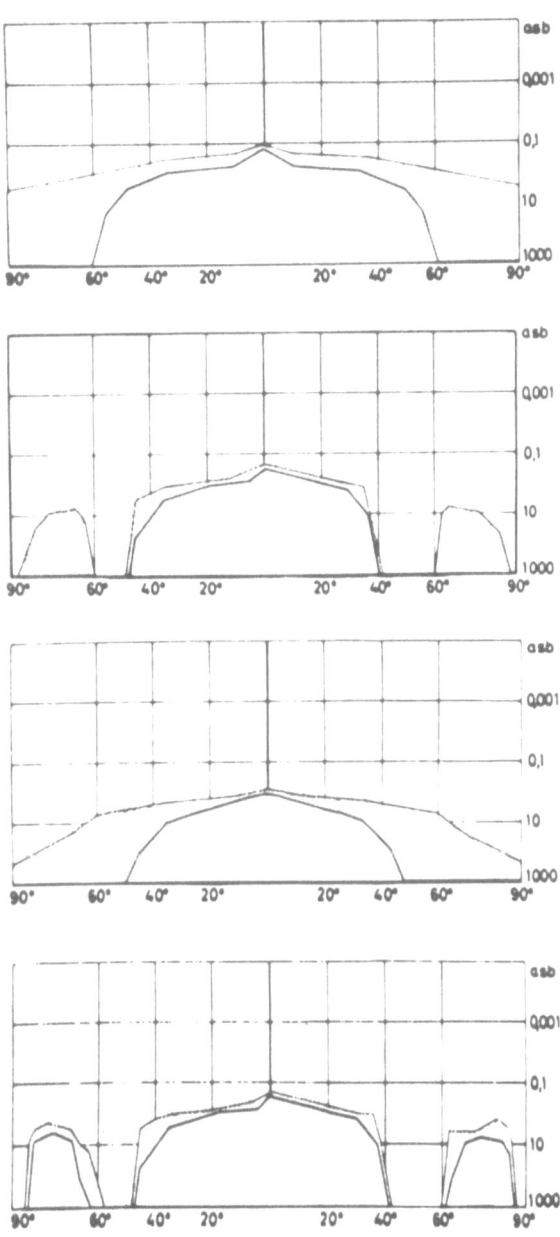

Fig. 5. Horizontal profiles of the detection (outer curves) and resolution (inner curves) binocular threshold sensitivities for the 116′ object of the Tübingen perimeter in (from above to below) normal vision, aphakic vision corrected by ordinary spectacles, aphakic vision corrected by contact lenses, and aphakic vision corrected by Jaeger's spectacles with side lenses. From Jaeger (1980).

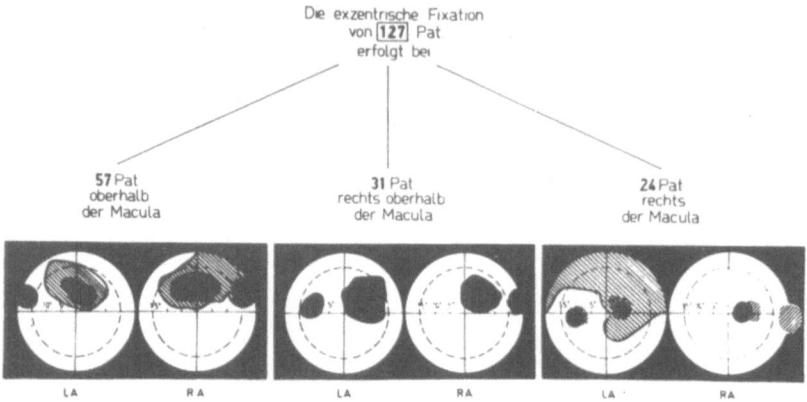

Fig. 6. Displacement of the central scotoma by eccentric fixation in maculopathy. From Aulhorn (1975).

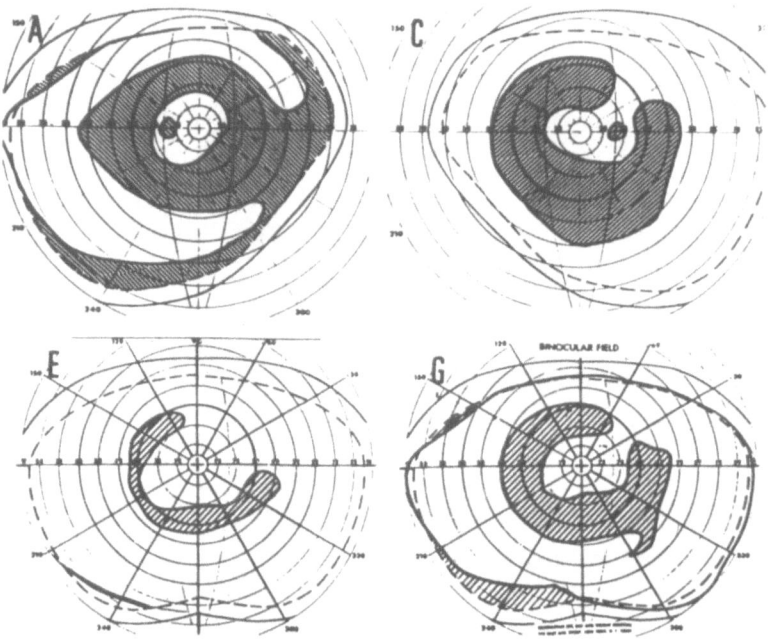

Fig. 7. Comparison, in a case of pigmentary retinopathy, of the left eye monocular field (A), of the right eye monocular field (C), of the true binocular field (E) and of the theoretical binocular field obtained by merging both monocular fields (G). From Esterman (1982).

multiple sclerosis temporal resolution is often affected (Galvin et al. 1976), and thresholds become elevated during the repeat static test, especially at high background luminances (Enoch et al., 1979). The functional visual field can also be affected by anomalies in saccadic eye movements displayed by patients with Parkinson's disease and myesthenia gravis, as well as multiple sclerosis.

In *posterior visual pathway lesions* (optic chiasm, optic tract, lateral geniculate body, optic radiations, visual cortex) facilitation and summation phenomena seem to prevail (Gandolfo et al., 1982). Visual neglect, in the absence of visual sensory deficits, is often produced by right parietal lobe lesions. In contrast, individuals with visual cortical damage may be able to localize stimuli within their scotomatous region. Such data are consistent with the concept that different neurological mechanisms are responsible for different aspects of visual perception and visually-guided behavior.

It is well known that *strabismic amblyopia* is characterized in monocular vision by a central scotoma and unsteady and/or eccentric fixation. The results obtained from binocular viewing are greatly dependent on the test procedure and the amount of dissociation achieved between the two eyes. Ophthalmologists have formerly used strong dissociating techniques to verify the role of the squinting eye in binocular vision. Their findings reveal large suppression scotomata in the visual field of the squinting eye, particularly in the homologous region corresponding to the fixation area of the non-squinting eye. With the use of non-dissociating techniques, it has recently been shown that, especially in small-angle strabismus, single vision is maintained with anomalous retinal correspondence throughout the binocular visual field, without suppression of the deviating eye (Campos, 1982; see Fig. 8). In large angle strabismus, suppression of the deviating eye prevails. Patients with esotropia or a history of esotropia show a suppression scotoma primarily within the nasal retina of the deviating eye (Jacobsen, Sandberg and Berson, 1983). Capris and Fava (1982) showed that while binocular sensitivities are better than monocular sensitivities in normal subjects, binocular sensitivities in squinting subjects should be equal to those of the better eye. Thus, individuals with anomalous binocular vision lack excitatory binocular interactions, although inhibitory interactions may continue to be present (Levi, Harwerth and Smith, 1980). In fact, there is a wide variety of intermediate levels between perfect binocular interaction and complete independence in subclinical cases (from partial or complete stereo-blindness to heterophoria and microstrabismus).

In adult subjects suffering from *hysteria, sinistrosis*, or *post-commotional syndrome* (even in uncomplicated cases) there is a concentric narrowing of the functional visual field by reduction of the span of attention and perception (similar to that found in normal children!). This phenomena has often been misinterpreted by clinicians as reflecting organically-based visual field loss, or as malingering. In many instances, the visual field progressively narrows during the perimetric test (producing a spiralling visual field, as shown in Fig. 9) and expands if incentives are provided. Another manifestation of such

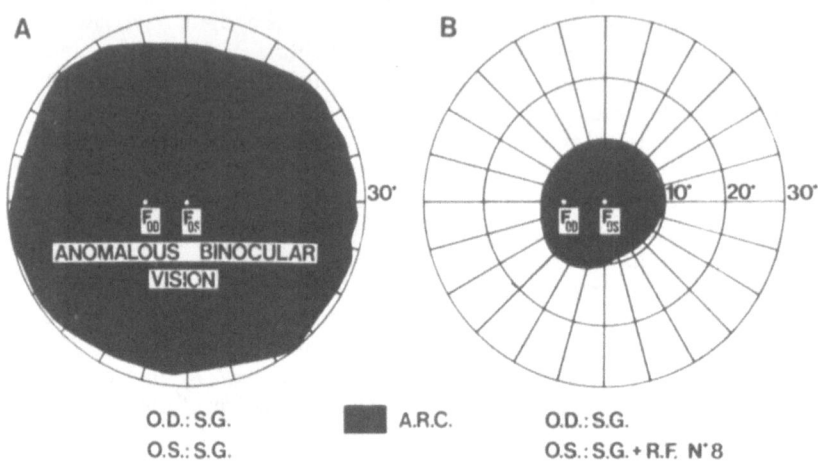

♀ 13
7° RIGHT ESOTROPIA
S.G.: A.R.C. - DIPLOPIA WITH BAGOLINI'S RED FILTER N° 11

A   B

30°   10° 20° 30°

ANOMALOUS BINOCULAR
VISION

O.D.: S.G.   A.R.C.   O.D.: S.G.
O.S.: S.G.   O.S.: S.G. + R.F. N° 8

STIMULUS: ∅ 0.3° 115 cd/m³ - BACKGROUND: 5 cd/m³

Fig. 8. A case of right small angle esotropia. Left (A): using striated glasses as a control for binocularity and a white light spot as the perimetric stimulus, a wide area of binocular single vision sustained by anomalous retinal correspondance is found; no suppression scotoma was detected. Right (B): in the same patient a red filter in front of the fixing eye causes a restriction of the area of binocular single vision. From Campos (1982).

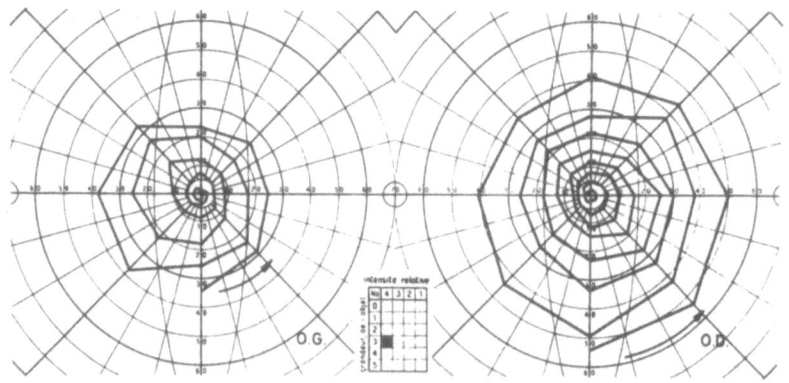

Fig. 9. Spiral visual field. Such a tracing is often obtained in subjects suffering from hysteria if the examiner's purpose is to determine kinetically the peripheral limits of the visual field by moving centripetally a given object on the successive meridians (here counterclockwise). From Verriest and Van de Casteele (1972).

functional visual field defects is that the eccentricity of disappearance of a target moving away from fixation is more central than the

290

eccentricity of appearance of the target as it moves towards fixation ('inversion of the limits': Kluyskens, 1948). Ravenstein et al. (1982) found that patients rehabilitating from brain injury showed reduced accuracy and slower responses for several driving tasks.

The effects of other factors should also be considered.

Drugs can affect the visual field by altering sensitivities, or in cases of chronic use, by the development of a central, pericentral or centrocecal scotoma or concentric visual field narrowing. Response latency (reaction time) can also be influenced by drugs. An example of paradoxical effects of drugs has been reported by Gandolfo (1983): at blood alcohol levels of 5 mg/ml, photopic and mesopic sensitivities in the central visual field are enhanced, while peripheral visual fields are constricted and angioscotomata are enlarged.

With regard to *hypoxia*, the visual field extent remains unaffected for decreases in oxygen pressure of up to 50% (corresponding to an altitude of 10 000 feet, or approximately 3000 meters). However, a reduction of 60% in oxygen pressure (12 500 feet, or approximately 3750 meters) produces a decrease in vidual field radius of about 10% (Nelson, 1983; a confirmation of older data). Guérin (1981) found no modification of the Friedmann analyzer results at 5500 m (about 18 000 feet).

Mild levels of *carbon monoxide* decrease performance in detecting peripheral moving targets, indicating some constriction of the visual field (Salvatore, 1974).

Verriest et al. (1984) described an increase in perimetrically-determined peripheral sensitivities during *mascular exercise*, and ascribed these changes to greater mental alertness.

When evaluating the effects of the *luminous environment* on visual field properties, the influence of glare and flicker must be considered. *Disability glare* can be expressed by the equivalent veiling luminance L_v calculated by means of Holladay's formula $L_v = K \cdot E/\theta^m$ (where E is the pupillary illumination provided by the glare source, θ is the angle between the glare source and the visual axis, and K and m are constants with values of approximately 10 and 2, respectively). This expression is true not only for the fovea, but also for all other parts of the visual field (provided that θ is regarded as the angle between the position of the glare source and the specific visual field location being considered). Indeed, the equivalent veiling luminance decreases symmetrically from the direction of the glare source (Enoch, Boynton and Bush, 1954; Ucke, 1973; Aulhorn, 1976). Disability glare can be augmented by both age-related and pathologic clouding of the ocular media (Verriest et al., 1983). The effects of *discomfort glare* must also be considered.

The critical *flicker* frequency can be higher in peripheral vision than in the central visual field, particularly for stimuli greater than 2 degrees (Lloyd, 1952). It is even possible that the flickering appearance of a bright fused foveal target is signalled by peripheral retinal elements stimulated by scattered light from a large distance away from fixation (Ronchi and Salvi, 1965). This may explain why part of a TV or VDU screen may seem to flicker while the centrally viewed portion remains steady. This type of flicker sensation has been reported to narrow the visual field (Tshernilovskaja, 1968) and to reduce foveal flicker fusion rate and visual acuity (Rey, 1975). The growing use of flickering lights to enhance the conspicuity of display items may also cause undue visual discomfort and stress.

Noise (Sanders, 1961) and *sleep loss* (Sanders and Reitsma, 1982) have been shown to have a greater disruptive effect on functional visual fields in the periphery than in central vision. Other physical stressors such as heat and humidity may also constrict peripheral vision (Bursill, 1958).

INTERFACES WITH VISUAL ERGONOMICS

Until recently, the functional visual field has not received much attention in visual ergonomics. This section will review some of the areas for which the functional visual fields are applicable.

An important feature of vision during *driving* is that every point in the visual environment is moving except for the 'focus of expansion', the point in the visual scene toward which the movement is directed. With increasing forward velocity and/or an increased angle from the focus of expansion, vision becomes progressively degraded because of increasing *speed smear* (due to the interaction of visual persistence and relative motion of the visual environment). This movement is the primary basis for kinetic narrowing of the functional visual field as described by Hockenbeamer (1952), Danielson (1957) and Kite and King (1961) (see Fig. 10). There is also a progressive narrowing of head movements (Åberg and Rumar, 1975) and gaze fields (Irving, 1965). Speed smear also accounts for the fact that as we go faster, we tend to look farther ahead of the car (Danielson, 1957).

Older publications (eg, Gibson et al., 1958) stressed the use of the focus of expansion as an optical cue for *heading direction*. In fact, perception of the focus of expansion lacks the precision necessary for accurate road driving (Johnston, White and Cumming, 1973). Vehicle guidance on a straight roadway (in spite of road irregularities, sidewinds, etc.) can be analyzed in terms of rapid corrections of the angle between the car axis and the road axis, and slower less frequent corrections of lateral positions of the car within the lane used. The role of peripheral vision for this tracking task has been investigated. Experimental restriction of the visual field by occluding parts of the windshield does not interfere much with such tracking behavior, due to compensation in the form of an increased frequency and amplitude of corrective movements (Riemersma, 1972; see Fig. 11). On the other hand, Blaauw (1974) demonstrated by means of eye movement recordings that only a small amount of fixation time is devoted to roadway markers on a straight highway; at least 27% of fixation time is

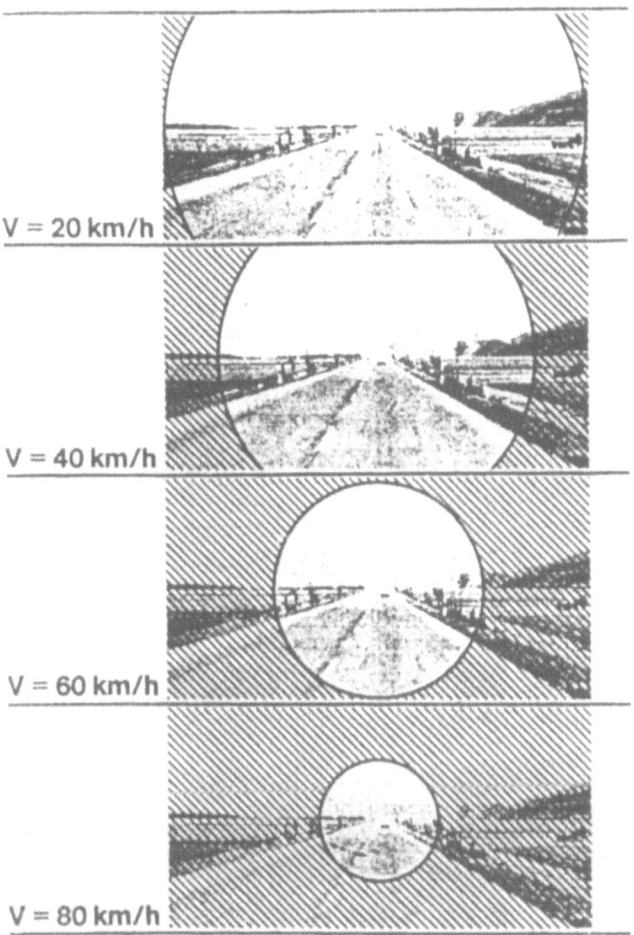

V = 20 km/h

V = 40 km/h

V = 60 km/h

V = 80 km/h

Fig. 10. Relation between narrowing of the functional visual fields and the vehicle forward speed. From Hirschberger and Miedel (1980).

above the horizon, and peripheral vision seems to be sufficient, since drivers prefer information about their lateral and longitudinal position on the road (as previously shown by Mourant and Rockwell, 1970). Asymmetrical movement patterns in the peripheral visual field have been found to shift the subjective position of 'straight ahead', which could have deleterious effects on tracking behavior (Olson and Moulden, 1972). When driving in curved sections of roadways, more foveal information about roadway conditions is necessary for accurate tracking (Blaauw, 1974).

When one car follows another, the driver of the following car makes

293

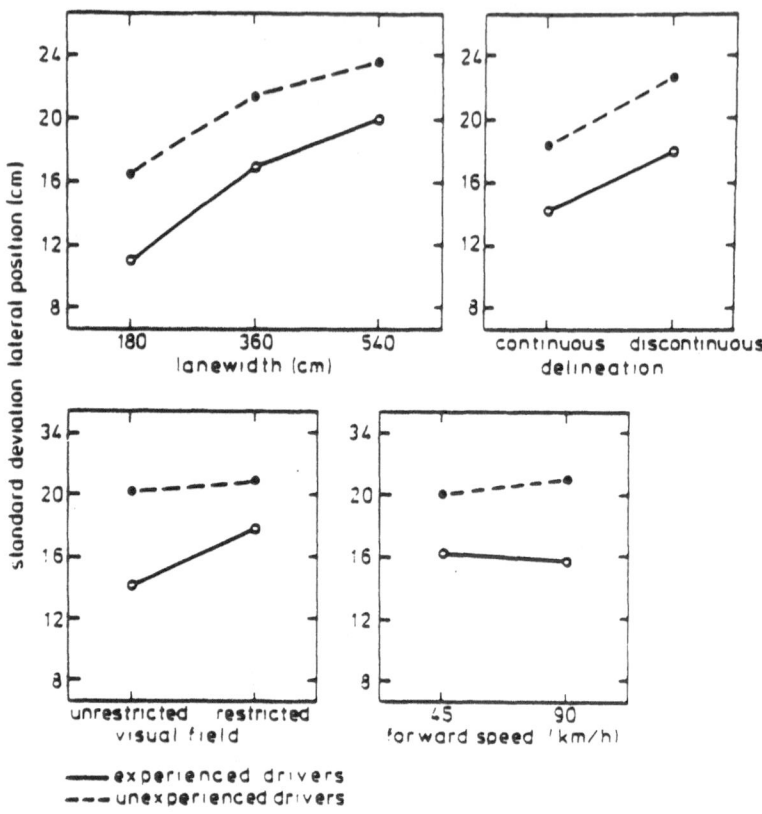

Fig. 11. Effects on the precision of driving of different factors, including available visual field. From Riemersma (1982).

spacing judgments based on observing the lead car within his field of vision. The same spacing appears greater for smaller forward obscuration (Evans and Rothery, 1976).

Peripheral information serves also *speed estimations* (Salvatore, 1968).

The functional visual field affects also *higher order aspects of driving behavior*, particularly decision-making behavior related to selection of roadways, changing lanes, passing other vehicles and other aspects of maneuvering a car (Blaauw, 1982). Noble and Sanders (1980) showed that when tracking and visual search tasks are performed concurrently (e.g. searching a traffic panel during driving), both tasks exhibit a performance decrement. This is particularly true if the identification of peripheral visual search targets is difficult.

The wearing of *spectacles* is usually recommended for drivers with large refractive errors, or those prone to eyestrain, although the effects

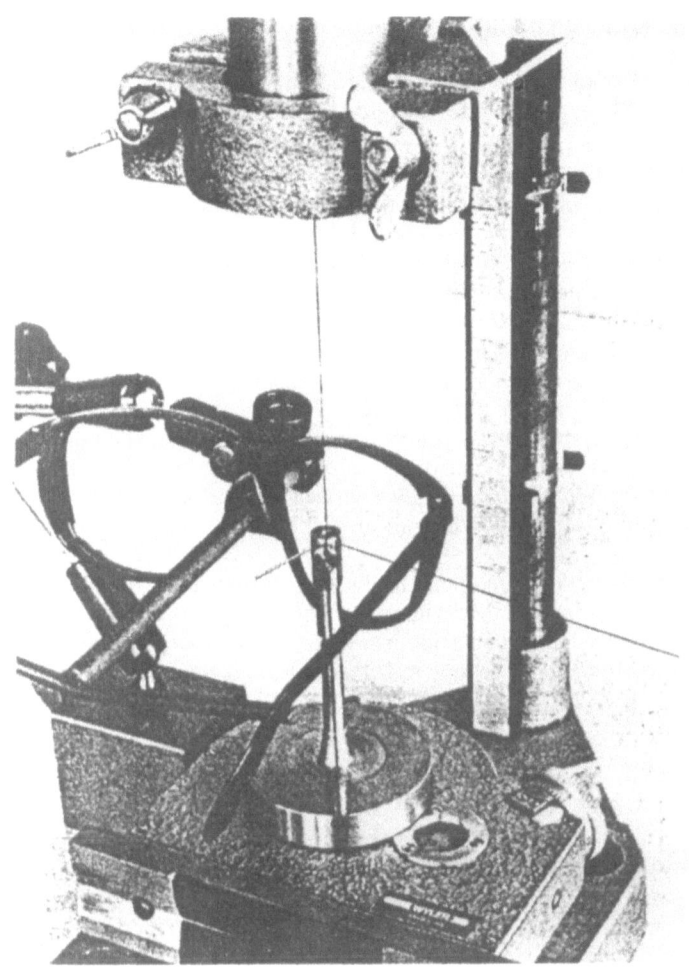

Fig. 12. Apparatus for measuring the visual field defects due to the spectacles frame. From Hirschberger and Miedel (1980).

of eyeglass frames on the field of vision must be considered. In Germany an instrument has been constructed for the purpose of measuring visual field defects due to spectacle frames (see Fig. 12), and a norm has been established for drivers' spectacles. According to this standard, only about 50% of the spectacles currently worn by drivers would meet such requirements (Hirschberger and Miedel, 1980). Large lenses are not an effective solution to this problem, since they have a great amount of prismatic distortion and oblique ray astigmatism. Chromatic aberration can disturb fixation through peripheral parts of a spectacle glass, so that some myopic drivers are obliged to turn the head instead of the eyes to look in the rear view mirror.

An automobile driver's view is not only limited by his spectacles, but also by the presence of any passengers and the limitations to visibility imposed by the structure of the car. This *'car field'* (Danielson, 1957) consists of a horizontal strip which varies most greatly in the vertical plane during changes in position of the driver's head in relation to the windshield and windows. The car field has been greatly improved since the 1950s. The location of drivers' eyes as a function of a vehicle's workspace geometry and percentile representation of driving population (the 'eyellipse': Meldrum, 1965; Gatchell and Miller, 1974; Miller and Gatchell, 1975) allows designers to minimize structures that interfere with a driver's vision to his environment. Other aids to visibility could also be implemented. For example, it has been estimated that 2% of highway traffic accidents could be avoided by the use of a second rear view mirror (Hirschberger and Miedel, 1980).

Vehicle handling characteristics as well as *road geometries* can be evaluated by means of driving performance models (Godthelp, Blaauw and Milgram, 1984).

As demonstrated mathematically by Byrnes (1967), peripheral vision becomes even more important for safety when vehicle *speed becomes lower*. This is particularly true for urban driving because of the many street crossings without traffic signals, and the presence of more

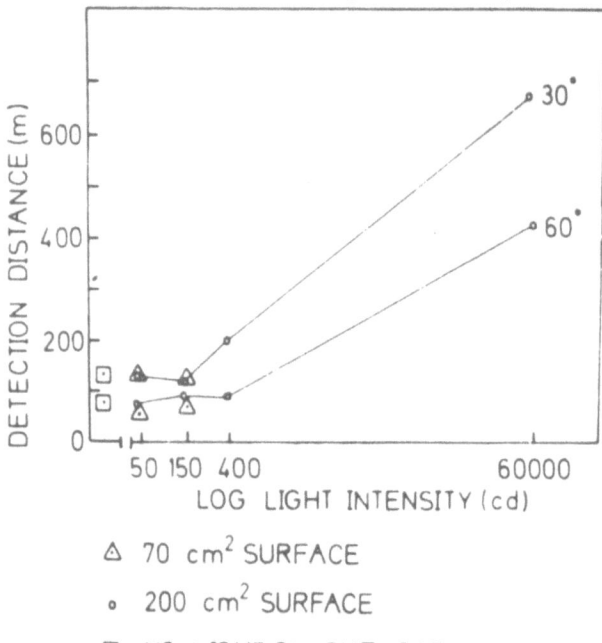

Fig. 13. Mean vehicle detection distance in daylight for two eccentricities in the visual field as a function of running light intensity. From Hörberg and Rumar (1979).

bicyclists, pedestrians and parked cars. Head movements become more important in urban driving (Åberg and Rumar, 1975), and it is for these conditions that ergonomics must be particularly concerned about unobstructed peripheral vision.

Highway traffic safety also depends on the conspicuity of *highway elements* such as route information, work-zone indicators, and reflectors, lines and other markers that delineate the geometry of the roadway. Godthelp and Riemersma (1980) reported that indicators of road geometry are more effective when they are positioned at height that is different from the eyes. The conspicuity of other vehicles (Hörberg and Rumar showed in 1979 that the mean daylight vehicle detection distance in peripheral vision is greatly improved by running lights: see Fig. 13) and the conspicuity of pedestrians (wearing retroreflective material greatly improves pedestrian safety) must also be taken into account. Rotating or flashing beacons can be very conspicuous in peripheral vision, but can also produce discomfort.

One of the reasons why the rates of *nighttime* accidents are higher than daytime accidents is the reduction of visual cues. Indeed at night

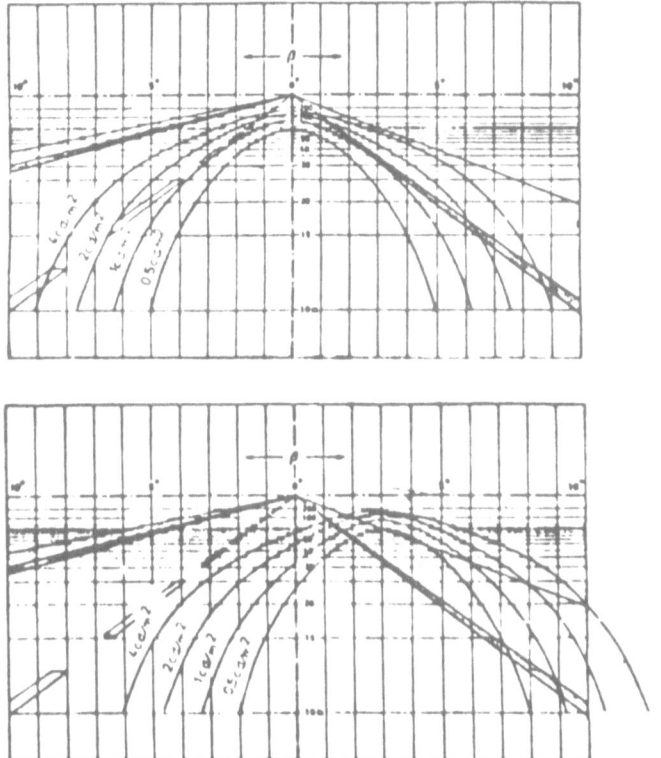

Fig. 14. Isoprobality detection contours per glimpse on a two lane road of 7 m width at various values of road surface luminance; height of eye position 1.25 m, target 20 × 20 cm, contrast 0.2, glimpse detection probability $P_g = 1$ (i.e. safe detection). Above: line of sight on lane axis. Beneath: 3 degree shift of the line of sight (driver looks at a traffic sign or at a pedestrian 35 m ahead). From Inditsky, Bodmann and Fleck (1982).

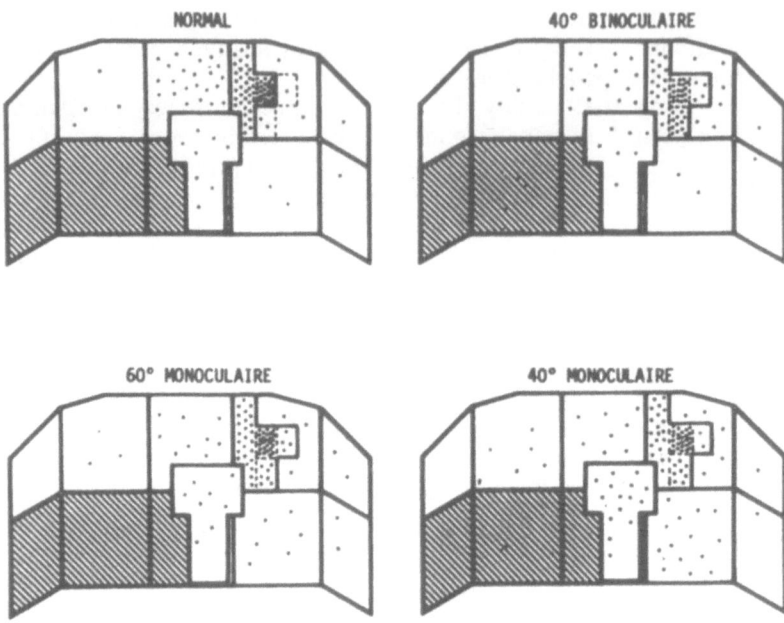

Fig. 15. Density of fixations of the pilot through the different parts of a helicopter window in normal conditions and when the visual field is restricted to 60° and to 40° in binocular and monocular vision. Each dot represents 1% of the total fixation time. From Papin, Menu and Santucci (1981).

the driver's eye movements concentrate in the area lighted by the head lamp beams (Rackoff and Rockwell, 1975). Moreover, Inditsky, Bodmann and Fleck (1982) showed that the conditions of drivers at night allow only small eye movements around the lane axis to maintain safe detection of possible obstacles (Fig. 14): detection ranges decreases by almost 50% for only 3° deviation. This can be improved by better lighting. For street and highway lighting, considerations of accident prevention should be given a higher priority than energy savings (Bauder, 1980).

Functional visual field studies are also important with regard to *learning to drive*. Evaluations of the scanning behavior of beginning drivers show that they tend to spend too much time looking at detailed information, with too many saccades and a shorter than optimal fixation time, thereby producing stress and preventing a general overview of the situation. In contrast, experienced drivers concentrate on useful features of road sections that are further away (3 or more seconds away from their current location). Saccadic eye movements are less frequent, and are most often from far-to-near or near-to-far (Hirschberger and Miedel, 1980). As with novice drivers, there is a perceptual narrowing in acute alcoholism and drowsiness due to a deficiency in lateral eye movements (Rockwell, 1972). Riemersma

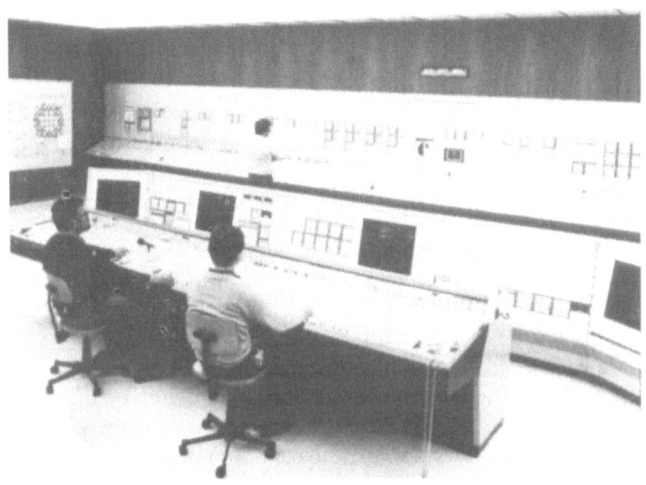

Fig. 16. Control task in a nuclear center. From Haubner (1983).

(1982) reported that artificial restriction of the visual field had an effect on the variability of lateral position, lateral speed and path angle, but only for experienced drivers (see Fig. 11). Thus inexperienced drivers gradually learn to use information from the peripheral visual field through practice, particularly the lateral speed cue.

The visual problems of *aircraft pilots* can be analyzed in the same manner as that of automobile drivers, although one must take into account the additional special problems of empty visual fields, glare from underlying clouds, accelerations during which the supersonic jet pilot cannot move his head, interactions between high speed flying and perceptual delays, etc. Direct visual information for large viewing angles is especially important for helicopter pilots (see Fig. 15). Representative visual studies in this area are related to cockpit design, special sunglasses, colors of aircraft, effects of reduction of the visual field by night vision image intensifier goggles (Papin, Menu and Santucci, 1981), and other factors.

With ongoing production and limited presentation time, *visual inspection* relies on off-axis detection of potential defects and thus will be improved with broader visibility lobes (Boyce, 1981). Indeed, Leachtenauer (1978) found a strong correlation between visual acuity field extent and performance for searching real objects in aerial photography using trained image interpreters.

For *prolonged control tasks associated with a large viewing display* (Fig. 16) the ergonomist must be aware of physiological factors such as lateral inhibition (see the first part of this report, or Sanders, 1967, for a discussion of peripheral discrimination of arrow directions),

299

progressive restriction of the functional visual field (Grass-Adamczek, 1981) and cyclic variations in perceptual probability of detection (Ronchi and Salvi, 1973). Performance decrements over time are more evident for vigilance tasks, during which observers respond at infrequent intervals, than for active or continuous reaction tasks (Sanders and Hoogenboom, 1969). Visual errors are more pronounced when the visual scene is too uniform or constant. Ergonomists have to evaluate color contrast, brightness, movement and flicker aspects of a visual display for each particular case in order to avoid local adaptation effects and increase perception probability. However paradoxical effects can occur: Gurevich and Steinschneider (1967) evidenced that higher field luminance increases recognition time of a small (1'5) embedded stimulus; foveal load can either decrease performance in detection of peripheral stimuli (see first part of this report) or increase this performance by arousing vigilance (Bartz. 1976).

The extent of the functional visual field in different directions has to be considered when *designing* helmets for motorists, headgears (Fig. 17), face masks, goggles, spectacle frames, multifocal or continuous curve lenses, and even curved windshields (since there have been complaints and accidents in auto races from the optical distortions introduced into the visual field by 'panoramic' windshields). Clear, unobstructed vision is essential for any worker or athlete (particularly those in contact sports) to be able to function at his best with the greatest amount of safety.

More communication should occur among ergonomists, ophthalmologists, optometrists and dispensing opticians to insure that *spectacle frames* are selected according to criteria other than just fashion and personal preference. To avoid annular scotomata, all convex lenses should be fitted into frames with either a small rim or no rim at all in the temporal and lower portion of the spectacle. Jaeger (1980) recommended detachable supplementary lenses on the sidepieces of cataract spectacles for better utilization of the temporal visual field (Fig. 5). For concave lenses, frames should be selected according to the lens power so that no diplopia ring is present (Hager, 1961b). For circumstances in which the visual field is important, pantoscopic frames have to be given preference over those which represent revivals of older fashions.

Illumination engineering is concerned with the allowable luminance levels and flicker rates of lighting in the surroundings of a job environment, and in the allowable luminance and color contrast levels between the surroundings and the specific visual task. The relationship of these factors to the visual field and functional visual field are of concern to ergoperimetry. Study of visual search behaviour can be useful in identifying the specific effects of various illumination designs on drivers performance (Rackoff and Rockwell, 1975). Devices which limit the visual field have been recommended for minimizing glare under conditions of bright surroundings and/or augmented intraocular scatter (e.g. honeycombs; Miller, Brooks and Wolf, 1976).

300

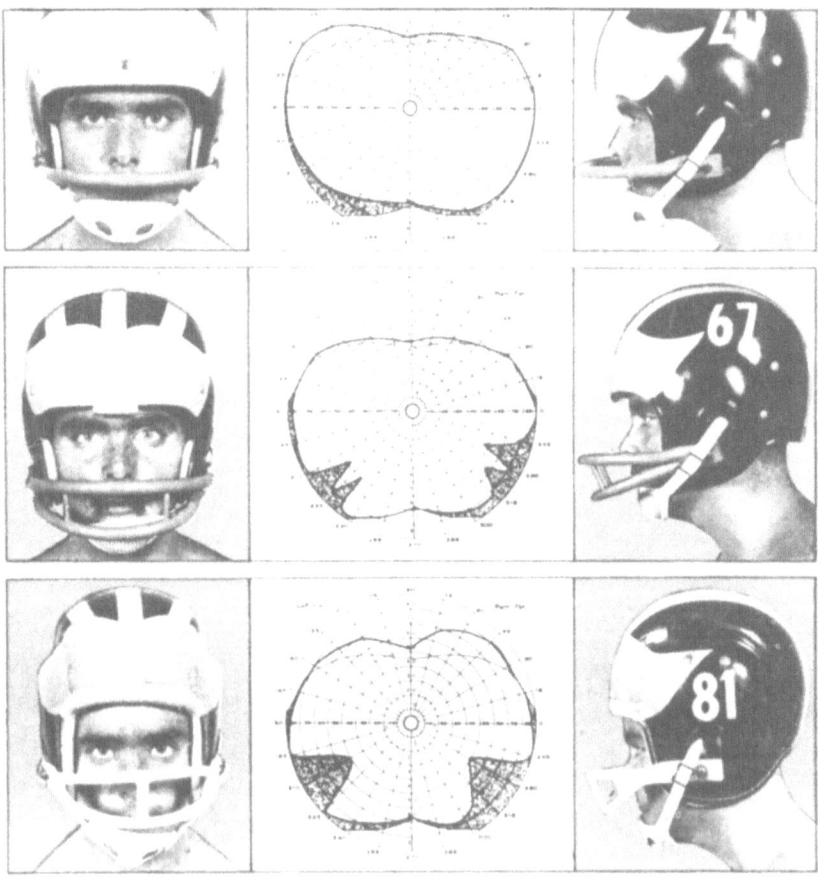

Fig. 17. Impairment of the binocular visual field by different types of american football face guards. From Schneider and Antine (1965).

The optimal extent of the field of view in *visual optical instruments* is also a problem related to the functional visual field. The (eyespace) field of view of an optical instrument is the angular area which is available to the observer at a given instant of time. Indeed, the transmitted bundle of rays reaching the retina depends on the intersection of the cones of rays from the object point through all aperture stops, including the observer's pupil. If vignetting is not avoided by the use of a proper field stop, there is a gradual fading of the image toward the periphery of the field of view due to the graded restriction of transmitted bundles of rays from off-axis object points. For an optical instrument with known abberrations and specifications, and/or a given position of the eye, the visual efficiency for each point in the visual field can be calculated as a ratio of the combined modulation transfer

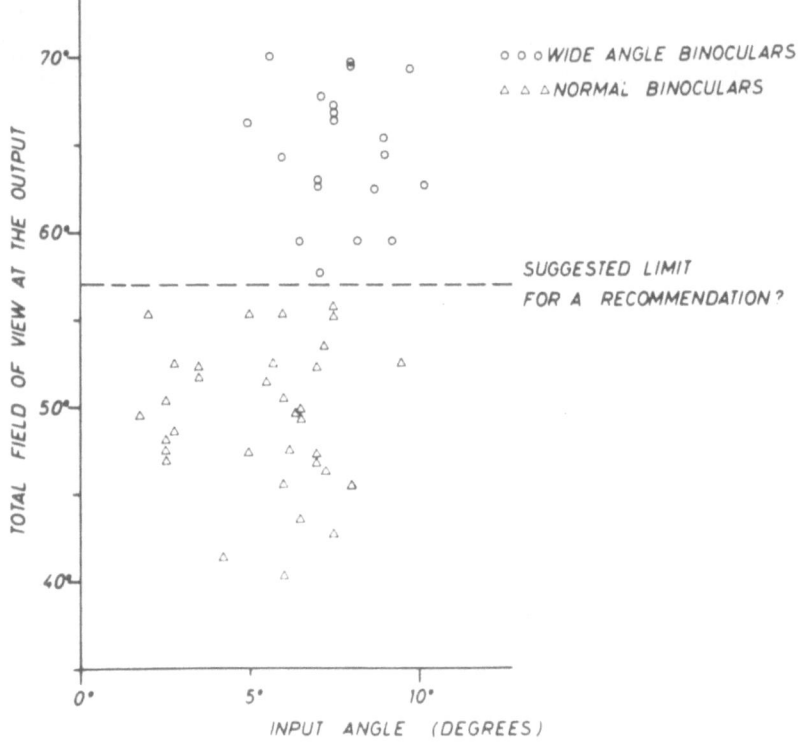

Fig. 18. Relationship between input and output angle in normal and wide angle binoculars. Unpublished data from L. Ronchi.

function of the optical system and eye together, to that of the eye alone (Overington, 1980). The available field of view is not only utilized by peripheral vision when viewing the central part of the field, but is also scanned by foveal vision through rotation of the eye. In general, a wide field of view, even one which is subject to vignetting, is preferable to a narrow field of view. When the field of view is restricted to less than 20 degrees on either side (a total field of view of 40 degrees), the observer has an impression of viewing through a tube (Zimmer, 1970). We may assume that this impression of looking through a tube is a psychological effect produced by the inability to make full use of peripheral vision and eye movement scanning behavior. However, predictive modelling of the effect of the field of view on visual search indicates that beyond 50 degrees field of view improvements are minimal, suggesting that wide angle binoculars (Fig. 18) could be a somewhat needless luxury. A total eyespace field of view of approximately 57 degrees could be recommended for visual search tasks, thus excluding instruments used for high precision central visual tasks (e.g., gunsight telescopes) for which a smaller field of view is

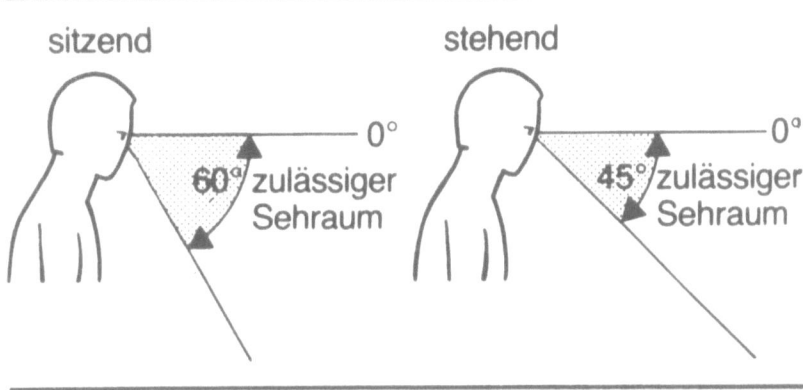

Fig. 19. Preferred and acceptable gaze field for VDU work. From Benz, Grob and Haubner (1981).

sufficient. In addition, a small field of view for some circumstances (e.g., very bright visual scenes) can be beneficial for minimizing disability and discomfort glare from sources surrounding the target, whereas a large field of view may be advantageous for attaining a more photopic state of adaptation when viewing dim, low contrast targets under minimal illumination. The topic of optical instruments will also be discussed in the section on visual impairment.

Since *visual display units* (VDUs) are widely used in many occupations for prolonged periods of time, the ergonomist must be concerned with the interaction with the functional visual field of display dimensions, viewing distance and the visual environment in which such display units are used. Glare from windows or other sources of light within the worker's peripheral field of view are one of the main causes of eye strain during VDU work. Targets which require frequent fixations should not be placed outside of an acceptable gaze field (Fig. 19). Specular reflections on the screen itself must be avoided. Non-essential letters or signs can seriously impair the ability to read other important letters (Mackworth, 1965). A somewhat unexpected finding has been reported by Bouma (1980) wherein interferring letters more peripheral to the target exhibit a stronger detrimental effect than inter-ferring letters placed near fixation. Color coding can often enhance performance for search or identification tasks (Christ, 1975) and should be used more in the future for such displays. However, symbol sizes smaller than 30' should not be used for color coding (Berggrund et al., 1984).

In recent years the use of *raster displays* for presentation of visual information has also become widespread (for example, television, thermal printers, etc.). Under some circumstances, an observer may perceive the raster lines more strongly than the letters or other information carried upon them. Biberman (1973) demonstrated that there is greater information transfer when the raster line is blurred and when the raster subtense is reduced. At the present time, there is very little information about the effects of the display angle. The prediction of models of raster display viewing suggest that these effects will be scaled such that an angle θ from the fovea a raster with a pitch subtense of $s(\theta + 1)$ 0.5 mrads will have spatial degrading effects that are similar to a foveally viewed raster of pitch subtense s mrads (Overington, 1983). Erikson (1978) computed equipment characteristics required to insure prescribed levels of target acquisition performance.

When *image data* needs to be transmitted, knowledge of the visual strategies associated with the target acquisition process may provide some clues for improving the presentation and efficiency of such tasks. Indeed, it should be possible to transmit a smaller picture area around the observer's fixation point to reduce the bandwidth of data transmission without loss of relevant information (Erikson, 1964; Schumacher and Korn, 1981).

INTERFACES WITH VISUAL IMPAIRMENT

Let us first consider *the appreciation of visual disability due to field loss*. Visual disability, with respect to specific jobs, will be discussed further in the section on job fitness. In this section, we will only describe the considerations of visual disability as related to daily activities or the general labor market (as defined for medico-legal purposes in many countries, especially in continental Europe).

Erroneous conclusions are still made, for example, by allotting equal values to all areas of the visual field, or by considering a complete bitemporal hemianopsia to be equal or more disabling than a complete homonymous hemianopsia. It is only gradually becoming an accepted concept that for most activities (and thus, also for appreciation of the amount of disability) the binocular field is the most important consideration. Furthermore, the central part of the visual field is more significant than the periphery, the lower field more valuable than the upper visual field, and the horizontal meridian more important than the vertical and oblique meridians for most visually related tasks. A more accurate functional evaluation of visual field loss corresponding to these concepts began at the end of the 19th century (Magnus, 1894; Groenouw, 1896) and has been refined in the new scoring system of Esterman (1982). This system is a simple procedure to obtain the functional visual efficiency of the entire visual field, expressed as a

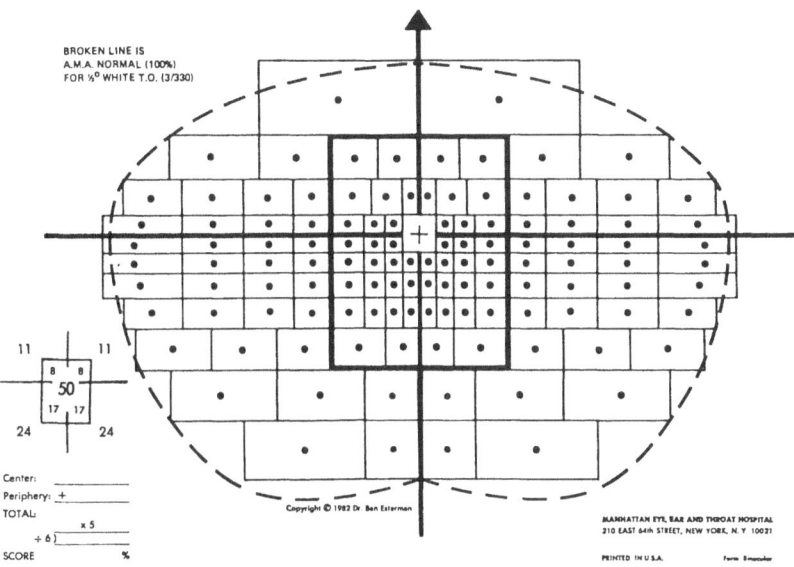

SCALE FOR BINOCULAR FUNCTIONAL FIELD

BROKEN LINE IS
A.M.A. NORMAL (100%)
FOR ½° WHITE T.O. (3/330)

Copyright © 1982 Dr Ben Esterman

MANHATTAN EYE, EAR AND THROAT HOSPITAL
210 EAST 64th STREET, NEW YORK, N. Y. 10021

PRINTED IN U.S.A.   Form: Binocular

Fig. 20. Binocular Esterman grid. From Esterman (1982).

percentage of the total normal functional visual field. It is sufficient to draw the peripheral visual field limit and scotomas present within the binocular visual field on a special chart (Fig. 20) consisting of 120 locations, count the dots which lie within the seeing portion of the binocular visual field, and multiply the total by 100/120.

Instead of using Esterman's unequally spaced dots in a conventional field representation, it should also be possible to adopt equally spaced dots into a convenient non-linear field projection (Dannheim, 1983; Furuno, 1983; Crick, Crick and Ripley, 1983: see Fig. 3 on p. 197 of the Proceedings of the 1982 IPS Symposium). In addition, each visual field unit that is represented by the stimulus as its center can be given a 'functional factor', which can itself be multiplied by a 'threshold factor' for taking into account relative scotomata. This would allow the inclusion of partial sensitivity losses for certain parts of the visual field, a factor that was not considered by Esterman for the sake of simplicity (Crick, Crick and Ripley, 1983: see Fig. 5 on p. 198 of the Proceedings of the 1982 IPS Symposium). Moreover, it could be beneficial to replace the usual sharp-edged target by a sine-bell stimulus because it minimizes the need to correct refractive error accurately (Crick and Crick, 1981) and because visual performance in many environments can be better predicted by such sine-wave contrast sensitivity assessments (Ginsburg, 1980).

The use of automated perimeters may allow this type of evaluation task to be performed in a much easier fashion, due to the computer's

305

ability to rapidly and accurately determine test results according to particular scoring or evaluation strategies.

A related problem is the specification of visual field extent in *definitions of low vision and blindness* for legal, social and statistical purposes. According to the World Health Organization and a number of national organizations, blindness is defined either as a visual acuity of less than 0.05, or a visual field of 10 degrees or less. A more complete set of definitions of include conditions ranging from low vision to complete blindness is needed as well as a concise description of the perimetric techniques to be used for such evaluations. In many of the documents reporting the definitions of legal blindness, there is no designation as to whether the minimum degrees of visual field extent refer to the radius or diameter of the visual field, nor along which meridional direction the diameter or radius should be measured.

As a combination of contrast sensitivity, near visual acuity and visual fields offers the best predictive relationship between visual disability and visual defect (Ross, Bron and Clarke, 1984) assessment of the (binocular) visual field in cases of low vision and incomplete blindness is important in *predicting functional abilities and designing treatment regimens.*

Low vision specialists such as Faye (1976) and Bailey (1978a) are aware of the distinction between standard clinical diagnostic visual field testing and functional field testing. They report that for functional visual field testing larger and unconventional perimetric targets may be used, while illumination conditions may be varied considerably. The functional visual field may be more reduced than standard clinical perimetric visual field determinations in cases of visual loss associated with neuro-psychological troubles such as mental retardation, visual deprivation, and other factors. The gaze field must also be considered, particularly in cases of nystagmus (Boissin, 1980). For the purposes of considering functional consequences and treatment options, it is often convenient to subdivide functional visual field loss into the categories of central scotoma, segmental loss and concentric narrowing.

A *central scotoma* may interfere with the perception of fine detail, however, static and dynamic orientation behavior may remain intact (Leibowitz, Post and Ginsburg, 1980). Telescopes can be helpful in distance detail vision, even when the individual is moving about as people with reduced vision have less trouble due to movement. Meire and De Laey (1984) found that children do not always use the telescope for distant vision before the eye with the best visual acuity, but often before the eye with the largest visual field. On the other hand, the type of magnification aid best suited to the reading needs of a low vision patient will usually be determined by considerations other than the extent of the field of view. Generally, a minimum magnification to produce the desired acuity level for reading is employed because of the diminishing field of view when optical power is increased. For any given type of magnification aid, it is desirable that the instrument field of view (and thus the number of letters seen at any one time) be as large as possible, particularly when a high-power magnification aid is

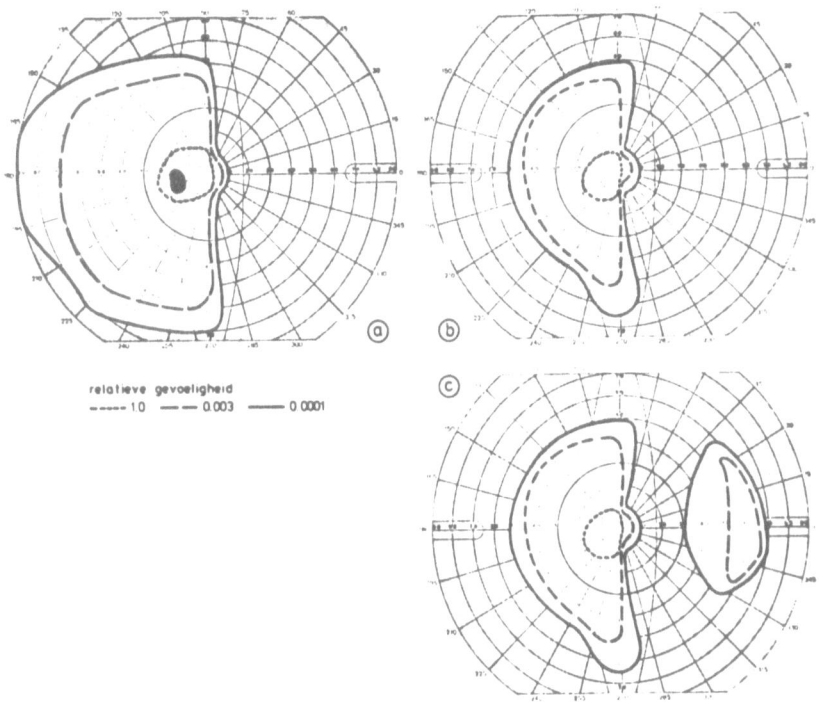

relatieve gevoeligheid
----- 1.0 — — 0.003 ——— 0.0001

Fig. 21. Vos' subject with right homonymous hemianopsia: visual field of the left eye (a), visual field of the right eye (b) and visual field of the right eye when equipped with the special mirror (c). From Vos (1974).

required (Sloan and Jablonski, 1959). One must also be concerned with peripheral aberrations such as oblique ray astigmatism and curvature of the field which can limit the usefulness of peripheral portions of the field of view (Bechtold, 1953). One of the advantages of closed-circuit television magnifiers is that the screen can be viewed from a normal reading distance. However, under such conditions, the field of view can be smaller than that of conventional reading aids (Sloan, 1974). Since patients with central visual field loss are often required to eccentrically fixate in order to achieve best resolution and visual efficiency, techniques for training eccentric viewing have been developed. The preferred degree and direction of eccentric fixation is often determined by the results of visual field testing (Inde and Blackman, 1975; Goodrich and Quillman, 1977).

Segmental field defects create significant impairments only when the field losses represent a substantial portion of the binocular visual field. Homonymous hemianopsias interfere significantly with mobility skills, driving safety and reading. Right hemianopsias are reported to cause more interference to the normal (occidental) reading process than do hemianopsias on the left side. Sometimes homonymous hemianopsias are treated through optical means by the use of mirror systems (Bailey, 1982) or prisms (Jose and Smith, 1976; Bailey, 1978; Hoeft, 1980) although the amount of success is far from universal (see Fig. 21). Hemianopic patients are likely to develop compensatory head rotations and larger, more frequent eye movements in order to examine the visual environment falling within the hemianopic side. Recently, there has been greater interest in evaluating and potentially utilizing the response properties and capabilities of sub-cortical visual pathways in patients with cortical disorders of vision such as hemianopic defects (Zihl and von Cramon, 1979).

The end stages of retinitis pigmentosa and glaucoma are the most common causes of *severe concentric visual field constriction*. In these cases, detection, orientation and mobility behavior are more affected than high resolution and fine detail visual tasks. The magnitude of visual field constriction and the degree of disability associated with it can be strongly dependent on the ambient illumination level. Faye (1976) suggested that 20 degree visual fields are required for maintaining a reasonable amount of mobility and visual search behavior. Marron and Bailey (1982) reported that field loss and reduced contrast sensitivity are of similar importance with regard to their effects on orientation and mobility of low vision patients. Optical compensation for constricted visual fields is sometimes provided by reversed galilean telescopes (the so-called 'field expanders': Drasdo, 1976; Bailey, 1978b; Keeney, 1978) or by Fresnel prisms (Hoeft, 1980; Ferraro, Jose and MacClain, 1982).

INTERFACES WITH JOB FITNESS

There are few *existing regulations* pertaining to the visual field extent necessary for specific jobs. Most of those which do exist are concerned with licensing provisions for various forms of transportation. A few examples will be presented.

Only 20 of the states in the U.S.A. perform any type of visual field examination for the licensing of drivers at the present time. Some of them specify a minimum horizontal extent for each eye and/or for both eyes, and in some instances require a greater horizontal extent for bus or truck drivers than for automobile or motorcycle drivers. However, they do not specify the conditions under which the limits of the visual field are measured. In Japan, there are no visual field requirements for any type of motor vehicle driver. Some of the European countries (such as Sweden) require automobile, truck and motorcycle drivers to have a binocular visual field which is equal to, or greater than, the size of a normal visual field in one eye alone, whereas taxi and bus drivers are required to have normal visual fields in both eyes (Hedin, 1981). Confrontation visual field testing is often recommended as the method of evaluating the visual field. Frequently the procedure for obtaining the test results are poorly defined. In Belgium, however, both eyes must have a visual field extent of 80 degrees temporally, 45 degrees nasally, 45 degrees superior and 50 degrees inferior to fixation as measured by a 10/300 target. In the Netherlands, automobile drivers must have a minimum visual field size of 80 degrees temporally and 40 degrees nasally for each eye, or 90 degrees temporally and 50 degrees nasally for one eye alone; the requirements for bus and truck drivers in 90 degrees temporally and 60 degrees nasally for each eye.

Two normal visual fields are often required for aviation pilots (ICAO Medical Manual), personnel on duty on the bridge in the Navy, and personnel working on railroad lines, although visual field examinations are frequently not performed. In the United Kingdom, a normal visual field is only required for civil aviation pilots with no indication as to the method of testing the visual field. For the Swiss military aviation, Goldmann I/4, I/3, I/2, and I/1 isopters are determined and compared with normal standards (Fankhauser, 1981).

Existing *regulations could be improved* and new regulations or guidelines for professional standards could be established by basing the visual field requirements on the opinions of experts in ergonomics and perimetry and by the results of empirical studies.

It can be *assumed* that there are: (a) Professions in which both a normal central and peripheral visual field are necessary. Automobile drivers, pilots, naval personnel working on the deck, officers, policemen, stage directors, and many other types of employment would fit in this category. (b) Professions in which the integrity of all or part of the central visual field is essential while the peripheral field is of little or no significance for the task. This would include professions requiring large amounts of reading, jewelers, engravers, watchmakers, surgeons, dentists, manicurists, hairdressers, tailors, electronic engineers, antique dealers, and many other types of employment. (c) Professions in which the integrity of the peripheral visual field is essential, whereas the central visual field is of little or no importance for performing the task. This would include stock breeders, shepherds, animal trainers, nursemaids, dancers, furniture movers, roofers, demolition experts, highway repairmen, longshoremen, and related types of employment. (d) Professions in which poor vision (including a degraded visual field) does not significantly affect performance. These professions might include farmers, gardeners, stable boys, packers, grave diggers, priests, basket makers, bartenders, cloakroom attendants, and other related professions. However, the visual field or other tests of visual performance are rarely used as a requirement for employment in these disciplines!

In sports, a visually impaired athlete has to compete with other athletes of a similar proficiency level. It can be assumed that a full field of vision is desirable for referees and for athletic participants that must check the position of other players or moving objects such as running, swimming, auto and boat racing, bicycling, tennis, cricket, polo, football, baseball, basketball, hockey, boxing, and fencing. In some instances, the critical visual field width is predictable on the basis of the geometry of the specific athletic activity. No strict visual field requirements need to be established for more individual sporting events such as long distance running and swimming, diving, gymnastics, archery, bowling, long jumping, discus, hammer throwing, or javelin throwing. It has to be taken into account that some athletes, as the swimmers, cannot wear glasses while competing. For wrestling the question was raised as to whether sight plays any part whatsoever when body contact is so intimate. This is perhaps an activity in which a totally blind individual is at no disadvantage to his sighted competitor (Douglas, 1984).

With regard to *observation*, the impact of a particular disability on performing a specific activity could be estimated by statistically comparing some type of average performance or the frequency of mishaps in a population affected by this disability with the performance characteristics or frequency of accidents in a normal control group (as attempted in the 1940's by Tiffin's group at Purdue University for many visual functions which were evaluated by means of a visual screening device). However, many handicaps can be compensated for by greater vigilance. The effect of such a handicap can be evaluated by starting a greater amount of a particular type of accidents or mishaps in the population with the handicap (Verriest et al., 1980). For visual field loss, there is the additional complication of numerous types of visual field defects and the differences in eperimental conditions, technical expertise and strategy employed in the evaluation of these defects. Some indications can be provided by comparing monocular individuals with a normal binocular population, although monocularity represents a condition that is somewhat greater than just visual field loss.

Finally, the functional visual field that is needed for a specific job can actually be *measured* by utilizing one of the techniques described in the last section of this report. However, it should also be remembered that professional training can augment the functional visual field to its optimal size (Steinschneider, 1968).

The basic pass/fail criterion could be replaced by an aptitude percentage, similar to Esterman's system but for a specific profession or job. Thus, Crick's suggestion of field units might be preferable, since for each professional group one could establish a different array of functional factors and cut-off sensitivities for each field unit. Considerable practical evaluation will be necessary to define such occupation-specific visual field requirements. Most of these functional visual field scores will need to be for binocular conditions to have practical meaning (although one eye can be occluded or neutralized during some occupational situations such as aiming and shooting a gun).

Since there are thousands of different industrial applications with numerous work patterns within each industry, it seems most reasonable to first consider a small group of environments and/or job related tasks in which visual function plays a critical role. Criteria and optimum test techniques applicable to these specific tasks can then be established and may be of value for general professional employment categories.

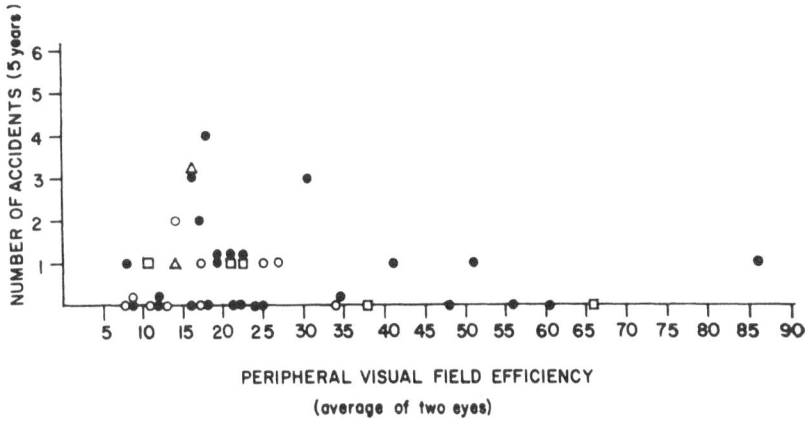

Fig. 22. Number of accidents vs. peripheral visual field efficiency (see text) in 42 patients with retinitis pigmentosa. From Fishman et al. (1981).

Driving is the human activity for which more appropriate fitness regulations are urgently needed. Although peripheral vision is undoubtedly necessary for driving (especially at lower speeds, as discussed in the section on ergonomics), the well known statistics of Henderson and Burg (1974), Council and Allen (1974), Shinar (1977) and Booher (1977) failed to find an obvious relationship between visual field size and the frequency of driving accident and/or conviction records. These negative findings can probably be attributed to the poor quality of perimetric techniques used for these studies, as compared to the standard procedures for visual field testing in clinical environments. Significant correlations between the status of the visual field and driving performance have recently been reported by Wolbarsht (1977), by Santucci et al. (1982) and also by Johnson and Keltner (1983). Using Fieldmaster automated perimetry to screen the visual fields of 10 000 California drivers, Johnson and Keltner found that individuals with binocular visual field loss had driving accident and conviction rates that were more than twice as high as those of an age and sex-matched control group (p < 0.001). Drivers with only monocular visual field loss did not show any difference in accident and conviction rates, as compared to their age and sex-matched control group.

However, previous studies (Kite and King, 1961; Gramberg-Danielsen, 1967; Keeney and Gravey, 1981) have shown that monocularity is associated with an increase in driving accident rates, particularly for pedestrian injuries and intersection accidents on the side of the missing or non-functional eye.

Fishman et al. (1981) found that retinitis pigmentosa patients with a visual acuity of 20/100 or better and various visual field defects had statistically slightly higher accident and conviction rates for driving as compared to an age and sex-matched control group of subjects with

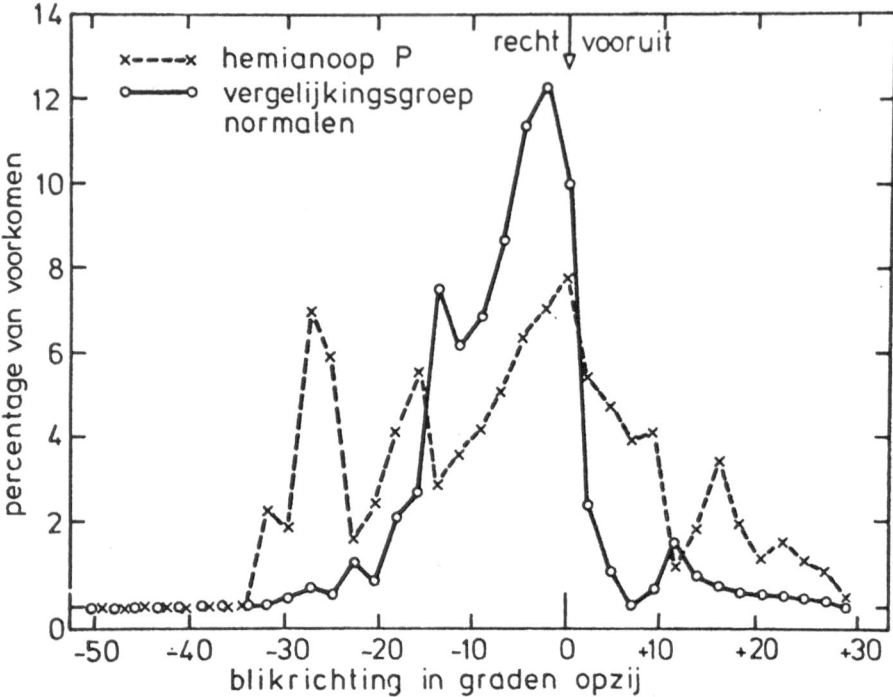

Fig. 23. Frequencies of the fixations in the different directions during driving in a group of normal subjects (continuous line) and in Vos' subject with right homonymous hemianopsia (dashed line). From Vos (1974).

normal visual fields. They found no relationship between the number of accidents and the peripheral visual field efficiency (erroneously calculated by averaging the visual field radius in the two eyes) (see Fig. 22). Although they have been used by individuals with low vision to pass the static visual acuity test for drivers' licensing, telescopic devices as centrally fixed telescopic attachments incorporates a higher risk factor for driving because they create an annular scotoma (Fonda, 1974; Lippmann, 1976; Keller and Eskridge, 1976; Hames, 1976). It is better to decenter such an attachment to the upper part of the spectacle glass, so that it is used only momentarily for reading inscriptions as that on traffic panels. The visual field defects which seem to have the greatest risk factors for driving are the bitemporal and homonymous hemianopsias. However, Danielson (1957) and Vos (1974) reported subjects with such visual field defects who drove very long distances without any difficulties encountered. Both of these authors reported that their subjects compensated for their handicap by a greater number of eye movements (Fig. 23). Moreover, Vos' subject wore a mirror.

In the section on ergonomics, we have already stressed that visual field defects are more dangerous when driving speed is slow than when it is fast. It can also be expected that when compared with Esterman's grid, driving is somewhat more concerned with the central area of the visual field within a radius of about 15 degrees including the road area beneath the fixation point (for example, for detecting irregularities in the driving surface), and with the horizontal sections in which traffic signals, crossing traffic and pedestrians most commonly appear (Rumar, 1981). Accordingly, individuals with defects in these areas (in binocular visual fields) should not be licensed for professional driving of emergency vehicles, school buses, or public transportation vehicles. However, after having examined normally sighted subjects and subjects with different visual field defects in a driving simulator, Loevsund (1982) concluded that it is impossible to say that with a certain type or size or defect a driver ought to be safe: indeed some subjects have a good compensatory mechanism while others do not. This will therefore be studied through eye and head movement recordings during driving*.

With regard to *aircraft pilots*, it has long been regarded that visual problems can be avoided by establishing a requirement of near-perfect eyesight and near-perfect standard visual functions. For example, in the United States pilots must leave at an early age because it is assumed that the reaction time becomes too long to detect movements in the far periphery as an individual grows older. However, the era of strict visual requirements appears to be dying out, since some companies now accept deuteranomalous individuals, contact lens wearers, and individuals with intraocular lens implants. The problem is now becoming one of testing relevant visual functions to establish job related visual standards.

TECHNICAL NOTES

Testing distance for behavior-related visual field evaluations should ideally be the same as the standard working distance (which at times could be different from the preferred testing distance). This is true not only because a shift from far to near distances involve changes in the optical aberrations and pupil size, but also because fatigue and performance for practical tasks over extended period of time often depends on the stresses associated with accommodation or relaxation of accommodation (Johnson, 1976).

*Cognitive factors related to vision and visual field are also important in judging driving aptitude. Indeed it is possible to recognize, e.g. by means of an embedded-figures test, field-independent drivers, who have the capacity to overcome embedding contexts in perceptual functioning, from field-dependent drivers, whose perception is dominated by the immediately given organization. There is evidence that field-dependent drivers do not quickly recognize developing hazards, are slower in responding to embedded road signs, have difficulties in learning to control a skidding vehicle, and fail to drive defensely in high-speed traffic (Olson, 1974; Goodenough, 1976). They are also less effective in their visual search pattern and require more time to process the available visual information (Shinar et al., 1978). It has to be noted that aged persons (60–70 years) took almost 7 times as long to find embedded figures than young (Mourant and Mourant, 1979), and that performance at Witken's embedded figure test is related to accident involvement (Harano, 1970).

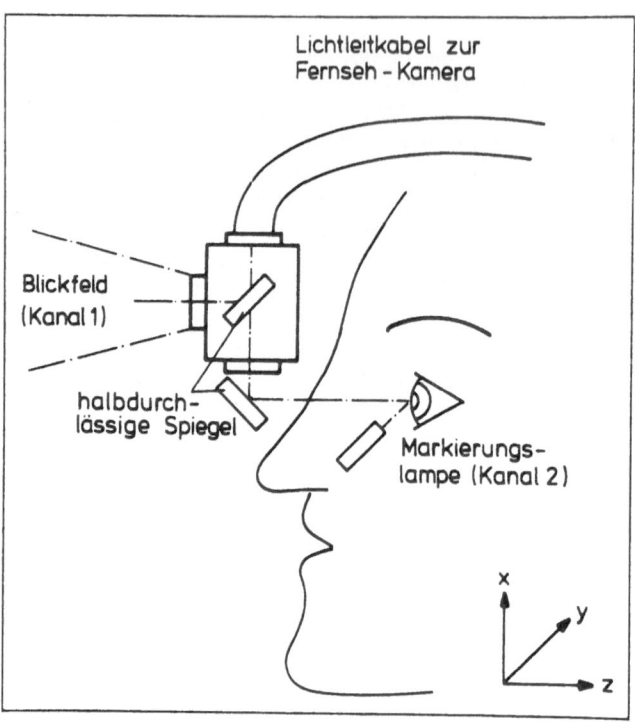

Fig. 24. Principle of the NAC-Eye-Mark-Recorder. From Enderle, Korn and Tropf (1982).

We have already emphasized several times that a realistic occupational visual field determination should generally be performed with *binocular vision*. Contrary to the procedures used in strabismus studies, occupational binocular perimetry should be performed without any dissociation between the two eyes. If the examiner uses a hemispheric perimeter bowl, the observer has to converge on the fixation point in the center of the bowl which can alter the binocular visual field: (1) by affecting lateral eccentricity estimates, (2) by reducing the lateral visual field extents, (3) by increasing the zone of overlap between the two monocular fields, (4) by creating diplopia when the perimeter bowl does not lie within Panum's fusional area, (5) by reducing binocular summation when the images of the target do not fall on exactly corresponding retinal points (see Home, 1978), and (6) by changing the angle of squint in cases of strabismus. Experience indicates that binocular perimetry is nonetheless usually performed by means of campimeters, Goldmann's perimeter and the Octopus and Dicon automatic perimeters without other problems than the eventual lack of fixation monitoring. Of course, a large radius is preferred. In cases of squint, one can ascertain which eye is responsible for detection by means of interposing Bagolini's striated lenses.

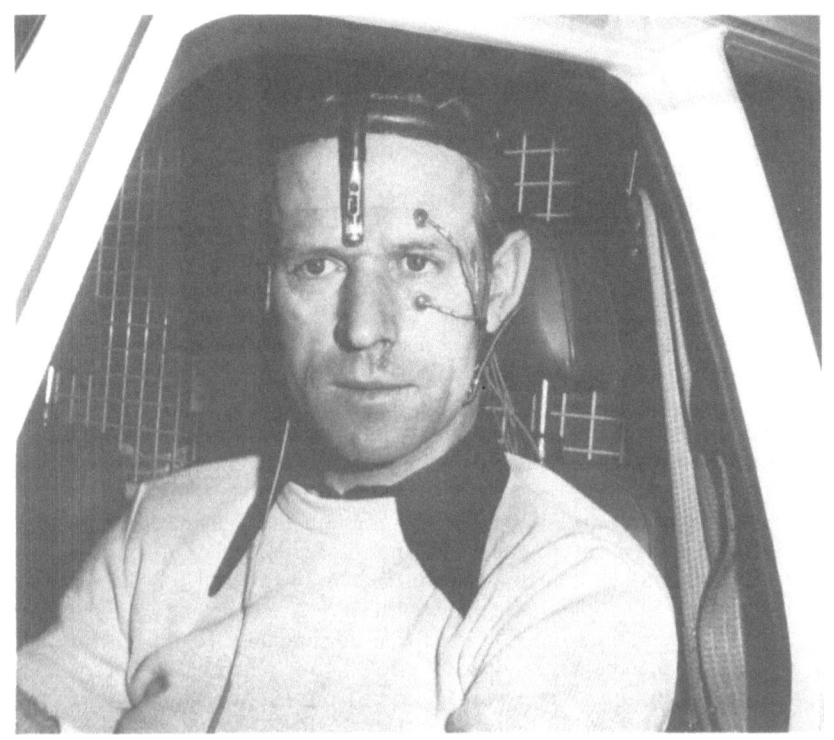

Fig. 25. Apparatus for recording gaze movements within the observed scene. From Blaauw.

Collecting eye movement data can be accomplished with electro-oculography (EOG), in which movements of the eye are determined from electrodes placed symmetrically about the eye. Another method of measuring eye movements is through the use of visible or infrared light reflected by the corneal surface or by means of a small mirror attached to a contact lens. In a new 'selspotsystem', small light-emitting diodes are attached to the contact lens. Resolution of better than 0.5 degrees usually requires a contact lens. Simple methods such as the EOG suffer from DC drifts.

The localization and tracking of the fixation point within an observed scene can be determined by means of special equipment. In the NAC-Eye-Mark-Recorder (Fig. 24), supported on the nose by means of a special type of spectacle frames, the first optical channel displays the frontal environment while a second channel follows the reflexion of a light source off of the cornea. This image can be adjusted to correspond to the visual axis. In a similar Dutch device the frontal environment is recorded by means of a television camera mounted on the subject's head by means of a helmet attachment, while the point of fixation in the visual field is measured by means of EOG electrodes and presented as a spot on the television display (Blaauw, 1974). In a newer device of the same author the television camera sees the frontal environment through fiber optics (Fig. 25). Both kinds of instruments are suitable for mobile use, as for example, in the measurement of eye movements of automobile drivers or airline pilots.

Head movements can be measured by means of different types of devices. The simultaneous measurement of eye and head movements is possible by the use of the 'Sensorsystem for Automation and Measurement' (S.A.M.) used by Schumacher and Korn (1981).

To assess the *dynamic functional visual field* of normal observers, it is necessary to restrict their field of view to a specific small area which maintains a constant relative position to the fovea in spite of eye movements. Subjects are than asked to carry out some type of visual task, such as sentence reading or pattern perception. The dynamic functional visual field is then determined by measuring the minimum visual performance occurs (for example, per cent correct or time for carrying out the task).

Three primary techniques for determining the dynamic functional visual field have been reported. The first consists of desensitizing retinal areas other than the portion that is to be used for the visual task by pre-adapting that region with very bright light (Kamiyama, 1976). This method has the advantage of simplicity in implementing and modifying the size and position of the restricted visual field, but has the disadvantages of a short period of time during which measurements are possible and being restricted to the use of very dim visual stimuli whose brightness must be continually adjusted so that they are only detected within the restricted portion of the visual field. A very small restricted visual field cannot be accomplished with this method.

The second method consists of limiting the visual field by fixing onto the subject's eye a special suction cup which has a small opening at its end (Andreeva, Vergiles and Lomov, 1972). It is possible with this method to restrict the visual field size to 0.5 degrees or less, but the suction cup has to be tightly fitted to the sclera and it is difficult to make many changes in field size for this reason.

The third method consists of using a TV screen and present a visual stimulus on a small area whose position coincides exactly with the visual axis despite eye movements made by the subject (Watanabe, 1971; McConkie and Rayner, 1975; Ikeda, Uchikawa and Saida, 1979; Schumacher and Korn, 1981) (see Fig. 17 on p. 180 of the first part of this report, 1983). This method has the advantages of ease in altering visual field size, changing stimulus conditions, and collecting simultaneous data on eye movements. However, it requires a precise alignment between the visual axis and the visual field on the TV screen regardless of any eye movement.

In addition, the influence of visual field defects on performance can be studied by means of driving simulators (Lovsund and Hedin, 1982), flight simulators, and simulators for general ergonomic purposes ('Sylvie' of Essilor).

The integration time necessary for pattern perception in the presence of a restricted visual field can be determined by displaying the pattern element by element (Ikeda and Uchikawa, 1978). For practical situations such as driving, the amount of visual information needed can be estimated by occluding both eyes and providing information elements only upon demand (Triggs, 1979; Fraser and Perry, 1980; Blaauw, 1981).

The last methodological issue that we will consider in this review is a very practical one consisting of the *detection of visual field defects in the context of industrial medicine and drivers' license requirements.*

The sophisticated manual perimeters used by ophthalmologists cannot be employed because: (1) they are very expensive, (2) they offer a homogeneous background that enhances annoying phenomena such as local adaptation, (3) they can only be used by skilled technical personnel, and (4) test time is quite long (even for a primitive arc perimeter!).

With regard to non-ophthalmologic multiphasic visual screening instruments, most of them, such as the Bausch & Lomb Ortho-Rater, the Titmus Vision Tester, the Essilor Visiotest, and the Rodenstock Instruments tester, can now be equipped with perimetric attachments which provide an approximate measurement of the horizontal extent of the binocular visual field for a gross test object (Fig. 26). However, the sole determination of horizontal visual field extent is insufficient if one wishes to detect the most frequent perimetric defects that are potentially incompatible with job performance. In pigmentary retinopathy, the patient often possesses temporal crescents while other remaining portions of the visual field are severely constricted. On the other hand, the most frequent disease process given rise to visual field defects, i.e., glaucoma, impairs the paracentral and nasal regions of the visual field long before the temporal portions of the visual field. In both disease processes, visual acuity is often minimally affected so that extensive visual field defects cannot be detected if vision is evaluated only by visual screeners such as those mentioned above, even with their perimetric attachment.

Better alternatives for rapid and reliable screening of the central and paracentral visual field are offered by the multiple pattern method of Harrington-Flocks (used by Danielson, 1957), by the multiple stimulus method of Friedmann (used by Chevaleraud and Perdriel, 1977), by the Central Field Screener of Otori, Hokki and Ikeda (1982) and especially by the Sine-Bell Screener of Crick and Crick (1981). All of these devices can be used by relatively unskilled technicians and require only a short time of testing. Many of them are also quite economical. The combination of using such a device for evaluating central and paracentral sensitivities with a device which evaluates the peripheral visual field limits by means of an arc perimeter or a perimetric attachment to a vision screener might be recommended for evaluation of individuals for whom a full visual field is a requirement for their profession.

Automatic perimeters could also be used for screening purposes. The

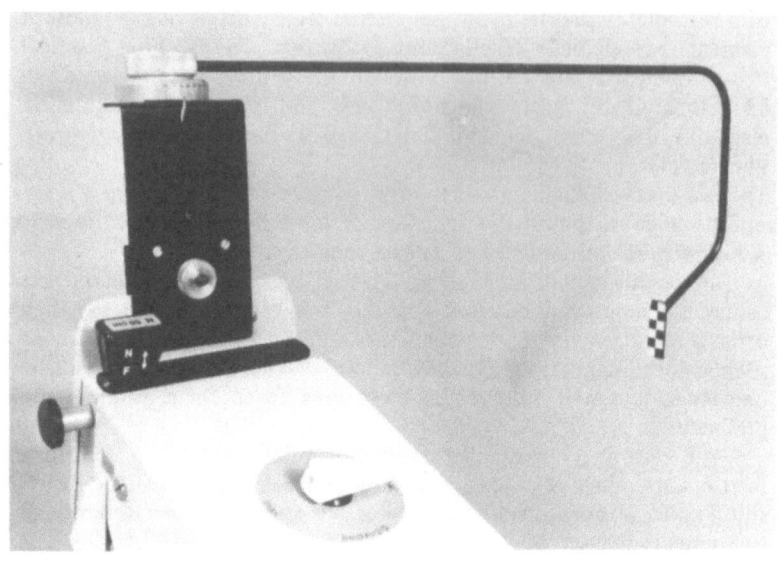

Fig. 26. Perimetric attachment of the Rodenstock multiphasic visual screener.

location of the stimuli is particularly convenient for ergonomic purposes in the Peritest (Rodenstock), in the Fieldmaster (Synemed), in the Ocuplot (Coherent) and, of course, in the Esterman program of the Dicon (Copper Vision), which automatically gives the percentage of effective visual field for the general labor market. However, an automatic perimeter is still too expensive for the examining room of an industrial physician.

It appears that we must develop for industrial physicians and examiners a perimeter which would be inexpensive, reliable, portable, have a calibrated background adaptation level, offer stimuli of fairly constant location and contrast, have a means of monitoring fixation, make minimum demands on the subject and the operator, and be adaptable to specific aspects of visual testing for ergonomic purposes.

Should the test be done with monocular or with binocular vision? Particularly in the case of squint, binocularity corresponds to the typical situation for most work conditions; however, a binocular test loses a great part of its value for detection of ophthalmic disease and technical problems also arise from convergence and testing distance.

The area of the visual field to be examined represents another fundamental decision process. Ophthalmologists now consider that the majority of visual deficits can be detected within the central visual field area, but the peripheral visual field is undoubtedly more important for job related activities than for ophthalmologic diagnosis.

318

Unfortunately, its evaluation excludes the sole use of a campimeter that could be folded up easily carried from location to location.

It must also be decided whether the spectacle correction worn at the job is to be used during the test. In this case, the peripheral scotomata introduced by the spectacle frames and/or lenses could be nullified by using large or double stimuli (Hedin, Rumar and Verriest, 1981). When the correction is not worn, the effects of refractive error can be minimized by using larger or sine-bell stimuli (Crick and Crick, 1981).

In order to decide the number and the location of the stimuli to be used, we must take into account all of the spatial localizations which are important from the ergonomic point of view and the location of the most frequent types of visual field defects. For this purpose, the Johnson and Keltner (1981) computer analysis of visual field loss could be performed again for binocular vision. However, mass screening for visual pathology vs. mass screening for effectiveness of an industrial or transportation task are two different issues.

Stimuli must be suprathreshold, but the intensities should be adjusted to correspond to the normal sensitivity gradient from the fovea towards the periphery. Gratings, or sine-bell stimuli, could be used because the quality of vision is better evaluated for targets larger than the resolution limits. The overall contrast could be adjusted to compensate for sensitivity losses associated with age (Hedin, Rumar and Verriest, 1981). Multiple stimuli could be used to reduce the duration of the test; however, incidence of visual field loss in an selected population is so low (about 3–3.5% between the ages of 16 and 60: Johnson and Keltner, 1983) that there is a great danger that the examiner would not pay attention to the presence of a definite area of visual field loss using these types of multiple stimulus procedures. A numerical scoring system could thus be helpful in reporting results or in categorizing subjects.

Additional topics for discussion with regard to visual field tests performed for industrial or transportation purposes would include the use of concentrated attention on the fixation point, a structured background, moving targets, and even allowing eye and head movements in order to determine the effective dynamic visual field. Hence, performance depends both upon what can be observed during a single fixation and the pattern of eye and head movements that are made, such experimental results might be somewhat ambiguous, particularly in the absence of eye movement recordings (Inditsky, 1980). However, it could be recommended that the presentation time of a static target corresponds to the mean interval between two successive ocular saccades (Bouma, 1980). Reaction time could also be readily measured.

Perimetry manufacturers who were approached about the possibility of making an industrial visual field device stated that there is little interest in visual field screening at the present time, and that the medical profession should oppose the use of such equipment by non-medical personnel. However, in visual ergonomics, all opinions change very rapidly. It appears that there is a greater potential demand for industrial perimeters than first thought. Many industries, state motor vehicle bureaux, school medical centers, worker's compensation boards, social security offices, military and aviation centers — all these will sooner or later be potential buyers of standard, simplified and less expensive perimeters.

BIBLIOGRAPHY

Abel, L.A., Troost, B.T. and Dell'Osso, L.F. The effects of age on normal saccadic chatacteristics and their variability. Vision Res. 23: 33–37 (1983).

Åberg, L. and Rumar, K. Headmovements of drivers, Equipment and exploratory study. Report 182, Department of Psychology, University of Uppsala, Sweden (1975).

Andreeva, E.A., Vergiles, J.Ju. and Lomov, B.F. On the functions of eye movements in the process of visual perception. Voprosy Phikhologii 18: 11–24 (1972).

Aulhorn, E. Die Gesichtsfeldprüfung bei macularen Erkrankungen. Ber. Dtsch. Ophthalmol. Ges. 73: 77–86 (1975).

Aulhorn, E. Funktionsprüfung des Auges zur Fesstellung der Kraftfahreignung. In: Straub W. (ed.): Die Ophthalmologischen Untersuchungsmethoden. Ferdinand Enke Verlag, Stuttgart (1976) (Bd. 2: 922–990).

Bailey, I.L. Visual field measurement in low vision. Optom. Monthly 69: 697–701 (1978a).

Bailey, I.L. Field expanders. Optom. Monthly 69: 813–816 (1978b).

Bailey, I.L. Prismatic treatment for field defects. Optom. Monthly 69: 1073–1078 (1978c).

Bailey, I.L. Mirrors for visual field defects. Optom. Monthly 72: 202–206 (1982).

Bartz, A.E. Peripheral detection and central task complexity. Human Factors 18: 63–70 (1976).

Bauder, R. SKS-Aktion 'Sehen und gesehen werden'. Schweizer Optiker 275–278 (1980).

Bechtold, E.W. An improved system of wide-angle magnifying spectacles. Opt. J. Rev. Optom. 40: 35–40 (1953).

Benz, C., Grob, R. and Haubner, P. Gestaltung von Bildschirm-Arbeitsplätzen. Verlag TUV Rheinland, Köln (1981).

Berggrund U., Derefeldt G., Hedin C. and Marmolin H. Colour coded vs. monochrome situational maps. NATO Workshop 'Colour Coded vs. Monochrome Electronic Displays', Farnborough (UK), 28.2–1.3.1984.

Biberman, L.M. Perception of displayed information. Plenum Press (1973) (Chapter 6.4).

Binkhorst, C.D. Pers. communication (1983).

Blaauw, G. J. Drivers' scanning behaviour on some curved and straight road sections. 1 er Congr. int. sur la Vision et la Sécurité Routière, 47–56 (1974).

Blaauw, G.J. Driver's internal representation and supervisory control: A first model verification in relation to driving experience, task demands and deteriorated vision. 1st Ann. Conf. on Human Decision and Manual Control, Delft 25–27.5.1981.

Blaauw, G.J. Ergonomie in het wegverkeer. Tijdschr. voor Ergonomie, Special ARBO 82, 11–19 (1982).

Boissin, J.P. Rôle de l'ophtalmologiste dans l'indication des aides visuelles. Vision ISSN 0151–2366 (1980).

Booher, H. NHTSA studies of new vision tests for state driver licensing exams. Traffic Safety 77: 26 (1977).

Bouma, H. Visual search and reading, Eye movements and functional visual field: A tutorial review. In: Nickerson R.S. (edit.): Attention and performance VIII. Lawrence Erlbaum Assoc., Hillsdale, New Jersey (1980).

Boyce, P.R. The visual detection lobe and visual inspection. Lux Europa, Granada, 1981.

Bronner, A., Baikoff, G., Charleux, J., Flament, J., Gerhard, J.P. and Risse, J.F. La correction de l'aphakie. Masson, Paris (1983).

Bursill, A.E. The restriction of peripheral vision during experiments to hot and humidity conditions. Quart. J. Exptl Psychol. 10: 113 (1958).

Byrnes, V.A. Vision and its importance in driving. Sight-Sav. Rev. 37: 87–91 (1967).

Calabria, G., Capris, P. and Burtolo, C. Investigations on space behaviour of glaucomatous people with extensive visual field loss. Docum. Ophthalmol. Proc. Ser. 35: 205–210 (1983).

Campos, E.C. Binocularity in comitant strabismus: Binocular visual field studies. Docum. Ophthalmol. 53: 249–281 (1982).

Capris, P. and Fava, G.P. Contribution to this paper (1982).

Chevaleraud, J. and Perdriel, G. L'intérêt du champ visuel central avec l'appareillage de Friedmann dans les expertises du personnel navigant. XXIe Congrès Int. Méd. Aéronautique et Spatiale, Munich 17–21 September (1973).

Christ, R.E. Review and analysis of color coding research for visual displays. Human Factors 17: 542–570 (1975).

Council, F.M. and Allen, J.A. A study of the visual fields of North Carolina drivers and their relationship to accidents. Report of Highway Safety Research Center, University of North Carolina, Chapel Hill, NC (1974).

Crick, R.P. and Crick, J.C.P. The sine-bell screener. Docum. Ophthalmol. Proc. Ser. 26: 233–237 (1981).

Crick, J.C.P. and Crick, R.P. The sine-bell stimulus in perimetry. Docum. Ophthalmol. Proc. Ser. 26: 239–246 (1981).

Crick, R.P., Crick, J.C.P. and Ripley, L. The representation of the visual field. Docum. Ophthalmol. Proc. Series 35: 193–203 (1983).

Cristiani, R. Gli occhiali (corettivi) colorati dal punto de vista ergo-oftalmologico. Atti Fond. G. Ronchi 36: 703–710 (1981).

Danielson, R.W. The relationship of fields of vision to safety in driving, with a report of 680 drivers examined by various screening methods. Am. J. Ophthalmol. 44: 657–680 (1957).

Dannheim, F. Non-linear projection in visual field charting. Docum. Ophthalmol. Proc. Ser. 35: 217–220 (1983).

Douglas, G.R. Pers. comm. (1984).

Drasdo, N. Visual field expanders. Am. J. Optom. Physiol. Optics 53: 564–567 (1976).

Enderle, E., Korn, A. and Tropf, H. Echtzeit-Registrierung von Blickbewegungen bei frei beweglichem Kopf. FhG Berichte 3: 12–15 (1982).

Enoch, J., Boynton, R. and Bush, W. Physical measures of stray light in excised eyes. J. Opt. Soc. Am. 55: 879–886 (1954).

Enoch, J.M., Campos, E.C. and Bedell, H.E. Visual resolution in a patient exhibiting a visual fatigue or saturation-like effect: Probable multiple sclerosis. Arch. Ophthalmol. 97: 76–78 (1979).

Erickson, R.A. Visual search performance in a moving structured field. J. Opt. Soc. Am. 54: 399–405 (1964).

Erikson, R.A. Line criteria in target acquisition with television. Human Factors 20: 573–588 (1978).

Esterman, B. Functional scoring of the binocular field. Ophthalmology 89: 1226–1234 (1982).

Evans, I. and Rothery, R. The influence of forward vision and target size on apparent inter-vehicular spacing. Transp. Sci. 10: 85–101 (1976).

Fankhauser, F. Contribution to this paper (1981).

Fankhauser, F. and Enoch, J. M. The effects of blur on perimetric thresholds. Arch. Ophthalmol. 68: 240–252 (1962).

Faye, E.E. Clinical low vision. Little & Brown, Boston (1976).

Ferraro, J., Jose, R.T. and Olsen McClain, L.M. Fresnel prisms as a treatment option for retinitis pigmentosa. Texas Optom. 38: 18–21 (1982).

Fishman, G.A., Anderson, R.J., Stinson, L. and Haque, A. Driving performance of retinitis pigmentosa patients. Br. J. Ophthalmol. 65: 122–126 (1981).

Fonda, G. Bioptic telescopic spectacles for driving a motor vehicle. Arch. Ophthalmol. 92: 348–349 (1974).

Fraser, P.J. and PE RY, E.R. The ARRB visual interruption apparatus. Australian Road Research Board Report 1980–02.

Furuno, F. Discussion part. Docum. Ophthalmol. Proc. Ser. 35: 223 (1983).

Galvin, R.J., Regan, D. and Heron, J.R. Impaired temporal resolution of vision after acute retrobular neuritis. Brain 99: 255–268 (1976).

Gandolfo, E. Perimetric changes cuased by ethyl alcohol. Docum. Ophthalmol. Proc. Ser. 35: 479–484 (1983).

Gatchell, S.M. and Miller, J.M. Prediction of drivers' eye location. Proc. 18th Ann. Meet. Hum. Factors Soc., 15–17.10.1974: 189–191.

Gibson, J.J., Olum, P. and Rosenblatt, F. Parallax and perspective during aircraft landings. Am. J. Psychol. 68: 372–385 (1958).

Ginsburg, A.P. Proposed new vision standards for the 1980's and beyond: Contrast sensitivity. AGARD Nr 310, pp. 9-1 to 9-15 (1980).

Gloria, E.M. and Sulli, R. Ergo-ophthalmological role of sunglasses. I. Influence on isopter perimetric response. Atti Fond. G. Ronchi 36: 155–158 (1981).

Godthelp, J., Blaauw, G.J. and Milgram, P. Supervisory behaviour in automobile driving: New approaches in modelling vehicle control. 20th FISITA Congr., Vienna, 6–11.5.1984.

Godthelp, J. and Riemersma, J.B.J. Werk in uitvoering op nietautosnelwegen. II: De bebakening en markering van het werkvak. Instituut voor Zintuigfysiologie TNO, Soesterberg, Rapport IZF C-20 (1980).

Goodenough, D.R. A review of individual differences in field dependence as a factor in auto safety. Human Factors 18: 53–62 (1976).

Goodrich, G.L. and Quillman, R.D. Training eccentric viewing. J. Vis. Impairm. Blindness 71: 377–381 (1977).

Gramberg-Danielsen, B. Sehen und Verkehr. Springer, Berlin (1967).

Grass-Adamczek, A. Research on influence of long-term vision task on the chosen functions of human vision organ. Prace Centralnogo Instytutu Ochrony (Warszawa) 110: 235–245 (1981).

Groenouw. Anleitung zur Berechnung der Erwebsfähigkeit bei Sehstörungen. Bergmann, Wiesbaden (1896).

Guerin, H. Electro-oculographie, campimétrie selon Friedmann, potentiels évoqués visuels en hypoxie à 5500 mètres d'altitude. Thèse med., Orléans-Tours (1981).

Gurevich, N.N. and Steinschneider, T.Y. The eye efficiency during the visual search (in Russian). All-Union Scientific Research Institute of Labour Safety in Leningrad, VCSPS, pp. 218–227 (1967).

Hager, G. Das Blickfeld, Gesichtsfeld und Umblickfeld von Brillenträgern sowie von Patienten mit kornealen Haftschalen und Patienten mit intraokularer Korrektur. Klin. Mbl. Augenheilk. 139: 317–338 (1961a).

Hager, G. Die Bedeutung von Gesichtsfeld und Blickfeldausfällen durch Brillenrahmen und Folgerungen für Billenrahmenherstellung und -Anpassung. Klin. Mbl. Augenheilk. 139: 543–553 (1961b).

Hames, L.N. Telescopic devices and driving. Traffic Med. 4: 66–67 (1976).

Harano, R.M. Relationship of field dependence and motor-vehicle-accident involvement. Percept Motor Skills 31: 272–274 (1970).

Haubner, P. Ergonomische Gestaltung der Mensch-Maschine-Kommunikation. LICHT-Forschung 5: 11–18 (1983).

Hedin, A. Contribution to this paper (1981).

Hedin, A., Rumar, K. and Verriest, G. Visual field testing of driving license applicants. 3rd Int. Congr. Ergophthalmol., Istanbul (1981).

Henderson, R.L. and Burg, A. Vision and audition in driving. Report No DOT-HS-801-265, Contract No DOT-HS-009-1-009. Prepared for U.S. Department of Transportation. National Highway Traffic Safety Administration, Washington, D.C. (1974).

Hirschberger, H.G. and Miedel, H. Sicht und Sehprobleme in der Fahrausbildung. Z. Verkehrssicherheit 26: 65–70 (1980).

Hockenbeamer, E.F. Side vision versus speed. Claims and Safety Dept., Pacific Gas and Electric C°, San Francisco (1952).

322

Hoeft, W.W. The management of visual field defects through low vision aids. J. Am. Optom. Assoc. 51: 863–864 (1980).

Home, R., Binocular summation: A study of contrast sensitivity, visual acuity and recognition. Vision Res. 18: 579–585 (1978).

Hörberg, U. and Rumar, K. The effect of running lights on vehicle conspicuity in daylight and twilight Ergonomics 22: 165–173 (1979).

Ikeda, F. Dynamic functional visual field of degeneratio pigmentosa retinae. In preparation (1983).

Ikeda, M. and Uchikawa, K. Integrating time for visual pattern perception and a comparison with the tactile mode. Vision Res. 18: 1565–1571 (1978).

Ikeda, M, Uchikawa, K. and Saida, S. Static and dynamic functional visual fields. Optica Acta 26: 1103–1113 (1979).

Inde, K. and Blackman, O. Visual training with optical aids. Hermods, Malmö (1975).

Inditsky, B. Contribution to this paper (1980).

Inditsky, B., Bodmann, H.W. and Fleck, H.J. Elements of visual performance, Contrast metric – visibily lobes – eye movements. Lighting Technol. 14: 218–231 (1982).

Irving, A. Visual acuity and driving. Road Research Laboratory, Laboratory Note No LN/819 and 915/AI (1965).

Jacobson, S.G., Sandberg, M.A. and Berson, E.L. Static fundus perimetry in amblyopia: Comparison with juvenile macular degeneration. Docum. Ophthalmol. Proc. Ser. 35: 421–427 (1983).

Jaeger, W. Abnehmbare Zusatzgläser an den Bügeln der Starbrille zur besseren Nutzung des temporalen Gesichtsfeldes. Klin. Mbl. Augenheilk. 176: 21–26 (1980).

Johnson, C.A. Effect of luminance and stimulus distance on accommodation and visual resolution. J. Opt. Soc. Am. 66: 138–142 (1976).

Johnson, C.A. and Keltner, J.L. Computer analysis of visual field loss and optimization of automated perimetric test strategies. Ophthalmology 88: 1058–1065 (1981).

Johnson, C.A. and Keltner, J.L. Incidence of visual field loss in 20,000 eyes and its relationship to driving performance. Arch. Ophthalmol. in press (1983).

Johnson, C.A. and Leibowitz, H.W. Practice, refractive error, and feedback as factors influencing peripheral motion thresholds. Perception & Psychophysics 15: 276–280 (1974).

Johnston, A.N. An investigation of some factors which impede the acquisition of visually displayed information. Thesis, Melbourne Univ. (1974).

Johnston, I.R., White, G.R. and Cumming, R.W. The role of optical expansion patterns in locomotor control. Am. J. Psychol. 86: 311–324 (1973).

Jose, R.T. and Smith, A.J. Increasing peripheral awareness with Fresnel prisms. Optom. J. Rev. Optom. 133: 33–37 (1976).

Kamiyama, T. Influence of visual field size for reading. Dissertation for Bachelor's Degree, Tokyo Inst. of Technology (1974).

Keeney, A.H. Field loss vs. Central magnification-telescopes and driving risk. Arch. Ophthalmol. 92: 273 (1974).

Keeney, A.H. Limiting factors in visual requirements for driving and suggestions concerning compensatory measures. In: Tengroth B. et al.: Current concepts in ergophthalmology, pp. 347–358. Edit. Societas Ergophthalmologica Internationalis, Stockholm, 1978.

Keeney, A. H. and Garvey, J. The dilemma of the monocular driver. Am. J. Ophthalmol. 91: 801–803 (1981).

Keller, J.T. and Eskridge, J.B. Telescopic lenses and driving. Am. J. Optom. Physiol. Opt. 53: 746–749 (1976).

Kite, C.R. and King, J.N. A survey of the factors limiting the visual fields of motor vehicle drivers in relation to minimum visual fields and visibility standards. Br. J. Physiol. Opt. 18: 85–107 (1961).

Kluyskens, J. L'inversion des limites du champ visuel et l'électro-encéphalographie, Importance du déplacement centrifuge du test en périmétrie. Bull. Soc. Belge Ophtalmol. 90: 529–539 (1948).

Kochhar, D.S. and Fraser, T.M. Peripheral visual performance in a simulated task, some quantitative aspects. First Int. Conf. on Driver Behaviour, Zürich, Oct. 1973.

Leachtenauer, J.C. Peripheral acuity and photointerpretation performance. Human Factors 20: 537–551 (1978).

Leibowitz, H., Post, R. and Ginsburg, A. The role of fine detail in visually controlled behavior. Invest. Ophthalmol. 19: 846–848 (1980).

Levi, D.M., Harwerth, R.S. and Smith, E.L. Binocular interactions in normal and anomalous binocular vision. Docum. Ophthalmol. 49: 303–324 (1980).

Lippmann, O. Driving with telescopic aids. Proc. 20th Conf. Am. Assoc. Automative Med., Atlanta, 1–3.11. 1976.

Lloyd, V.V. A comparison of critical fusion frequencies for different areas in the fovea and in the periphery. Am. J. Psychol. 65: 346 (1952).

Lövsund, P. Traffic safety effects caused by drivers with visual field defects. First Nordic Congr. on Traffic Med., 8–11.6.1982, Linkoeping, Sweden: 185–187.

Lövsund, P. and Hedin, A. A method for evaluation of the influence of visual field defects on driver performance. 9th int. Ergophthalmol. Symp., San Francisco (1982).

McConkie, G.W. and Rayner, K. The span of the effective stimulus during a fixation in reading. Perception & Psychophysics 17: 578–586 (1985).

Mackworth, N.H. Visual noise causes tunnel vision. Psychonomic Science 3: 67–68 (1965).

Magnus, H. Leitfaden für Begutachtung und Berechnung von Unfallsbeschädigung der Augen. Kern, Breslau (1894).

Marron, J.A. and Bailey, I.L. Visual factors and orientation and mobility performance. Am. J. Optom. Physiol. Optics 59: 413–426 (1982).

Meire, F. and De Laey, J.J. How do visually handicapped children use their low vision aids? Bull. Soc. Belge Ophthalmol., in press (1984).

Meldrum, J.F. Driver eye position. Ford Motor C°, Dearborn, Mich.: TR No. 5-65-3 (1965).

Meur, G. L'acuité visuelle périphérique chez l'aphake et le pseudophake. Bull. Soc. Belge Ophtalmol., in press (1983).

Miller, D., Brooks, S.M. and Wolf, E. The effect of the honeycomb on glare function. Arch. Ophthalmol. 94: 451–454 (1976).

Miller, J.M. and Gatchell, S.M. A research design to collect data for a second generation eyellipse. Automotive Eng. Congr. and Exhib., Detroit, 24–28. 2. 1975.

Mourant, R.R. and Mourant, R.R. Driving performance of the elderly. Accid. Anal. & Prev. 11: 247–253 (1979).

Mourant, R.R. and Rockwell, T.H. Mapping eye-movement pattern to the visual scene in driving: An exploratory study. Human Factors 12: 81 (1970).

Nelson, W. The effects of reduced partial pressures of oxygen (hypoxia) on the size of the visual field in humans. Thesis, Durham (N. Carolina), 1983.

Noble, N. and Sanders, A.P. Searching for traffic signals while engaged in compensatory tracking. Human Factors 22: 89–102 (1980).

Olson, P.L. Aspects of driving performance as a function of field dependance. J. Appl. Psychol. 59: 192–196 (1974).

Olson, R. A. and Moulden, J. V. Interactions of peripheral and central visions. Pennsylvania Transp. and Traffic Safety Center, Techn. Note 45 (1972).

Otori, T., Hohki, T. and Ikeda, M. Central Field Screener: A new tool for screening and quantitative campimetry. Stencyl (1982).

Overington, I. Modelling of visual threshold performance with imperfect imagery. Br. Aerospace Dynamics Group, Bristol Division, Rep. N° ST 23214 (1980).

Overington, I. Limitations of spatial-frequency-based criteria for assessment of raster display systems. SPIE Proceedings 399 (1983).

Papin, J.P., Menu, J.P. and Santucci, G. Vision monoculaire et vol tactique sur hélicoptère. pp. 21-2 to 21-14 in the Conference Proceedings N° 312 'The impact of new guidance and control system on military aircraft cockpit design'. AGARD, Neuilly-sur-Seine (1981).

Post, R. and Leibowitz, H. The effect of refractive error on central and peripheral motion sensitivity at various exposure durations. Perception & Psychophysics 29: 91–94 (1981).

Rackoff, N.J. and Rockwell T.H. Driver search and scan patterns in night driving. In:

Moore M. (ed.), Driver Needs in Night Driving, TRB Special Report 156, Washington (1975).

Ravestein, R., Veling, I.H. and Gaillard, A.W.K. De rijgeschiktheid van revalidanten met een diffuse hersenbeschadiging: Een probleemoriëntatie. Rapport nr. IZF 1928-16, RVO-TNO, Soesterberg (1982).

Rey, P. Lumière intermittente et sécurité routière. 1er Congr. int. Vision Sécurité Routière, Paris, 239–248 (1975).

Riemersma, J.B.J. Analyse van de rijtaak. TNO-Nieuws 27: 218–220 (1972).

Riemersma, J.B.J. Perceptual cues in vehicle guidance on a straight road. 2nd Eur. Ann. Conf. on Hum. Decision Making and Manual Control, Bonn (1982).

Rockwell, T.H. Eye movement analysis of visual information acquisition in driving: An overview. 6th Conf. Australian Road Res. Board, 316–331 (1972).

Ronchi, L. and Salvi, G. Capacity of the visual system, CFF, and entoptic straylight. Atti Fond. G. Ronchi 20: 735–742 (1965).

Ronchi, L. and Salvi, G. Performance decrement under prolonged testing across the visual field. Ophthalmic Res. 5: 113–120 (1973).

Ross, J.E. The functional effects of visual disorder. Thesis, Oxford (1983).

Ross, J.E., Bron A.J. and Clarke, D.D. Contrast sensitivity and visual disability in chronic simple glaucoma. Br. J. Ophthalmol., in press (1984).

Rumar, K. Contribution to this paper (1981).

Salvatore, S. The estimation of vehicular velocity as a function of visual stimulation. Human Factors 10: 27–31 (1968).

Salvatore, S. Performance decrement caused by mild carbon monoxide levels on two visual fonction. J. Saf. Res. 6: 131–734 (1974).

Sanders, A.T. Aandachtverschuiving en lawaaihinder. Ned. Tijdschr. Psychol. 16: 460 (1961).

Sanders, A.F. and Hoogenboom, W. Mental blocking in continuous serial performance. 19th Int. Congr. Psychol., London (1969).

Sanders, A.F. and Reitsma, W.D. The effect of sleep-loss on processing information in the functional visual field. Acta Psychol. 51: 149–162 (1982).

Santucci, G.F., Menu, J.P., Batejat, D. and Barrault, B. Acuité visuelle, champ visuel et accident automobile. Stencyl, L.C.B.A. Divition Psychophysiologie de la perception visuelle, Paris (1982).

Schneider, R.C. and Antine, B.E. Visual field impairment related to football headgear and face guards. J. Am. Med. Assoc. 192: 616–618 (1965).

Schumacher, W. and Korn, A. Automatic evaluation of eye and head movements for visual information selection. Conf. of the Eur. Group of Eye Movement Res., Bern (1981).

Serra, A. Quantitative isopter constriction under image degradation by defocus. Docum. Ophthalmol. Proc. Ser. 35: 289–293 (1983).

Shinar, D. Driver visual limitations, diagnosis and treatment. Report No. DOT-HS-803-260, Contact No. DOT-HS-5-01275. Prepared for US Department of Transportation, National Highway Traffic Safety Administration, Washington, DC (1977).

Shinar, D., MacDowell, E.D., Rackoff, N.J. and Rockwell, T.H. Field dependence and driver visual search behavior. Human Factors 20: 553–559 (1979).

Sloan, L.L. Area and luminance of test object as variables in examination of the visual field by projection perimetry. Vision Res. 1: 121--138 (1961).

Sloan, L.L. Evaluation of closed-circuit television magnifiers. Sight-Sav. Rev. 123–133 (1974).

Sloan, L.L. and Jablonski, M.D. Reading aids for the partially blind. Arch. Ophthalmol. 62: 465–484 (1959).

Steinschneider, T. The visual search influence on the visual field (in Russian). Sbornik Nauchnye Raboty Institutov Okhrany Truda VZSPS (Profizdat) 51: 58–61 (1968).

Surwillo, W.W. Frequency of the 'alpha' rhythm, reaction time and age. Nature (Lond.) 191: 823–824 (1961).

Tshernilovskaja, F.M. Lighting of industrial buildings and man's working ability. Rep. Min. Publ. Health, Leningrad (1968).

Ucke, C. Streulicht im Auge. Thèse, Munich (1973).

Triggs, T.J. Visual sampling by drivers in different visibility conditions. Ergonomics 22: 764 (1979).

Verriest, G. (ed.), Barca, L., Dubois-Poulsen, A., Houtmans, M.J.M., Inditsky, B., Johnson, C., Overington, I., Ronchi, L. and Villani, S. The occupational visual field. I. Theoretical aspects. The normal functional visual field. Docum. Ophthalmol. Proc. Ser. 35: 165–185 (1983).

Verriest, G., De Landtsheer, A., Uvijls, A., Claeys, P., Cobbaut, L. & Van Langenhove, M. Muscular activity and perimetric thresholds. Int. Ophthalmol. 7: 37–43 (1984).

Verriest, G., Dela Ruye, J., Uvijls, A., Roucour, J., Bayet, R. and Porteman, A. Etude comparative des effets sur la vision d'un vitrage non teinté et de trois vitrages teintés de pare-brise. Bull. Soc. Belge Ophtalmol. 193: 213–229 (1981).

Verriest, G., Neubauer, O., Marre, M. and Uvijls, A. New investigations concerning the relationships between congenital colour vision defects and road traffic security. Int. Ophthalmol. 2: 87–99 (1980).

Verriest, G. and Uvijls, A. Spectral increment thresholds on a white background in different age groups of normal subjects and in acquired ocular diseases. Docum. Ophthalmol 43: 217–248 (1977).

Verriest, G. and Van De Casteele, J. Le champ visuel clinique. Acta Belg. Arte Med. Pharmac. Milit. 18: 35–205 (1972).

Verriest, G., Van Laethem, J., Benozzi, J. and Uvijls, A. La measure de la luminance équivalente de voile en ophtalmologie. I. Introduction. Bull. Soc. Belge Ophtalmol. 201: 127–142 (1982).

Vos, J.J. On the traffic behavior of a man with homonymous hemianopsia of the right half of the visual field. Inst. Percept. RVO-TNO nr. IZF-1974-3 (1974).

Watanabe, A. Fixation points and the eye movements. Oyo Butsuri 40, 330–334 (1971).

Weale, R.A. Physical changes due to age and cataract. In: Ducan G. (ed.) Mechanisms of cataract formation in the human lens. Academic Press, London pp. 47–70 (1981).

Wolbarsht, M.L. Tests for glare sensitivity and peripheral vision in driver applicants. J. Safety Res. 9: 128–139 (1977).

Zihl, J. and Von Cramon, D. Restitution of visual function in patients with cerebral blindness. J. Neurol. Neurosurg. Psychiat. 42: 312–322 (1979).

Zimmer, H.G. Geometrical optics. Springer, Berlin 1970).

DETERIORATION IN READING WITH NARROWED VISUAL FIELDS

F. IKEDA, M. IKEDA, S. SHIOIRI and M. TAKAO

(*Tokyo and Yokohama, Japan*)

ABSTRACT

The recognition time for a test stimulus of 80 degrees diameter of Japanese hiragana was measured for 39 subjects and found to vary from 0.1 sec to more than 600 sec, depending on the residual area of the visual field. A formula relating the recognition time to visual field size was determined from normal subjects by artificially narrowing their visual fields and was used to estimate the patients' functional visual fields. In one patient with an extremely narrow visual field, the functional visual field was only 3 degrees in diameter, which was about 50 degrees in normal subjects.

INTRODUCTION

Earlier Ikeda and his colleagues showed by artificially narrowing of the visual field of normal subjects that a wide visual field is indispensable to achieve a normal pattern perception and that a serious deterioration takes place when the visual field is narrowed, resulting in great prolongation of recognition time or even in inability to perceive any meaningful pattern (1, 2). It was expected that such a deterioration also takes place in patients with narrow visual fields, and it will be shown in the present paper that such is indeed the case.

RECOGNITION TIME

Experimental arrangement: To assess the ability of patients to perceive patterns we measured the recognition time for Japanese phonetic 'hiragana' letters. An example of the letter stimulus is shown in Fig. 1. A letter drawn with a bush was transferred onto a polka dots sheet to digitize the letter so as to make it harder to read. The subject sat down at a certain distance from a rear screen to observe monocularly a letter which was projected from behind the screen with a slide projector installed with a shutter. The stimulus diameter was 1 meter when projected, corresponding to a visual angle of 80 degrees when viewed from a distance of 60 cm. A total of 131 stimuli were

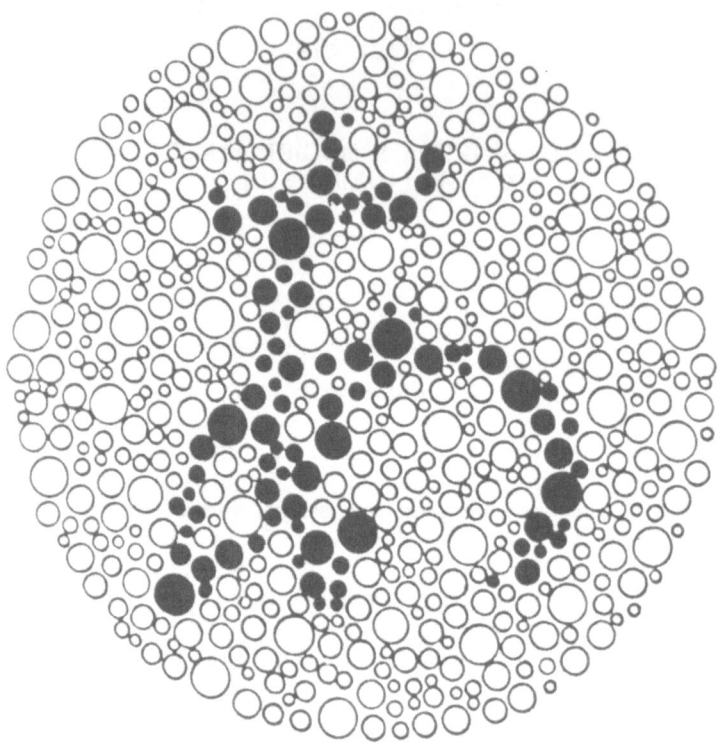

Fig. 1. An example of the test stimulus. The Japanese phonetic letter 'a'.

prepared and presented sequentially to the subject using three prefixed durations in random order. The subject responded to each stimulus by reading the letter or saying 'no' when he could not recognize the stimulus. He could move his eyes freely and turn his head, but not move it back and forth from the screen. The percentage of correct answers was obtained for each of the three durations and the recognition time corresponding to the point of 50% of the answers correct was determined.

A total of 39 subjects participated in the experiment — 14 normal, 13 with glaucoma, 10 with pigmentary degeneration, 1 with macular hole, and 1 other. Results: Fig. 2 shows the recognition time T logarithmically plotted against the stimulus size α in degrees. Some subjects were tested at two or three different distances giving two or three experimental points in the figure. These points are connected by straight lines. The slopes of these lines average about 3 as represented by the thick line at the bottom, which implies the relation T/α^3 is constant. The smaller the test stimulus, the shorter the

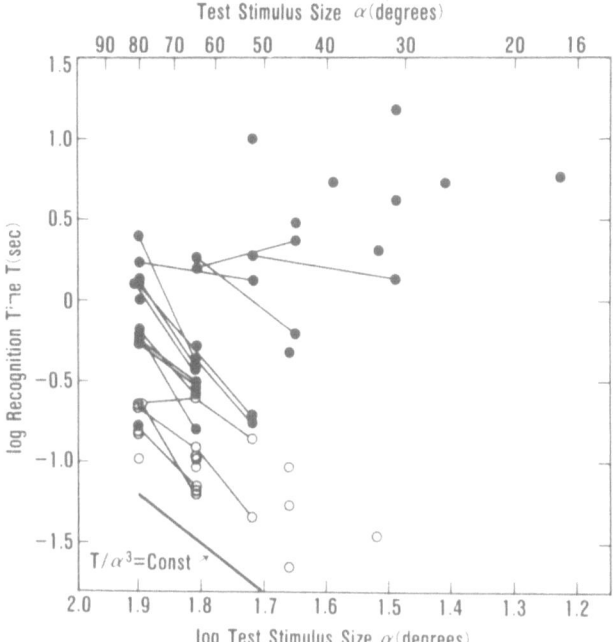

Fig. 2. Plots of recognition time versus stimulus size. Open circles are for normal subjects and filled ones are for patients with narrowed visual fields.

recognition time. Open circles are from normal subjects and filled ones from patients. In normal subjects the recognition time T is short even with a large stimulus size, while in patients with narrowed visual field, T is longer for a stimulus of the same or even of smaller size. Deterioration in pattern perception is quite evident.

To compare the capability for pattern recognition directly among subjects, the recognition time for a test size of 80 degrees was estimated for each subject by utilizing the formula $T/\alpha^3 =$ constant. For subjects who provided more than one experimental point the averaged recognition time was used for the estimation. The results are shown in Fig. 3. It is to be noticed that it took only 0.2 seconds or so for normal subjects to recognize a Japanese hiragana, while it took as much as 600 seconds for a glaucoma patient.

FUNCTIONAL VISUAL FIELD

Experimental arrangement: To estimate the functional visual field size of each subject, first a formula to relate the recognition time to the functional visual field size was obtained by artificially narrowing the visual fields of normal subjects by utilizing a masked television monitor (1). The same

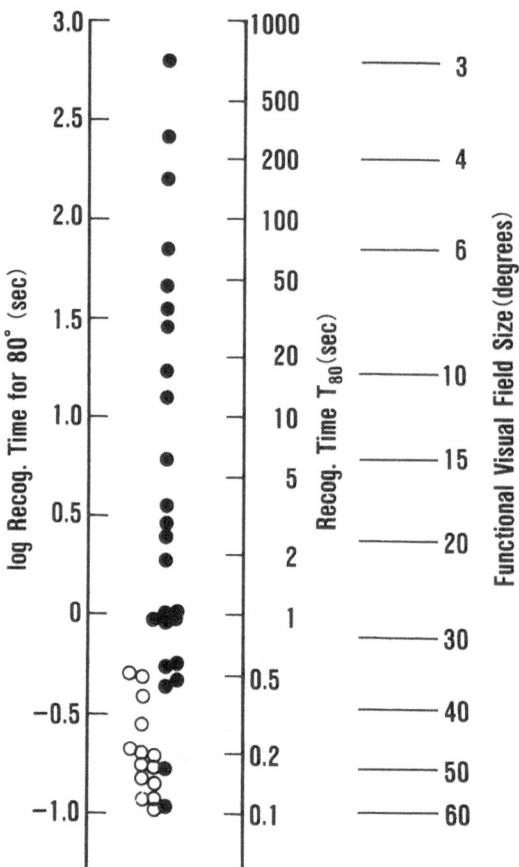

Fig. 3. Recognition time for stimulus size of 80 degrees and the functional visual field diameter.

Japanese hiragana stimulus as before was presented on a TV monitor. However the entire letter was not shown, but only a square portion of a certain size. The subject's eye movement was detected by the corneal reflection method so precisely as to control the position of the square, which eventually coincided exactly with the visual axis of the subject wherever he viewed, thus effectively narrowing his visual field down to the size of the square. Three normal subjects participated in the experiment.

Results: The following formula was obtained,

$$\log T = -2.69 \log P_{FVF} + 4.06$$

where T represents the recognition time and P_{FVF} the percentage of functional visual field diameter relative to the stimulus size.

If, therefore, the recognition time was T_α when a patient observed the

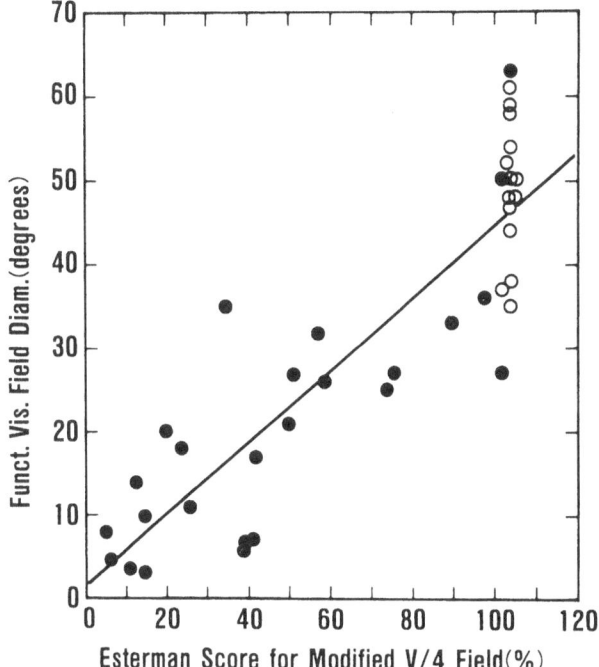

Fig. 4. Plots of the functional visual field diameter versus Esterman score for the modified V/4 isopter.

stimulus at an angle α, then P_{FVF} is obtained by inserting the T_α into the T in the formula, and his functional visual field diameter is calculated by the formula

$$\alpha_{FVF} = P_{FVF}\alpha/100.$$

This calculation was done for all 39 subjects. The righthand scale in Fig. 3 was constructed from this data. The functional visual fields varied from 60 degrees down to 3 degrees.

The final remark is on the relation of the present result to work of others, particularly to that of Esterman (3). Fig. 4 is the plot of the present functional visual field versus the Esterman score obtained for the isopter V/4, which was modified so as to discount from the calculation any area not connectable to the fovea by a straight line passing through all points of which are in the usable visual field, because the pattern in such an area cannot meaningfully connect to that seen in the fovea. Thus areas on the other side of a large scotoma from the fovea or 'cut off' from the fovea by an 'inlet' in the isopter were discounted. 5% was given to the central area. The straight line shows the regression line of

$$\alpha_{FVF} = 0.43\,S_E + 1.57$$

where S_E denotes the Esterman score. The correlation coefficient is 0.88.

REFERENCES

1. Ikeda, M., Uchikawa, K. and Saida, S. Static and dynamic functional visual field. Optica Acta 8: 1103–1113 (1979).
2. Verriest, G., Barca, L., Dubois-Poulsen, A., Houtmans, M.J.M., Johnson, C., Overington, I., Ronchi, L. and Villani, S. The occupational visual field. I. Theoretical aspects: the normal functional visual field. Doculmenta Ophthal. Proc. Series 35: 165–185 (1983).
3. Esterman, B. Grids for scoring visual fields. II. Perimeter. Am. Arch. Ophthal. 79: 400–406 (1968).

Authors' address:
Drs. F. Ikeda and M. Takao
Dept. of Ophthalmology
Kanto Teishin Hospital
Higashi-Gotanda, Shinagawa, Tokyo 141
Dr. M. Ikeda and S. Shioiri
Dept. of Information Processing
Tokyo Inst. Technology
Nagatsuta, Midori-ku, Yokohama
Japan

COMPUTERIZED SCORING OF THE FUNCTIONAL FIELD PRELIMINARY REPORT

B. ESTERMAN, E. BLANCHE, M. WALLACH and A. BONELLI

(New York, U.S.A.)

ABSTRACT

The new computerized Autoperimeter has now been programmed to include the Functional Relative-Value Scale. This combination simultaneously performs automated perimetry and ergoperimetry: it plots the field, either monocular or binocular, and instantly prints the Functional score. The score is called 'functional' because it measures more than merely area; it assesses the total field's usefulness and expresses it in percent or simple fraction — as does the Snellen Scale for *central* acuity. Thus, consultants for industry or government now have a standard scale to help determine job fitness, driver safety, social security disability, worker's compensation, etc and to do this automatically, quickly, impersonally and as accurately as subjective testing will permit.

This year, the American Medical Association has adopted the Scale as standard for the U.S. with its publication of the 1984 edition of the official 'A.M.A. Guides to Impairment — The Visual System.'

As part of more extensive trials performed at the suggestion of the President of the International Ophthalmological Council, preliminary tests have already calibrated the combined Autoperimeter and Relative-Value Scales so that scores match those of the standard Goldmann. Certain problems arose. Their solution yielded some interesting fundamental biological observations; also ideas for monitoring (by the I.P.S.) of the Scales' manufacture and, if necessary, their future modification.

The method for determining the usefulness of a patient's visual field by means of relative value scales has been described elsewhere (1–3). More recently, during the past year, there have been two new developments: (1) these scales have been adopted by the American Medical Association; and (2) they have been computerized.

Last month (April 1984) the Scales became standard for the United States by their publication in the latest edition of the official 'A.M.A. Guides to Impairment — The Visual System' (4).

In America, the Scales are already available as software on the Cooper Vision/Dicon Automated Perimeter (as you have seen in today's commercial exhibit). And from Switzerland, Prof. Fankhauser has written me that he intends to incorporate them into his Octopus perimeter.

Heijl, A. and Greve, E.L. (eds.), Proceedings of the 6th Int. Visual Field Symposium.
© 1985, Dr W. Junk Publishers, Dordrecht, The Netherlands. ISBN 978-94-010-8932-6

The newly devised combination of automated testing and automated scoring has produced certain advantages: It has made assessment of the functional field less tedious, faster, more repeatable, more objective, more accurate and less dependent on highly trained personnel. At the same time it raised an immediate question of validity, the answer to which revealed a new concept of perception.

The immediate question was: Do the automated scores match those heretofore obtained conventionally on the standard Goldmann perimeter? The answer is: They do now. They did not, at first − not until adjustments were made in the light intensities of the automated test-objects. This led to some interesting revelations.

MATERIAL AND METHODS

As a preliminary to more extensive investigation, 422 perimetries were performed on patients routinely referred from other hospital departments.

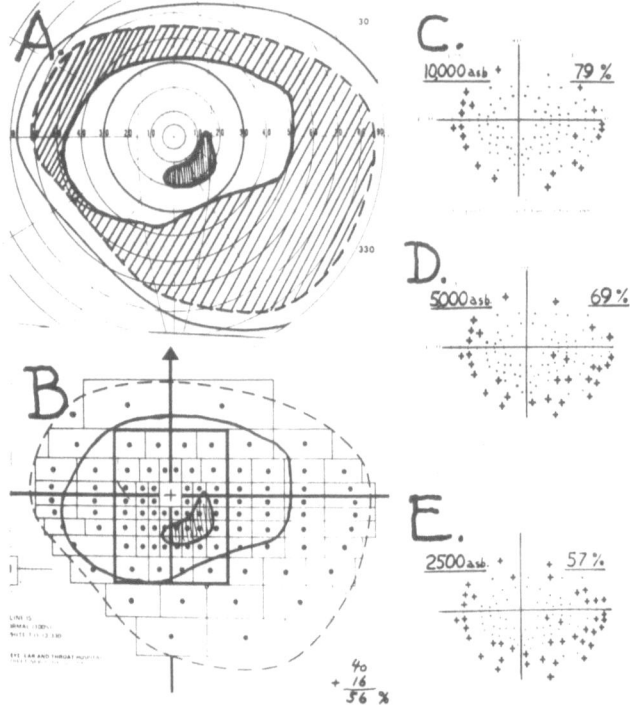

Fig. 1. Monocular field O.D. A: Plotted on Goldmann perimeter at standard III 4 e. B: Scored at 56% by the relative value scale on reverse of the Goldmann chart. C, D, E: plotted and scored automatically and simultaneously on the Cooper Vision Autoperimeter at 3 different intensities (10 000 asb = 79%; 5000 asb = 69%; 2500 asb = 57% − matching Goldmann score of 56%).

Each field was first plotted conventionally on a carefully calibrated Goldmann perimeter; it was then scored by means of the standard functional relative-value scale imprinted on the reverse side of that Goldmann chart. This double procedure was next repeated on the Cooper Vision/Dicon Autoperimeter, which automatically performs both the plotting and the scoring simultaneously and does it much more quickly. The Goldmann and the Dicon scores were then compared. The goal was for each pair of scores to match within ten percent. (10% is a reasonably acceptable match, considering the subjective nature of the test). Figs. 1 and 2.

Illumination of the test-stimulus on the Goldmann was kept constant at III 4e because that has long been the accepted standard. Similarly, the Dicon was at first set at III 4e, calibrated by the manufacturer as 10 000 asb. When the resulting Dicon scores proved much too high, we tried reducing the intensity to 5000 asb., then to 2500 asb. (See Table 1).

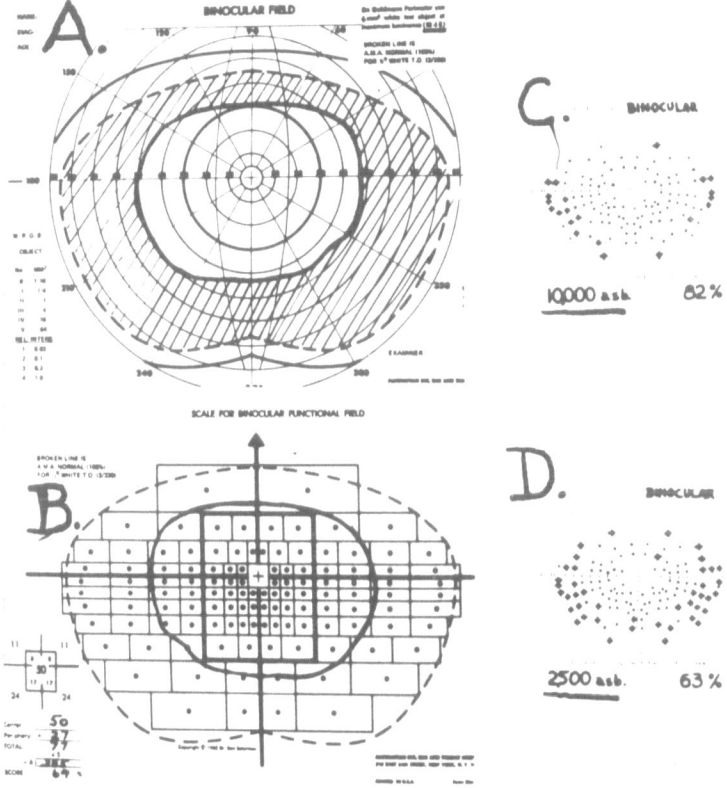

Fig. 2. Binocular field. A: Plotted on Goldmann perimeter at standard III 4 e. B: Scored at 64% by relative-value scales on reverse of Goldmann Chart. C and D: plotted and scored on Autoperimeter at 10 000 asb (82%) and 2500 asb (6%).

Table 1. The matching of scores on autoperimeter vs. Goldmann. All Goldmann scores at standard illumination of III 4 e automated (Cooper vision) at 10000 asb, 5000 asb, 2500 asb.

Illumination in asb.	Total number of fields	Discard (more than 21%)	Total number of valid fields	Disparities			
				0%–5%	6%–10%	11%–15%	16%–20%
10 000	122	7	115	40 (35%)	30 (26%)	32 (28%)	13 (11%)
5000	72	2	70	33 (47%)	21 (30%)	14 (20%)	2 (3%)
2500	228	13	215	162 (75%)	34 (16%)	14 (7%)	5 (2%)
	422	22	400		196 (91%)		

Summary

Illumination in asb.	Total number of valid fields	Disparities	
		0%–10%	11%–20%
10 000	115	70 (61%)	45 (39%)
5000	70	54 (77%)	16 (23%)
2500	215	196 (91%)	19 (9%)

Out of the total, 22 pairs of scores were discarded because their disparities were over 20% – indicating either inadequate cooperation, fixation, comprehension or perception – too poor to be counted as meaningful.

Of the remaining 400: among those tested at 10 000 asb on the Dicon, 39% of the scores were more than 10% too high. At 5000 asb, disparities dropped to 23%. At 2500 asb, 91% matched the Goldmann within 10%.

Based on these findings and aware that they are preliminary, we feel that 2500 asb on the Dicon is reasonably equal to the accepted standard of III 4 e on the Goldmann and therefore valid for functional scoring.

We might add that the original suggestion for these tests came from Professor Francois and Professor Drance in 1982, after they saw the prototype of the computerized scale at the San Francisco Scientific Exhibit of the International Congress of Ophthalmology.

THE CALIBRATION OF PERIMETERS

The above calibration took much time and work in repeated perimetries, but the adjustments were made easily, thanks to the flexibility and precision of the Dicon instrument. However, the effort was not wasted. The search for the cause of the original disparity between scores on the Dicon and on the Goldmann led to an important realization: that it was due to a difference in perception between *emitted* and *reflected* light. Light *emitted* in a direct line from a naked diode (as on the Dicon) was more readily perceived than light *reflected* and *diffused* by the *un*polished surface of the Goldmann bowl. Merely reducing the *area* and the duration of the Dicon's test stimulus has not quite compensated for its greater 'perceivability.'

Because perception is what perimetry is all about, and because the newly automated scale now enables us to quantitate that perception, we would do well to heed this concept in the future design and calibration of perimeters. We should measure the actual total light energy as it reaches the eye, rather than at the source or at the point of reflection. The Dicon engineers tell me they place a sensitive light-meter not on the bowl but at the position of the subject's eye. This should be accurate and ought to eliminate the need to calibrate by plotting and scoring hundreds of patients.

CONTROL OF STANDARDS

When standards are established, they must be monitored. For the past fifteen years, this writer has monitored the functional relative-value scales by personally supervising their printing and manufacture before the Manhattan Eye and Ear Hospital distributed them to American ophthalmologists. Now that they are more widely used and are official standards and, in addition, incorporated into computerized perimeters, this monitoring has become too important to entrust to a single individual. Such monitoring should now be transferred to a committee of the International Perimetric Society.

COMMENT

How reliable is perimetry? The new automated perimeter-plus-scale now enables us to answer this question more quantitatively. Experienced perimetrists have always suspected that perimetry is not as reliable as we would like to believe.

Perimetry is still a basically subjective test. Now that all the other measuring tools — the instrument, the scale, the illumination, even the computerized technique — can be kept standard and constant, the only factor not consistently repeatable is the patient himself, due to individual variations in perception, fixation, attention, alertness, fatigue and motivation. Until the test can be made more objective, perhaps by perfection of the diagnostic scanning laser, the only way to quantitative petients' perimetric reliability (or unreliability) is by scoring them *against themselves*, i.e. by studying the *repeatability* of their own scores.

We have started a series of such repeatability comparisons at different levels of competence, age, illumination. We hope to establish basic standards of reliability analagous to the isopters set down perimetrically for the general population by Ferree and others early in the century.

Will all this call into question the usefulness of perimetry? Not at all. For diagnosis, a dependable field is one of our most important aids. For the assessment of functional competence or disability, scoring is now quantitative and meaningful. Our awareness of its reliability or lack of it will simply make our evaluation of patients more realistic. The more this helps our judgment, the better is the ophthalmology we practice.

PROSPECT

Our new capacity to score by computer has led to other interesting paths of investigation, some of which have already been started. Because time is limited, mere mention of them must suffice; they will be published subsequently.

They include studies on the reliability of perimetry in general and its significance in diagnosis; comparison between manual and automated perimetry with repeatability as the criterion; studies of the deterioration of visual efficiency (expressed quantitatively, in percent) resulting from fatigue, from relative anoxia, or from smoking — or from all three combined, as measured among airline pilots during long flights; and some suggestions for the future of automated perimetry.

SUMMARY

The newly devised combination of the relative-value scale and the computerized perimeter is a satisfactory tool for assessing the percentage of usable field. It is fast, repeatable and as accurate as the subjective nature of the patient's responses will allow. When properly calibrated, its functional scores. In calibrating the instensity of the test stimuli, we must be aware of the difference in perception between direct (emitted) light and indirect (reflected and diffused) light and be guided solely by measuring the total amount of light energy *which reaches the eye* being tested.

Automation eases perimetry by lessening drudgery; also, mechanizing technique has made fields more consistently repeatable. But the computer has no capacity for thought, reasoning or judgment, therefore cannot replace the human perimetrist in the Diagnostic process. Functional assessment, on the other hand, is better without these human attributes. It is precisely the *impersonal* nature of the machine that best enables it automatically to measure the peripheral effectiveness (ergoperimetry) revealed by the patient's responses *without* the influence of the examiner's technique or wishful thinking.

REFERENCES

1. Esterman, B. Grid for Scoring Visual Fields I Tangent Screen A.M.A. Arch. Ophth. 77: 780–786 (1967).
2. Ibid. Grid for Scoring Visual Fields II Perimeter. A.M.A. Arch. Ophth. 79: 400–406 (1968).
3. Ibid. Binocular Scoring of the Functional Field Ophthalmology 89: No. 11 1226–1234 (1982).
4. 'Guides to Evaluation of Impairment – The Visual System' Amer. Med. Assoc. – Chicago 1984 2nd Edition.

LIGHT EMITTING DIODES IN EXTRAFOVEAL VISION: AN ERGOPERIMETRIC PROBLEM

LUIGI BARCA, FRANCO PASSANI and VANNA GALASSI PRINCIPE

(*Firenze, Italy*)

ABSTRACT

An experiment is performed where is measured the effectiveness of LEDs used as coloured sources is suprathreshold perimetry. A number of observers have been requested to quantify, by the use of a color-naming technique, the eccentricity dependence of the coloured aspect of the source, consisting of a raster of eight red or green LEDs.

In good agreement with previous works on classical (say non-LED) sources, the red perception is more resistant than green to peripheral degradation of colour vision. In spite of individual differences a normal behaviour can be assessed in various meridians; limited to our selected experimental conditions for background and target illuminance. We found that green percept reduces to 50%, compared to that in the fovea, within about 30–40 degrees of eccentricity, while the red one remains higher for almost all eccentricities and orientations. A reduction of exposure time from 800 to 32 ms does not lead to appreciable differences in our luminance range.

The test seems to be of interest for testing patients, e.g. with a previous history of optic neuritis, which are known to exhibit a generally desaturated foveal colour vision.

AIM OF THE WORK

Light Emitting Diodes (LEDs) (1) are modern, relatively narrow band sources based on the phenomenon of semiconductor's electroluminescence. Their performances are similar, when not better, to others normal lamps for luminous efficacy and heat dissipation. There is a wide range of applications for single sources: they can indicate the presence of operating conditions such as in test instruments or in the usage of a line in a key telephone; as warning signals such as in the dashboard of modern cars or in control panels, where they are multicoloured. All these applications require that the 'on' and 'off' states and small colour differences be clearly distinguishable in spite of the little size of the source, even if the operator is not fixating the LED. Another device using typically LEDs is calculator's and instrument's display, in which they are employed not as single source but in a few arrays such as seven

Heijl, A. and Greve, E.L. (eds.), Proceedings of the 6th Int. Visual Field Symposium.
© *1985, Dr W. Junk Publishers, Dordrecht, The Netherlands. ISBN 978-94-010-8932-6*

bars or 5 x 7 dots matrix. Studies have been made to optimize shape, colour and brightness of single display. Presently red and green are the most used colours.

A number of authors (2–4) have recently assessed the visuophotometric implications of LEDs in foveal vision. The present report aims at recording some data on extrafoveal vision, which might be of interest from the ergonomical stand point. In fact peripheral colour vision is of relevance to speed the search process (5).

It is known that colour vision is less developed in the periphery than in the fovea; for the centrally normal trichromat the periphery shows deutan-anomalous and/or -anopic tendencies (6). However the quality of colour vision in the periphery has been found to depend critically on stimulus size. If the target is 'large' and sufficiently bright the foveal-peripheral differences are of small entity; on the other hand small targets appear desaturated and in much the same way across the retina, apart from the case of red ones (7).

One single LED has 'per se' a small size; a skilled observer perceives its small source desaturation also in foveal vision. On the other hand a matrix of LEDs may have even a large size. Briefly we wonder how they appear to observers at different locations in their visual field. Of course the validity of our findings is limited to the experimental conditions adopted by us as far as intensity of the source and background adapting luminance are concerned.

MATERIALS AND METHOD

The source used in this experiment is a 4 x 4 matrix consisting either of red LEDs or of green ones; these are the HLMP0500 green LED and the HLMP0300 red LED. Their size in total is approximately 4.4 degree to the eye. The matrix is fastened to the center of a bowl, whose internal wall is covered by white paper. The illuminance (fluorescent daylight) is 1.7 lux. The observer, at a viewing distance of 33 cm, is instructed to fixate at a cross placed at a variable eccentricity along a chosen meridian of the visual field. The minimum step in eccentricity is 10°. The orientations considered are: horizontal (0°), oblique (45°), vertical (90°).

The observer, fully preadapted to background luminance, having directed his gaze to the wanted fixation point, delivers a flash by pushing a button. In the main experiment the duration is of 800 ms, but some sessions were also devoted to the effect of a change in duration.

The intensities of the current feeding the LEDs are so arranged as to produce matched illuminances at the eye, accordingly to the foveal photometry, for either red or green LED, say of 10^{-2} lux. The task consists in specifying the appearance of colour through a color-naming technique.

EXPERIMENTAL FINDINGS AND DISCUSSION

We tested a number of people healthy and normal from the ophthalmological stand point, aging from 13 to 65 years; colour discrimination in central vision has been previously assessed by the use of F.M. 100-Hue Test.

Starting tests were in monocular vision and we checked that, together with the expected nasal-temporal asymmetry, the perception of green drops out before than red and in addition peripheral vision is well predisposed toward the 'yellow' percept (8). In the following sessions however we addressed our attention essentially to binocular vision because we thought this condition much more common from an ergo ophthalmological stand point in practice. Accordingly we adopted 800 ms as a reasonably long exposure time, and suprathreshold source intensity.

A synthetic view of our results in binocular vision is shown in Figs. 1–6, where the average color-naming score across six normal observers is plotted versus eccentricity for every inspected meridian and for each colour, the single total score being estimated by the use of Boynton et al's method (9). Of course the far peripheral regions are viewed only monocularly by either eye.

The known trend met in monocular vision is fully confirmed: at all positions red percept is superior to the green one. Nevertheless, in addition to peripheral degradation, the responses obtained up to eccentricities of 30° exhibit strong inter-individual and inter-meridian variability, so as a poor intraindividual reliability. This renders difficult to draw definite conclusions about a standard 'normal' response. Note that the entity of standard deviation shows a larger variability for green than for red, at least for some orientations.

The comparison among single observer's data shows that the reduction of principal colour is accompanied by an increase of yellow response for some-one, and of white or achromatic response for others.

The plots of flashes of 100 ms at all eccentricities have substantially similar shapes as for the 800 ms flashes. However the response variability seems to increase.

In Figs. 7 and 8 the time dependencies of green and red responses are shown, the flash duration being reduced from 800 to 32 ms. In this case the eccentricity is fixed at 40° along the right horizontal meridian.

Apart from individual differences, more enhanced for green than for red, the red flash practically exhibits the same amount of 'redness' whatever is duration in the explored range; on the other hand the amount of 'green-ness' drops out as duration decreases. The transition from durable to instan-taneous sensation clearly occurs at about 100 ms.

We attempted to test patients suffering from eye diseases affecting the extent of visual field, e.g. retrobulbar neuritis. If the patient is cooperative the test can be performed giving rise to valid results. Unfortunately we did not have the opportunity and the time to test a sufficient number of patients. Our preliminary results confirm that these subjects present an a-specific general desaturation of colour vision (10). On the other hand retrobulbar neuritis is an unpredictable illness and in several occasions its ultimate result does not show any appreciable difference from normality.

343

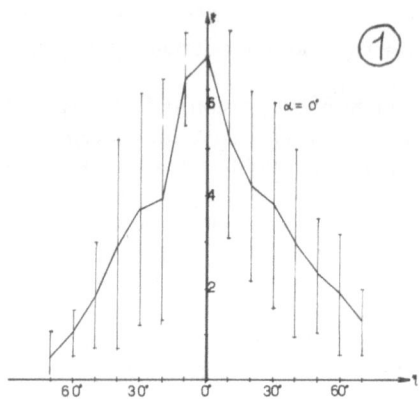

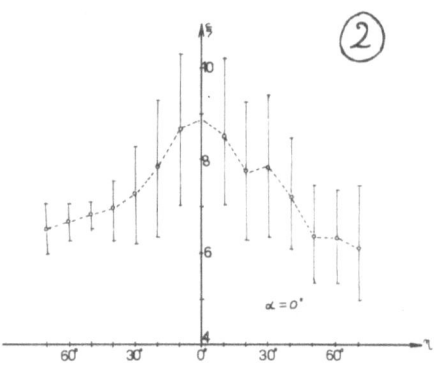

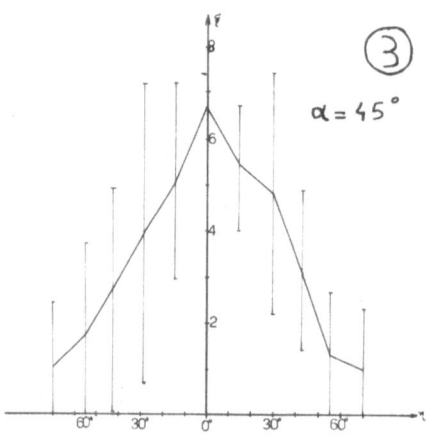

344

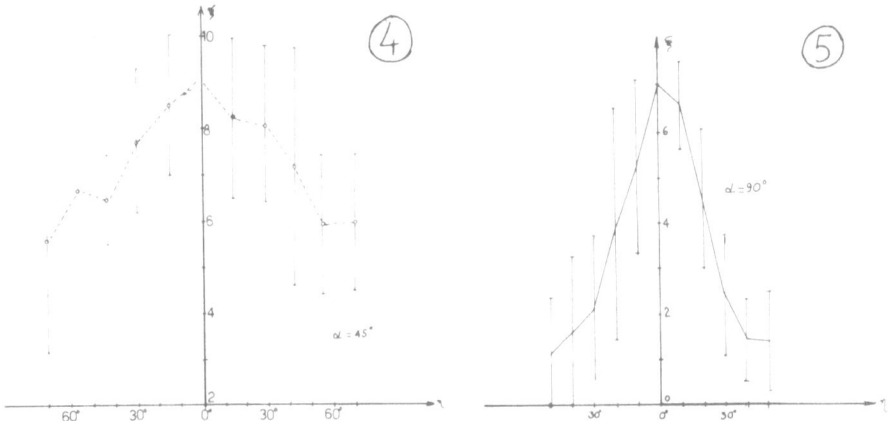

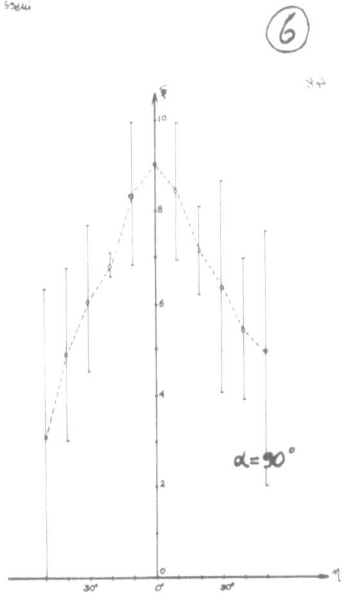

Figs. 1—6. Average percept across six normal observers. Abscissae: retinal eccentricity. Ordinates color-naming score. Meridional orientation is indicated by α. Full line for green flash, broken line for red one. Vertical straight lines are S.D. for repeated variability.

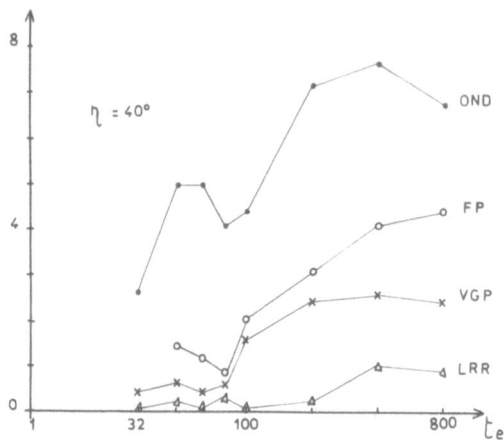

Fig. 7. Effect of reducing exposure time of green flash, at a fixed eccentricity (40°). Abscissae: duration of flashes in ms. Ordinates: color-naming score. Labels denote the observers.

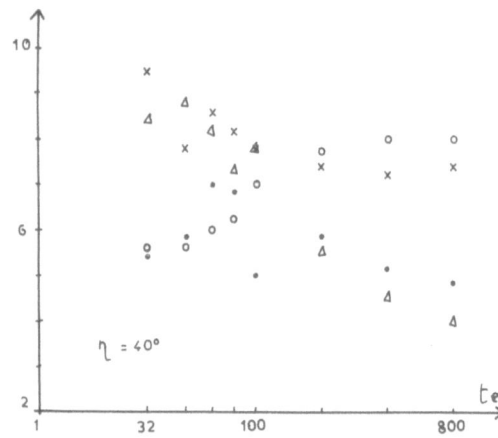

Fig. 8. Effect of reducing exposure time of the red flash at a fixed eccentricity (40°). Abscissae: duration of flashes in ms. Ordinates: color naming score. Observers and marks are the same as Fig. 7.

REFERENCES

1. Bergh, A.A. and Dean, P.J. Light Emitting Diodes, Clarendon Press, Oxford (1976).
2. Ronchi, L., Macii, R. and Stefanacci, S. Some experiments on the brightness-luminance discrepancy for Light Emitting Diodes, Optica. Acta. 27, 671–682 (1980).
3. Ronchi, L., Macii, R., Stefanacci, S. and Bassan, M. Brightness and luminance of Light Emitting Diodes: influence of size and defocus, Color Res. Appl. 5(4), 207–211 (1980).
4. Booker, R.L. Luminance-brightness comparison of LED alphanumeric sources at suprathreshold levels, J.O.S.A. 68, 949–952 (1978).

5. Christ, R.E. Review and analysis of color coding research for visual displays, Human Factors 17, 542–570 (1975).
6. Uchikawa, P.K., Kaiser, P. and Uchikawa, K. Color-discrimination perimetry, Color Res. Appl. 7(3), 264–270 (1982).
7. Gordon, J. and Abramov, J. Color vision in the peripheral retina II: Hue and saturation, J.O.S.A. 67, 202–207 (1977).
8. Ronchi, L. and Tittarelli, R. Does the best signal exist?, Atti Fond. G. Ronchi, XXI 3, 468–504 (1966).
9. Boynton, R.M., Gordon and Bezold-Brücke, J. Hue shift measured by color-naming technique, J.O.S.A. 55, 78–86 (1965).
10. Verriest, G. Les déficiences acquises de la discrimination chromatique, Mem. de l'Academie Royale de Medecine de Belgique II serie, tome IV, 5, 205–206 (1964).

Authors' address
Prima Clinica Oculistica,
Università di Firenze,
50100 Firenze,
Italy

ERGOPERIMETRY IN PATIENTS WITH SEVERE VISUAL FIELD DAMAGE

GIOVANNI CALABRIA, ENRICO GANDOLFO, MAURIZIO ROLANDO,
PAOLO CAPRIS, CARMEN BURTOLO

(*Genoa, Italy*)

Patients with similar severe visual field damage of different nature often have different difficulties in environmental behaviour.

In a previous paper (1), in order to explain this phenomenon, we have studied the visual performances of patients with severe perimetric defects. For an ergonomic evaluation we examined binocular visual field, reaction times and critical fusion frequency. In that research we were able to note that all the patients demonstrated good integration of the two monocular visual fields, but the sensitivity summation was less efficient in glaucomatous patients: the phenomenon was significant, but not sufficient to justify the greater behaviour difficulties that those patients demonstrate.

Therefore we have tried to investigate the actual absolute peripheral limits of the field of visual perception in patients with large visual field defects attempting to study what Ikeda (3) calls the sensation visual field. We define the sensation (or perception) visual field as 'the portion of space inside which a subject can perceive the presence of an object'.

The investigation was carried out using a very simple method involving easily seen objects of large size and high contrast: our aim was to identify and measure the absolute limits of the field of visual preception, because we believe that these limits do not correspond to the so called absolute limits of clinical perimetry.

MATERIAL AND METHODS

20 patients with serious visual field defects in at least one eye (generalized concentric contraction, tubular visual field, hemianopia etc.) were studied.

Perimetric alterations were due to varied diseases (16 glaucomas, 2 pigmentary retinal degeneration, 2 chiasmal disturbances).

All patients previously underwent a standard kinetic monocular and binocular Goldmann perimetric examination using targets of maximum size and luminance.

The patients and the patients' relatives were interviewed concerning difficulties in environmental behaviour. The patients were then observed performing a simple task, moving in an every day setting, and consequently divided in 3 groups:

Heijl, A. and Greve, E.L. (eds.), Proceedings of the 6th Int. Visual Field Symposium.
© *1985, Dr W. Junk Publishers, Dordrecht, The Netherlands. ISBN 978-94-010-8932-6*

1) patients with very serious difficulties
2) patients with serious difficulties
3) patients with modest difficulties

In order to reproduce experimentally conditions closest to that of every day setting, but with measurable and reproducible parameters, we utilized rolled black screens. The unrolling in the center of a room or against a white background. The screens were progressively unrolled so the screen edge was brought closer to the fixation point (while the 'object' gradually increased in size). Four directions of screen movement were used. When exploring a fairly binocular visual field, four diagonal screen directions were also used for better comparison with clinical perimetry. The fixation target was represented by a black round object of 3 degrees of diameter. The experiences were carried out in normally lighted room (about 200 lux candles against the walls).

The eccentricity of the perceived screen edge was recorded. The perception visual field was then reported as a quadrangular or hexagonal area.

For a functional scoring of the binocular field the Esterman binocular grid was used (2). The residual field score represented as a percentage based on the 120 units of the grid.

RESULTS

When compared with the clinical visual field the perception field was always greater in all explored meridians. The evaluation of the obtained data demonstrated, in all cases, a direct unequivocal relationship between visual perception constriction and the patient's difficulties in environmental behaviour.

The score of the clinical visual field limits do not always correspond to the degree of the patient's difficulties. These results emerge from the analysis of the scores of each individual case and the three different groups. (Table 1–3). Only in the group of patients with very serious difficulties in environmental behaviour one notes how both the perception and visual field score are seriously compromised in homogeneous manner. When patients with less serious or modest difficulties are examined a discrepancy is often observed between the visual and perception scores. Only the percentual performance is always in agreement with the patients environmental behaviours.

DISCUSSION

Verriest et al. (4) in the official I.P.S. report on the occupational visual field have noted that Ikeda's definition of the sensation field corresponds in the last analysis to the traditional definition of the absolute limits of the visual field. Fundamentally we agree with this concept: we think that with our method we have measured the actual limits of the peripheral visual field. But we also think that perhaps with our examination method we were able to measure something different than the mere absolute limits of the visual field

Table 1. Group 1. Patients with very serious behaviour difficulties.

Patients	Diagnosis	Binocular score	
		Perception field	Visual field
L.G.	Glaucoma	2.5	0.8
N.B.	Glaucoma	5	2.5
L.A.	Pigmentary retinopathy	5.8	3.3
P.B.	Glaucoma	6.6	5.0
C.R.	Glaucoma	7.5	1.6

Table 2. Group 2. Patients with serious behaviour difficulties.

Patients	Diagnosis	Binocular score	
		Perception field	Visual field
P.C.	Glaucoma	21.6	13.3
M.Z.	Glaucoma	23.3	6.6
R.S.	Glaucoma	26.6	21.6
C.B.	Glaucoma	30	5.8
M.M.	Glaucoma	33.3	26.6
V.R.	Glaucoma	35	7.5

Table 3. Group 3. Patients with modest behaviour difficulties.

Patients	Diagnosis	Binocular score	
		Perception field	Visual field
G.B.	Glaucoma	32	14
G.C.	Glaucoma	51.6	26.6
P.R.	Glaucoma	55.0	51.6
W.C.	Glaucoma	56.6	50
R.M.	Hemianopia	63.3	58.3
L.S.	Glaucoma	63.3	60
R.Z.	Pigmentary retinopathy	66.6	38.4
T.V.	Glaucoma	71.6	35
F.R.	Hemianopia	76.6	68.3

and possibly something closer to the functional visual field: the close relationship between our results and the patient's environmental behaviour seems to demonstrate it.

In the future, to emphasize this ergoperimetric possibility, our investigation can be performed in different environments or surroundings with the subject performing different tasks. The simple shape of perception field usually allows an easy and accurate evaluation by means of the Esterman grid. To better simulate objects disappearance from the peripheral visual field that occurs in the subject movement, the examination can also be performed using centrifugal movement. In testing normal individual or patients with minimal visual field disturbances the object contrast can be varied using different grey screens.

In spite of the fact that our method appears fairly simple, we believe that it offers the possibility of simulating a large number of every day obstacles that an individual encounters (steps, ceiling, doors edge etc.) Testing individual with severe visual field defect we were able to note the functional importance of some residual visual field areas often neglected or underestimated (e.g. temporal areas of glaucomatous patients, peripheral inferior visual field in hemianopia etc.): these areas of the visual field were important to obtain a larger perception field therefore allowing a subject to be included in a group of better environmental behaviour.

The actual absolute limits of the binocular perception visual field are studied in patients with large field defects. The binocular perception field was always greater than the clinical visual field. A direct unequivocal relationship between visual perception constriction and patient difficulties in environmental behaviour was noted.

Possibilities for utilization of this method for perception field scoring in ergoperimetry are discussed.

ACKNOWLEDGEMENTS

This study was supported from a Grant of the Consiglio Nazionale delle Ricerche, Progetto Finalizzato Medicina Preventiva e Riabilitativa, sotto-progetto Malattie Degenerative, Obbiettivo N. 47a, Rome, Italy.

REFERENCES

1. Calabria, G., Capris, P. and Burtolo, C. 'Investigations on space behaviour of glaucomatous people with extensive visual field loss', Fifth I.V.F. Symposium Documenta Ophthalmologica Proc. 35: 205–210 (1983).
2. Esterman, B. 'Functional scoring of the binocular field' Documenta Ophthalmol. Proc. 35: 187–192 (1983).
3. Ikeda, M., Uchikawa, K. and Saida, S. 'Static and dynamic functional visual field' Optica. Acta. 8: 1103–1113 (1979).
4. Varriest et al. 'The occupational visual field' Doc. Ophthalmol. Proc. 35: 165–185.

Author's address:
Dr. G. Calabria
University Eye Clinic
Viale Benedetto XV, 5
16132 Genoa, Italy

EXPERIMENTS OF PERIPHERAL VISION IN RELATION TO DISTORTION OPERATED BY MULTIFOCAL LENSES

A. SERRA

(*Cagliari, Italy*)

ABSTRACT

Recently, multifocal lenses are being used by some people with various degrees of presbyopia. Their meridional distribution of optical power may produce a distortion which has a counterpart in the estimate of the visual field.

Data recorded by us, on a number of skilled and cooperative individuals reveal an isopter constriction as well as a loss in peripheral vernier acuity.

AIM OF THE WORK

The lenses for presbyoptic eyes exhibiting a 'continuous' variation in optical power from their horizontal meridian down to the bottom are a tool relatively presented to the layman.

The question arises as to which is their ergo-ophthalmological relevance. Indeed, they exhibit a complex meridional dependence in optical power, which is likely to produce an unusual distribution of blur in the visual field. However, the prolonged use of lenses (for near vision) with a progressive change in power may lead to 'adaptation' to the new situation.

In this connection, it might be of interest to recall that first Stratton, at the end of the last century, and more recently Kohler (1) concluded that humans can adjust both perceptually and motorwise either to inversion or to right-left reversal in the visual field, but some days are required before the complete adjustment is attained.

Kohler's conclusion was that in reversed or inversed visual fields the performance may even become equal to that found in normal vision. This optimistic conclusion is contradicted by others, who assert that a residual impairment persists for some critical distortions at least.

Now, the ophthalmological practice indicates that some patients soon become adapted to the new situations, others, adapt in a reasonable time, but there are some people who at last refuse the progressive lenses in the end.

Heijl, A. and Greve, E.L. (eds.), Proceedings of the 6th Int. Visual Field Symposium.
© *1985, Dr W. Junk Publishers, Dordrecht, The Netherlands. ISBN 978-94-010-8932-6*

MATERIALS AND METHOD

Our subjects were first tested by the use of Goldmann perimeter (target II/2d), under three different conditions:

(a) by naked eye
(b) by wearing a spherical dioptric for near vision
(c) by wearing lenses with progressive change in power.

Next we used a set of tests designed by us to inquire about the 'distortion' of visual imagery operated by the spectacles for near vision. One is based on the trapeze vs rectangle paradigm, the other is based on extrafoveal vernier acuity.

Subjects

Our subjects are six cooperative individuals aged around fifties (requiring 2 dt additional power for near vision). They are well 'adapted' to the spectacles with the continuous variation in power, having worn them for several months (4 to 16, according to the individual).

EXPERIMENTAL FINDINGS

Isopter perimetry

All our subjects exibit a narrower isopter when wearing the lens with continuous variation in power than in the case of spherical lens or naked eye. An example is shown in Fig. 1.

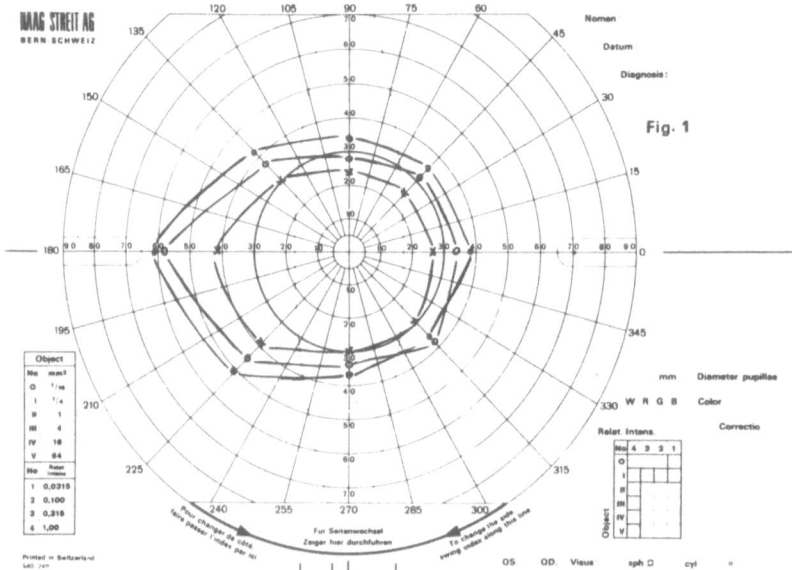

Fig. 1. A sample of narrower isopter when wearing the progressive lens: Full points: naked eye; open circles: spherical lenses; crosses: progressive lenses.

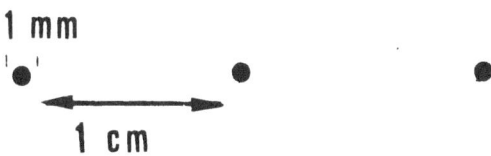

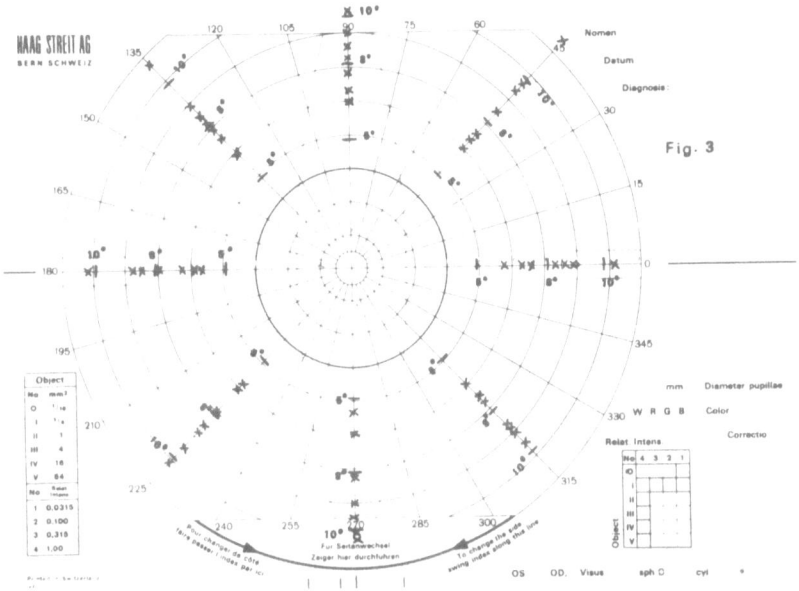

Fig. 2. The target used in our experiments to investigate the peripheral vernier acuity.

Fig. 3. Results of three dot target test: each cross refers to response of each subject.

This finding might be explained in terms of relative 'refraction scotoma', due to the change in lens power across various meridians.

Three dot target

We presented the target shown in Fig. 2 consisting of three dots, 1 mm diameter, 1 cm apart from one another, well mutually aligned.

We shifted them across the visual field, and stopped when the observer judged this target free of distortion and curvature. The result of this test, performed by subjects wearing their variable power lens, is shown in Fig. 3.

In spite of the inter-individual variability we may consider as distortion free the region of the visual field within, say 8°. This finding may serve as a basis for the test described in the next section.

355

Pairs of dots to be completed

This test is shown in Fig. 4. The task consists in adding one dot to the pairs of dots at the same distance and aligned.

The histogram (Fig. 5) shows the difference in mm between the distance between dots when wearing spherical lens and that wearing progressive lens.

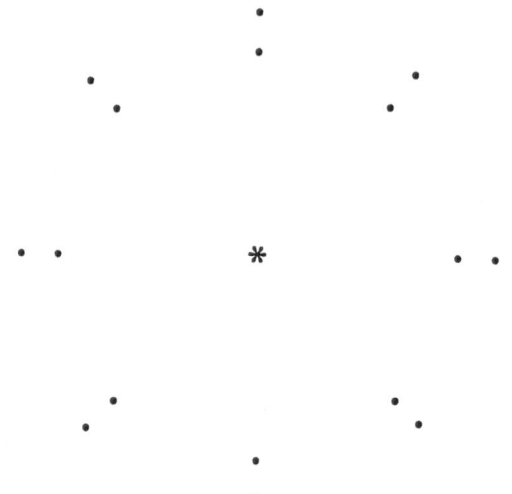

Fig. 4. Pairs of dots to be complete. The distance from the fixation point (asterisk) is 7°.

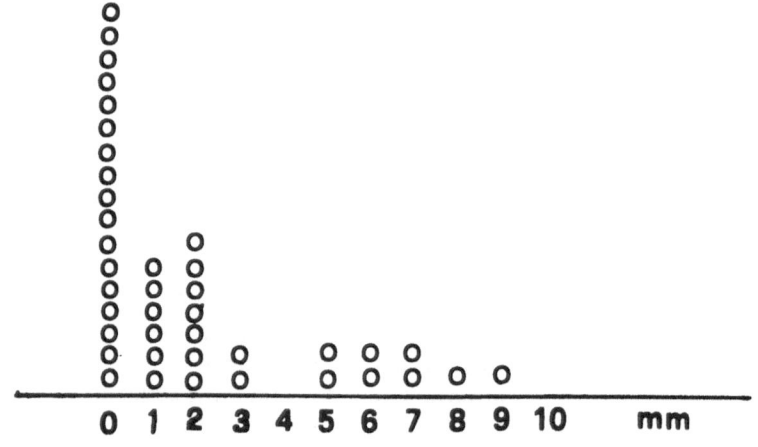

Fig. 5. Histogram of the estimate of the difference in mm (abscissae) between the distance when wearing spherical lens and that wearing progressive lens.

Table 1.

Difference (degrees) between the lines distance at the top and at the bottom	Number of observers judging parallel the two lines	
	With progress. lenses	With spherical lenses
+ 2°	0	0
+ 1°.67	1	0
+ 1°.33	1	0
+ 1°	1	0
+ 0°.67	3	1
+ 0°.33	4	3
0°	4	5
− 0°.33	3	4
− 0°.67	3	3
− 1°	3	2
− 1°.33	2	1
− 1°.67	0	0
− 2°	0	0

Trapezoid

This test consists in a sheet with two vertical straight lines 230 mm (38°.33 visual angle) apart at the top and with variable distance on the bottom.

The subject is requested to judge if these are parallel, divergent or convergent.

The results are shown in Table 1.

The concluding remarks which we can take into account are the following: For the 'naked eye' we considered an inborn distortion to which the individual is adapted. For the use of classical spherical lens, we have a prismatic effect at the border, which situation causes an image re-evaluation, thus adaptation in needed.

With new multifocal and progressive power lens we have an unusual distortion (for near vision only!) to which the individual becomes adapted. The question arises as to whether differential simultaneous adaptation for far and near vision, respectively, has an ergonomical relevance.

The problem belongs surely to Ergophthalmology, possibly involving eye adaptability.

REFERENCES

Kohler: quoted by Rhule, W. and Smith, K.V. Effects of inversion of the visual field on human motions. J. Exp. Psychol., 57, 358 (1959).

Wittemberg, S. Field study of a new progressive addition lens. J. Am. Optom. Ass., 49, 1013–1021 (1978).

ACUITY PERIMETRY: A SENSITIVE TEST FOR THE DETECTION OF GLAUCOMATOUS OPTIC NERVE DAMAGE

CHARLES D. PHELPS, PIERRE BLONDEAU and BENITA CARNEY

(Iowa City, U.S.A.)

ABSTRACT

Acuity perimetry differs from conventional perimetry in that peripheral visual acuity, not light sensitivity, is the visual function measured. We propose that acuity perimetry is more sensitive than conventional perimetry for the detection of early glaucomatous optic nerve damage.

Early field defects plotted by conventional perimetry are accompanied by profound impairment of peripheral acuity. Acuity may be impaired in the opposite hemifield, or in the fellow eye, when these are normal by conventional perimetry. Patients with ocular hypertension but asymmetric disc cupping usually have corresponding asymmetry of peripheral acuity. Three eyes were observed to devleop defects to conventional perimetry several years after defects were detected by acuity perimetry.

INTRODUCTION

With our acuity perimeter, we test peripheral visual acuity at selected visual field points located between fixation and 20 degrees eccentricity (6). The acuity target is a laser interference fringe grating which is round, one degree in diameter, and variable in spatial frequency and orientation. The individual light and dark stripes of the grating can subtend visual angles ranging from 0.75 to 20 minutes. The target is presented briefly, and the patient is requested to identify the grating's orientation. In previous studies, we determined the optimal background illumination and stimulus presentation time for testing peripheral acuity and measured acuities in a large number of normal subjects of varying ages (1, 5).

In the present study we tested peripheral acuity in patients with glaucoma and ocular hypertension. Our purpose was to determine if acuity perimetry is more sensitive than conventional perimetry for the early diagnosis of glaucoma.

MATERIALS AND METHODS

Fifty-two patients with primary open-angle glaucoma and 35 patients with ocular hypertension were tested with acuity perimetry and conventional

Heijl, A. and Greve, E.L. (eds.), Proceedings of the 6th Int. Visual Field Symposium.
© 1985, Dr W. Junk Publishers, Dordrecht, The Netherlands. ISBN 978-94-010-8932-6

light sensitivity perimetry. Conventional visual field testing was done with either the Goldmann perimeter (using the Armaly suprathreshold static technique for screening) or the Octopus perimeter (using Program 32). Bilateral visual field loss was present in 24 of the glaucoma patients. The other 28 patients had visual field defects in only one eye and a normal visual field in the other eye. One of the ocular hypertensive patients was blind in one eye from non-glaucomatous reasons. Thus, the study material consisted of 76 eyes with glaucomatous visual field defects by conventional perimetry, 28 fellow eyes without visual field defects, and 69 eyes of patients with high intraocular pressures but no visual field defect in either eye. The majority of the glaucomatous visual field defects were minimal, either small nasal steps or isolated paracentral scotomas.

Optic disc stereophotographs were examined to determine the amount and the type of glaucomatous disc cupping. Glaucomatous eyes were classified according to whether the disc cupping was localized to only one pole or was generalized. Fellow eyes and ocular hypertensive eyes were classified as 'probably normal' or 'suspicious' on the basis of the appearance of the neuro-retinal rim. Thinning, notching, absence, hemorrhage, or abnormal trans-lucency of the rim was considered suspicious. Ocular hypertensive patients were classified as having asymmetric cupping if the horizontal cup:disc diameter ratio in the two eyes differed by 0.2 or more.

Acuity perimetry was done with a background illumination of 4.3 apostilbs, a target presentation time of 1/4 second, and a forced choice response. Threshold was defined as the minimal angular separation at which the patient responded correctly to three of five presentations, including three or four of the target orientations. Acuity was measured at 5, 10, 15, and 20 degrees eccentricity along the 45, 90, 145, 225, 270, and 315 degree meridians. Other locations were tested in some patients, especially 15 degrees above and below the nasal meridian and adjacent to locations with poor acuity.

An acuity determination was considered abnormal if the minimal angle of resolution was at least two standard deviations above the mean value for the normal observers at that location (1, 6). The values for the six loci 20 degrees from fixation were disregarded in the analysis because of the difficulty some normal observers had at this eccentricity. Thus, only 18 test locations were used when evaluating the patients' acuity fields. An acuity field was considered abnormal if two adjacent test loci were abnormal or if three loci somewhere in the field were abnormal. Acuity fields in patients with ocular hypertension were considered asymmetric if the two eyes had acuities at 5, 10 or 15 degrees eccentricity that differed by 2, 2.5, or 4.1 minutes of arc, respectively.

RESULTS

All eyes with glaucomatous visual field defects by conventional perimetry had corresponding defects of peripheral acuity. In areas of absolute scotoma on conventional field testing the patients, of course, were also unable to see

Table 1. Grating contrast sensitivity levels.

Cyl/Deg	0.2	0.4	0.8	1.6	3.2	6.4
Normal data mean age 34	11.5	10.0	11.5	11.5	10.0	9.0
30 normal subjects mean age 35	9.0	8.5	10.0	9.5	9.5	8.75
Open angle glaucoma	14.4 ± 2.2	12.8 ± 1.5	15.3 ± 2.0	15.9 ± 2.5	18.1 ± 4.3	23.2 ± 5.5
Ocular hypertension	13.8 ± 1.8	12.0 ± 1.9	14.1 ± 1.0	14.8 ± 0.6	17.8 ± 4.8	21.5 ± 6.4

Table 2. Relationships with intraocular pressure.

I.O.P.	>22	22–25	26–29	30 +
% Field loss	40%	23%	11%	29%
M.T.	15	13	20	12
Arden grating score	17 SD 2.4	17.5 SD 1.7	14.3 SD 0.7	14.2 SD 0.7

Table 3. Field loss and contrast sensitivity.

Scale of loss	100–80	79–60	59–40	< 40	OHT
% Glaucoma field loss	8%	27%	49%	63%	Nil
M.T.	17.8	13.9	14	12.5	14.8
Arden grating score	15.9	19.1	18.6	16.5	15.3

Table 4. Age correlation.

Age	> 59	60–69	70–79	80 +
% Glaucoma field loss	21%	29%	43%	38%
Macular threshold	18.3 SD 1.8	15.4 SD 1.8	15.4 SD 2.6	11.5 SD 4.1

the acuity stimulus. In areas of relative scotoma the patients were able to see the acuity stimulus light but were often unable to resolve the striped pattern, even when tested with the coarsest of the available gratings.

The loss of peripheral acuity often involved a more extensive area of the visual field than did the defect as plotted by conventional perimetry. Areas of relative loss of acuity surrounded the areas which had no acuity.

Some eyes in which the field loss by conventional perimetry was confined to the upper or lower half of the visual field had acuity defects in the opposite hemifield as well. These eyes usually had generalized enlargement of the optic cup. In other eyes the acuity defect was sharply localized to the area defective to conventional perimetry. These eyes had focal disc cupping.

Twenty-four glaucoma patients had unilateral visual field loss when tested by conventional perimetry. Acuity perimetry disclosed abnormalities of peripheral acuity in both eyes of 12 of these patients. In each of these 12 patients the optic disc in the fellow eye was thought to be 'suspicious'.

Of the 65 eyes (33 patients) with ocular hypertension, 17 eyes (15 patients) were abnormal by acuity perimetry. Twelve of these 17 eyes had 'suspicious' appearing optic discs. In the other five eyes, the discs did not look glaucomatous but had some cupping.

All in all, 19 of the ocular hypertensive eyes had optic discs that appeared 'suspicious'. Twelve (63.2%) of these eyes had abnormal acuity fields. The optic discs appeared normal in 50 eyes. Only five (10.0%) of these eyes had abnormal acuity fields ($X^2 = 18.2$, $p < 0.001$).

Fourteen of the ocular hypertensive patients had asymmetric disc cupping, and 20 had symmetric disc cupping. (One patient had only one eye.) Asymmetry of acuity fields in the predicted direction was present in 10 (71.4%) of the patients with disc asymmetry and in 5 (25.0%) of the 19 patients without disc asymetry ($X^2 = 5.44$, $p = 0.02$). One patient with asymmetric cupping had asymmetry of acuity fields in the opposite direction! This one discrepancy remains unexplained.

Three ocular hypertensive eyes with abnormal acuity fields (including both eyes of one patient) developed visual field defects by conventional perimetry two years later. In each instance, conventional fields were normal on several occasions preceding the acuity field and at least once after the acuity field, before the conventional field became abnormal.

DISCUSSION

This study provides evidence that acuity perimetry is more sensitive than conventional perimetry for the detection of early glaucomatous optic nerve damage. The rationale for undertaking this study was based on two hypotheses, which are, in part, substantiated by its results. The first hypothesis is that the acuity at any location in the visual field is limited by the concentration of ganglion cells in the corresponding area of the retina (2, 3, 8, 9). In other words, the visual system's ability to resolve two image points requires, as a minimum, that a message be sent from the retina to the brain along two activated channels (i.e., ganglion cell-nerve fiber units) which are separated by at least one silent channel. In support of this theory, peripheral acuity has been shown to correlate better with ganglion cell density than with photoreceptor density (3, 8, 10).

The second premise is that in early glaucomatous optic nerve damage the loss of ganglion cells and axons in some patients is widespread but scattered, and that with scattered axon loss the visual field as tested by conventional perimetry may remain normal. Many clinicians have observed that in early glaucoma the cup of the optic disc may enlarge before a visual field defect can be detected with conventional perimetry (4). Histopathologic studies suggest that the cause of this early cupping is a loss of nerve fibers (7). The probable reason that axons can be lost without causing a visual field defect is the relatively large size of the test lights used in conventional perimetry. The size I test stimulus on the Goldmann perimeter is 7.7×5.4 minutes and the size III stimulus is 15.4×10.8 minutes. These relatively large lights stimulate many receptive fields in the normal retina. Only if glaucoma destroys most of the axons from a given area of the retina will a visual field defect occur. If, instead, the axon loss is sparsely scattered throughout the optic nerve, the receptive fields of the remaining axons will still overlap sufficiently the stimulus light will be seen. However, the reduced number of axons may cause a loss of acuity.

In general, acuity perimetry is easy to perform, and we have shown in other studies that it gives reproducible results (1). The test has some drawbacks that limit its widespread clinical use. It requires a somewhat more intelligent patient than conventional perimetry. A few patients cannot remain correctly aligned for acuity perimetry. The test is time-consuming: about 30 minutes per eye is required to measure acuity at 24 locations with the thresholding method that we employed in this study. Thus, although acuity perimetry is a sensitive method for detecting early glaucomatous damage, more work is needed to speed up the testing and to make the examination easier for the patient before it can be recommended for routine diagnostic use.

ACKNOWLEDGEMENTS

We are indebted to the National Institutes of Health for their support of this research through Grants EY03330 and R59.

This study comprises part of a thesis prepared for the American Ophthalmological Society by Dr. Phelps as part of the requirements for membership.

REFERENCES

1. Blondeau, P. and Phelps, C.D. Peripheral acuity in normal subjects. To be published in Documenta Ophthalmologica Proceedings Series (this issue).
2. Clemmensen, V. Central and indirect vision of the light-adapted eye. Acta. Physiol. Scand., 9 (Suppl. 27): 1–206 (1944).
3. Frisón, L. and Frisón, M. A simple relationship between the probability distribution of visual acuity and the density of retinal output channels. Acta. Ophthalmol., 54: 437–444 (1976).
4. Pederson, J.E. and Anderson, D.R. The mode of progressive disc cupping in ocular hypertension and glaucoma. Arch. Ophthalmol., 98: 490–495 (1980).
5. Phelps, C.D. Acuity perimetry and glaucoma. To be published in the Trans. of the American Ophthalmological Society.
6. Phelps, C.D., Remijan, P.W. and Blondeau, P. Acuity perimetry. Doc. Ophthalmol. Proc. Series 26: 111–117 (1981).
7. Quigley, H.A., Addicks, E.M. and Green, W.R. Optic nerve damage in human glaucoma. III. Quantitative correlation of nerve fiber loss and visual field defect in glaucoma, ischemic neuropathy, papilledema, and toxic neuropathy. Arch. Ophthalmol., 100: 135–146 (1982).
8. Ten Doesschate, J. Visual acuity and distribution of percipient elements on the retina. Ophthalmologica, 112: 1–18 (1946).
9. Weber, E.H. Der Tastsinn u. das Gemeingefühl. In Wagner, R., ed. Handwörterb. d. Physiol. Braunschweig: Bd. 3, 2., 1846 (cited by Clemmensen [58]).
10. Weymouth, F.W. Visual sensory units and the minimal angle of resolution. Am. J. Ophthalmol., 46(II): 102–113 (1958).

Author's address:
Charles D. Phelps, M.D.
Department of Ophthalmology
University of Iowa Hospitals
Iowa City, Iowa 52242, USA

THE SHORT-TERM EFFECT OF LASER TRABECULOPLASTY ON THE GLAUCOMATOUS VISUAL FIELD

ANDERS HEIJL and BOEL BENGTSSON

(*Malmö, Sweden*)

ABSTRACT

Several earlier studies have shown improvement of glaucomatous visual fields after pressure reduction achieved by acetazolamide or filtering surgery while other studies have given conflicting results. In the present study laser trabeculoplasty was used to reduce IOP in 42 eyes with glaucomatous visual field defects. The visual field was tested with the Competer perimeter before and one month after the laser trabeculoplasty. Although good pressure reduction (mean: 10.3 mm Hg) was achieved no general regression of field defects was observed. The changes of the visual field were not correlated to the degree of pressure reduction. Deterioration and improvement were equally common and it is likely that the registered visual field changes were due simply to random variation. The results do not support the hypothesis that glaucomatous field defects are reversible when the IOP is reduced.

The full article will be published in Acta Ophthalmologica.

Author's address:
The University of Lund,
Department of Ophthalmology,
Malmö, Sweden

Heijl, A. and Greve, E.L. (eds.), Proceedings of the 6th Int. Visual Field Symposium.
© *1985, Dr W. Junk Publishers, Dordrecht, The Netherlands. ISBN 978-94-010-8932-6*

THE EFFECT OF ARGON LASER TRABECULOPLASTY ON THE VISUAL FIELD OF PATIENTS WITH GLAUCOMA

CARLO E. TRAVERSO, GEORGE L. SPAETH, RONALD L. FELLMAN, RICHARD J. STARITA, KEVIN C. GREENIDGE and EFFIE PORYZEES

(*Philadelphia, USA*)

ABSTRACT

Argon laser tarabeculoplasty (ALT) was performed on 232 eyes of 168 patients. Indication for treatment was progression of visual field loss due to glaucoma, despite maximum tolerated medical treatment. Mean percentage IOP change was -21.6% ($\pm$ 19); mean F.U. was 9 months (3–21). Visual field were obtained with an Octopus computerized perimeter, using programs 31 or 32. Quantitative analysis of functional results was done only on eyes without significant amount of false answers or visual acuity changes or pupil size changes. 113 eyes met these requirements. IOP variations secondary to ALT were similar to those observed in the total group of treated eyes. Mean F.U. was 10 months (4–21). A visual field change was considered significant when a 15% variation of the mean quadrantic sensitivity was observed and the initial mean sensitivity was greater than 10 dB. When initial mean sensitivity was less than 10 dB a 40% change was required to be considered significant. In our sample visual fields improved in 17% of patients, remained unchanged in 55% and worsened in 28%. Although visual field changes and IOP changes did not overlap always as expected there is a good correspondence between hydrodynamic and functional success. Patients with less advanced disease were more likely to have good functional results. The last decades have witnessed much debate regarding how, when, and, even, whether elevated intraocular pressure is responsible for glaucomatous optic nerve damage. Traditionally, treatment has largely been based on lowering intraocular pressure to a level which will no longer compromise an eye. Since the report of Wise and Witter argon laser trabeculoplasty (ALT) has been used successfully to decrease intraocular pressure in patient affected by primary open angle glaucoma (POAG) (7–10). The long-term effect of ALT on the natural history of glaucomatous disease, that is, on the functional visual ability of patients with POAG is, however, not established. We report here information regarding the course of visual field changes in patients undergoing ALT. The data are analyzed to determine possible relationships between change in IOP and change in the visual field.

Heijl, A. and Greve, E.L. (eds.), Proceedings of the 6th Int. Visual Field Symposium.
© *1985, Dr W. Junk Publishers, Dordrecht, The Netherlands. ISBN 978-94-010-8932-6*

PATIENTS AND METHODS

After informed consent was obtained, ALT was performed on 232 eyes of 168 patinets with primary open-angle glaucoma, pigmentary glaucoma or glaucoma associated with the exfoliation syndrome. All patients were phakic. Indication for treatment was progression of visual field loss due to glaucoma despite maximum tolerated medical therapy. The Wise technique was used, but with a more anterior placement of the burns. Pre- and post-laser examinations included disc drawings and/or stereo photographs of the optic disc. Visual fields were obtained with an Octopus computer-assisted perimeter, using programs 31 or 32. In order to quantify visual field changes after treatment we considered only eyes with pupil size changes of less than 0.6 mm, visual acuity changes of less than 3 Snellen lines, and less than 25% false answers as defined by the perimetric examination program.

One hundred and thirteen eyes met these requirements. A visual field change was considered significant when variation of the mean quadrantic sensitivity was greater than 15% and the initial mean sensitivity was greater than 10 dB. When initial mean sensitivity was less than 10 dB a 40% change in sensitivity was required for the alteration to be considered significant.

Mean follow-up was 10 months (maximum 21, minimum 4). For purposes of analysis the latest visual field and intraocular pressure were compared to the pre-treatment examination of field and pressure.

In all cases the pre-treatment visual field was determined no earlier than one month prior to the date of the argon laser trabeculoplasty. IOP was measured immediately after every visual field examination.

A 'better' IOP was defined as a decrease of IOP (pre-ALT minus post-ALT) greater than 2 mmHg. A worse IOP was considered to occur when IOP rose following ALT by more than 2 mmHg. Cases in which the differences between the pre- and post-ALT IOP was less than plus or minus 3 mmHg. were considered unchanged.

Patients were staged arbitrarily upon entering this study, being divided into two groups, one with less advances and the other with more advanced disease; the criteria for staging were a clinical impression of the extent of disc damage and visual field loss.

RESULTS

The effect of ALT on IOP of the cases in our sample is summarized in Tables 1 and 2. Tables 3 and 4 show the behaviour of the visual field.

DISCUSSION

Previous works have shown that Octopus Computerized Perimetry is an effective way to obtain reliable and reproduceable visual fields (1, 3, 5, 6). Furthermore, since results are given in a numerical format, data analysis is facilitated.

Table 1. Intraocular pressure (IOP) changes after argon laser trabeculoplasty.

N	Pre treatment IOP (*) mean (SD)	Post treatment IOP (*) mean (SD)	Mean percentage change pre treatment level (IOP%)
113	21.0 (± 5)	16.7 (± 5)	− 19.6 (± 18.8)

* = mmHg by Goldmann applanation.

Table 2. Distribution of eyes with improvement of IOP less than 10% or greater than 19%.

	IOP improvement less than 10%	IOP improvement greater than 19%
Cases acceptable for study n = 113	25 (22%)	73 (65%)
All cases treated n = 232	49 (21%)	145 (63%)

Table 3. Visual field changes after argon laser trabeculoplasty*.

	No. of eyes	No. of expected variations*	No. of unexpected variations (%)
Worse	32	24 (75)	8 (25)
Unchanged	62	57 (92)	5 (8)
Better	19	18 (95)	1 (5)
Total	113	99 (88)	14 (12)

Mean F.U. 10 months (max 21, min 4).
*See text for definitions of unchanged, better, worse, expected and unexpected.

Table 4. Visual field changes after argon laser trabeculoplasty related to stage of the diesase

	Early + medium[1]	Advanced + far advanced[2]	Total
Worse	7	25	32
Unchanged	35	27	62
Better	6	13	19
Total	48	65	113

x^2: p < 0.01
[1] = Mean IOP improvement (percentage) = 19 (± 19).
[2] = Mean IOP improvement (percentage) = 20 (± 18).

In order to enhance the likelihood that the observed visual field changes are 'real' a standardization of method and conditions of the tests is essential. Therefore, we attempted to employ the same settings and the same strategies for pre- and post-treatment examinations wherever possible. Where this was not feasible, patients were excluded from this study. Thus, all patients included not only met the criteria described in the section on patients methods, but also had field examinations in which the entire testing event was as similar as possible. Although this study was prospective by design, the final calculations were made on a non-randomized sample: the reliability of the Octopus visual field test was no forseeable beforehand.

In our groups of patients the intraocular pressure response to ALT was similar to that reported by other authors (7−10). The effect of ALT in the total population studied, and in the smaller sample selected for visual field analysis, was highly similar (Table 2). That is, the smaller sample appears to be an accurate representation of the effect of ALT on the entire group. For purposes of analysis we compared the behaviour of the visual field with the behaviour of the intraocular pressure. The visual field and IOP were considered 'better', 'unchanged', or 'worse', as defined in the patients and materials section. If it is assumed that there is a causal relation between IOP and visual field loss in glaucoma then it would be expected that the course of visual field change would be different in those in whom the intraocular pressure was worse from those in whom the intraocular pressure was better. An 'expected' result would, therefore, be a result in which (1) IOP and visual field both got 'better', or (2) IOP got 'better' but visual field remained 'unchanged' (recall that in all present cases visual field was in a deteriorating state), or (3) IOP was 'unchanged' and the visual field was 'worse', or (4) IOP was 'worse' and visual field was 'worse'. 'Unexpected' results would be those in which (1) IOP was 'better' and visual field was 'worse', or (2) IOP was 'unchanged' and visual field 'better', or (3) IOP and visual field were both 'unchanged', or (4) IOP was 'worse', the visual field was 'better', or (5) IOP was 'worse' and the visual field was 'unchanged'. Examination of Table 3 shows that the majority of patients behaved in an 'expected' manner. The strongest correlation was between those who had improvement in both IOP and visual field. The poorest relation was seen in those with a deterioration of visual field despite apparent improvement of IOP. The explanation for the poor correlation in this group may be that the patients needed a greater pressure lowering effect than we arbitrarily defined as 'better'. It may well be that some patients need a pressure fall far greater than 3 mmHg. In order to permit restoration of normal physiology. In this regard four of the 'unexpectedly worse' cases had far-advanced optic nerve damage, suggesting that they needed a greater fall in IOP than was obtained.

In addition, one of the other four 'unexpectedly worse' cases had an acute pressure elevation after ALT. Thus, there were three cases in which the 'unexpected' result is not readily understandable.

The 'unexpectedly stable' cases included three eyes with a minimum follow-up (four months), one eye with borderline visual field changes, and another eye which maintained low pressures for eight months, after which a substantial increase of pressure occurred. Thus, all five of these cases have a reasonable explanation for the 'unexpected' results.

Table 4 shows that the result of IOP, in terms of effect on visual field, is directly related to stage of disease. The better results being obtained with those with less advanced disease.

We chose a definition of 'improvement' in visual field (as described in patients in method six) that probably represents a change greater than expected to occur as a result of short- and long-term fluctuations (1−3). However, even if we were wrong in this assumption, the direction of the results of analysis *would not* be significantly affected. The reason for this is as follows. The inclusion of fields whose actual change differed from our description of that change would add 'noise' to the analysis. But, unless the noise systematically favored one direction or the other (improvement or deterioration) the addition of such noise would serve only to lessen the apparent significance of the results, but would not affect the direction of the results. Thus, though the *extent* of statistically significance of our results will be decreased by the extent to which observed visual field changes do not reflect actual changes, the direction of change will *not* be affected. In fact, quite to the contrary; the greater the noise, the greater is the biological significance of the results, because the elimination of the noise would result in clearer separation of the two groups.

In conclusion we believe that visual field changes in this study have reflected the intraocular pressure changes. Patients with more advanced diseases had poorer functional response to ALT than patients with less advanced disease. The cause for this poorer response was not a function of relation between the stage of disease and the effect of ALT on IOP. The poorer response is presumably a factor either of (1) need for greater intraocular pressure fall in patients with advanced disease in order to prevent continuing deterioration, or (2) inexorable course of the disease in patients with advanced optic nerve damage.

REFERENCES

1. Bebie, H., Fankhauser, F. and Spahr, J. Static perimetry: accuracy and fluctuations. Acta. Ophthalmol. 54: 339–348 (1976).
2. Flammer, J. Drance, S.M. and Schulzer, M. The estimation and testing of the components of long-term fluctuation of the differential light threshold. Doc. Ophthalmol. Proc. Ser. 35: 383–389 (1983).
3. Gloor, B., Schmied, V. and Fässler, A. Changes of glaucomatous field defects. Int. Ophthal. 3, 1: 5–10 (1983).
4. Heijl, A. and Drance, S.M. A clinical comparison of three computerized automatic perimeters in the detection of glaucoma defects. Doc. Ophthal. Proc. Series, 26: 43–48 (1981).
5. Li, S.G., Spaeth, G.L, Schatz, N.J. et al. Clincical experiences with the use of an automated perimeter (Octopus) in the management of patients with glaucoma and neurological disease. Ophthalmol. 85: 74 (1978).
6. Schmied, U. Automatic (Octopus) and manual (Goldmann) perimetry in glaucoma. In: Proc. Int. meeting automated perimetry system Octopus. Interzeag. publ., Schlieren Switzerland (1979).
7. Schwartz, A. and Kopelman, J. Four-years experience with argon laser trabecular surgery in uncontrollated open-angle glaucoma. Ophthalmology 90: 771–780 (1983).
8. Thomas, J., Simmons, R. and Belcher, D. Argon laser trabeculoplasty in the presurgical glaucoma patient. Ophthalmology 89: 187–197 (1982).
9. Wilensky, J.T. and Jampol, L.M. Laser therapy for open angle glaucoma. Ophthalmology 88: 213–217 (1981).
10. Wise, J. Long-term control of adult open angle glaucoma by argon laser trabeculoplasty. Ophthalmology 88: 197–202 (1981).

Author's address:
The William and Anna Goldberg Glaucoma Service and
Research Laboratory,
Wills Eye Hospital,
Ninth and Walnut Sts.,
Philadelphia 19107 PA, U.S.A.

THE VISUAL FIELD BEFORE AND AFTER ARGON LASER TRABECULOPLASTY. REGRESSION ANALYSIS BASED ON COMPUTERIZED PERIMETRY

CATHARINA HOLMIN and C.E.T. KRAKAU

(*Lund, Sweden*)

ABSTRACT

15 eyes with glaucomatous visual field defects were followed with computerized perimetry (Competer) before and about 13 months after argon laser trabeculoplasty. The pressure reduction amounted to on an average 33% (8.5 mm Hg). Regression analysis based on series of visual fields did not reveal any influence of the pressure reduction on the rate of visual field decay.

INTRODUCTION

The efficiency of therapy in glaucoma is usually judged on the basis of its pressure reducing capacity. In this respect argon laser trabeculoplasty (ALT) has turned out to be a most valuable method. For instance, from a long term study on open angle glaucoma Wise reported a rate of IOP control by ALT equivalent to that following trabeculectomy but with far fewer complications (4).

A different problem is whether the trabeculoplasty will control the glaucoma even in the sense that the visual field will be protected from further deterioration. In a long term study of cases with increased intraocular pressure 'a deterioration of the visual field could be noted even in eyes where pressure was considerably reduced', though in most cases the progression of the field defect seemed to be checked (3). Manual perimetry was used and for some of the patients only one visual field was available after the trabeculoplasty.

The establishment of a possible favourable effect of a treatment on the glaucomatous visual field is attended with some specific difficulties. For instance, an admixture to the material of ocular hypertensives, with a low risk of developing defects, may seemingly give an impression of successful therapy. Furthermore, the occurrence of the sometimes considerable spontaneous variations in the glaucomatous field make an evaluation based on a too limited number of fields rather unreliable.

By using a computerized perimeter which furnishes results in numerical form it is possible to condense the result into a single number. With a sufficient number of consecutive fields, it makes sense to calculate the linear regression coefficient as an expression of the trend (1).

Heijl, A. and Greve, E.L. (eds.), Proceedings of the 6th Int. Visual Field Symposium.
© *1985, Dr W. Junk Publishers, Dordrecht, The Netherlands. ISBN 978-94-010-8932-6*

The tools for a study of the trend in visual field development before and after a pressure reduction are available and therefore this enterprise may be expected to shed some light on a crucial question in glaucoma research.

MATERIALS AND METHODS

The material comprises 15 eyes with glaucomatous field defects (15 patients, age 61–79) in which argon laser trabeculoplasty was performed. The indications for treatment were either a progression of the visual field loss or pressure readings of ≥ 30 mm Hg, or both. In the case of all eyes but one, pressure reducing therapy was already provided and was continued unchanged after the trabeculoplasty was performed.

The computerized perimeter Competer was used for the visual fields. With this method the threshold values at 64 points inside 20 degrees are determined and given as numerical values. A high value corresponds to a high sensitivity. A 'performance' value (P) is calculated as the sum of the 64 threshold values and used in the calculation of the regression coefficient (b) of performance (P) on time.

In all cases at least 6 pre-operative fields obtained for more than one year and under the same test conditions were available. Postoperatively the visual fields have so far been checked five times; the first about one month, the 2nd about 3 months after treatment, and the following at an interval of about 3 months.

The regression coefficients (b) were calculated on the last 6 pre-operative fields and on the 5 post-operative fields, respectively. The IOPs are mean values based on single applanation tonometry readings obtained in connection with the visual field testing.

RESULTS

IOP

Preoperatively the mean IOP for the whole group was 25.7 mm Hg (range 18–32) and the IOP level exceeded 20 mm Hg in all cases but one. In the post-operative period the mean IOP had fallen to 17.3 mm Hg (range 13–23) and thus a pressure reduction of on an average 33 per cent (8.5 mm Hg, s.e.m. 0.77) had been achieved. The mean post-operative IOP and the pressure reduction for each eye appear from Fig. 1. The pressure effect remained during the post-operative follow-up.

Visual field

The progression rate of visual field loss, expressed as the *mean* regression coefficient (b) for the whole group, was the same before as after ALT, or −3.5 P-units/month, s.e.m. 0.75 and 0.84 respectively (both significantly (p < 0.001) different from zero). In all eyes 3 the *individual* post-operative

372

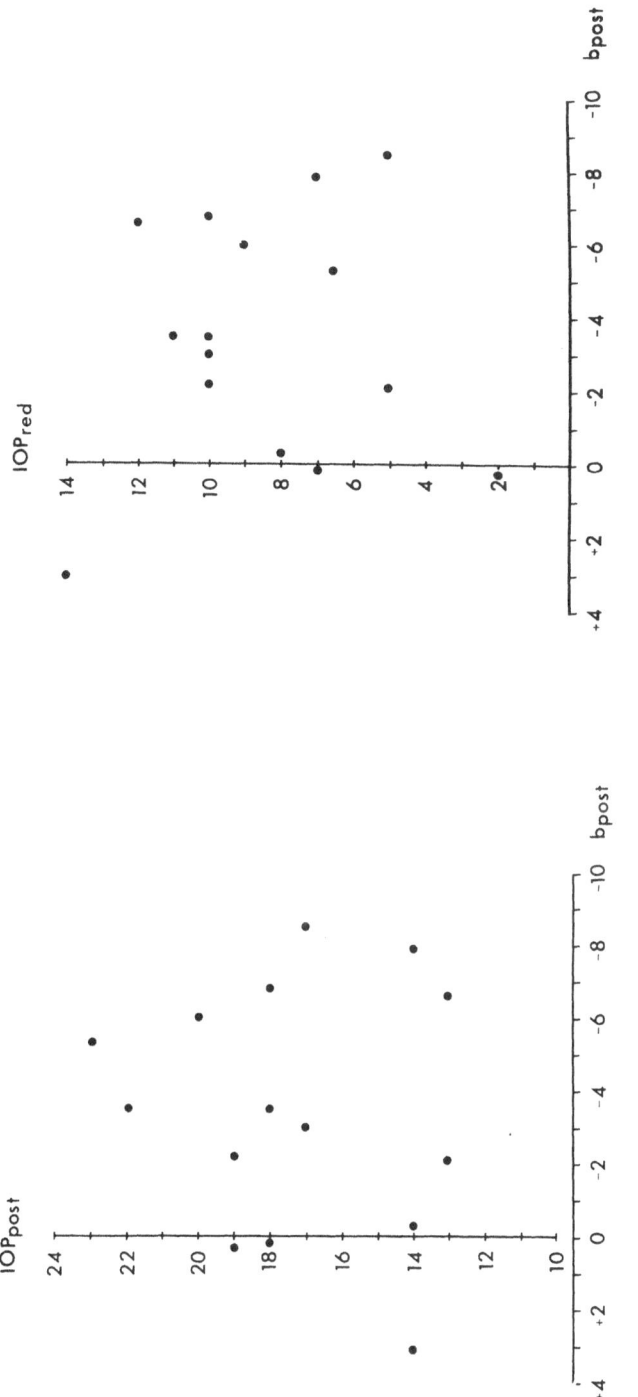

Fig. 1. The regression coefficients (b = P-units/month) from the postoperative period plotted against the mean IOP (left) and the IOP reduction achieved by the trabeculoplasty (right). The IOP's are given in mm Hg.

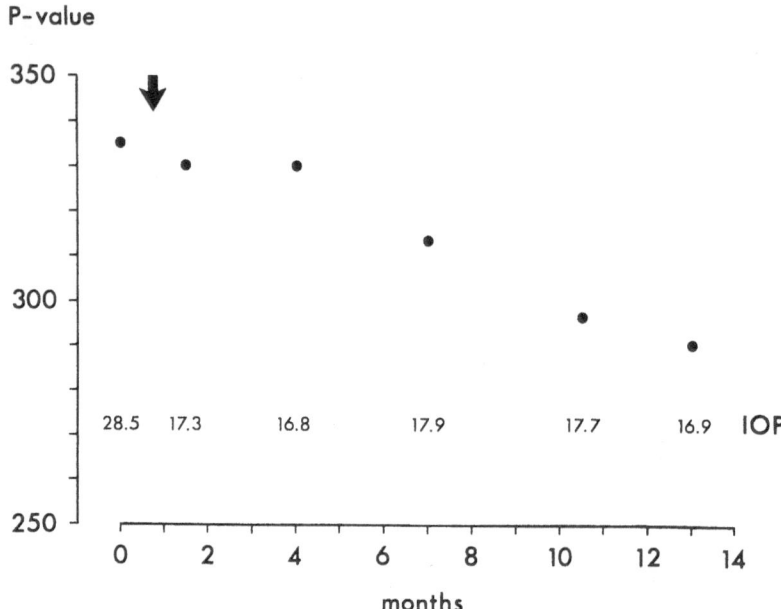

Fig. 2. Mean values for the visual field performance (P) and the IOP obtained at the last pre-operative and the 5 post-operative observations. The trabeculoplasty is indicated by the arrow.

regression coefficient was negative. Five of these had a significant ($p < 0.05$) progression of field loss. None of the 3 positive regression coefficients was significantly > 0.

The post-operative field decay is demonstrated in Fig. 2, which shows the mean P-values from the last pre-operative and the 5 post-operative check ups. Due to less regular intervals, it was not possible to treat the other observations in the pre-operative period in the same way.

No correlation between either the post-operative pressure level or the amount of the pressure reduction and the rate of the visual field loss could be demonstrated (Fig. 1).

DISCUSSION

The effect of the laser treatment on the IOP was on the whole quite satisfying and of about the same order as that reported from other clinics (3, 4).

Despite this pressure reduction no effect on the rate of visual field decay could be traced during the follow up. Most cases had a trend towards deterioration, just as before the intervention, and the mean regression coefficient was the same after the trabeculoplasty as before.

Hypothetically a substantial but transitory improvement of the visual field following immediately after the treatment might influence the regression coefficient during a relatively short follow up by giving high 'start values' in the series of P-values. However, neither in the present material nor in a larger group which included the present material could any support for the existence of such short-term effect be demonstrated (2).

To conclude, in this group of eyes with glaucomatous field defects a regression analysis of series of visual fields did not reveal any influence of pressure reduction by laser trabeculoplasty. A slight effect might of course be obscured by random fluctuations, but this might have been a tendency towards increased deterioration as well as towards improvement, an in any case no very dominating influence can be assumed.

ACKNOWLEDGEMENTS

This work was supported by the Swedish Medical Research Council (project No. B84-04X-5 202-07C) and H. and L. Nilsson's Foundation.

REFERENCES

1. Holmin, C. and Krakau, C.E.T. Automatic perimetry in the control of glaucoma. Glaucoma 3: 154–159 (1981).
2. Holmin, C. and Bauer, B. Computerized perimetry before and after trabeculoplasty. A study of the short term effect. Doc. Ophthalmol. Proc. Ser. Acc f. publ.
3. Pohjanpelto, P. Late results of laser trabeculoplasty for increased intraocular pressure. Acta Ophthalmol (Copenh) 61: 998–1008 (1983).
4. Wise, J.B. Long-term control of adult open angle glaucoma by argon laser treatment. Ophthalmology 88: 197–202 (1981).

Author's address:
Department of Experimental Ophthalmology
University Eye Clinic, S-221 85, Lund, Sweden.

PERIPHERAL NASAL FIELD DEFECTS

R.P. LeBLANC, A. LEE. and M. BAXTER

(*Halifax, Nova Scotia, Canada*)

ABSTRACT

Visual field assessment using the Octopus Perimeter was carried out on 96 eyes with early P.O.A.G. The central visual field was assessed quantitatively using programmes 31 and 32 while the peripheral field was assessed using a two-step suprathreshold screening programme (07).

In all cases, central field changes were noted while in 80 eyes peripheral nasal field changes were present. No cases were found with isolated nasal field defects in this series.

The assessment of the peripheral nasal field as an integral part of the visual field examination of glaucoma patients, has been the subject of several reports in the literature since 1971 (1–3, 5, 6, 8, 9). Prior to 1970 little was written about this subject, although the peripheral nasal step had been well described by Rönne or Rønne (6) at the end of the last century. Several of the reports which have appeared during the past decade have confirmed the importance of *isolated* nasal steps as an early sign of glaucomatous damage (1, 5, 6, 8). Most authors agree that the incidence of this sign is inversely proportional to the quality of the central field examination. Nonetheless, the incidence of this sign remains at a significant level (4 to 8%) even when the central field is tested with static techniques using the Goldmann perimeter.

With the increasing use of automated perimetry, particularly for the quantitative assessment of the central field, it is of interest to re-assess the value of the peripheral nasal field in the diagnosis of glaucomatous field loss. The purpose of this study was to assess the significance of the nasal field in patients having visual field assessment using automated quantitative perimetry.

MATERIALS AND METHODS

A retrospective review of all records of primary open angle glaucoma patients followed in the Nova Scotia Eye Centre was carried out. All patients were carefully followed regularly and were diagnosed as primary open angle

Heijl, A. and Greve, E.L. (eds.), Proceedings of the 6th Int. Visual Field Symposium.
© *1985, Dr W. Junk Publishers, Dordrecht, The Netherlands. ISBN 978-94-010-8932-6*

glaucoma on the basis of ophthalmological and perimetric assessment. Excluded from review were all cases of secondary glaucoma, angle closure glaucoma and pseudoexfoliative glaucoma. Cases of advanced field loss were also excluded to allow this study to consider only early or moderate field loss cases.

Ninety-six (96) eyes were retained for assessment each having had initial and follow-up visual field examination on the Octopus 201 Perimeter. All eyes had peripheral field testing carried out using Programme 07 (spatially related suprathreshold screening) while the central visual field was assessed using a programme from the 30 Series (Figs. 1 and 2). Each visual field examination was independently assessed to consider the presence or absence of (a) a central field defect, (b) a peripheral nasal defect and (c) the concomitant

OCTOPUS®

Correction, (sph., cyl., + axis):	+ 2.00	+ 0.00	+ 0
Diameter of pupil, headposition:	5.00	06	
Size of stimulus:	3		
Fixationring:			
Program number:	07		

Number of questions:	206	Number of repetitions:	2	Date of printout:	3.04.1984
False positive answers (%):	0(0/20)	False negative answers (%):	0(0/ 0)		

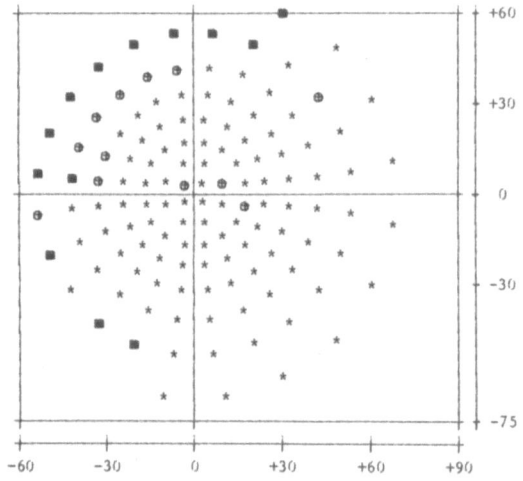

LEGEND: * NORMAL
         ⊕ RELATIVE DEFECT
         ■ ABSOLUTE DEFECT

Fig. 1. Two level suprathreshold screening (Program 07) using Octopus perimeter showing nasal contraction with step accompanied by superior arcuate scotoma.

378

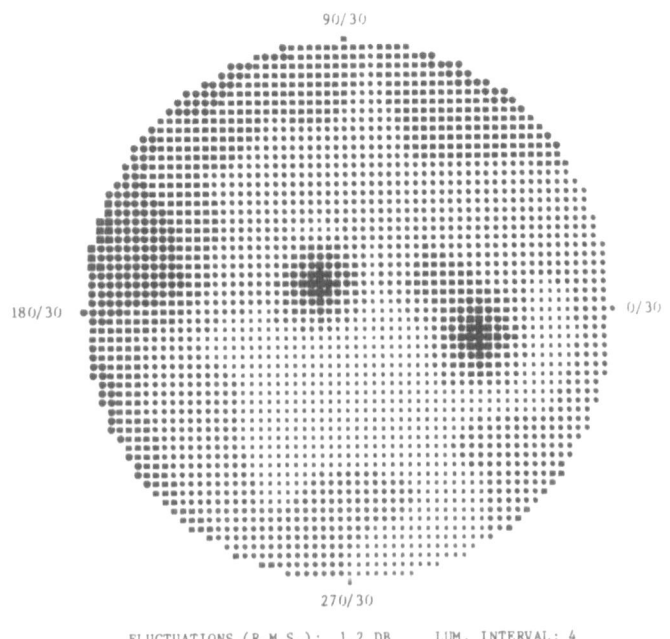

OCTOPUS®

Correction, (sph., cyl., + axis):   + 2.00   + 0.00   + 0
Diameter of pupil, headposition: 5.00   06
Size of stimulus: 3
Fixationring:
Program number: 32

Number of questions: 394
False positive answers (%):   0(0/ 9)   Number of repetitions: 2   Date of printout   3.04.1984
                                            False negative answers (%):   0(0/10)

90/30

180/30   0/30

270/30

FLUCTUATIONS (R.M.S.): 1.2 DB   LUM. INTERVAL: 4

Fig. 2. Program 32 – Static quantitative thesold measurement confirming superior arcuate scotoma.

presence of a central defect and a peripheral defect. The criteria used to determine the presence or absence of such defects have been previously described (4).

RESULTS

Eighty (80) of the 96 eyes tested demonstrated a peripheral nasal field defect on the 07 Programme, an incidence of 83% of eyes tested, while 16 eyes (17%) showed no peripheral defect but did have a central defect consistent with the diagnosis of primary open angle glaucoma. In non of the 80 eyes demonstrating a peripheral nasal defect was the central field normal.

379

In twenty-nine (29) of the eyes assessed, the original perimetric assessment was performed using the 07 screening programme (whole field) combined with the 03 suprathreshold screening programme for the central field. In each case this was followed by a repeat test using the 07 Programme combined with the 30 Series quantitative assessment. In all cases, there was complete correlation between the central screener and the quantitative assessment of the central field.

DISCUSSION

It is clear from several studies in the literature that the peripheral nasal field defect is an important marker for glaucomatous damage, being reported in up to 50% of cases showing visual field loss. In most of the studies, the field was analyzed using kinetic techniques, often with markedly suprathreshold targets. The intensity with which the central field was analyzed varied greatly in these different studies and seemed to influence the incidence of the peripheral defect found as an *isolated* finding. It is clear that the incidence of isolated peripheral nasal steps will be higher in those patients in whom the central visual field examination has been less than absolutely thorough. In this context we have advocated that the peripheral nasal step is an easy marker to detect in patients with open angle glaucoma in whom the central visual field may show but the earliest of visual field changes.

With the use of automated quantitative static perimetry, it is felt that the central visual field is being assessed at a level beyond the scope of manual suprathreshold static perimetry. In this context, it is possible that the search of the central visual field is so thorough that all patients with peripheral nasal field defects may in fact show central defects as well. This current series would seem to support this view in that none of the 96 eyes in this study had a peripheral nasal defect in the absence of a central field defect. It is clear however that suprathreshold screening of the peripheral field may not be sensitive enough to pick up early nasal scotomas, particularly in view of the 15° grid in this programme. If cases with normal central fields and early nasal scotomas had been surveyed, they could have been missed. To avoid this eventuality, a *quantitative* programme for nasal field assessment would have been more appropriate and such a programme with a tight grid pattern can be developed using Sargon software (1). It was the author's view however that to address this question with existing programmes was an important initial assessment.

Our results suggest that for diagnostic purposes a meticulous search of the central visual field may be sufficient and additional time spent searching the peripheral field might not be necessary. However, while the testing of the peripheral field with suprathreshold screening techniques is adequate to define the presence or absence of a nasal step, this approach may fail to detect earlier changes, i.e., small scotoma, in the peripheral field which may precede central field changes. Thus further studies correlating quantitative peripheral field assessment to quantitative central field assessment are needed.

CONCLUSION

It appears to these investigators that when using well-controlled *sensitive* techniques to examine the central visual field (i.e., the Goldmann perimeter/ Drance Armaly Screener) approximately one out of eight to ten cases of primary open angle glaucoma may be detected by means of the nasal step only. It is therefore of paramount importance to investigate the nasal step in this context.

When using *less sensitive* techniques, the value of the nasal step as a marker of primary open angle glaucoma increases markedly and must be assessed in each and every patient.

When using *very sensitive* techniques, such as automated quantitative assessment of the central field with an Octopus System, nasal step defects as detected by suprathreshold techniques are accompanied by central defects in all cases and do not add diagnostic value to the central field assessment.

Further 'studies correlating quantitative peripheral field assessment to quantitative central field assessment are currently under way in several laboratories and should help define the correlation of these findings.

REFERENCES

1. Caprioli, J. The Peripheral Visual Field in Glaucoma. Presented at the Third Octopus Users' Society Meeting, Denver, Colorado, March (1984).
2. de Oliveira Bassi, Marcia and Shields, Bruce. Crowding of the Peripheral Nasal Isopters in Glaucoma. American Journal of Ophthalmology 94: 4–10 (1982).
3. Hart, William M. and Becker, Bernard. The Onset and Evolution of Glaucomatous Visual Field Defects. Ophthalmology, 89: 268–279 (1982).
4. LeBlanc, Raymond P. Abnormal Static Threshold Values in Computerized Visual Fields, edited by Whalen and Spaeth, Charles B. Slack, Inc, in press.
5. LeBlanc, Raymond P. Peripheral Nasal Field Defects. Doc. Ophthalmol. Proc. Series 14: 131–133 (1977).
6. LeBlanc, Raymond P. and Becker, Bernard. Peripheral Nasal Field Defects. American Journal of Ophthalmology, Vol. 72: 415–419 (1971).
7. Rønne, H. Über das Gesichtfeld beim Glaukom. Klin. Mbl. Augenheilk, 47: 12–33 (1909).
8. Werner, Elliot B. and Beraskow, Jane. Peripheral Nasal Field Defects in Glaucoma. Ophthalmology, 86: 1875–1878 (1979).
9. Zingirian, M.D., Calabria, M.G. and Gandolfo, E. The Nasal Step in Normal and Glaucomatous Visual Fields. Canadian Journal of Ophthalmology, 14: 88–94 (1979).

Author's address:
R. LeBlanc, M.D.
Nova Scotia Eye Centre
1335 Queen Street
Halifax, Nova Scotia
B3J 2H6 Canada

THE NATURE OF VISUAL LOSS IN LOW TENSION GLAUCOMA

ANDERTON, S.A., COAKES, R.C., POINOOSWAMY, S., CLARKE, P.,
and HITCHINGS, R.A.

(*London, UK*)

ABSTRACT

A retrospective review of visual fields in fifty-six patients with Low Tension Glaucoma is described. This review shows that the upper and lower halves of the visual field behaved in a semi independent fusion. With a mean follow-up of 10.5 years 60% of visual fields did not progress. Of those fields that did show progression it may take years (mean 4.4) to occur. If progressions occurs there is a one in two chance of an already damaged visual field being further damaged but only a one in four chance of it occurring in a previously normal field. The progression occurs over a 60% chance of repeated episodes of visual field loss occurring within the same 10.5 year follow-up period.

INTRODUCTION

Low Tension Glaucoma is a common type of glaucoma accounting for approximately one third of all the primary open angle glaucomas. Patient so classified should have an intraocular pressure less than or equal to 21 mm. Hg off treatment, glaucomatous type of visual field defect, glaucomatous cupping and an open angle. The clinical importance lies in the number of these patients whose visual field defects progresses despite 'normal' intra-ocular pressures. Frequently, eyes with such progressive field loss are offered treatment. In order to assess the efficacy of treatment it is essential to under-stand the rate and type of visual field loss seen in this disease. As yet the pattern of visual field loss in Low Tension Glaucoma is uncertain (1). Chumbley and Brubaker (2) reviewed thirty-four eyes of seventeen patients who had more than one visual field examination and who had been followed for four months to twelve years. They found that 41% of these patients showed visual field progression. Levene in his review article (1) also noted a 41% progression in thirty-four eyes of twenty-three cases. There is however little information on the rate of progression and the nature of the visual field defects in this type of condition.

This paper reviews the visual fields of patients with Low Tension Glaucoma seen at Moorfields Eye Hospital.

Heijl, A. and Greve, E.L. (eds.), Proceedings of the 6th Int. Visual Field Symposium.
© *1985, Dr W. Junk Publishers, Dordrecht, The Netherlands. ISBN 978-94-010-8932-6*

MATERIAL AND METHODS

The visual field charts of patients with Low Tension Glaucoma were reviewed. Low Tension Glaucoma was considered to be present when the intraocular pressure was less than or equal to 21 mm Hg off treatment during a 24 hour period of in-patient phasing together with glaucomatous cupping and visual field loss in patients with an open angle and no evidence for other ocular disease.

The visual fields were charted on the Goldmann bowl perimeter and were kinetic fields. The I-4 isopter was used. The central 30° of each visual field chart was used for the analysis. To obtain a figure for percentage visual field loss a planometer (map reader) was used to calculate the total length of the 24 radii on the chart. Thus for each individual fields the planometer was used to calculate the extent (length) of the radii involved in the visual field defect. A percentage involved for each individual field of vision was calculated as was the percentage for the upper and lower visual field calculated.

RESULTS

Fifty-six patients had their charts reviewed. Thus 112 visual fields or 224 hemi fields were available for analysis. (A hemi field was the upper or lower part of the visual field.)

The minimum follow-up was 3.5 years, the maximum 26 years mean 10.5 years.

Each patient had on average 1.5 visual field examination per year.

A normal hemi field was considered to be ⩾ 47.5%.

A clinically significant visual field defect was one of 5° across. Depending on the position in the visual field the percentage visual field loss was 5° would vary (for the closer to fixation the closer the radii were together and therefore the greater visual field loss) however 5° on average was equivalent to 5% visual field loss.

Visual field progression was either *sudden* loss, defined as ⩾ 5% loss between two visual field tests or *gradual* loss defined ⩾ 2% loss per annum.

At the outset 224 hemi fields were analysed, 120 were 'normal', 54 upper, 66 lower.

120 hemi fields were normal at the outset. After a mean 10.5 year follow-up 37 upper fields and 54 lower fields remain normal. 17 upper and 22 lower fields developed visual field defects.

25% of *normal hemi fields* developed a visual field defect during the period of follow-up.

Abnormal hemi fields. 104 were abnormal at the outset. After a mean follow-up of 10.5 years 28 upper and 24 lower hemi fields were unchanged. 32 upper and 22 lower hemi fields worsened, i.e. 50% chance of developing a worsening of the visual field defect developed. 93 of the 224 hemi fields or 41% progressed.

Onset of progression. 81 hemi fields progressed with sudden visual field loss.

12 hemi fields showed gradual decline. Of the 81 hemi fields with sudden visual field loss the time until progression occured was mean 4.4 years. The size of the new visual field defect was 10% in the upper field, 8.7% in the lower field.

Number of episodes of visual field progression:

(a) One only 18 upper fields 7 lower fields (25).

(b) > 1 22 upper, 29 lower fields (51).

Nature of progress. It would appear that progressive visual field defects did not effect the two hemi fields or the two eyes simultaneously. It would also appear that the visual field progression was not associated with relative increases in intraocular pressure.

The following four comments can be made:

1. At presentation there is a 60% chance of no further progresssion of the visual field occurring (with a mean follow-up of 10.5 years).
2. If progression does occur it may take years to develop (mean 4.4 years).
3. If progression occurs there is a one in two chance of it occurring in an already damaged hemi field and a one in four chance of it occurring in a previously normal hemi field.
4. If progression occurs there is a 60% chance of further progression occurring during the mean 10.5 year follow-up period.

DISCUSSION

A longitudinal all be it retrospective study such as this goes some way towards outlining the natural history of visual field loss in Low Tension Glaucoma. It should be noted that the patients included in this study had intraocular pressures of ≤ 21 mm Hg off all treatment during a 24 hour period of phasing together with visual field defect in at least one eye. These patients may have tried topical anti-glaucoma therapy at some stage during their follow-up period but it was not persisted with because it had no effect on the intraocular pressure. Any patients originally diagnosed as suffering from Low Tension Glaucoma who subsequently showed an elevation of intraocular pressure exceeding 21 mm Hg were not included in this study.

The visual fields were analysed using a single 1–4 isopter on a kinetic Goldmann field. Incomplete information on the visual field state would have been analysed but the isopter was common to all the fields included. In a retrospective study not all observations could have been made regularly however the patients were seen in a Low Tension Glaucoma follow-up clinic and as such had on average 1.5 visual fields per year.

The data presented shows that it is possible to divide the visual field into upper and lower halves. It would appear that the two halves behave independently for progression of a visual field defect is more likely to occur in a hemi field already abnormal rather than to develop de novo in a previously normal hemi field. Progression of the visual field defect did not seem to be associated with a relative pressure spike on a recurring basis.

Long term follow-up shows that the visual field may remain 'static' for (mean 4.4) years.

This means that the effects of (surgical) treatment should be treated with caution. If however progression is documented then there seems to be a 60% chance of more than one episode of progression occurring. With these previsors it would appear reasonable to offer treatment designed to limit further progression in such eyes.

The treatment required to limit further progression of visual field loss would appear to be limited to insuring optimum perfusion pressure at the optic nerve head either by attending to the patients general health and/or by lowering intraocular pressure. The latter may require fistulising surgery.

ACKNOWLEDGEMENT

We would like to thank Mrs. Kay Mills for typing the manuscript.

REFERENCES

1. Chumbley, L.C. and Brubaker, R.F. Low Tension Glaucoma. Amer. J. Ophth. 81: 761–765 (1976).
2. Levene, R.Z. Low Tension Glaucoma; a critical review and new material. Survey Ophth. 24: 621–664 (1980).

THE MODE OF PROGRESSION OF VISUAL FIELD DEFECTS IN GLAUCOMA

FREDERICK S. MIKELBERG and STEPHEN M. DRANCE

(*Vancouver, Canada*)

ABSTRACT

In order to study the pattern of progression of visual field defects in glaucoma we performed a retrospective study of 48 eyes of 48 patients with glaucoma. In those eyes showing progression the scotomas became denser in 79% whereas enlargement occured in 52% and 50% developed new scotomas. 63% of eyes maintained a defective single hemifield during the entire follow up. Patients with a longer follow up were more likely to show progression while age and mean or maximum IOP were not related to progression or non progression.

INTRODUCTION

The classical visual field defects seen in patients with glaucoma have been well documented (1). The mode of progression of glaucomatous field defects has attracted little attention. Hart and Becker published the only large quantitative study to look at the evolution of field defects in glaucoma (2). They have shown progression in 73% of glaucoma eyes with 10 years of follow up. 22% of eyes with initial single hemifield involvement involved both hemifields by the end of 10 years. The mean IOP was not related to the final extent of the visual field defects.

Holmin and Krakau described the rate of progression of field loss in glaucoma patients using a P value of overall retinal sensitivity obtained on the Competer perimeter but they did not address the mode of progression of individual scotomas (3, 4). No relationship between mean IOP and rate of loss of visual field function or differential threshold was found.

We performed a retrospective study in an attempt to determine the following points: How do glaucomatous visual field defects progress? What proportion of eyes with visual field defects develop new defects in a previously unaffected hemifield? What is the relationship of age, duration of follow up and IOP to progression of visual field defects?

Heijl, A. and Greve, E.L. (eds.), Proceedings of the 6th Int. Visual Field Symposium.
© 1985, Dr W. Junk Publishers, Dordrecht, The Netherlands. ISBN 978-94-010-8932-6

METHODS

The charts of glaucoma patients in whom a computerized record was available were reviewed. Only chronic open angle glaucoma patients were selected for analysis. To qualify for study they had to have paracentral or arcuate defects within the central 30 degrees and two or more years of follow up after the development of field defects. The fields were recorded by kinetic and static visual field measurements on the Tubinger perimeter since such field records are large enough to be easily planimetrized. The initial visual acuity had to be 6/9 or better and final acuity of 6/12 or better.

All the visual field records were measured using planimetry with a MOP video plan to determine the area of the scotomas within the central 30 degrees, the area of the central and peripheral isopters, the area under the static profile curve as well as the areas of the scotomas measured on the static profile. The foveal sensitivity was recorded.

Visual field progression occurred when a scotoma increased in area or depth, or a fresh scotoma developed. The size of scotomas were divided into four categories: $25-250 \text{ mm}^2$, $351-1000 \text{ mm}^2$, greater than 1000 mm^2 and finally a peripheral breakthrough. A scotoma was judged to have increased in area if it changed category and had also at least doubled its initial area.

The depth of scotomas was divided into three groups: shallow — 32 apostilbs or less, moderate — 64 to 640 apostilbs, or dense — 1000 apostilbs as measured on the Tubinger perimeter with a ten minute target. An increase in scotoma depth meant a change in category or an increase in area of an existing nucleus within the existing outer boundaries of the already present scotoma. All but two of the scotomas defined as having increased in depth had deepened by at least one log unit.

A new scotoma was deemed to have developed if it was not present initially and was present at the last follow up visit.

RESULTS

48 eyes of 48 patients comprising 28 males and 20 females were available for analysis. The age at development of scotomas ranged from 35 to 84 years with a mean of 61.5 ± 9.0 years and a median of 62.0 years. The duration of follow up ranged from 2 to 15 years with a mean of 8.0 ± 3.5 years and a median of 7.5 years.

Although our study was not designed to determine the frequency of progression in patients with glaucoma we found that 42 (87.5%) of eyes progressed, 5 (10.4%) were stable and 1 (2.1%) improved. The patterns of progression of the 42 eyes showed that 79% developed denser scotomas, 52% developed enlargement of scotomas and 50% developed new scotomas (Table 1).

Of the 48 eyes of 48 patients, 35 started with single hemifield involvement and 13 started with both hemifields involved. Of the 35 with initial single hemifield involvement 25 affected the superior field and 10 affected the inferior hemifield. At the completion of follow up 22 (63%) still had

Table 1. Mode of progression of field defects.

Denser, Larger, New Scotoma	11	26%
Denser only	10	24%
Denser, Larger	8	19%
New Scotoma only	6	14%
Denser, New Scotoma	4	9%
Larger only	3	7%

Table 2. Relationship of follow up duration and intraocular pressure to progression or non-progression of visual field defects in patients with glaucoma.

	Years of follow up		IOP mm Hg	
	Mean ± S.D.	Median	Mean ± S.D.	Max ± S.D.
Non-Progression	6.2 ± 2.7	6.1	19.2 ± 3.2	25.7 ± 5.3
Progression	8.2 ± 3.6	8.0	18.9 ± 2.7	27.7 ± 8.3
	p > 0.05		N.S.	N.S.
No New Scotoma	6.5 ± 2.5	6.7	18.6 ± 2.2	28.9 ± 8.4
New Scotoma	9.9 ± 3.7	10.3	19.2 ± 3.1	26.5 ± 8.1
	p = 0.001		N.S.	N.S.
Single Hemifield	7.5 ± 3.4	7.1	18.7 ± 2.3	27.0 ± 7.7
Both Hemifields	9.2 ± 3.8	10.1	20.1 ± 3.5	27.5 ± 9.9
	p > 0.05		N.S.	N.S.

N.S. = No statistically significant difference.

only single hemifield involvement whereas 13 (37%) had both hemifields involved.

The age at the time of the development of a scotoma was not statistically significantly different in the group who progressed.

The length of available follow up was related to the chance of development of fresh scotomas but did not achieve statistical significance when related to progresssion of visual field damage or to the change to involvement of the other hemifield (Table 2).

No relationship between the mean IOP or the maximum recorded IOP and progression could be established (Table 2).

DISCUSSION

We have looked at the progression of established field defects in patients with glaucoma. 79% of visual fields that progress show an increase in scotoma depth, whereas in 52% the area of the scotoma increases and 50% develop new scotomas. These patterns of progression indicate that in monitoring patients with glaucoma it is essential to quantify scotoma depth in addition to careful delineation of the area of a scotoma. Unaffected areas of the visual field must be fully examined to search for the development of new scotomas.

63% of patients with single hemifield involvement initially remain so over the duration of the follow up. The longer the follow up duration the more likely the patient is to show progression.

In this study, progression or non progression did not appear to relate to either the mean IOP or the maximum recorded IOP over the duration of the follow up. This is not meant to imply that control of IOP is unimportant in the management of patients with glaucoma. There are some possible explanations for this finding and some of them are inherent in a retrospective study. Patients showing progression of their field loss may have had more vigorous treatment of their IOP; the effect of different drugs was not evaluated; there may have been a selection bias due to the referral nature of the practise from which the patients were drawn.

Nevertheless this unexpected finding is consistent with the results reported by Hart and Becker (2) who found no relationship between the final extent of visual field loss and mean IOP in their patients with established glaucoma. Holmin and Krakau (3–4) found no relationship between IOP and the rate of loss of overall retinal sensitivity in patients with glaucoma. Careful study of the relationship of IOP to progressive damage is warranted. We will be reporting the relationships of the rates of progression of visual field damage to IOP separately.

The implications for perimetry of field defects in glaucoma are that threshold information of disturbed points in a scotoma or its quantification with kinetic perimetry are necessary if the commonest mode of progression, which indicates deterioration of the disease is going to be detected.

REFERENCES

1. Drance, S.M. The Early Field Defects in Glaucoma. Invest. Ophthalmol., 9: 84–91 (1969).
2. Hart, W.M. Jr. and Becker, B. The Onset and Evolution of Glaucomatous Visual Field Defects. Ophthalmol., 89: 268–279 (1982).
3. Holmin, C. and Krakau, C.E.T. Visual Field Decay in Normal Subjects and in Cases of Chronic Glaucoma. Albrech V. Graefes Arch., Klin. Exp. Ophthalmol., 213: 291–298 (1980).
4. Holmin, C. and Krakau, C.E.T. Regression Analysis of the Central Visual Field in Chronic Glaucoma Cases. Acta. Ophthalmol., 60: 267–274 (1982).

Author's address:
Frederik S. Mikelberg,
Department of Ophthalmology,
University of British Columbia,
Vancouver, Canada

THE GLAUCOMATOUS VISUAL FIELD IN DETAIL AS REVEALED BY THE OCTOPUS F-PROGRAMS

J. STÜRMER, B. GLOOR and H.J. TOBLER

(*Basle, Switzerland*)

ABSTRACT

Meridional profile perimetry was performed in the central field of 20 patients with chronic simple glaucoma and mild to severe field loss. 229 F_2-programs consisting of 30° long profiles with 1° resolution and double measurements of light sensitivity threshold were analyzed. Additionally selected areas of the field of one patient were examined over $1\frac{1}{2}$ years with F_4-programs (threshold measurements four times at one point).

There is a strong correlation between mean loss and mean short term fluctuations: short-term fluctuations tend to be larger with increasing loss of sensitivity. Analysis of the F_2-programs showed 12 different patterns of disturbance. The most frequent found 'increased scatter with normal sensitivity' appears to be the earliest perimetric sign of glaucoma. Progression of the glaucomatous damage produces the so-called relative scotoma, which is rather a grey area of increased scatter with a poorly defined lower and upper threshold.

The data show why it is so difficult, if not impossible, to define progression of field loss over a relatively short period of time in patients with established glaucoma, despite repeated examinations. Only long-terms follow-up over years will establish a definite trend in a single patient.

INTRODUCTION

Long-term fluctuations as well as a grid which is too coarse may hide visual field defects. Therefore we addressed ourselves to the question to what extent concealed features of glaucomatous fields could be revealed by making use of the program with the finest grids offered by the Octopus 201, the so-called F-programs.

PATIENTS AND METHODS

Out of 500 patients who had already been examined with Octopus perimetry because they either were glaucoma suspects or had glaucoma, 20 patients (10

Heijl, A. and Greve, E.L. (eds.), Proceedings of the 6th Int. Visual Field Symposium.
© *1985, Dr W. Junk Publishers, Dordrecht, The Netherlands. ISBN 978-94-010-8932-6*

men and 10 women; mean age = 65.1 ± 8.8 years; median = 66 years) were chosen for this study. They had to fulfill the following criteria: willingness and ability for good collaboration, established chronic simple glaucoma with mild to severe visual field loss documented with the combination of Octopus programs 31 and 32 at least once. If the field loss was mild, it had to be present at least once. The patient also had to show an open angle, intraocular pressure above 22 mm Hg without therapy, cup/disc-ratio of ≥ 0.5, visual acuity ≥ 0.7 with optimal correction, ametropia ≤ ± 3.0 Dpt., pupil ≥ 2 mm, good fixation, no eye surgery in the past, no cataract.

In all these patients except one only 1 eye was examined.

The central visual field was tested with the Octopus programs 31 and 32. The mean of the total loss of differential light sensitivity threshold ('sensitivity') was determined with program Delta 'change' to provide a criterion dividing the eyes into 3 groups:

group 1: 6 eyes, no sensitivity loss in the actual 31 and 32 programs or not more than 10 dB in one single point

group 2: 7 eyes, total loss of sensitivity between 20 and 200 dB

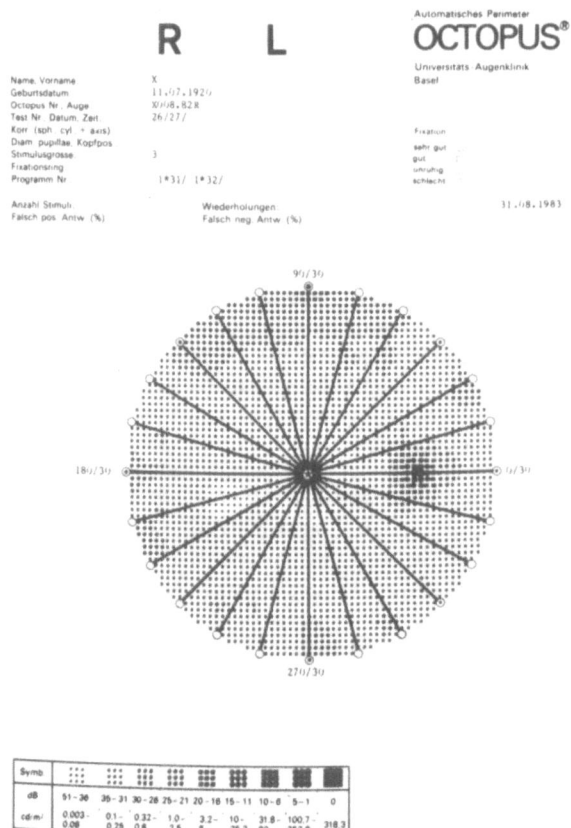

Fig. 1. Topography of the profiles for the F_2-programs.

group 3: 8 eyes, total loss of sensitivity between 201 and 900 dB

After classification of these eyes into groups, their central visual fields were investigated with F_2 programs consisting of 30° long profiles, 1° resolution, test object III (0.43°), angle between the meridians 15°. Figure 1 shows the arrangement of the profiles in the 30° field. Because it takes 12 hours to perform 24 such F_2 profiles, only 4 patients performed the whole test program. In the other 16 the sector with the largest loss of sensitivity was tested (at least 1 quadrant). This resulted in 229 F_2 profiles in which numerous parameters were evaluated. In this abbreviated communication only the following 2 parameters are considered:
- weighted fluctuations (RMS fluctuations) defined according to Bebie and Fankhauser (2) as

$$\sigma^2 = \frac{1}{\Sigma(n_i - 1)} \cdot \Sigma (n_i - 1) \cdot \sigma_i^2$$

- aspect and frequency of the deviations of sensitivity and fluctuations from the norm ('deformations')

In one extremely cooperative patient (50 years old male) selected areas of the field were investigated repeatedly with F_4-programs over a period of $1\frac{1}{2}$ years (length of profile 10°, resolution 0.5°, test object 0.43°, light sensitivity threshold determinations 4 times at one point) to get precise information on short- and long-term fluctuations in an area of so-called relative scotoma.

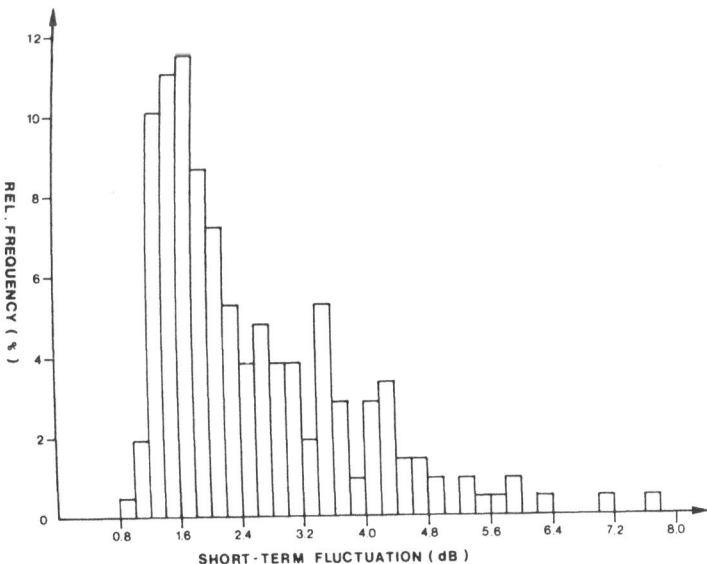

Fig. 2. Relative frequency distributions of RMS fluctuations in all of the 229 F_2-programs.

RESULTS

Figure 2 shows a frequency distribution of RMS fluctuations in all of the 229 F_2-tests. The frequency maximum is at 1.7 dB, the mean is 2.6 dB ± 1.24, the minimum 1.0 dB, the maximum 7.8 dB.

As Fig. 3 shows, there is good correlation (r = 0.83) of RMS fluctuations as revealed in the F_2 profiles on the x-axis and log mean loss as revealed by programs 31 and 32 on the y-axis with the cubic equation $y = -7.50 + 7.04x - 1.68x^2 + 0.14x^3$. This high correlation is confirmed in the histograms of Fig. 4, in which the relative frequencies are shown in the different sub-groups of patients with almost no field loss in the first, loss of 20–200 in the second, and loss of 201–900 dB in the third group. The more disturbed the visual field is, the more frequent are elevated RMS fluctuations.

If the 30° long profiles are divided into 10° sections and if all the normal sections with a mean RMS fluctuation of 1.18 dB are excluded, 12 different types of deviation from normal can be found. The most frequent deviation (30%) from normal is an increased fluctuation in regions of normal sensitivity (Fig. 5). The second most frequent deviation is absolute scotoma (Fig. 6). The 2 third most frequent deviations (11% each) are normal RMS fluctuations in an area of reduced sensitivity adjacent to increased fluctuations in an area of reduced sensitivity in a profile section of 10° (Fig. 7) and, as shown in Fig. 8, normal RMS fluctuation with normal sensitivity adjacent to decreased sensitivity and increased RMS fluctuation.

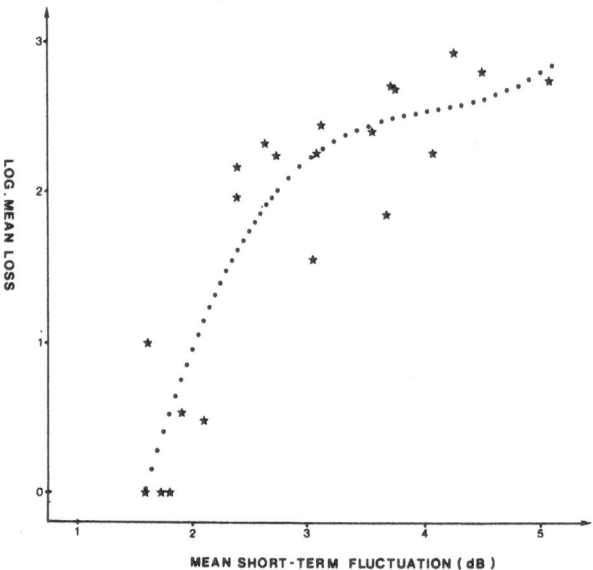

Fig. 3. Correlation between RMS fluctuation (x-axis) and log mean loss, as revealed with programs 31 and 32 (y-axis). Good correlation (r = 0.83) with the equation $y = -7.5 + 7.04x - 1.68x^2 + 0.14x^3$. (Each * is a patient).

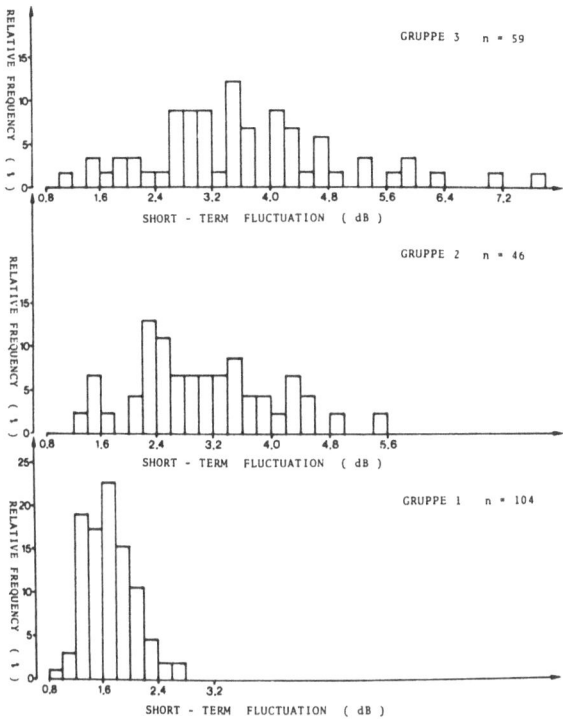

Fig. 4. Relative frequency distribution of RMS fluctuations of the F_2-programs in the 3 groups with different amount of field loss (below group 1: no loss of sensitivity, in the middle group 2 with $20 - 200$ dB loss and above group 3 with $201-900$ dB loss).

F_4-*programs*: From the multiple F_4 programs performed at 5 different dates over a period of $1\frac{1}{2}$ years, the $10°$ long profile passing above the blind spot $12°$ away from the horizontal meridian is chosen. If Fig. 9 the results of the 5 consecutive examinations are shown. Note that the relative scotoma has no clearly defined threshold, but is an area of more or less increased fluctuation. The surface area is largest in the examinations of November 1982 and November 1983. The worst patient performance was found in November 1983 thereafter an increase of the mean sensitivity can be seen again.

In fig. 10 the total sensitivity reached during each test run through one profile (F_1, F_2, F_3, F_4.) of the five examinations performed at different dates are shown. The number of stimuli necessary for all four test runs at each examination, the false positive, the false negative answers, the value of RMS fluctuations, and the intraocular pressure at the date of examination are also shown. There is no spectacular change of sensitivity from the first to the fourth test run at the examinations 4 and 5 (in February and in April 1984) when the sensitivity threshold was fairly high, but there is a rather

395

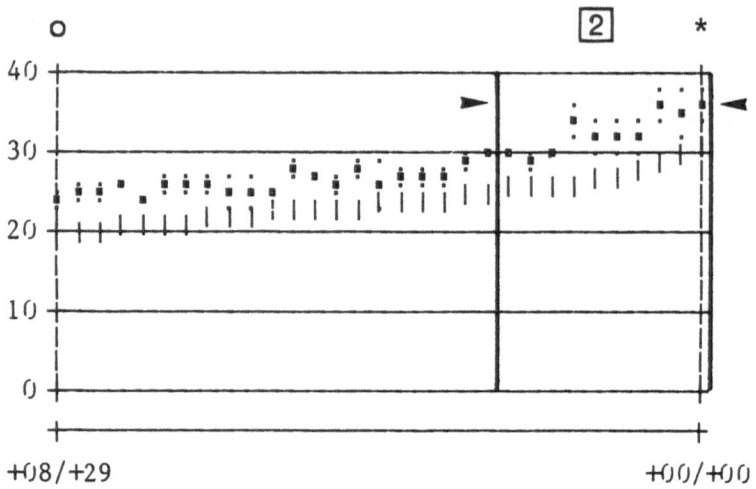

Fig. 5. The most frequent deviation from the norm (30%) was the increased RMS fluctuation in a region of normal sensitivity as here in the central 10° of the profile.

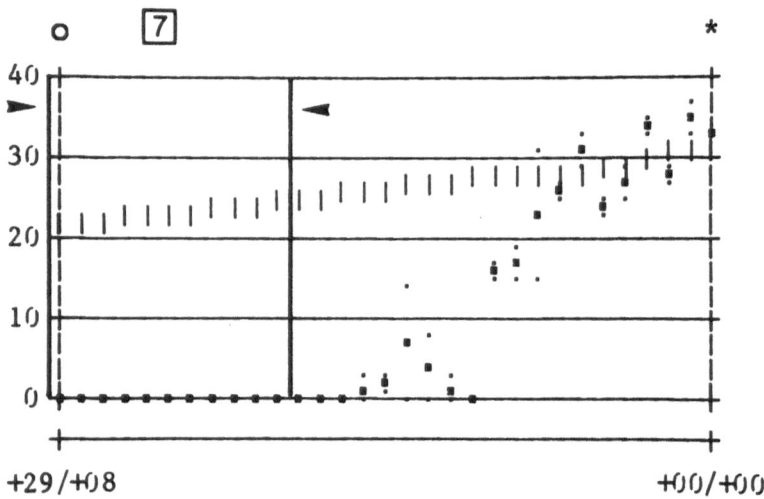

Fig. 6. The second frequent deviation from the norm (17%) was the absolute scotoma as shown here in the peripheral section of the 30° profile.

strong impression, that there is an effect of fatigue at the other dates (examination 1, 2 and 3) when the sensitivity threshold was low. There is a high linear correlation between mean sensitivity of the 4 test runs in one examination and the number of stimuli necessary for threshold determination (Fig. 11).

396

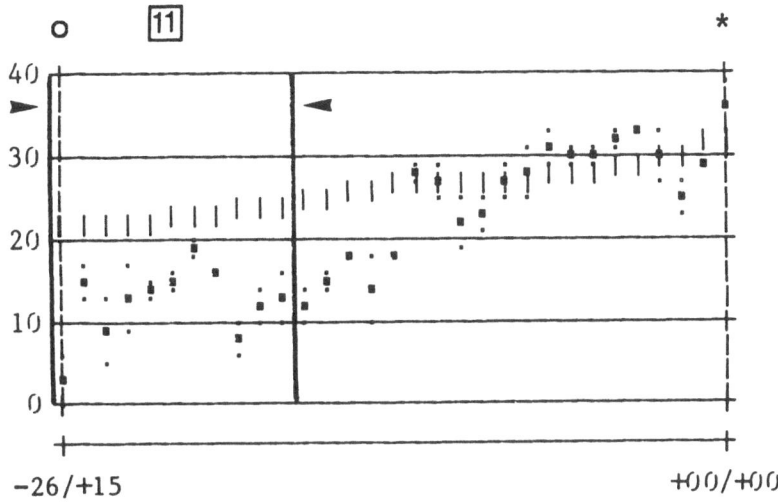

Fig. 7. Eleven percent showed normal fluctuation adjacent to increased fluctuations in zones of reduced sensitivity.

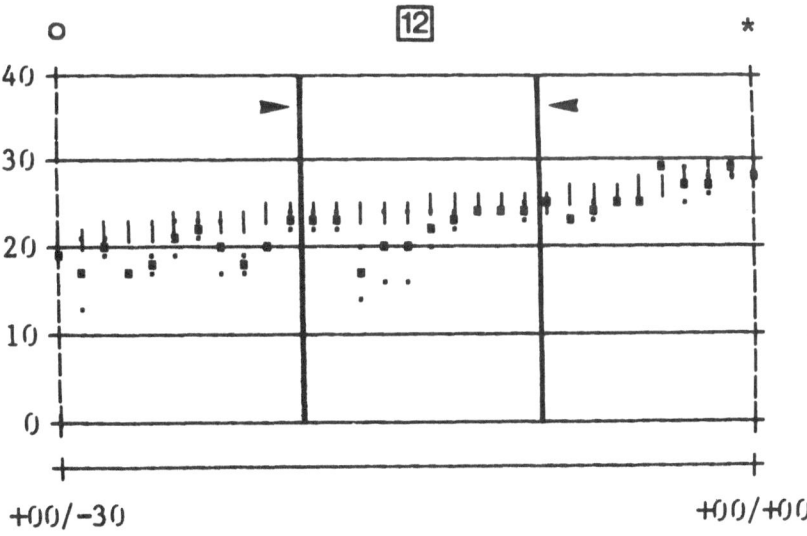

Fig. 8. Eleven percent showed normal fluctuation in zones of normal sensitivity adjacent to increased fluctuations in zones of decreased sensitivity. Note that the profile diameter of this disturbance is not more than 5°.

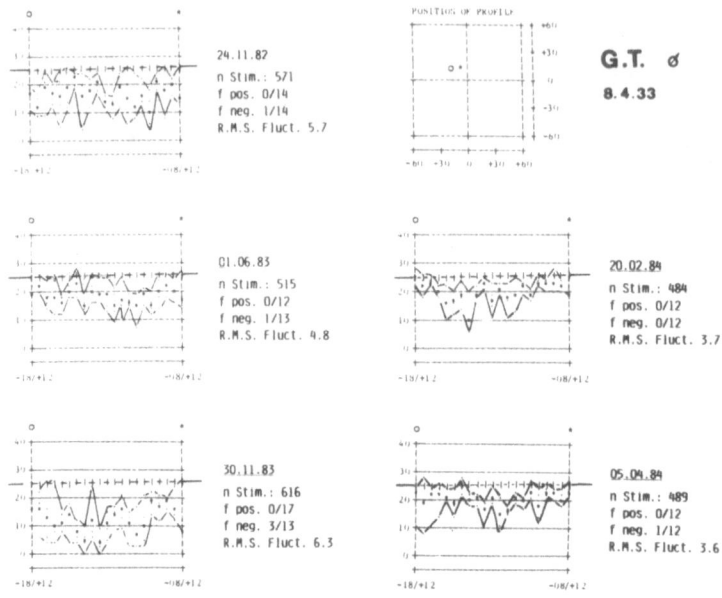

Fig. 9. F_4-programs: determination of the profile 4 time in a row. The localisation of the profile is shown in the right upper corner of the figure. Five examinations have been performed from 1982–1984. RMS fluctuations are highest when the mean sensitivity is the worst. The threshold became depressed from the first to the third examination and then again increased.

TOTAL SENSITIVITY IN ONE PROFILE IN FOUR CONSEQUENT EXAMINATIONS ($F_1 - F_4$)

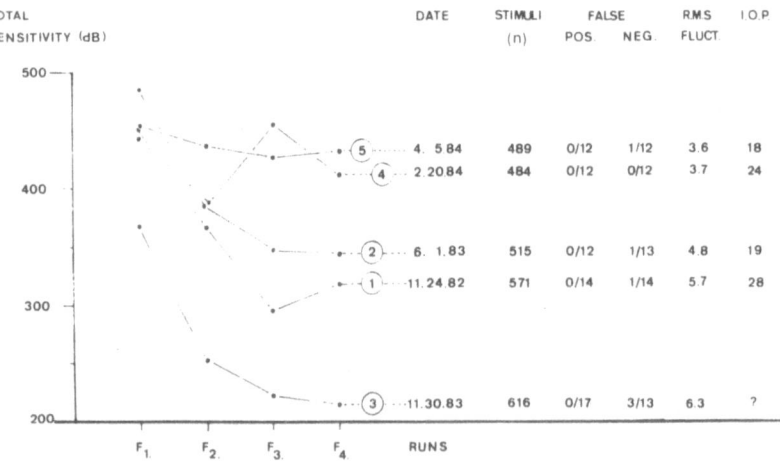

Fig. 10. Performance of whole sensitivity changes from one test run to the other. These changes are highest in examinations 3, 1 and 2 and lowest in examinations 4 and 5.

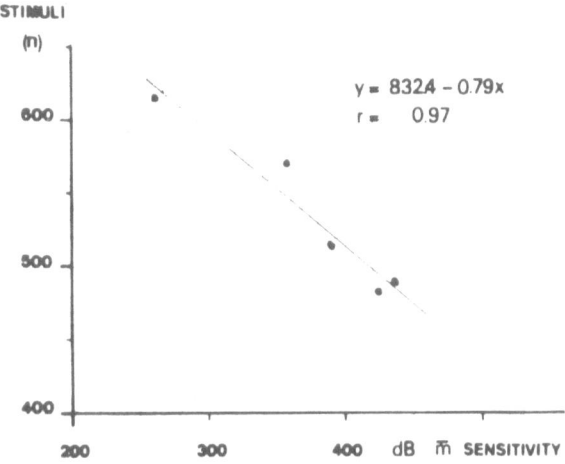

Fig. 11. There is a good linear correlation between mean sensitivity and the number of stimuli which had to be presented for threshold determination.

DISCUSSION

The data presented here confirm recent reports, that increased fluctuations of differential light sensitivity threshold may be the earliest findings of glaucomatous damage (7, 8, 15, 17). There is a considerable overlap between normal and pathological (16), but RMS fluctuations over 2.5 dB are highly suspicious (16). Because Rabineau et al. (16) found the highest fluctuations in the central 10° circle, this area needs further investigation. But even if there is a clear mathematical correlation between mean short-term fluctuations and log mean loss, this is not obligatory for each area of field disturbance. Decreased sensitivity may be present without increased RMS fluctuation (as can normal threshold with increased fluctuations), at least as long as the threshold is determined only twice. Disturbed areas in one profile can be very small e.g. 4—5° in diameter. This demonstrates how easy such zones may escape detection if we look for glaucomatous changes with a relatively coarse grid.

Because short-term fluctuations are a characteristic finding of glaucomatous fields, to a smaller amount in areas with normal threshold, and to a much larger amount in disturbed areas, we can now explain, why we are confronted with such a tremendous amount of long-term fluctuations as present earlier (7—11).

In the F_4-programs the chosen profile is tested four times in sequence (F_1, F_2, F_3, F_4.). Therefore discrimination between local scatter, which is fatigue-dependent, and local scatter which is fatigue- (and time-) independent, seems to be possible that the following questions can be answered satisfactorily:

1. Are the sensitivities determined in the first half of the F_4-program (F_1 and F_2) in the 5 examinations statistically different from those in the second half (F_3, F_4 and F_5)? — Yes, they are ($p = 0.048$; Wilcoxon-Mann-Whitney-U-Test).
2. Is one of the 4 test runs (Fig. 10) statistically worse or better than the others? — F_1 is better than either F_2 ($p = 0.038$) or F_4 ($p = 0.0143$).
3. Is the performance in one of the 4 test runs (F_1 or F_2 or F_3 or F_4) statistically better than one immediately adjacent? F_1 is better than F_2, but there is no difference between F_2 and F_3 and between F_3 and F_4.
4. Is there a difference between the results of examinations no. 4 and 5 and the group of examinations no. 1, 2 and 3? — Yes, this difference is highly significant ($p = 0.0044$).

The statistically significant difference between the performance in the first and in the second half may indicate that fatigue plays a role. But fatigue can not explain the whole thing because from one run to the next there is a significant difference between first and second run, but not between second and third and third and fourth run. Because there is a significant difference between the two groups of examination four and five and the examinations one, two and three, it seems reasonable to state, that fatigue becomes more and more a critical factor as the sensitivity is decreased, and this would be in good agreement with Heijl and Drance (14). But even so we have to be careful: this fatigue effect may be enhanced through the fact, that the more the threshold is lowered the larger the scatter is, the more stimuli have to be presented for threshold determination using the F_4 program. Today we have no means to determine whether most of the stimuli are lost in the first (F_1) or in the last (F_4) test run of the F_4-program, even if we know that for the first test run the program starts from normal values and in the subsequent runs restarts from that which was determined in the previous run.

In summary, differential light sensitivity is one of the simplest retinal functions that may be investigated, much simpler than contrast sensitivity or visual acuity as tested with letters or numbers. Nevertheless, the details we have to consider in evaluation the influences on this differential light sensitivity threshold in glaucoma is still a hard nut to crack. However, we hope that bringing these details to light will finally enable us to work out a glaucoma program, which does not only look for defect, but takes other parameters, such as RMS fluctuations, the topography of the most affected areas (13) and the effect of fatigue into consideration. Even so, a visual field can not be the only parameter by which we evaluate the situation of a patient with glaucoma or a so-called glaucoma suspect; measurement of (state) the neuroretinal rim and the intraocular pressure are at least as important (1, 3–6, 11, 12).

REFERENCES

1. Balasi, A.G., Drance, S.M.., Schulzer, M. and Douglas, G.R. The area of the neuro-retinal rim in glaucoma suspects and early chronic open-angle glaucoma. Arch. Ophthalmol. (in print).

2. Bebie, H., Fankhauser, F. and Spahr, J. Statistic perimetry: Accuracy and fluctuations. Acta Ophthalmol. 54: 339–348 (1979).
3. Betz, Ph., Camps, F., Collignon-Brach, C., Lavergne, G. and Weekers, R. Biometry study of the disc cup in open angle glaucoma. Albrecht v. Graefe's Arch. Klin. exp. Ophthalmol. 218: 70–74 (1982).
4. Betz, Ph., Camps, F., Collignon-Brach, C. and Weekers, R. Photographie stéréoscopique et photogrammétrie de l'excavation physiologique de la papille. J. Fr. Ophthalmol. 4: 193–203 (1981).
5. Dimitrakos, S.A., Fey, U., Gloor, B. and Jäggi, P. Correlation or Non-correlation between glaucomatous field loss as determined by automated perimetry and changes in the surface of the optic disc? In E. Greve and W. Leytheckes, ed. The Second symposium of the European Glaucoma Society, Hyomkia 1984 (in print).
6. Drance, S.M. and Balaszi, A.G. Die neuroretinale Randzone. Klin. Mbl. Augenheilk. 184: 271–273 (1984).
7. Flammer, J., Drance, S.M. and Zulauf, M. The short- and long-term fluctuation of the differential light threshold in patients with glaucoma, normal controls and glaucoma suspects. Arch. Ophthalmol. (in print).
8. Flammer, J., Drance, S.M., Fankhauser, F. and Augustiny, L. The differential light threshold in automated static perimetry. Arch. Ophthalmol. (in print).
9. Gloor, B. Die Computerperimetrie in der langfristigen Beurteilung des Glaukoms. Krieglstein, G.K., Leydhecker, W. Medikamentöse Glaukomtherapie. J.F. Bergmann Verlag München. 59–72 (1982).
10. Gloor, B. and Vökt, B. Long-term fluctuations versus definite field loss in glaucoma patients. ARVO suppl. to Investigative Ophthalmol. and Visual Science Vol. 24 No. 3: 103 (1983).
11. Gloor, B., Stürmer, J. and Vökt, B. Was hat die automatisierte Perimetrie mit dem Octopus für neue Kenntnisse über glaukomatöse Gesichtsfeldveränderungen gebracht? Klin. Mbl. Augenheilk. 184: 249–253 (1984).
12. Gloor, B., Jäggi, P. and Stürmer, J. Wo steht die Perimetrie im Verlaufe des Glaukoms? Bücherei des Augenarztes (in print).
13. Gramer, E., Gerlach, R. Krieglstein, G.K. and Leydhecker, W. Zur Topographie früher glaukomatöser Gesichtsfeldausfälle bei der Computerperimetrie. Klin. Mbl. Augenheilk. 180: 515–523 (1982).
14. Heijl, A. and Drance, S.M. Changes in differential threshold in patients with glaucoma during prolonged perimetry. British Journal of Ophthalmol. 67: 512–516 (1983).
15. Langerhorst, C.T., van den Berg, T.J.T.P. and Greve, E.L. Schätzung der verschiedenen Fluktuationsfaktoren bei der Computerperimetrie von Glaukompatienten. Neuere Entwicklungen in der Ophthalmologie. ed. Merté, H.J. und Mertz, M. Beihefte Klin. Mbl. Augenheilk. (in print).
16. Rabineau, P.A., Gloor, B.P. and Tobler, H.J. Fluctuations in threshold and effect on fatigue in automated static perimetry (with the Octopus 201). Documenta Ophthalmol. Proc. Series.
17. Stürmer, J., Gloor, B. and Tobler, H.J. Wie sehen Glaukomgesichtsfelder wirklich aus? Klin. Mbl. Augenheilk. 184: 390–393 (1984).

Author's address:
J. Stürmer,
Department of Ophthalmology,
University of Basle,
Switzerland

PERIPAPILLARY ATROPHY AND GLAUCOMATOUS VISUAL FIELD DEFECTS

ANDERS HEIJL and CHRISTIAN SAMANDER

(*Malmö, Sweden*)

ABSTRACT

It has been suggested that the conformation of the peripapillary tissues helps determine which portion of the disc and field will be affected by glaucomatous damage (1). We studied 62 consecutive glaucomatous field loss. There was a statistically highly significant correlation between the location of the widest peripapillary atrophy and the direction of the field defect. Thus it was more common that eyes showed field defects in the opposite direction of the peripapillary atrophy than in the same direction. The results were the same if only pigmented or both pigmented and non-pigmented atrophies were taken into consideration, and also if all or only larger atrophies were analyzed. Further studies are necessary to explain this correlation.

Peripapillary atrophy and peripapillary haloes are associated with glaucoma (e.g. 3, 5). At the 1982 IPS meeting in Sacramento to Dr Douglas R. Anderson suggested 'that the conformation of peripapillary tissues help determine how susceptible a particular disc is to pressure-induced damage, and also which portion of the disc (and field) will be most affected' (1).

We decided to study, in a quantitative way, whether there was any correlation between the location of peripapillary changes and the location of visual field defects in eyes with glaucoma.

METHODS

A large number of consecutive fields, stored on floppy discs, and tested with the Competer computerized perimeter at the glaucoma out-patient department in Malmö were printed out and reviewed. Fields showing unidirectional field loss (i.e. fields with damage occurring in only the superior or the inferior, but not in both, halves of the field) were selected. The corresponding patient records were studied. There were 62 eyes with an unquestionable diagnosis of glaucoma and unidirectional field loss, where (monocular) disc photographs had been obtained within a few months of the field test.

The disc photographs from these eyes were projected and the peripapillary atrophy was measured in six sectors around the disc circumference (from 1 to 3 o'clock, from 3 to 5 etcetera). The width of the maximum peripapillary

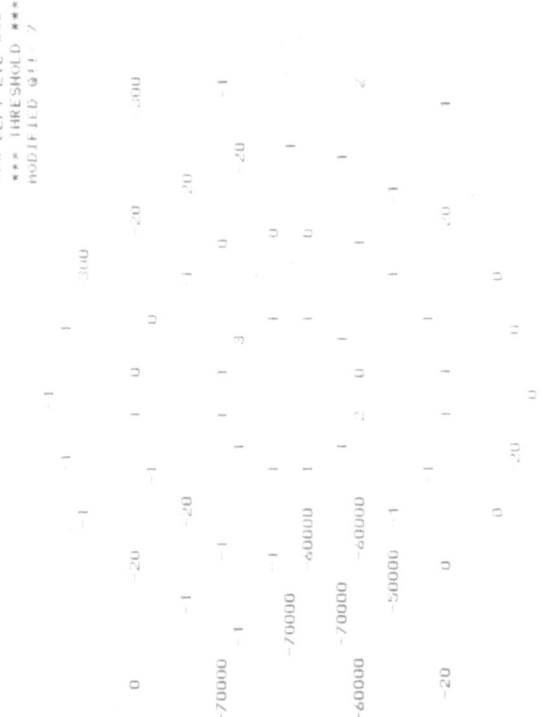

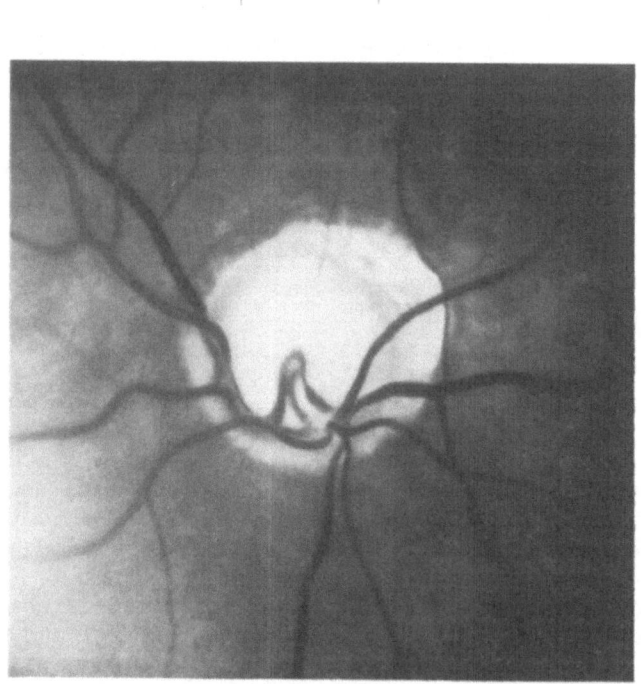

Fig. 1. The disk photograph and Competer field chart of one of the studied eyes. The peripapillary atrophy is widest at the inferior temporal margin of the disk. The field chart shows a shallow defect in the superior nasal area.

atrophy within each sector was measured with a ruler, perpendicularly to the disk margin. The mm measurements were converted into disc diameters (DD). All imperfections in the alignment of the peripapillary tissues and the disc leading to a white or pigmented peripapillary crescent or halo with a width = > 0.05 DD were defined as peripapillary atrophy. Originally we had planned to distinguish between peripapillary atrophies and peripapillary haloes, but we found it extremely difficult to maintain an objective separation between haloes and other nonpigmented peripapillary changes covering a large part of the disc circumference, and we therefore had to abandon the effort to make such a distinction. It is almost impossible to distinguish between all the various possible misalignments of the retina, pigment epithelium and the choroid at the disc margin. Even determining the exact borders of the disk and the peripapillary changes can often be difficult. However, a separation between peripapillary nonpigmented changes and lesions with pigmentation can usually be maintained without too much subjectivity.

The assessment of the peripapillary changes was performed blindly, without access to the visual fields. We did not try to mask the disk, but we disregarded the conformation of the cupping.

Tables were made showing the width of the peripapillary atrophy in the various sectors. This was done taking into account:
1. All peripapillary atrophy.
2. Only atrophy with at least some pigmentation.
The fields were then inspected in order to determine whether the largest (widest) atrophy was present in the same (superior or inferior) direction as the field direction or in the opposite direction.

RESULTS

The results are shown in Table 1. Peripapillary atrophy is more common in the opposite direction of the field defects than in the same direction. This,

Table 1. Correlation between the location of peripapillary atrophy and the glaucomatous field defect. Atrophies grouped according to width (in disc diameters = DD).

Peripapillary changes	Number of eyes			
	All atrophy > 0.05 DD	Pigm. atrophy > 0.05 DD	Atrophy > 0.1 DD	Atrophy > 0.3 DD
Same direction as VFD	11	9	6	2
Opposite direction of VFD	47	47	31	14
Same width up and down	4	2	0	0
Atrophy below stipulated limit	0	4	25	46
Statistical significance (sign test)	$p < 0.001$	$p < 0.001$	$p < 0.001$	$p < 0.001$

of course means that the peripapillary changes predominantly occur in the same direction as the glaucomatous nerve fibre damage. This association is highly statistically significant, but exceptions are common. The results are the same whether all atrophy or only pigmented atrophy is taken into account.

DISCUSSION

It is remarkable that we have found some degree of atrophy to be present in all cases. Also Primrose found peripapillary changes to be very common in glaucoma (3). It is possible that we have been too generous when defining non-perfect alignments of peripapillary tissues as peripapillary atrophy. However, the clear correlation between the direction of the field defects and peripapillary changes remain even when milder forms of misalignments are disregarded (Table 1).

This correlation cannot be explained at this time. We do not even know whether the peripapillary changes precede the changes of the optic disc leading to the glaucomatous visual field loss, or whether the disc and the peripapillary tissues are damaged at the same time. The disk is often situated in watershed zones of the choroidal circulation (2). In glaucoma hypoperfusion both of the disk and of the adjacent peripapillary tissues can often be demonstrated with fluorescein angiography (4). A concurrent damage of the disc and the peripapillary tissues is logical. It should be possible to study the time course through retrospective inspection of disc photographs taken over long time periods in patients with ocular hypertension, who later developed glaucoma. If the peripapillary changes could be shown to precede the glaucomatous field loss, the presence of peripapillary atrophy could have a certain predictive value in glaucoma suspects — although, of course the changes in the disc and in the peripapillary tissues could have the same vascular etiology even if the damage started a few years earlier in one of the locations.

If Dr Anderson's observation that peripapillary changes seem to be more common in patients with low tension glaucoma than in patients with glaucoma and high pressures can be confirmed through controlled studies, his theory that the peripapillary configuration is a factor in determining whether a particular disc, or part of a disc, is susceptible to elevated pressure seems very plausible. This theory could be further supported if it could be shown that the peripapillary changes are present much earlier than any signs of glaucoma.

ACKNOWLEDGEMENT

This study was supported by the Järnhardt foundation.

REFERENCES

1. Anderson, D.R. Correlation of the peripapillary anatomy with the disc damage and field abnormalities in glaucoma. Documenta Ophthalmol. Proc. Series 35: 1–10 (1983).
2. Hayreh, S.S. Segmental nature of the choroidal vasculature. Brit. J. Ophthalmol. 59: 631–48 (1975).
3. Primrose, J. Early signs of the glaucomatous disc. Brit. J. Ophthalmol. 55: 820–825 (1971).
4. Raitta, C. and Sarmela, T. Fluorescein angiography of the optic disc and the peripapillary area in chronic glaucoma. Acta Ophthalmol. 48: 303–308 (1970).
5. Wilensky, J.T. and Kolker, A.E. Peripapillary changes in glaucoma. Amer. J. Ophthalmol. 81: 341–345 (1976).

Author's address:
Department of Ophthalmology
Malmö General Hospital
S-21401 Malmö
Sweden

RETINAL NERVE FIBRE LAYER AND VISUAL FIELD FUNCTIONS IN GLAUCOMA

P. JUHANI AIRAKSINEN, STEPHEN M. DRANCE and
MICHAEL SCHULZER

(*Vancouver, B.C., Canada*)

ABSTRACT

Semi-quantitative retinal nerve fibre layer (RNFL) scores given separately to diffuse and localized RNFL damage were correlated with visual field indices calculated from 49 thresholds of the Octopus program JO. The indices have been developed to differentiate between generalized reduction (mean damage) and localized disturbance (corrected loss variation) of the retinal sensitivity. RNFL damage scores and visual field indices correlated statistically highly significantly and approximately 50% of the variation of the indices could be accounted for by the RNFL abnormality. The best fit of data was achieved with a quadratic function, suggesting that there may be a latency between the appearance of structural changes and the disturbances of retinal sensitivity.

INTRODUCTION

Overall reduction of light sensitivity as manifested by a generalized contraction of isopters and baring of the blind spot in kinetic perimetry are well known in glaucoma. Such changes occur in depressions of the visual field induced also by many other states and are therefore non-specific and difficult to interpret and quantitate. Localized visual field defects have therefore been genrally accepted as the classical glaucomatous visual field defects.

New photographic techniques have made it possible to demonstrate structural changes in the retinal nerve fibre layer (RNFL) corresponding to the localised visual field defects (3, 9) and there are indications that RNFL photographs of glaucoma patients with various patterns of optic nerve head damage have shown that besides the localised RNFL defects generalized reduction of nerve fibres can also be detected (1, 5).

We undertook the present study in order to correlate the semiquantitative evaluation scores of diffuse and localized RNFL damage with some new visual field indices of the Octopus program JO (6) which, utilizing data reduction, are thought to be capable of differentiating between a diffuse reduction of light sensitivity and localized disturbances of the visual field (7).

Heijl, A. and Greve, E.L. (eds.), Proceedings of the 6th Int. Visual Field Symposium.
© *1985, Dr W. Junk Publishers, Dordrecht, The Netherlands. ISBN 978-94-010-8932-6*

MATERIAL AND METHODS

All the patients had a full clinical examination including monochromatic nerve fibre layer photography with a 60 degree wide-angle fundus camera. In addition black-and-white stereo photographs of the optic discs including large areas around the disc were obtained to have a more magnified, three dimensional view of the peripapillary retina. A detailed description of the peripapillary retina. A detailed description of the photographic methods has been given previously (4). Enlarged paper prints were made of all negatives with a 1:9 negative-to-print magnification. One eye of each patient was randomly selected for the study, the optic discs were masked and photographs of all patients were evaluated in random order with no knowledge of the clinical information. For RNFL evaluation the optic disc circumference was divided in 10 sectors (1) and in each sector a score from 0 to 4 was given separately for diffuse and localized RNFL damage. It was shown previously that reproducibility of this RNFL assessment is good (1). For statistical analyses the sum of the diffuse damage scores and localized damage scores were calculated as well as the sum of the two subtotals to give the total nerve fibre layer damage score.

Ten patients (7%) had to be excluded because of poor or missing photographs. The remaining 132 patients included 29 normals, 52 ocular hypertensives and 51 patients with glaucoma. The mean ages between groups were not statistically significantly different (Table 1).

All patients had their visual field examined with the Octopus perimeter using program JO (8). Using formulas presented by Flammer et al. (7) we calculated from the 49 measured thresholds the visual field indices namely the mean damage compared to Octopus normal values and the corrected loss variation.

Regression analyses of mean damage and corrected loss variation on diffuse, localized and total RNFL damage scores were carried out. In

Table 1. Distribution of patients into different clinical groups and the mean ages.

Group	No. of patients	Age (Yrs +/− SD)
Normal	29	54 +/− 16.9
Ocular hypertension	52	57 +/− 12.7
Glaucoma	51	62 +/− 20.5

Table 2. Regression of visual field indices on total retinal nerve fibre layer (RNFL) damage score.

	Mean damage index	Log corrected loss variation index
Correl. coeff.	0.67	0.74
R^2 (%)	44.7 (p = 0.0000)	55.2 (p = 0.0000)
Total RNFL damage score	0.19 (p = 0.0000)	0.049 (p = 0.0000)
(Total RNFL damage score)^2	0.0059 (p = 0.0119)	0.0019 (p = 0.0004)
Constant	1.38	0.90

410

addition, mean damage and corrected loss variation as dependent variables were correlated with diffuse and localized damage scores entered jointly into multiple regression analyses in order to examine the relative contribution of the two nerve fibre layer scores. The corrected loss variation values were not normally distributed and therefore a logarithmic transformation was used.

RESULTS

In the linear regression analysis both mean damage and corrected loss variation were statistically highly significantly correlated with total RNFL damage score. A quadratic function improved the fit of the data statistically significantly so that 44.7% and 55.2% of the variation of mean damage and corrected loss variation, respectively, were accounted for by the nerve fibre layer damage score (Table 2; Figs 1 and 2).

In the multiple regression of mean damage of the visual field on diffuse and localized nerve fibre layer scores the diffuse damage score accounted for twice as much of the correlation as the localized damage score which did not significantly add to the correlation. 42.6% of the variation of mean damage could be accounted for by loss of nerve fibres (Table 3).

Multiple regression of corrected loss variation on diffuse and localized nerve fibre layer damage scores showed that both were statistically significantly correlated with corrected loss variation index but in this instance the localized RNFL damage score provided 1.7 times as much information as the diffuse damage scores (Table 3). 51.4% of variation of the corrected loss variation values could be accounted for by the nerve fibre layer abnormality.

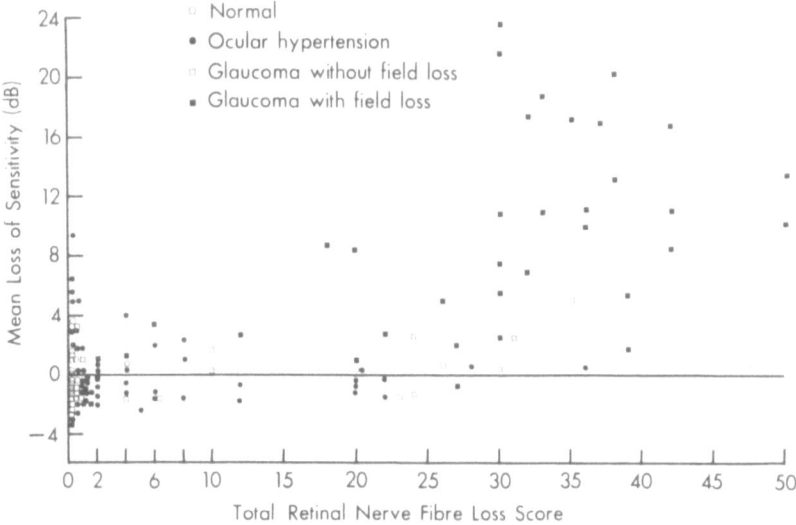

Fig. 1. A scattergram showing relationship between the total nerve fibre layer damage score and the mean damage index in 4 clinical groups.

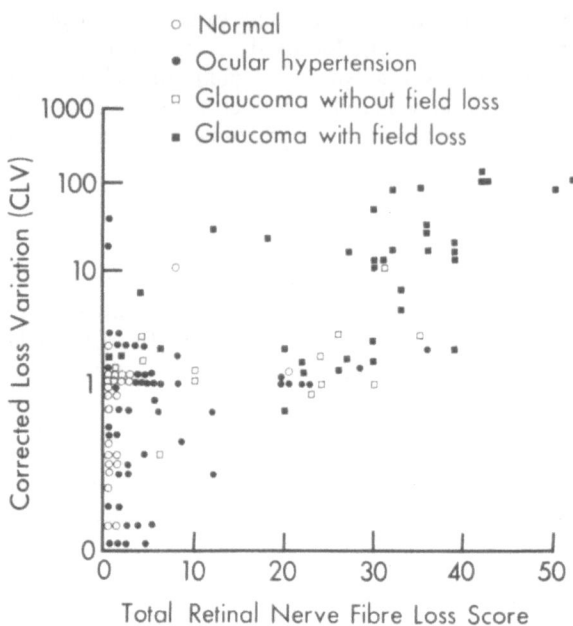

Fig. 2. A scattergram showing relationship between the total nerve fibre layer damage score and the log of corrected loss variation index in 4 clinical groups.

Table 3. Multiple regression of visual field indices on diffuse and localized nerve fibre layer damage score.

	Mean damage index	Log corrected loss variation index
Multiple correl. coeff.	0.65	0.72
R^2 (%)	42.6 (p = 0.0000)	51.4 (p = 0.0000)
Localized RNFL damage score	0.149 (p = 0.0864)	0.102 (p = 0.0000)
Diffuse RNFL damage score	0.281 (p = 0.0000)	0.064 (p = 0.0000)
Constant	−0.49	0.35

DISCUSSION

This study shows a statistically highly significant correlation between neural structure of the retina as observed with nerve fibre layer photographs and visual function measured with the new visual field indices calculated from the 49 thresholds of the Octopus program JO.

The index which expresses overall loss of retinal sensitivity was related to diffuse nerve fibre loss in the retina whereas the index expressing localized disturbances of the retinal functions while related to both diffuse and localized retinal damage was considerably better related to the estimates of localized loss. This strengthens the theoretically developed background of these indices and may allow one to attach more clinical significance to hitherto non-specific, overall loss of retinal sensitivity in relationships to the early diagnosis of glaucoma.

Linear regression did not provide the best possible fit of the visual field indices on the RNFL damage score but a non-linear function improved the coefficient of determination (R^2) statistically highly significantly. The non-linearity of the regression suggests that there can be a substantial amount of generalized RNFL damage without accompanying effect on retinal sensitivity and after a certain level of structural damage has been reached further damage in retinal nerve fibre layer is associated with an increasing, steep reduction of light sensitivity. This might be a reflection of the fact that early psychophysical abnormalities which are currently measured in cases of glaucoma may be preceeded by changes in the retina.

The regression analyses in the present study were performed without any reference to the patients' clinical diagnoses but normals, ocular hypertensives and glaucoma patients can be identified by their symbols in Figs 1 and 2. The majority of abnormally high values of mean damage and corrected loss variation occurred in patients with established glaucoma. Among the ocular hypertensives may patients had abnormal RNFL findings but the vlaues of their visual field indices were within the normal range. Some ocular hypertensives and normal individuals with normal nerve fibre layer showed slightly abnormal visual field values.

It was quite heartening that the results of a visual field examination expressed with mathematical functions to distinguish between generalized and localized reduction of differential retinal threshold were in such good agreement with the semi-quantitative assessment of generalized and localized nerve fibre layer changes in the retina. Further research is now needed to ascertain how these findings can be used in the detection of early glaucomatous damage which would allow earlier and more rational therapeutic intervention where needed.

ACKNOWLEDGEMENTS

This study was supported in part by the Medical Research Council of the Academy of Finland, Government of Canada Award, the E.A. Baker Foundation for the Prevention of Blindness, and Medical Research Council of Canada Grant No. MT 1578.

REFERENCES

1. Airaksinen, P.J., Drance, S.M., Douglas, G.R. and Mawson, D.K. Diffuse and localized nerve fibre loss in glaucoma. Am. J. Ophthalmol. Submitted for publication (1984).
2. Airaksinen, P.J. and Heijl, A. Visual field and retinal nerve fibre layer in early glaucoma after optic disc haemorrhage. Acta Ophthalmol. 61: 186–194 (1983).

3. Airaksinen, P.J., Mustonen, E. and Alanko, H.I. Optic disc haemorrhages precede retinal nerve fibre layer defects in ocular hypertension. Acta Ophthalmol. 59: 627–641 (1981).
4. Airaksinen, P. J., Nieminen, H. and Mustonen, E. Retinal nerve fibre layer photography with a wide angle fundus camera. Acta Ophthalmol. 60: 362–368 (1982).
5. Airaksinen, P.J. and Tuulonen, A. Early glaucoma changes in patients with and without an optic disc haemorrhage. Acta Ophthalmol. 62: 197–202 (1984).
6. Flammer, J. and Bebie, H. The concept of visual field indices. Albrecht von Graefes Arch. Ophthalmol., in press (1984).
7. Flammer, J., Drance, S.M., Augustiny, L. and Funkhouser, A. Quantification of glaucomatous visual field defects with automated perimetry. Invest. Ophthalmol., in press (1984).
8. Flammer, J., Drance, S.M., Jenni, A. and Bebie, H. JO and STATJO: programs for investigating the visual field with the Octopus automatic perimeter. Can. J. Ophthalmol. 18: 115–117 (1983).
9. Quigley, H.A., Miller, N.R. and George, T. Clinical evaluation of nerve fiber layer atrophy as an indicator of glaucomatous optic nerve damage. Arch. Ophthalmol. 98: 1564–1571 (1980).

Authors' addresses:
Dr. P.J. Airaksinen
Department of Ophthalmology,
University of Oulu,
SF-90220 Oulu 22, Finland

Dr. S.M. Drance
Department of Ophthalmology,
University of British Columbia,
2550 Willow Street,
Vancouver, B.C., Canada
V5Z 3N9

FLUORESCEIN ANGIOGRAPHY OF THE OPTIC DISC AND VISUAL FIELD DEFECTS IN OPEN-ANGLE GLAUCOMA AT THE INITIAL STAGE

CLAUDIO AZZOLINI and PAOLO BRUSINI

(*Udine, Italy*)

ABSTRACT

The vascularization of the optic disc in 55 eyes affected with open-angle glaucoma at the initial stage was studied by fluorescein angiography. The fluorescein filling defects of the optic disc were divided into absolute and relative defects. The visual field examination was performed with a Goldmann perimeter in all cases, and in 15 eyes also with the Perimetron automatic perimeter. A positive correlation between the fluorescein angiography data and perimetric defects was found in 45.7% of the eyes with absolute fluorescein defects. We think that fluorescein angiography of the optic disc still has limitations which in its current state makes it of doubtful value in chronic glaucoma in the initial stage.

INTRODUCTION

The deficiency of blood perfusion is currently considered the main cause of campimetric glaucomatous damage (5). It can manifest itself with more or less extensive alteration of the choroidal circulation or with partial changes of the vascularization of the optic nerve head.

In this report we studied the vascularization of the optic disc by fluorescein angiography in patients with incipient open-angle glaucoma comparing fluorescein filling defects with visual field defects.

MATERIALS AND METHODS

55 eyes of 30 patients, 18 male and 12 female, affected with open-angle glaucoma at the initial stage were studied. The visual acuity was 20/20 in 51 cases, slightly reduced because of initial opacity of the lens in 4 cases. All cases had an open anterior chamber angle. In all cases repeated tonometry and at least one tonography were carried out.

We also studied a control group of 28 normal eyes of 19 voluntary subjects, 10 male and 9 female. We used a Carl Zeiss fluoretinograph equipped with interference filters, Ilford film FP4 125 ASA and Ilfospeed

Heijl, A. and Greve, E.L. (eds.), Proceedings of the 6th Int. Visual Field Symposium.
© *1985, Dr W. Junk Publishers, Dordrecht, The Netherlands. ISBN 978-94-010-8932-6*

paper. Mydriasis was obtained through instillations of tropicamide 1%. The examination was performed with a rapid injection into the anticubital vein of the arm of 5 ml of 20% sodium fluorescein. The frequency of photograms was one frame per second during the initial stages of the examination and one each minute during the following 5 minutes.

The areas of hypofluorescence were divided into absolute defects (present in all phases of the angiographic examination) and relative defects (evident only in the initial phases of the examination). We intentionally ignored the late hyperfluorescence of the optic disc because of its uncertain clinical meaning. We did not take into account unclear or very small areas of hypo-fluorescence of the optic disc.

The visual field examination was carried out with a Goldmann perimeter (31.5 asb background). All patients were examined with kinetic perimetry and suprathreshold static perimetry between isopters. Profile static perimetry and circular static perimetry along the 15° parallel were used to better demonstrate and quantify the perimetric defects observed.

The Perimetron automatic perimeter was used in 9 patients (15 eyes) employing program 10 (3–5 isopters kinetic perimetry + blind spot delimitation + static testing of 129 points within 25°).

RESULTS

In 47 eyes (85.5%) there were more or less marked fluorescein filling defects. Among these, there were absolute defects in 35 eyes (74.5%) and relative defects in 12 eyes (25.5%) (Fig. 1). In the remaining 8 eyes no perfusion defects of the optic disc was found.

In the control group of 28 normal eyes we found fluorescein filling defects in 20 eyes (71.4%). Among these there were 12 relative (60%) and 8 (40%) absolute defects.

The visual field examination demonstrated only small glaucomatous defects, isolated paracentral scotomas, nasal steps and barings of the blind

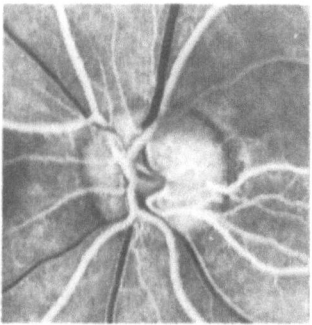 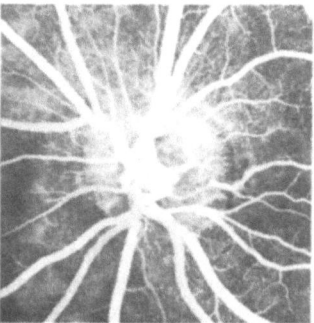

Fig. 1. Typical case of relative fluorescein filling defect from 12 to 2 o'clock, present only in the initial phases of the examination.

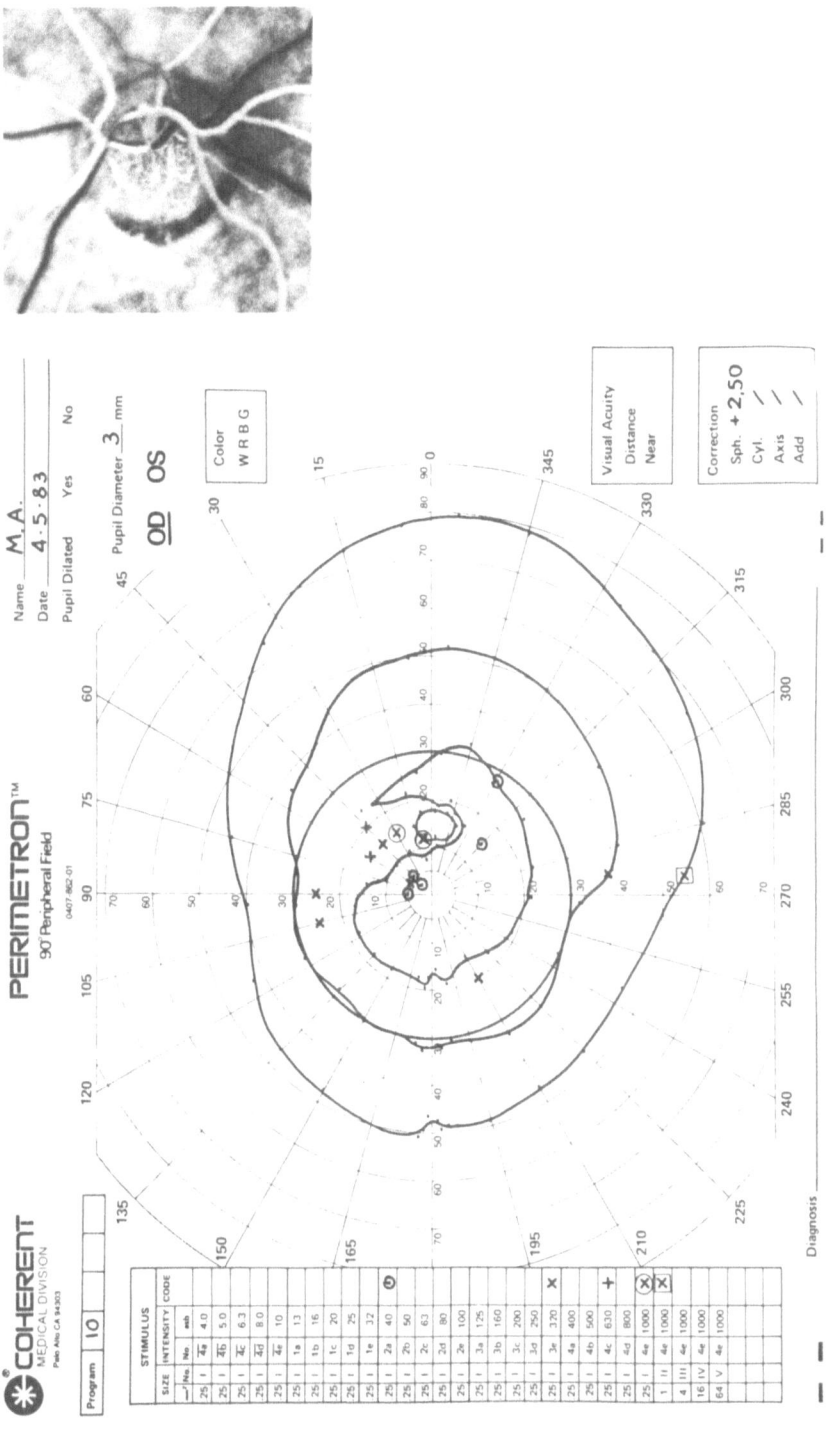

Fig. 2. Positive correlation between absolute fluorescein filling defect and visual field defects. Hypofluorescence of the nasal rim from 3 to 7 o'clock present in all phases of angiographic examination. Arcuate superior scotoma and small paracentral scotoma with the Perimetron.

417

spot. In 6 eyes the Perimetron found small paracentral scotomas, not identified by manual perimetry, but later quantified with static profile perimetry.

Bearing in mind the classic model of the pathways of the nerve fibres in the optic nerve and retina, we have compared the fluorescein filling defects of the optic disc with visual field defects in the glaucomatous eyes. In 35 eyes with absolute fluorescein filling defects we found a positive correlation in 16 eyes (45.7%) (Fig. 2); in 12 eyes with relative defects there was a correspondence in 2 eyes (16.7%).

DISCUSSION

Many papers have demonstrated absolute and relative fluorescein filling defects in glaucomatous, hypertensive, and normal eyes (6, 7, 9). Late disc hyperfluorescence in glaucomatous eyes has also been reported (3, 8, 10).

The importance of relative defects is not yet completely clear, while the absolute defects are generally interpreted as ischemic areas. This is in accordance with the vascular theory of glaucomatous visual field loss. A positive correlation between absolute fluorescein defects and glaucomatous visual field defects has already been demonstrated (1, 4).

Our aim has been to find the relationship between fluorescein and perimetric defects in eyes with open-angle glaucoma at the initial stage. The use of automatic perimetry is very useful to detect small glaucomatous defects in very early glaucoma. Such defects are not often found using manual perimetry. If program 10 is used, the Perimetron permits early diagnosis in patients with good collaboration.

In this material the percentage of positive correlation (45.7%) between absolute fluorescein defects and visual field defects in glaucomatous eyes is lower than the percentage found by other authors (4). This may be due to the fact that, as other papers have pointed out, in glaucoma at the initial stage the fluoroangiographic alterations without campimetric findings could precede the visual field defects (1, 7). Also, in the initial phases of the illness the vascular papillary alterations, like the field changes, are presumably discrete and difficult to find.

The meaning of relative defects is not clear. Some authors think that they could be a normal variation of the vascularization of the optic disc and that they could become absolute defects in hypertensive eyes (7). The low percentage of cases with significant correlation between relative fluorescein defects and visual field defects makes this kind of fluorescein alterations of little interest in eyes with open-angle glaucoma at the initial stage.

The fluorescein angiography alterations in the control group are probably due to physiologic variations of blood supply at the papillary level.

The study of the vascularization of the optic disc is yet difficult because of some technical and interpretative limits:
- the excitation and barrage filters do not yet permit us to totally eliminate the pseudofluorescence of the optic disc. Only recently the utilization of special interference filters has resolved this problem;
- the superimposition of the fluorescence of different focal planes makes a selective analysis of the various capillary districts difficult;

418

— anatomical vascular alterations can alter the reading of a fluorescein angiography;
— unsatisfactory results can sometimes be due to the high number of photograms which must be carried out in a few seconds;
— ocular media may not be clear;
— finally, the data can be fogged by subjectivity of the reading.

We think that in the future an exact interpretation of the hypofluorescence disc areas, often with slight contrast, may be possible with the diffusion of computerization of fluoroangiographic data, already introduced experimentally by Brancato et al. for retinal angiography (2). Besides it is useful, as it has already been suggested (4), to apply planimetry or still more sensitive methods in order to quantify the optic disc fluorescein defects. Finally, a standardization of criteria and of terminology for interpretation of fluorescein angiograms is useful.

In conclusion, fluorescein angiography of the optic disc still has limitations which currently makes it of doubtful value in incipient open-angle glaucoma.

REFERENCES

1. Bonnet, M., Baserer, T. and Grange, J.D. Angiographie fluoroscéinique de la papille dans l'hypertension oculaire et le glaucome. J. Fr. Ophthalmol. 2: 239–246 (1979).
2. Brancato, R., D'Amore, A., Del Caro, L., Ravalico, G. and Sicuranza, G. An attempt towards a new technique for the computer analysis of fluorescein angiography. Bull. of Hellen Ophthalmol. Soc. 45: 529 (1975).
3. Cardillo Piccolino, F., Capris, P. and Selis, G. Capillary hyperpermeability of the optic disc and functional evolution in glaucoma. Doc. Ophthalmol. Proc. Series 35: 75–80 (1983).
4. Fishbein, S.L. and Schwartz, B. Optic disc in glaucoma. Topography and extent of fluorescein filling defects. Arch. Ophthalmol. 95: 1978–1979 (1977).
5. Hayreh, S.S. Pathogenesis of optic nerve damage and visual field defects in glaucoma. Doc. Ophthalmol. Proc. Series 22: 89–109 (1980).
6. Loebl, M. and Schwartz, B. Fluorescein angiography defects of the optic disc in ocular hypertension. Arch. Ophthalmol. 95: 1980–1984 (1977).
7. Schwartz, B., Rieser, J.C. and Fishbein, S.L. Fluorescein angiographic defects of the optic disc in glaucoma. Arch. Ophthalmol. 95: 1961–1974 (1977).
8. Talusan, E.D., Schwartz, B. and Wilcox, L.M. Fluorescein angiography of the optic disc. A longitudinal follow-up. Arch. Ophthalmol. 98: 1579–1587 (1980).
9. Tenner, A. Fluorescent angiography of the papillary region in glaucoma. Adv. Ophthalmol. 32: 35–51 (1976).
10. Tsukahara, S. Hyperpermeable disc capillaries in glaucoma. Adv. Ophthalmol. 35: 65–72 (1978).

Author's address:
Divisione Oculistica
Ospedale Civile 33100 Udine
Italy

FLUORESCEIN FILLING DEFECTS OF THE OPTIC DISC AND FUNCTIONAL EVOLUTION IN GLAUCOMA

F. CARDILLO PICCOLINO, G. SELIS, D. PEIRE', G.C. PARODI and
G. RAVERA
(*Genoa, Italy*).

ABSTRACT

A computerized system of image analysis allowed us to identify and measure areas of hypoperfusion and areas of non perfusion on the optic disc of glaucoma patients. A significant inverse correlation was observed between the disc areas of non perfusion and the extension of visual field. A significant direct correlation was revealed between the increase of non perfusion areas and the decrease of visual field. The results of our study support the assumption that the optic disc perfusion defects may precede functional deterioration in glaucomatous eyes.

INTRODUCTION

Many studies confirm that fluorescein filling defects of the optic disc are associated with perimetric alterations in glaucoma patients (4, 6–8). A topographic correspondance has been demonstrated between the location of visual field loss and the site of absolute filling defects of the optic disc (1, 3).

A significant correlation between the percent areas of filling defects and the degree of visual field loss has also been observed (5). In this study a sophisticated method to analyze quantitatively the areas of disc hypofluorescence in glaucomatous eyes was used. Hypofluorescent areas were compared to the extension of the residual field. A further purpose of our study was to determine the relationship between papillary and perimetric changes on long-term follow-up.

MATERIALS AND METHODS

Thirty-two eyes with chronic open angle glaucoma of 27 patients 45 to 52 years of age were included in our study. The follow-up ranged from 2 to 5 years. All the selected cases had fluorescein angiograms of the optic disc performed at the same time as visual field examination with kinetic method on the Goldmann perimeter.

At the first observation 18 eyes had advanced visual field loss, 14 had normal (4) eyes or almost normal (10 eyes) visual fields. During follow-up

Heijl, A. and Greve, E.L. (eds.), Proceedings of the 6th Int. Visual Field Symposium.
© *1985, Dr W. Junk Publishers, Dordrecht, The Netherlands. ISBN 978-94-010-8932-6*

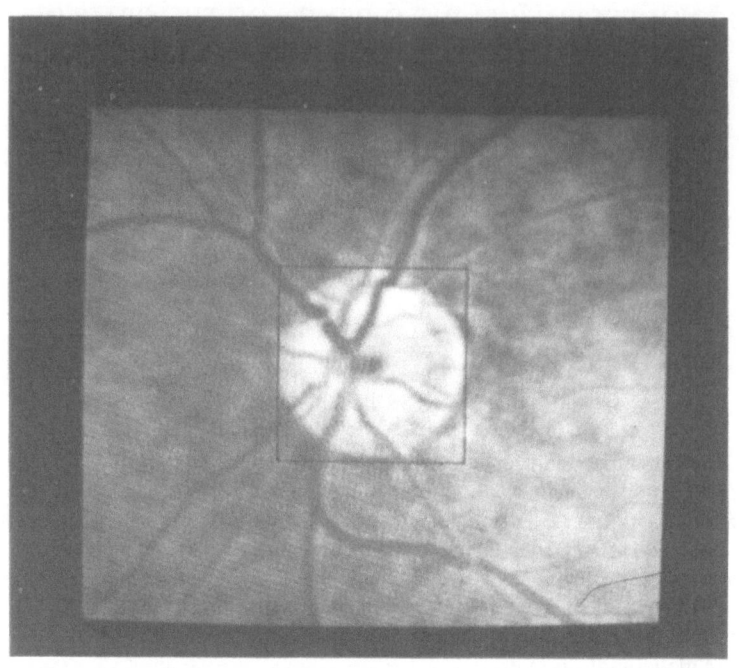

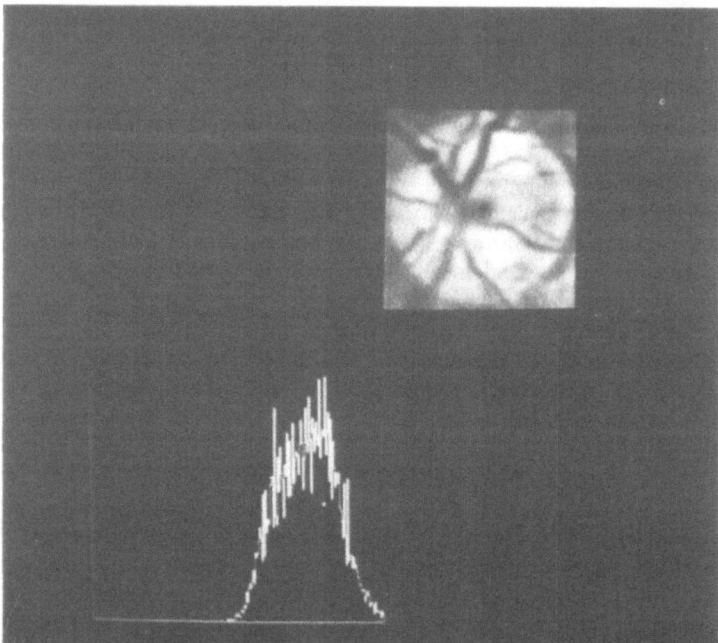

Fig. 1. (a) the disc image displayed on the monitor and 'extracted' for analysis. (b) the histogram of grey levels vs number of pixels on the disc area.

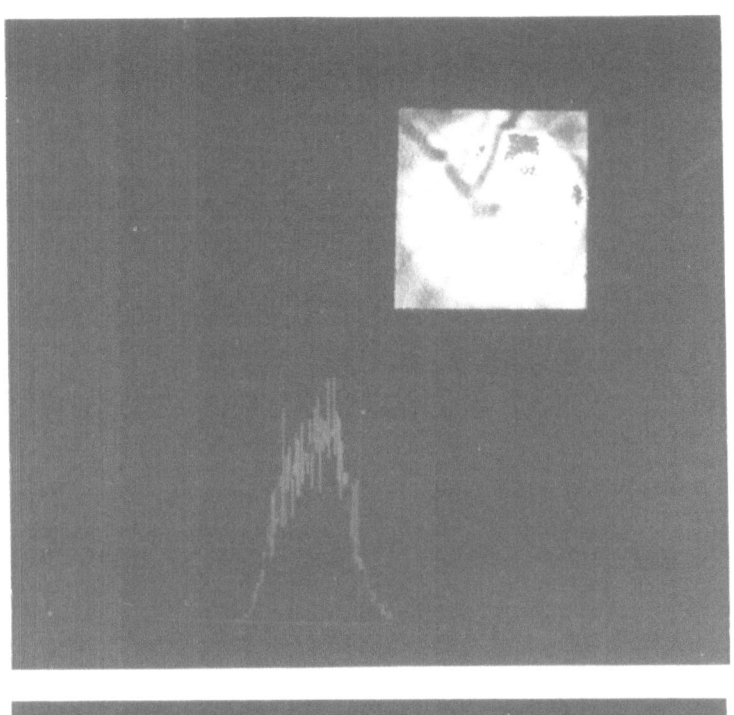

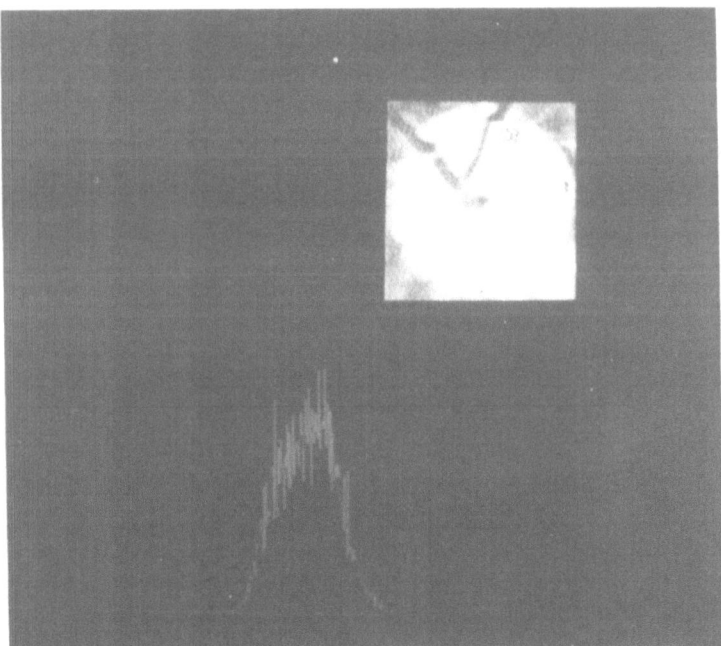

Fig. 2. (a) the display of disc area of hypoperfusion by selecting the highest intensity band of a 5 bands grey scale. (b) the display of disc area of non perfusion by selecting the highest intensity band of a 10 bands grey scale.

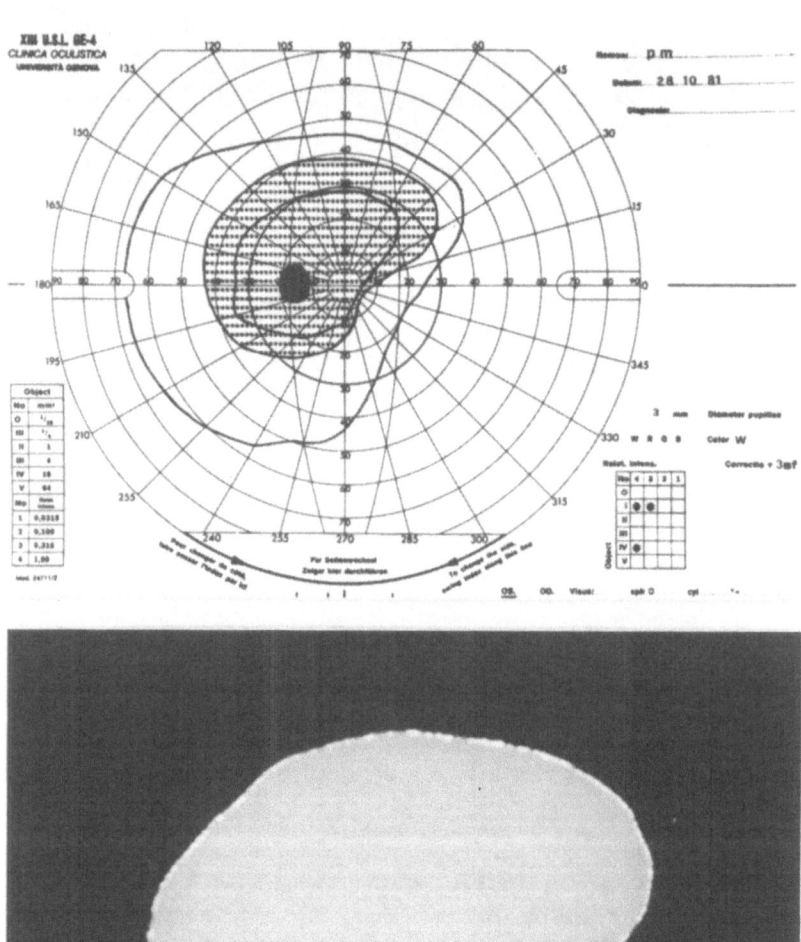

Fig. 3. (a) a visual field showing the isopter (I-4-e) chosen for analysis. (b) the area of visual field elaborated by the image processor.

the visual field deteriorated in 22 eyes it showed no or minimal changes in 10 eyes.

Areas of absolute filling defect of the optic disc and areas of visual field were measured using a system of image analysis (ACTA 500) able to store and to elaborate a TV image by a computer (HP 1000).

The disc image on the negative angiogram was 'extracted' for analysis by using a 'window' programmable for size and position (Fig. 1a). The number of picture-points (pixels) included in the 'window' was arbitrarily considered the area of the optic disc (Fig. 1b). The grey scale of the disc image was divided in 5 bands so that the band of higher intensity corresponded to the area of filling defect on the fluorescein angiogram. When this high intensity band was selected the number of pixels measured the area of the whole filling defect. We called this area 'disc area of hypoperfusion' (DAH) (Fig. 2a).

A further subdivision of the grey scale in 10 bands allowed to display pixels corresponding to the deepest hypofluorescence in the same area of filling defect. We called this area 'disc area of non perfusion' (DANP) (Fig. 2b).

The measurements of the DAH and the DANP in an optic disc were expressed as a percentage of the area of the disc.

The same system of image analysis permitted measurement of the area of visual field. This determination was made for the I-4-e isopter, which was examined in each case under contant testing conditions (Fig. 3a, b).

The Spearman rank correlation (r_s) was used for the following evaluations (2):
1. Relationship between the DAH and the areas of visual field (at the first observation).
2. Relationship between the DANP and the areas of visual field (at the first observation).
3. Relationship between increase of DAH and decrease of areas of visual field (during the follow-up).
4. Relationship between increase of DANP and decrease of areas of visual field (during the follow-up).

A p level $\leqslant 0.05$ was considered as significant.

RESULTS

Spearman correlation coefficients for each evaluation are shown in Tables 1 and 2.

Table 1. Spearman correlations (r_s).

	r_s	N	P
DHA vs visual field	− 0.6532	32	< 0.001
DNAP vs visual field	− 0.7794	32	< 0.001
Δ DAH vs Δ visual field	0.5974	32	< 0.001
Δ DANP vs Δ visual field	0.6294	32	< 0.01

DAH = disc area of hypoperfusion.
DNAP = disc area of non perfusion.

425

Table 2. Spearman correlations (r_s) for DANP vs area of visual field.

	r_s	N	P
Advanced visual field loss	− 0.8431	18	< 0.001
Normal or almost normal visual field	− 0.2307	14	> 0.05

A significant inverse correlation was obtained between both the DAH and DANP and the areas of visual field.

A significant direct correlation was obtained between the increase of both the DAH and DANP and the decrease of the visual field. The highest values of r_s resulted when the DANP and its increase were correlated with the areas and to the decrease of visual field respectively. These relationships are shown in Figs. 4 and 5. Different degrees of correlation with the DANP were obtained by separate evaluation of cases with advanced visual field loss and cases with normal or almost normal visual field (Table 2). A very high value of r_s existed between the DANP and the areas of largely altered visual fields. A non-significant relationship resulted between the DANP and areas of slightly altered visual fields.

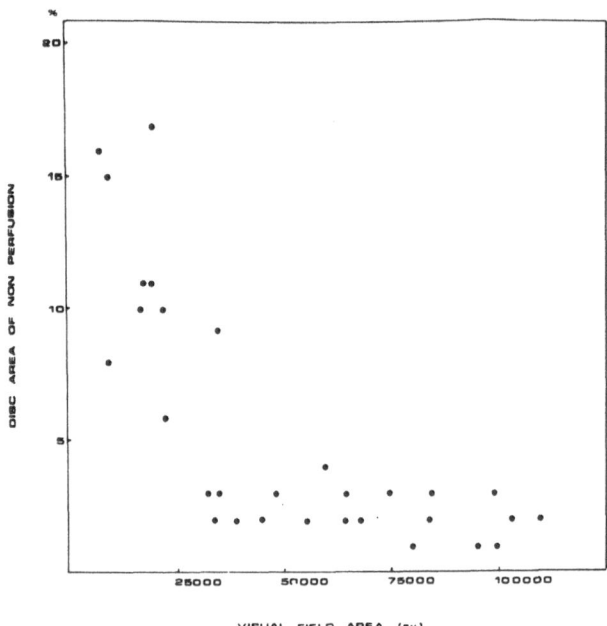

Fig. 4. The relationship between disc area of non perfusion and area of visual field in glaucomatous and ocular hypertensive patients.

426

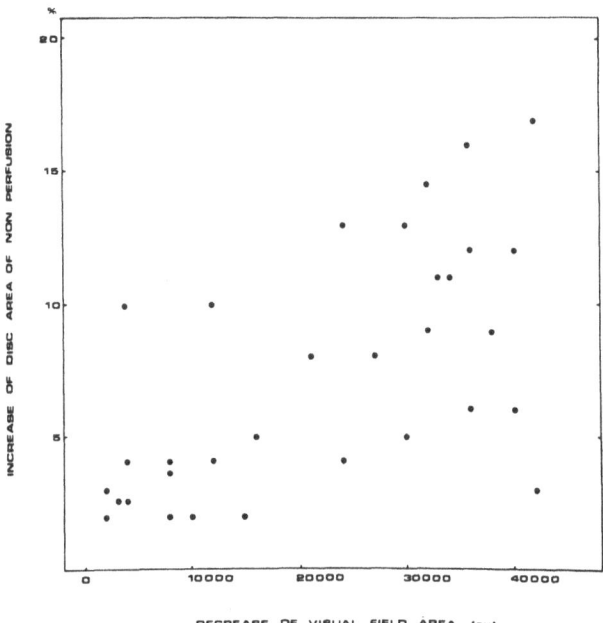

Fig. 5. The relationship between increase of disc area of non perfusion and decrease of visual field area in glaucomatous patients.

COMMENTS

The results of our study confirm the negative correlation of the percent area of filling defect with the area of visual field in glaucoma as already observed by Nanba and Schwartz (5).

Our system of image analysis allows the identification of areas with different degrees of filling defect on the optic disc: the DAH, corresponding to the total absolute filling defect as evaluated in fluorescein angiography, and the DANP, corresponding to a more limited area of deep hypofluorescence.

The DANP was better correlated with the visual field than the DAH. The highest values of correlation were observed in cases with advanced visual field loss. These results indicate that areas of disc filling defect may precede functional deterioration in glaucoma patients.

We can suppose that areas of hypoperfusion on the optic disc progressively change into areas of non perfusion. The visual field loss seems to be directly related to the progression of this non perfusion phenomenon of the optic disc.

ACKNOWLEDGEMENT

This study was supported by a grant from Consiglio Nazionale delle Ricerche, Roma, Italy.

REFERENCES

1. Cardillo Piccolino, F., Parodi, G.C. and Beltrame, F. Optic disc analysis by computerized image subtraction and perimetry. Doc. Ophthalmol. Proc., 35: 87–91 (1983).
2. Daniel, W.W. Applied nonparametric statistics. Boston, Houghton Mifflin Company (1978).
3. Fishbein, S.L. and Schwartz, B. Optic disc in glaucoma. Topography and extent of fluorescein filling defects. Arch. Ophthalmol., 95: 1975–1979 (1977).
4. Hayreh, S.S. Pathogenesis of optic nerve damage on visual field defects in glaucoma. Doc. Ophthalmol. Proc., 22: 89–109 (1980).
5. Nanba, K. and Schwartz, B. Fluorescein angiographic defects of the optic disc in glaucomatous visual field loss. Doc. Ophthalmol. Proc., 35: 67–73 (1983).
6. Oosterhuis, J.A. and Gortzak-Moorstein, N. Fluorescein angiography of the optic disc in glaucoma. Ophthalmologica 160: 331–353 (1970).
7. Schwartz, B., Rieser, J.C. and Fishbein, S.L. Fluorescein angiographic defects of the optic disc in glaucoma. Arch. Ophthalmol. 95: 1961–1974 (1977).
8. Spaeth, G.L. Fluorescein angiography: its contribution towards understanding the mechanism of visual loss in glaucoma. Trans. Am. Ophthalmol Soc. 73: 491–553 (1975).

Authors' addresses:
Dr. F. Cardillo Piccolino
Dr. G. Selis
Dr. D. Peirè
Dept. Of Ophthalmology
University of Genoa
Viale Benedetto XV, 5
16132 Genoa, Italy

G.C. Parodi
Dept. Of Biophysical and Electrical Engineering
University of Genoa

Dr. G. Ravera
Medical Statistics and Biometry Institute
University of Genoa

DIURNAL VARIABILITY OF THE VISUAL FIELD AS MEASURED BY THE OCTOPUS PERIMETER

SATOSHI MIZUTANI and AKIHIRO SUZUMURA

(*Aichi, Japan*)

ABSTRACT

Although it is known that intraocular pressure (IOP) fluctuates diurnally and that these variations are great in glaucomatous patients, little is known about the diurnal variability of the visual field. In this study we used an Octopus automatic perimeter (program No. 31) to measure diurnal variability of the visual field in normal controls, ocular hypertensive patients and glaucomatous patients. As a result of demonstrating the normal diurnal variations of the visual field and comparing them with those of ocular hypertension (OH) and primary open angle glaucoma (POAG), clear differences in sensitivity variation were observed. Cases of OH which have large diurnal sensitivity variation are therefore thought likely to develop into POAG. As result of our research, we considered the above method of determination as having the potential to become a diagnostic method for OH and to facilitate early diagnosis of glaucoma.

INTRODUCTION

As the automatic perimeter has been developed for examination of the visual field, early diagnosis of glaucoma and changes of the visual field in other diseases are being reviewed. The Octopus automatic perimeter has the advantage of high reliability and repeatability, and the fact that the sensitivity of the visual field is expressed in numerical values. Making use of these characteristics, other applications of the Octopus perimeter were considered. One of these is the measurement of diurnal variability in the visual field.

MATERIALS AND METHODS

Subjects used as the controls were 32 eyes of normal intraocular pressure (IOP) belonging to 17 normal individuals aged 22–45. Program No. 31 to measure the visual field three times a day:morning (8:00–9:00 am); afternoon (1:00–2:00 pm); evening (5:00–7:00 pm). Diurnal variations of IOP

Heijl, A. and Greve, E.L. (eds.), Proceedings of the 6th Int. Visual Field Symposium.
© 1985, Dr W. Junk Publishers, Dordrecht, The Netherlands. ISBN 978-94-010-8932-6

were determined at the same time. The test subjects included 31 eyes (16 individuals) with ocular hypertension (OH) and 18 eyes (9 individuals) with primary open angle glaucoma (POAG). They were investigated in the same way as the controls and then compared with them. Taking into consideration the training effect on patient measurement, only subjects with previous octopus perimeter examination experience were used (3).

CLINICAL RESULTS

1. Diurnal variations of normal

Sensitivity was determined as the loss at each point, calculated from the total of differences between actual results and those of the normal visual field for the subject's age group; the blind spot was omitted. In the controls the average loss of sensitivity at one point was 1.4 dB and the average IOP was about 15 mmHg (Fig. 1). The variation in both IOP and sensitivity was small. The average number of points where the sensitivity difference in the three test's results exceeded 5 dB (points of large change) was 2.3 ± 2.0 (Table 2).

2. Diurnal variations of OH and POAG

Case 1: A 21-year-old male with ocular hypertension, who complained of eye pain and eye fatigue. On first examination the patient's IOP was 22 mmHg in the left eye, loss of sensitivity was small, but over the three tests, a difference of greater than 5 dB was recorded for 17 points. The change in both ocular pressure and sensitivity was also great (Fig. 2).

Case 2: A 49-year-old woman with main complaint of eye fatigue. On first examination the patient's IOP was 22 mmHg in the right eye and 25 mmHg in the left (Fig. 3-2). Sensitivity loss was observed in the upper part, within

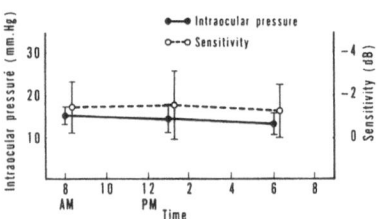

MEAN SENSITIVITY LOSS		CONTROLS	OH	POAG
WHOLE FIELD		0.46	0.77	6.17
QUADRANT UPPER NASAL		0.47	0.94	9.40
LOWER NASAL		0.31	0.41	2.47
UPPER TEMP.		0.67	0.95	8.43
LOWER TEMP.		0.24	0.57	0.90
ECCENTRICITY	0 - 10	0.49	0.42	11.30
	10 - 20	0.57	0.31	7.23
	20 - 30	0.39	1.17	4.13
				[dB]

Table 1. Whole field mean sensitivity loss and area sensitivity loss in controls, ocular hypertension and primary open angle glaucoma.

Fig. 1. The relationship between intra-ocular pressure and sensitivity of visual field in average results of all normal controls.

	VARIATION OF IOP (mmHg)	VARIATION OF SENSITIVITY(dB)	NUMBER OF POINTS WITH DIFFERENCE OVER 5dB (points)
CONTROLS	3.86 + 0.97	0.59 + 0.27	2.3 + 2.0
OH	7.20 + 2.29	1.28 + 0.95	11.7 + 9.0
POAG	8.80 + 1.17	1.54 + 1.26	13.0 + 3.2

Table 2. Diurnal variation of intraocular pressure and sensitivity, and number of points where difference in sensitivity was more than 5 dB in controls, ocular hypertension and primary open angle glaucoma.

		CONTROLS	OH	POAG
QUADRANT	UPPER NASAL	3.8	10.2	33.3
	LOWER NASAL	0.5	8.2	7.7
	UPPER TEMP.	3.0	12.3	12.8
	LOWER TEMP.	0.5	14.5	12.1
ECCENTRICITY	0 10	0	5.2	3.7
	10 20	3.5	10.5	22.2
	20 30	4.2	20.3	17.6

[%]

Table 3. The ratio of number of points where sensitivity difference was over 5 dB, to number of test points in each area in controls, ocular hypertension and primary open angle glaucoma.

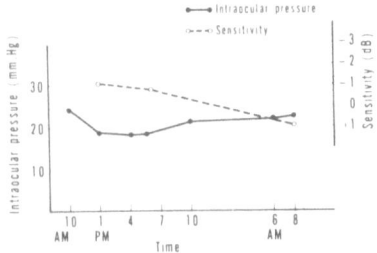

Fig. 2. The relation between intraocular pressure and sensitivity of right visual field in ocular hypertension (case 1). Sensitivity here is the loss at each point calculated from the total of differences between actual results and the normal visual field for the subject's age group. The blind spot is omitted.

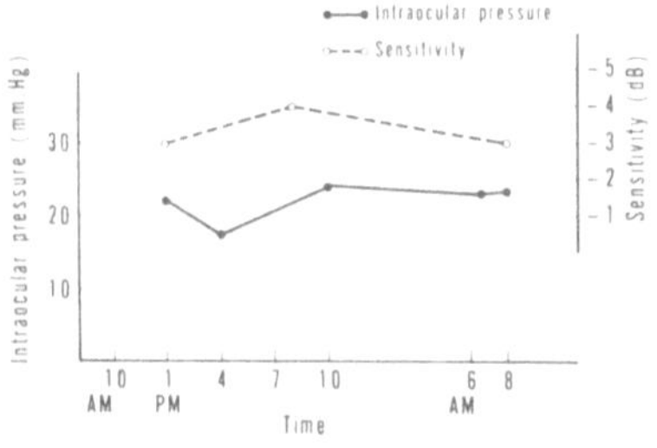

Fig. 3-1. The relation between intraocular pressure and sensitivity of left visual field in early primary open angle glaucoma (case 2).

the range of 10 to 30 degrees. Scotoma was not detected by Goldmann perimeter. A difference of greater than 5 dB was recorded for 14 points. In this case, sensitivity of visual field changed with IOP variations (Fig. 3-1).

There was no change in the whole field mean loss between the controls

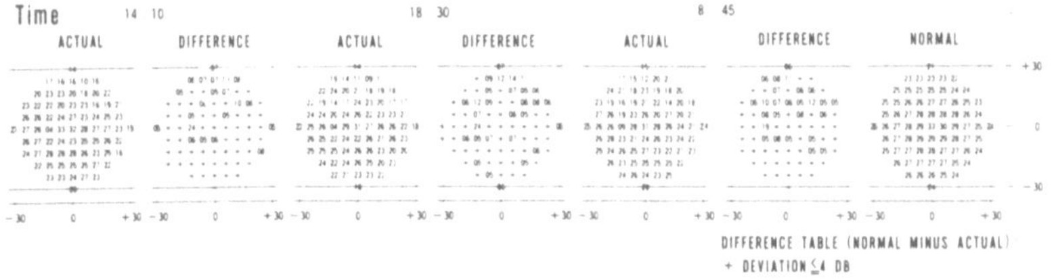

Fig. 3-2. Comparative display of POAG. Each pair is the result of afternoon, evening and following morning testing.

and ocular hypertensive patients. In the case of POAG, sensitivity loss was great. Sensitivity loss was common in the 20–30 degree region in OH and in the upper part of the 0–20 degree region in POAG. These results corresponded to the change in the visual field associated with glaucoma (Table 1). Table 2 shows the variation in IOP and sensitivity, and the average number of points where the sensitivity difference in the three test's results exceeded 5 dB.

Comparison of diurnal variability in the visual field among the controls, OH and POAG revealed to clear difference in sensitivity variation. Regions where the greatest change was observed were the upper nasal field, the upper and lower temporal fields, and between 20 and 30 degree in the case of OH. In POAG, it was the upper nasal field and between 10 and 20 degrees (Table 3).

DISCUSSION

Visual field testing for early diagnosis of glaucoma is very important. Recently, as a result of prospective studies of OH, some (about 15%) ocular hypertensive patients have been recognized to develop glaucoma (1). Therefore, it is important that ocular hypertensive patients who are likely to develop glaucoma are determined early and preventive treatment initiated. To this end, we measured diurnal variation of the visual field by program No. 31.

In the controls, the variation in both IOP and sensitivity was small (Table 2). This result indicates that the octopus perimeter has high reliability and repeatability. In consideration of the experimental results and errors of measurement (2), the normal controls were considered as follows;

1) diurnal variation in intraocular pressure within 5 mmHg,

2) a difference of more than 5 dB recorded at less than 5 points,

3) variation in sensitivity not exceeding about 1 dB.

As a result of determining the normal controls and comparing them with OH and POAG, large variations were observed.

Since some ocular hypertensive patients had little variation in sensitivity, the ocular hypertensive patients who had large variation were considered as likely to develop glaucoma. The areas with points of great change were the same areas as visual field loss in early glaucoma. Therefore, in ocular hypertension, the areas with points of large change will become gradually larger, and there will be sensitivity loss. Finally, scotoma will be observed in the same area. As a result, the authors consider this method of determination has the potential to become a diagnosis of ocular hypertension and an early diagnosis for glaucoma.

REFERENCES

1. Ikuo Azuma. Ocular hypertension and glaucoma, Jpn. J. Clini. Ophthalmol., 34(5): 625–633 (1980).
2. Harrington, D.O. The visual fields. A text book and atlas of clinical perimetry, Fourth edition, The C.V. Mosby, Saint Louis (1976).

3. Yoichi Inoue and T. Ioue. Evaluation of campimetry by computerized perimetry bracket (Octopus), Jpn. J. Clini. Ophthalmol., 36(9): 1149–1154 (1982).

Authors' address:
Satoshi Mizutani and Akihiro Suzumura
Dept, of Ophthalmology
Aichi Medical University
Nagakute-cho, Aichi-gun
Aichi Pref., 480-11
Japan

PRACTICAL USE OF AREA COMPUTATION FOR ASSESSMENT OF VISUAL FIELDS: ANALYSIS OF THE RESULTS OF MECOBALAMIN THERAPY FOR VISUAL FIELD DEFECTS IN CHRONIC GLAUCOMA

HIROSHI KOSAKI, HAJIME NAKATANI, IKUO AZUMA KAZUYUKI SAKAGUCHI

(*Osaka, Japan*)

ABSTRACT

We reported at the previous IPS symposium that we had developed a method of calculating isopter areas on kinetic Goldmann field charts using a computer, which was very useful in the assessment of clinical progress of visual field defects. In the present study, this method was used to assess the results of mecobalamin therapy for visual field defects in glaucoma. The method proved to be useful. Mecobalamin tablets, each containing 500 μg of the drug, were administered T.I.D. for 6 months to 160 patients with 298 eyes with chronic primary glaucoma. Recovery of the visual field was assessed by the isopter area computation method which we had developed. The following conclusions were drawn:
1) Visual field recovery was seen in about 50% of the eyes.
2) Visual field recovery was better in young patients than in the middle aged or old patients.
3) Changes in visual field defects were greater at a C/D ≤ 0.6 and in the early stages of the disease.
4) The isopter area computation method was excellent for assessing clinical progress of visual field defects.

INTRODUCTION

Visual fields are genrally assessed directly from field charts for diagnostic purposes, and this assessment is not difficult. However, when the disease is followed, minute changes are more rapidly detected with numerical assessment than with assessment for field charts alone, and statistical analysis is easier. For this reason, we developed a computerized method of measuring isopter areas (3) and presented it at the previous IPS symposium.

In our present study, mecobalamin tablets, each containing 500 μg of the drug, were given orally at 3 tablets daily for 6 months to 160 patients with 298 eyes with chronic primary glaucoma. In these patients, the intraocular pressure had been controlled at 21 mmHg or less for more than 3 months. The visual fields improved in about 50% of these eyes. Our area computation method was used to analyze the results of the therapy.

Heijl, A. and Greve, E.L. (eds.), Proceedings of the 6th Int. Visual Field Symposium.
© *1985, Dr W. Junk Publishers, Dordrecht, The Netherlands. ISBN 978-94-010-8932-6*

435

PATIENTS AND METHODS

160 patients presenting 298 eyes of chronic primary glaucoma with visual field defects, in whom intraocular pressure had been controlled at 21 mmHg or less for more than 3 months, are admitted to the study. The patients were 17 to 79 years old (mean age: 59.2 years). Ninety-one (166 affected eyes) were male, and 69 (132 affected eyes) were female. 248 eyes were of the POAG type, and 38 of the PCAG type. 112 eyes were in the early stages (up to Stage IIb in Kosaki's Classification (5)), 85 in the middle stages (stages IIIa and IIIb), and 75 eyes in the terminal stages (Stage IV and high stages). The C/D ratio was up to 0.6 in 91 eyes, 0.7 to 0.8 in 62 eyes, and 0.9 to 1.0 in 53 eyes.

Mecobalamin was administered to these patients, $3 \times 500 \mu g$ tablets daily. Kinetic Goldmann perimetry was conducted before treatment and after 3 and 6 months of treatment. Thirty-four clinics participated in this study program.

ANALYSIS

The areas of isopters V_4, I_4 and I_3 on visual field charts were calculated by a computer using the method we presented at the 5th IPS Symposium in 1982 (3). These values (Fig. 1 in our report in the 1st IPS Symposium in 1980 (4)) were calculated as percentages relative to normal standard values of each age group (i.e. the residual rate of the visual field: R, recovery range of the visual field: ΔS). The difference in the percentages between the pre-treatment and post-treatment levels was analyzed statistically.

$R_0 (\%) =$ Pre-treatment isopter area/normal standard of the relevant age group $\times 100$

$R_6 =$ Isopter area after 6 months of the treatment/normal standard of the relevant age group $\times 100$

$\Delta S = R_6 - R_0$

RESULTS

(1) Frequency distribution of visual field recovery range, ΔS:

The frequency distribution of each isopter is shown in Fig. 2. In all isopters examined, $\Delta S = 5$ was the most frequently seen. The frequency of this level of ΔS was highest in Isopter I_3.

(2) Visual field recovery by isopter:

The visual field recovery range, ΔS, was classified into 9 grades, each grade representing a change in ΔS of an additional 10 units. Each grade was then calculated as a percentage of all the groups and represented by a bar graph as shown in Fig. 3. Visual field recovery was seen in about 50% of the eyes, but it differed between isopters and was more frequent in the outer isopters with 55.9% in Isopter V_4, 45.6% in Isopter I_4 and 42.0% in Isopter I_3.

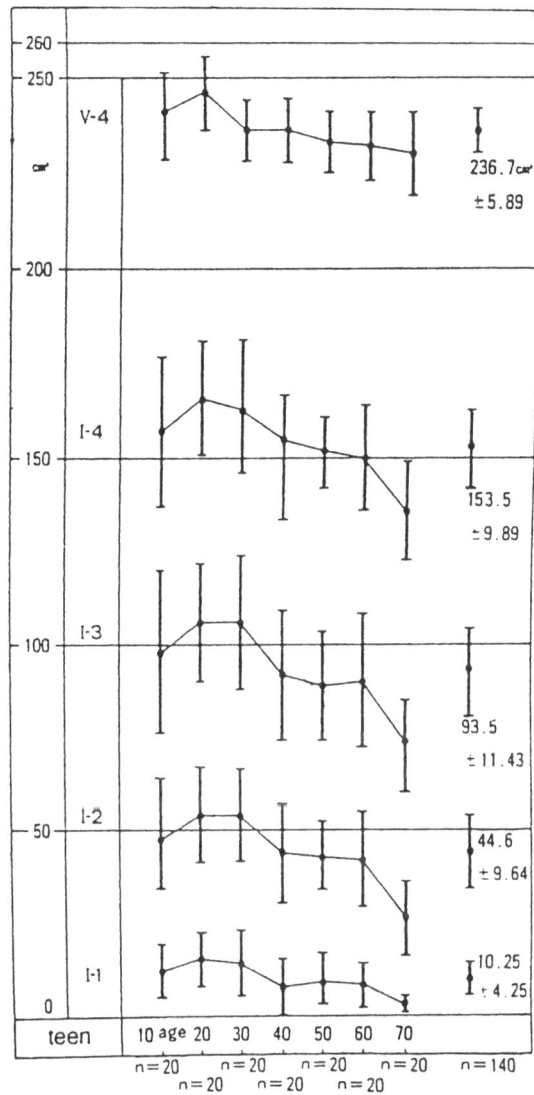

Fig. 1. Normal values of isopter area.

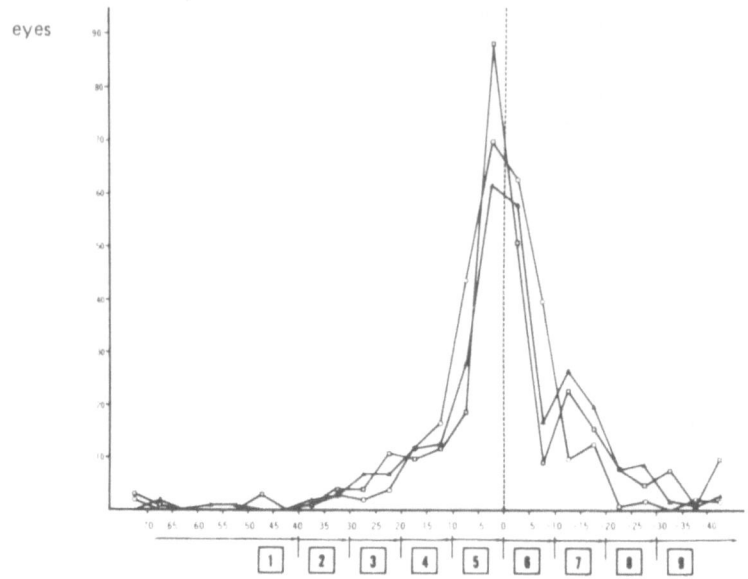

Fig. 2. Frequency curve for the recovery range: ΔS of visual fields.

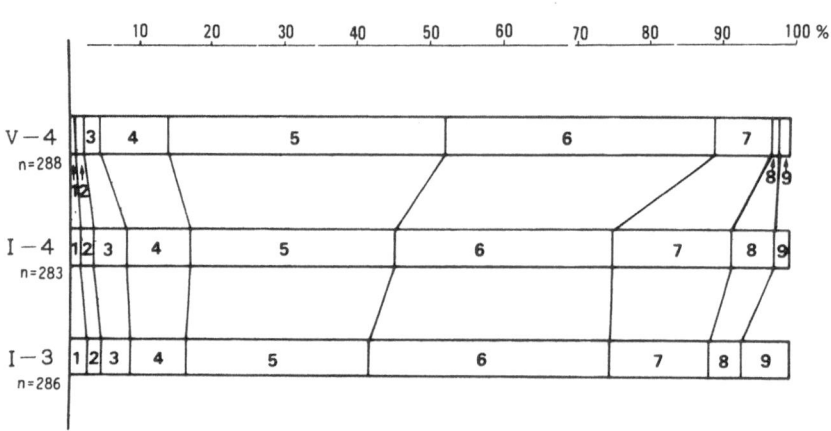

Fig. 3. Visual field recovery by isopter.

(3) Visual field recovery range, ΔS, in relation to age:

The recovery of Isopter I_3 in relation to age is shown in Fig. 4. Visual field recovery was not related to age.

The distribution of visual field recovery range in Isopter I_3 was analyzed in 3 age groups, up to 39 years, 40 to 59 years, and 60 years or more, and shown by bar graphs in Fig. 5. Visual field recovery was significantly ($P < 0.001$) better in the young patients than in the older ones.

438

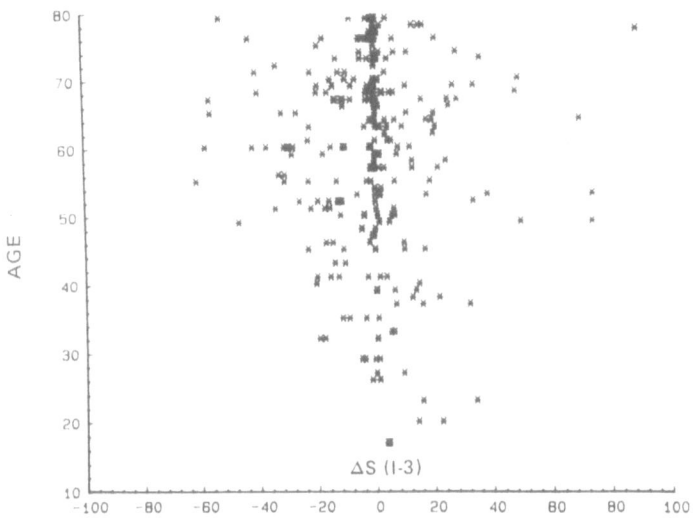

Fig. 4. Recovery range of visual fields: ΔS relative to age (Isopter I-3).

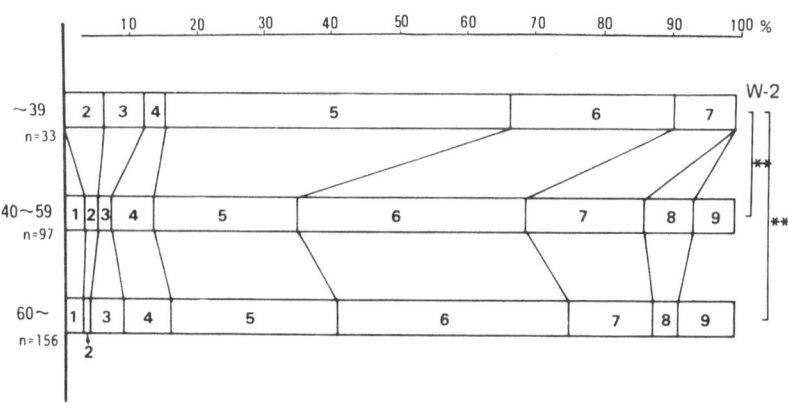

Fig. 5. Visual field recovery by age group: ΔS (I-3).

(4) Visual field recovery by sex:
   Visual field recovery did not differ between sexes.
(5) Visual field recovery by disease type:
   Visual field recovery did not differ between POAG and PCAG.
(6) Visual field recovery by C/D:
   The distribution fo visual field recovery in Isopter I$_3$ in 3 groups of C/D, one with a C/D of up to 0.6, the second with a C/D of 0.7 to 0.8, and the third with a C/D of 0.9 to 1.0, is represented in bar graphs in Fig. 6. Visual field recovery was better (P < 0.1) with C/D ratios ≦ 0.6.

439

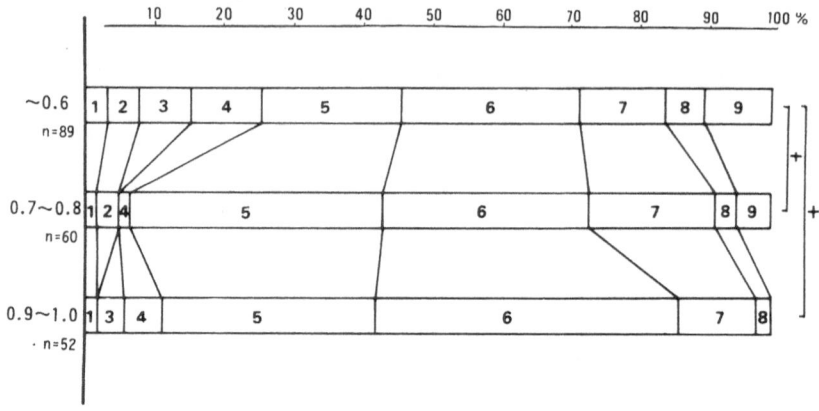

Fig. 6. Visual field recovery by C/D: ΔS (I-3).

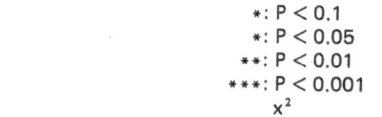

*: P < 0.1
*: P < 0.05
**: P < 0.01
***: P < 0.001
x^2

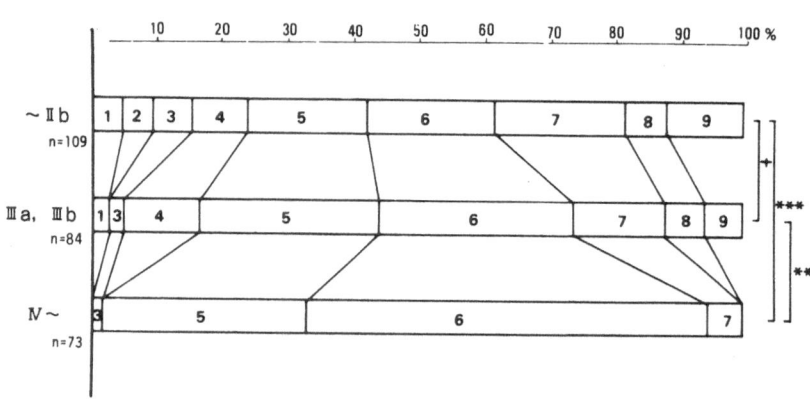

Fig. 7. Visual field recovery by disease stage: ΔS (I-3).

(7) Visual field recovery by disease stage:
The distribution of visual field recovery range in Isopter I_3 in each of the 3 stages (early stages of Stage IIb or less according to Kosaki's Classification, middle stages of IIIa and IIIb, and terminal stages of IV or more) was analyzed and represented by bar graphs in Fig. 7. Changes in the visual field were greater (P < 0.001) in the early stages than in the middle and terminal stages.

440

DISCUSSION

There have been several attempts to follow clinical progress by making quantitative assessments of visual fields. Esterman (1, 2) presented a method, in which the visual field was divided into a network. Each section of the network was given a different weighting, and thus, the visual field defect in the center was expressed as greater damage than that of the same area in the periphery.

In Fisher's method (7), the visual field was shown as the product of the number of longitude lines and degrees of latitude. In visual fields of 40° or less, for example, the normal value was defined as 960, that is, the product of 24 lines of longitude and 40° of latitude. If there was any visual field defect, the number of longitude lines equivalent to the length of the defect was counted, and the residual visual field was expressed as the difference between the total number of longitude lines minus the number of lines, corresponding to the defect, and the total number of lines, as a percentage. In this method, again, the defect in the center was shown as greater damage than that in the periphery even if the area of the defect was the same.

Another method is the use of Kosaki's Classification of Disease Stages by Visual Fields (5). However, this method was developed for diagnosis of disease stages, based on kinetic Goldmann perimetry. Since the disease was in only 10 stages, it was too rought to follow clinical progress of visual fields, and minor changes could not be detected.

The method of expressing the visual field in volume by assuming that the visual field is a three dimensional island seemed to be rational, and we presented a method based on this concept (6). However, calculations were slightly complicated, and most importantly, changes in the central visual field not accurately reflected in the figures.

The isopter area method (3) which we used in the present study is very easy to use, becasue all calculations are made by a computer. All values are automatically related to normal standard values. Objective assessment is possible with this isopter area computation, even minor changes are detectable, and statistical analysis is readily made as shown by the results of the present study.

REFERENCES

1. Esterman, B. Grid for scoring visual fields, I. Tangent Screen. Arch. Ophth., 77: 780–786 (1967).
2. Esterman, B. Grid for scoring visual fields, II. Perimeter. Arch. Ophth., 79: 400–406 (1968).
3. Kosaki, H. and Nakatani, H. Computer analysis of kinetic field data determined with a Goldmann perimeter. Doc. Ophthalmol. Proc. Series 35: 473–477 (1983).
4. Kosaki, H. and Higashitarumizu, K. Normal kinetic visual field topography of the Japanese by Goldmann Perimeter. 1st Japanese Perimetric Society Symposium. Tokyo, 14 December, (1980).
5. Kosaki, H., Nakatani, H., Tsukamoto, H. and Nakauchi, M. Topographical studies of field defects in various stages of perimetry chronic glaucoma. Doc. Ophthalmol. Proc. Series 14: 121–130 (1977).

6. Kosaki, H. and Nakatani, H. A New method for numerical expression of visual field. Acta Soc. Ophthalm. Jap., 78 (11): 1202–1207 (1974).
7. Smith, R.J.H. Medical versus surgical therapy in glaucoma simplex. Brit. Ophth., 56: 277–283 (1972).

Author's address:
H. Kosaki
Kosaki Eye Hospital,
1-15-10 Hannan-Cho, Abeno-Ku,
Osaka 545, Japan

A COMPARISON OF CONTRAST SENSITIVITY FUNCTION AND FIELD LOSS IN GLAUCOMA

V.J. MARMION

(*Bristol, UK*)

ABSTRACT

Contrast sensitivity function was measured in 27 patients with early glaucomatous visual field defects and 6 patients with ocular hypertension. Defects were found at 3.2 and 6.4 cycles per degree and to a lesser extent at 0.2 cycles per degree as measured by the Arden Gratings. The error score produced by these defects was compared with the percentage reduction in the visual field and macular threshold. This suggests that contrast sensitivity function loss is an early defect in open angle glaucoma.

INTRODUCTION

The Arden Plates provide a specific series of spatial contrast sensitivity gratings which permit a measurement of the contrast sensitivity function. The range is limited at the higher end to 6.4 cycles per degree, (cpd). It is suitable for clinical practise and should be particularly helpful as a screening technique in glaucoma. (Arden 1978). The relationship between this measurement of spatial contrast sensivity function and other quantified standard measurements of visual impairment in glaucoma could be particularly interesting as indicated by Bodis-Wollner (1980). The work of Atkin et al. and Tyler does not clearly separate the effect of flicker or look at a range of spatial frequencies. This should be a pre-requesite before determining which is the optimum level for further investigation in depth. The comparison of a precise measurement achieved by contrast sensitivity function should be paralleled by a precise level of visual field loss. Recently developed computer programmes, Dallas 1984, permit the quantification of field loss. The present study of a group of glaucomatous subjects has been designed to clarify the relationship between age, intraocular pressure, field loss and the special contrast sensitivity function as measured by the Arden Plates.

MATERIALS AND METHODS

Twenty seven subjects with proven open angle glaucoma were studied. Eyes with an acuity of less than 6/9 N5 were excluded as were those with opacities

Heijl, A. and Greve, E.L. (eds.), Proceedings of the 6th Int. Visual Field Symposium.
© 1985, Dr W. Junk Publishers, Dordrecht, The Netherlands. ISBN 978-94-010-8932-6

Table 1. Grating contrast sensitivity levels.

Cyl/Deg	0.2	0.4	0.8	1.6	3.2	6.4
Normal data mean age 35	11.5	10.0	11.5	11.5	10.0	9.0
30 normal subjects mean age 35	9.0	8.5	10.0	9.5	9.5	8.75
Open angle glaucoma	14.4	12.8	15.3	15.9	18.1	23.2
	+2.2	+1.5	+2.0	+2.5	+4.3	+5.5
Ocular hypertension	13.8	12.0	14.1	14.8	17.8	21.5
	+1.8	+1.9	+1.0	0.6	4.8	+6.4

Table 2. Relationship with intraocular pressure.

I.O.P.	> 22	22–25	26–29	30 +
% Field loss	40%	23%	11%	29%
M.T.	15	13	20	12
Arden grating score	17	17.5	14.3	14.2
	SD 2.4	SD 1.7	SD 0.7	SD 0.7

Table 3. Field loss and contrast sensitivity.

Scale of loss	100–80	79–60	59–40	<40	OHT
% Glaucoma field loss	8%	27%	49%	63%	Nil
M.T.	17.8	13.9	14	12.5	14.8
Arden grating score	15.9	19.1	18.6	16.5	15.3

Table 4. Age correlation.

Age	>59	60–69	70–79	80 +
% Glaucoma field loss	21%	29%	43%	38%
	18.3	15.4	15.4	11.5
Macular threshold	SD 1.8	SD 1.8	SD 2.6	SD 4.1
	15.6	16.2	16.3	18.8
Arden grating score	SD 1.6	SD 1.4	SD 2.3	SD 1.6

in the media. Therefore, thirty-six eyes were available for comparison. Six subjects with ocular hypertension were studied. This group comprises twelve eyes. All measurements were made while off treatment or before treatment had started. The intraocular pressure levels used were those recorded at the time of diagnosis – the first out-patient visit. Friedmann fields were estimated from above threshold and the threshold for each eye was determined centrally at the start of the examination. The computer programme for the Friedmann visual fields estimates the depth and area of the defects found at steps of four units below the threshold. The macular threshold was determined using the standard procedure.

The Arden Plates were viewed at a distance of 57 cm with an illumination of one hundred foot candles and the full plate was exposed over a period of 15 sec. The total score to the individual plates were calculated. The total score for the six plates for individual eyes were summated and then averaged to produce a composite score.

All examinations of the Arden Plates and the visual field, as measured by the Friedmann Analyser Mark II were undertaken with the optimum optical correction and were performed in mid-afternoon.

The results of the spatial contrast sensitivity grating examination indicate clearly a significantly lower contrast sensitivity for the finest pattern in the glaucomatous subjects. The reverse of the trend observed in normal subjects. A similar trend was noted in ocular hypertension. (Table 1).

A comparison between the percentage visual field loss, macular threshold and spatial contrast grating sensitivity in relation to the intraocular pressure revealed no clearcut correlation between these three parameters. (Table 2). The degree of field loss correlated quite well with the level of macular threshold. The relationship between field loss and the contrast grating scores was the reverse of that anticipated. (Table 3). In this table it can be seen that ocular hypertension provides a distinct group.

A close correlation exists between age and all three parameters as demonstrated by Table 4.

DISCUSSION

Previous reports, (Atkin 1979 and 1980, Tyler 1981, and Bodis Wollner 1982), have concentrated more on the temporal than the spatial element of grating sensitivity and their results should be compared with those obtained from plate 5 of the Arden tests, the point at which the variation from normal is becoming most apparant. A moderate variability was noted in Plate 2 the closest proximity to normal occurred with plate 3 and it was in this particular sector that the most uniformity appeared. The overall pattern of results corresponds with the findings of Arden and Jacobson and, like theirs, shows a divergence from the normal score commencing at Plate 5.

The absence of a clear relationship between the intraocular pressure level and any of the three parameters measured suggest that elevated pressure per se, is not responsible for the defects observed. This concurs with the observation of Atkin 1979 and 1980. The report of Tyler indicates, in only four cases a difference between the eye with greater pressure and its fellow eye, and this is a peripheral loss at a particular temporal frequency. In this report the field loss is not quantified.

The work of Arden and Jacobson indicates that sensivity for the fine gratings is likely to deteriorate with age and the results from this study would support this observation. Age alone does not explain the marked overall change which existed and it will be noted that at 0.2 cpd there was quite a marked variability.

A difference does exist between those patients with field loss of minimal degree and those with more than 20% field loss. This could suggest that once the disease has reached an established stage deterioration in spatial contrast sensitivity is to be expected and further studies during the course of the disease in individual patients is indicated.

ACKNOWLEDGEMENT

This work has been considerably facilitated by the availability of the computerised visual fields made available by courtesy of Mr. N.L. Dallas.

REFERENCES

Arden, G.B. and Jacobson, J.J. A simple grating test for contrast sensitivity. Preliminary results indicate value in screening for glaucoma. Invest. Ophthalmol. Visual Sci. 17: 23 (1978).

Atkin, A., Bodis-Wollner, I., Wolkstein, M., Moss, A. and Podos, S. Abnormalities of central contrast sensitivity in glaucoma. Amer. J. Ophthal. 88: 205–211 (1979).

Atkin, A. Wolkstein, M., Bodis-Wollner, I., Anders, M., Kels, B. and Podos, S.M. Intraocular comparison of contrast sensitivities in glaucoma patients and suspects. Brit. J. Ophthal. 66: 11, 858–862 (1980).

Bodis-Wollner, I. and Camisa, J.M. Contrast sensitivity measurement in clinical diagnosis. Neuro-Ophthal. A series of critical surveys of the international literature. Vol. 1 (1980).

Bodis-Wollner, I. Methodological aspects of contrast sensitivity measurements in the diagnosis of optic neuropathy and maculopathy. Documenta Ophth. Proc. Series 35: 225–237 (1983).

Dallas, N.L. Computerised Visual Field Analysis in Glaucoma. European Congress in Ophthalmology, Helsinki (1984).

Author's address:
73 Pembroke Road,
Bristol
England, UK

RESPONSE OF MACULAR CAPILLARY BLOOD FLOW TO CHANGES IN INTRAOCULAR PRESSURE AS MEASURED BY THE BLUE FIELD SIMULATION TECHNIQUE

BENNO PETRIG, ELLIOT B. WERNER, CHARLES E. RIVA and
JUAN GRUNWALD

(*Philadelphia, USA*)

ABSTRACT

The effect of induced elevations of intraocular pressure on the velocity of the leukocytes in the macular capillaries was studied in six normal subjects using a suction cup to elevate the intraocular pressure (IOP). Subjects were studied over a range of intraocular pressures from baseline to 45 mm Hg. The velocity of the leukocytes was measured using a computer simulation of the Blue Field Entoptic Phenomenon. The subjects compared and matched the speed of simulated particles displayed on a CRT screen to that of their own entoptically perceived leukocytes.

In most subjects the velocity of the particles was maintained at or near baseline up to an IOP of about 30 mm Hg. Above this pressure the velocity fell in a linear fashion proportional to the IOP. The results indicate that the macular microcirculation is auto-regulated over a range of perfusion pressures, but that autoregulation fails to maintain baseline blood flow at intraocular pressures which are still well below diastolic retinal artery pressure. The blue field simulation technique may form the basis of a clinical test to evaluate autoregulation in glaucoma, vascular retinopathies, and other diseases. The blood supply of the eye is unique in that the intraocular blood vessels are subjected to a significant extrinsic hydrostatic pressure, the intraocular pressure (IOP). This tends to reduce the net perfusion pressure in the eye compared to other vascular beds. Despite this stress, however, the blood flow of the retina and optic nerve shows fairly efficient autoregulation over a wide range of perfusion pressures. A variety of techniques and animal models have demonstrated this (1–3, 5–8, 10, 11, 19, 20).

Studies of ocular blood flow autoregulation in humans are scarce due to the difficulties in studying blood flow using available non-invasive techniques. There have been attempts using fluorescein angiography (4), static perimetry (2) and the blue field entoptic phenomenon (BFE) (12–14, 16–18).

The development of the blue field simulation technique (15) now allows the measurement of the macular capillary blood flow in a quantitative fashion. We have studied the autoregulatory capacity of this microvascular bed in response to acute elevation of IOP.

Heijl, A. and Greve, E.L. (eds.), Proceedings of the 6th Int. Visual Field Symposium.
© *1985, Dr W. Junk Publishers, Dordrecht, The Netherlands. ISBN 978-94-010-8932-6*

Table 1. Ages of the six normal male subjects studied and the maximum IOP at which blood flow was autoregulated.

Subject	Age	IOP_{max}
1	27	32
2	32	30
3	38	31
4	45	29
5	32	25
6	29	31
Mean ± 1 S.D.	35.5 ± 5.8	29.2 ± 2.5

MATERIALS AND METHODS

Six healthy adult male subjects experienced in the technique volunteered for the experiment (Table 1). Each subject was placed in the blue field simulator so that he observed his own blue field entoptic phenomenon with his left eye and the simulator screen with the right eye. Shutters allowed the subject to alternately view either his own blue field entoptic particles or the particles on the simulation screen. Using knobs on a control panel, the subjects were asked to adjust the velocity, pulsatility and number of simulation screen particles as seen with the right eye until they matched the velocity, pulsatility and number of the entoptically perceived particles of the left eye.

A computer recorded the subjects' simulation screen setting and stored the results. At the beginning of each experimental session, the subject made 5 baseline adjustments. The brachial blood pressure was measured. The baseline intraocular pressure and all subsequent IOP readings were measured using a Goldmann applanation tonometer. The intraocular pressure in the left eye was elevated to a predetermined level using a suction cup applied to the sclera near the outer canthus (9).

The subject was then asked to make repeated measurements matching simulation screen particles to entoptically seen particles over a period of 12 to 15 minutes. Every 2 or 3 minutes, the intraocular pressure was measured and the suction on the scleral cup was increased as required to return the intraocular pressure to the predetermined level. In this way it was possible to make measurements at a fairly constant level of intraocular pressure.

Over the course of five experimental sessions performed by each subject, measurements were made over an IOP range of 20 to 45 mm Hg. The level of IOP at the beginning of each session was randomized and unknown to the subject.

RESULTS

Figure 1 shows the results for two of the subjects. The mean particle velocity is shown as a function of intraocular pressure. The velocity values have all been normalized to the baseline value so that baseline velocity is one.

448

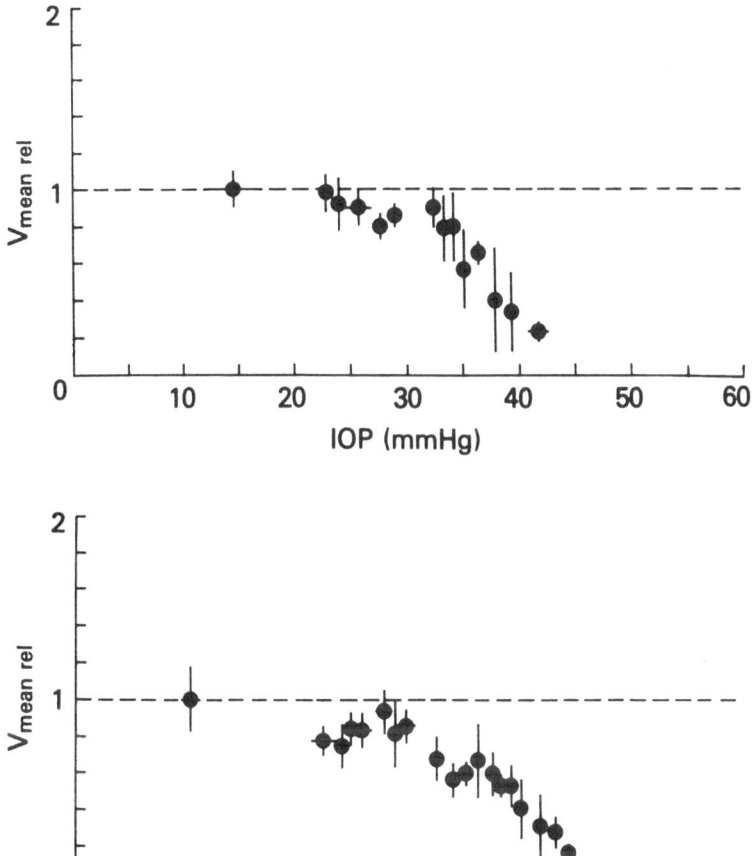

Fig. 1a and 1b. Results from two of the subjects. The mean relative particle velocity represents the mean velocity of the particles on the simulation screen, normalized to the baseline, as adjusted by the subject to match his own entoptically perceived leukocytes. A biphasic response is noted with blood flow as reflected by particle velocity remaining fairly constant at or near baseline until the autoregulation begins to fail at an IOP of 32 mm Hg for subject 1 (Figure 1a) and 30 mm Hg for subject 2 (Fig. 1b). Above this IOP, a linear decrease in blood flow is seen as IOP increases.

In each case a biphasic response is noted. At relatively low IOP's the simulation particle velocities remained at or near baseline, showing little tendency to decrease as IOP was raised. Above a certain IOP level, however, velocity tended to fall in a linear fashion as a function of increasing IOP. By visual inspection of the results, we estimated the maximum IOP (IOP$_{max}$) at which the system seemed to autoregulate. The results for the 6 subjects are shown in Table 1.

DISCUSSION

The blue field entoptic phenomenon (BFE) is generated by light passing through the leukocytes moving through the macular capillaries. The velocity of the particles seen against the blue background (wavelength 430 nanometer) reflects, therefore, the velocity of the blood flowing in the macular capillaries. Since retinal capillaries probably do not dilate or constrict, they behave like rigid tubes. Total blood flow in this bed, therefore, is proportional to the velocity and changes in blood flow will be directly reflected as changes in velocity, assuming no change in the number of perfused capillaries.

In our subjects, the maintenance of relatively constant velocities at levels of IOP above normal is evidence of autoregulation of blood flow in the macular microcirculation in the face of elevated IOP. At levels of IOP above IOP_{max}, however, the ability of the vascular bed to autoregulate is overcome and blood flow decreases as IOP is raised further.

The IOP at which this occurs in our normal subjects is about 30 mm Hg, a figure which agrees well with results reported by Riva, Sinclair and Grunwald (16) using a qualitative technique for estimating BFE particle velocity.

Animal studies of retinal blood flow have usually been interpreted as showing autoregulation over a wide range of IOP, nearly up to levels of diastolic retinal artery pressure (11, 19). Our study suggests, however, that the range of autoregulation in the macular micro-circulation is much more restricted and begins to break down at IOP levels well below diastolic retinal artery pressures.

In conclusion, the blue field entropic phenomenon can be used to demonstrate autoregulation of macular capillary blood flow in normal subjects and may prove useful to study the effects of disease on auto-regulation (19).

REFERENCES

1. Alm, A. and Bill, A. The oxygen supply to the retina. I. Effects of changes in intra-ocular and arterial blood pressures, and in arterial pO_2 and PCO_2 on the oxygen tension in the vitreous body of the cat. Acta. Physiol. Scand. 84: 261 (1972).
2. Alm, A. and Bill, A. The oxygen supply to the retina, II. Effects of high intraocular pressure and of increased arterial carbon dioxide tension on uveal and retinal blood flow in cats. A study with radioactively labelled microspheres including flow determinations in brain and some other tissues. Acta. Physiol. Scand. 84: 306 (1972).
3. Alm, A. and Bill, A. Ocular and optic nerve blood flow at normal and increased intraocular pressures in monkeys (Macaca irus): a study with radioactively labelled microspheres including flow determinations in brain and some other tissues. Exp. Eye Res. 15: 15 (1973).
4. Archer, D.B., Ernest, J.T. and Krill, A.E. Retinal, choroidal, and papillary circulations under conditions of induced ocular hypertension. Am. J. Ophthalmol. 73: 834 (1972).
5. Armaly, M.F. and Araki, M. Optic nerve circulation and ocular pressure: contribution of central retinal artery and short posterior ciliary arteries and the effect on oxygen tension. Inv. Ophthalmol. 14: 475 (1975).

6. Dollery, C.T., Henkind, P., Kohner, E.M. and Paterson, J.W. Effect of raised intra-ocular pressure on the retinal and choroidal circulation. Inv. Ophthalmol. 7: 191 (1968).
7. Ernest, J.T. Pathogenesis of glaucomatous optic nerve disease. Tr. Am. Ophth. Soc. 73: 366 (1975).
8. Ernest, J.T. Optic disk oxygen tension. Exp. Eye Res. 24: 271 (1977).
9. Ernest, J.T., Archer, D. and Krill, A.E. Ocular hypertension induced by scleral suction cup. Inv. Ophthalmol. 11: 29 (1972).
10. Ffytche, T.J., Bulpitt, C.J., Kohner, E.M., Archer, D. and Dollery, C.T. Effect of changes in intraocular pressure on the retinal microcirculation. Brit. J. Ophthalmol. 58: 514 (1974).
11. Geijer, C. and Bill, A. Effects of raised intraocular pressure on retinal, prelaminar, laminar and retrolaminar optic nerve blood flow in monkeys. Invest. Ophthalmol. Visual Sci. 18: 1030 (1979).
12. Riehm, E. and Podestá, H.H. Verhalten der retinalen Kapillardurchblutung bei Augeninnendrucksteigerungen. Adv. Ophthalmol. 29: 150 (1975).
13. Riehm, E., Podestá, H.H., and Bartsch, C.: Untersuchungen über die Durchblutung in Netzhautkapillaren bei intraokularen Drucksteigerungen. Ophthalmologica. 164: 249 (1972).
14. Riva, C.E. and Loebl, M.: Autoregulation of blood flow in the capillaries of the human macula. Invest. Ophthalmol. Visual Sci. 16: 568 (1977).
15. Riva, C.E. and Petrig, B. Blue field entoptic phenomenon and blood velocity in the retinal capillaries. J. Opt. Soc. Am. 70: 1234 (1980).
16. Riva, C.E., Sinclair, S.H. and Grunwald, J.E. Autoregulation of retinal circulation in response to decrease of perfusion pressure. Inv. Ophthalmol. Visual Sci. 21: 34 (1981).
17. Sinclair, S.H., Grunwald, J.E., Riva, C.E., Brunstein, S.N., Nichols, C.W. and Schwartz, S.S. Retinal vascular autoregulation in diabetes mellitus. Ophthalmol. 89: 748 (1982).
18. Sint, M., Riehm, E. and Podestá, H.H. Untersuchungen über die Beziehungen der zentralen kapillaren Retinadurchblutung zur Augendruckhöhe bei Glaukom-patienten mit hilfe der entoptisch sichtbaren Blutbewegung. Klin. Mbl. Augenheilk. 171: 743 (1977).
19. Sossi, N. and Anderson, D.R.: Effect of elevated intraocular pressure on blood flow. Occurrence in cat optic nerve head studied with Iodoantipyrine I 125. Arch. Ophthalmol. 101: 98 (1983).
20. Weiter, J.J., Schachar, R.A. and Ernest, J.T. Control of intraocular blood flow. I. Intraocular pressure. Inv. Ophthalmol. 12: 327 (1973).

Author's address:
Department of Ophthalmology,
Scheie Eye Institute,
University of Pennsylvania,
Philadelphia,
PA 19104, USA

EARLY MACULAR DAMAGE IN GLAUCOMA AND SUSPECTED GLAUCOMA PATIENTS

A. POLIZZI, E. GANDOLFO, N. GRILLO and G. CALABRIA

(*Genoa, Italy*)

ABSTRACT

Ten glaucoma and 16 suspected glaucoma patients were examined by traditional kinetic perimetry, automated kinetic-static glaucoma screening (Perikon), and threshold-related static perimetry (Peritest). In these patients macular recovery after photostress was tested by Goldmann-Weekers adaptometry, and colour discrimination was tested by Farnsworth 100 hue and Panel D 15. Ten normal subjects were examined as controls.

The results of the macular function tests in both glaucoma and suspected glaucoma patients were significantly different from those of the normals. In patients with glaucoma or ocular hypertension (IOP > 24 mmHg) the macular function appeared disturbed in a significantly higher percentage than in normal subjects. The correlation between visual field changes and macular function alterations is discussed.

INTRODUCTION

Early alterations of macular function in suspected glaucoma patients have been recently reported by several authors. In particular modifications in spatial contrast sensitivity (2, 10) and chromatic sense (1, 3, 4, 7–9) have been described. Such alterations in macular function have been seen when perimetric defects were not demonstrable by traditional Goldmann perimetry.

With the aim of demonstrating eventual macular functional damage in glaucoma and suspected glaucoma patients, we carried out the macular recovery test after photostress using the Goldmann-Weekers adaptometer and examined chromatic sense with the Farnsworth 100 hue and Panel D 15 tests. We then compared these results with those of traditional Goldmann perimetry, automatic perimetry 'Genoa glaucoma screening' program (PERIKON) (5, 12) and automatic static perimetry (PERITEST) (6).

Heijl, A. and Greve, E.L. (eds.), Proceedings of the 6th Int. Visual Field Symposium.
© *1985, Dr W. Junk Publishers, Dordrecht, The Netherlands. ISBN 978-94-010-8932-6*

MATERIALS AND METHODS

16 suspected glaucoma patients, averaging 47 years of age (34–63), 10 patients with open angle glaucoma, averaging 40 years of age (37–55), and 10 subjects without ophthalmological diseases whose ages ranged from 40 to 50 were examined. All the patients had natural or corrected 20/20 visual acuity.

The untreated suspected glaucoma patients had intraocular pressures ranging from 20 to 24 mmHg. Glaucomatous patients, under Timolol maleate therapy, and tonometric values varying from 18 to 21 mmHg.

The optic discs examined under mydriasis by direct ophthalmoscopy and Goldmann's contact lens revealed, in suspected glaucomatous patients, minor morphological alterations: increased C/D ratio $\geqslant 0.6$, baring of the circumlinear vessels and margin anomalies in 12 eyes (40%). In glaucomatous patients disc examination revealed typical early glaucomatous damage in all cases.

Macular recovery after photostress

We followed the methods proposed by Zingirian et al. (11) using a Goldmann-Weekers adaptometer, provided with a special Snellen chart, under mesopic illumination (0.30 asb).

After a 5' adaptation at 2100 asb, the time required by the patient to reach his best mesopic visual acuity was evaluated with a stopwatch. After another period of 5' at 2100 asb, macular photostress was performed with a lamp (125 asb) for 60 seconds, and the time that the patient needed to reach his best mesopic visual acuity was again measured. Each eye (20/20 V.A.) was corrected for near vision and had a mesopic visual acuity of 8/20.

Macular recovery time is the difference (in seconds) between the time needed to read the chart, before and after macular photostress.

Chromatic tests

Chromatic sense was examined by the Farnsworth 100 hue and Panel D 15 tests. For the Panel D 15 test box n°2 from the Lantony-Munsell test was used.

The patients were examined in binocular vision and standard illumination conditions.

Perimetric methods

The following techniques were used:
— traditional perimetric examination with the Goldmann perimeter (kinetic method: 4 isopters), performed with the aim of early detection of glaucomatous defects;
— static-kinetic examination, specific for demonstrating glaucomatous alterations (Genoa glaucoma screening program), using the automated Goldmann perimeter 'Perikon';

454

— over-threshold static, automatic, computerized perimetry with 'Peritest'.

RESULTS

The average macular recovery times were:
— 134.18 seconds (SD 56.44) in suspected glaucoma patients (30 eyes)
— 211.24 seconds (SD 38.50) in glaucomatous patients (17 eyes)
— 70.12 seconds (SD 32.40) in normal subjects (20 eyes).
The average total score for the Farnsworth 100 hue was the following:
— 299.34 (SD 63.20) in suspected glaucoma patients
— 322.75 (SD 60.22) in glaucomatous patients
— 230.17 (SD 50.21) in normal subjects.
Most of the errors were localized along the tritan axis. The Panel D 15 test revealed:
— tritan axis errors in 60% of suspected glaucoma patients
— tritan axis errors in 80% of glaucomatous patients (in these patients other axis errors were present in 40% of the cases)
— normal subjects never showed tritan axis errors.
In suspected glaucoma patients:
— traditional kinetic Goldmann perimetry revealed early glaucomatous alterations in 5 eyes (18.6%)
— Perikon examination showed typical glaucomatous defects in 18 eyes (60.3%)
— Peritest examination revealed visual field defects in 10 eyes (33.3%).
In glaucomatous patients, all three perimetric methods revealed visual field defects with the same degree of sensitivity. True glaucomatous visual field alterations were found in 80% of the patients.

DISCUSSION

Macular recovery time and colour test score were found to be different in glaucomatous and suspected glaucoma patients, when compared with normal subjects. Statistical analysis was significant for the macular recovery time ($P < 0.01$) and Panel D 15 errors ($P < 0.001$) and less significant for the total Farnsworth 100 hue score ($P < 0.05$).

Macular recovery time and colour tests responses in suspected glaucomatous patients did not differ significantly from those found in open angle glaucoma patients ($P = N.S.$). The prolonged macular recovery time and the tritan axis alterations in the majority of cases were associated with early perimetric alterations, in particular those revealed by PERIKON.

Minimal alterations of macular sensitivity seem to precede the typical perimetric visual field defects, when traditional kinetic Goldmann perimetry is used.

Although the tests used in our study specifically analyse the macular function, we do not think that our results are due to elective lesions of the macula, in agreement with Drance (3). Our findings may represent a sign of widespread depression of the overall retinal sensitivity, more easily evaluated at the macular level.

In our opinion the extended visual acuity preservation, showed by traditional methods in glaucomatous patients, does not disagree with our finding concerning early alterations of macular function in suspected and glaucomatous patients. It is possible that ocular hypertension itself can cause metabolic stress of retinal cells.

CONCLUSION

The results of our research at present indicate that in the screening of patients with ocular hypertension with a risk of developing glaucomatous damage, macular function tests, together with sophisticated perimetric techniques, can be used early in high risk detection patients.

REFERENCES

1. Adams, A.J., Radic, R., Husted, R. and Stamper, R. Spectral sensitivity and color discrimination changes in glaucoma and, suspected glaucoma patients. Invest. Ophthalmol. Sci. October: 516–584 (1982).
2. Atkin, A., Bodis-Wollner, I., Wolkstein, M., Moss, A. and Podos, S. Abnormalities of central contrast sensitivity in glaucoma. Am. J. Ophthalmol. 88: 205–211 (1979).
3. Drance, S.M., Lakowski, R., Schulzer, M. and Douglas, G.R. Acquired color vision changes in glaucoma. Arch. Ophthalmol. 99: 829–831 (1981).
4. Fishman, G.A., Krill, A.E. and Fishman, M. Acquired color defects in patients with open angle glaucoma and ocular hypertension. Mod. Probl. Ophthalmol. 13: 335–338 (Karger, Basel) (1974).
5. Gandolfo, E., Zingirian, M. and Capris, P. Computerized perimetric program for detection of early glaucomatous defects. Doc. Ophthalmol. Proc. in press.
6. Greve, E.L. and Dannheim, F. The Peritest, a new automatic perimeter. Int. Ophthalmol. 5: 201 (1982).
7. Lakowski, R., Bryett, J. and Drance, S.M. A study of colour vision in ocular hypertensives. Canad. J. Ophthalmol. 7: 86–95 (1972).
8. Marmion, V.J. The colour deficiency in open angle glaucoma. Mod. Probl. Ophthalmol. 19: 305–307 (Karger, Basel) (1978).
9. Poinoosawmy, D., Nagasubramanian, S. and Gloster, J. Colour vision in patients with chronic simple glaucoma and ocular hypertension. Brit. J. Ophthalmol. 64: 852–857 (1980).
10. Tagami, Y., Onuma, T., Mizokami, K. and Isayama, Y. Comparison of spatial contrast sensitivity with visual field in optic neuropathy and glaucoma. Doc. Ophthalmol. Proc. Series 26: 147–153 (1981).
11. Zingirian, M., Castellazzo, R. and Trillo, M. Il test del recupero maculare dopo abbagliamento nei soggetti normali. Standardizzazione del metodo. Boll. Oculist. 47: 833–848 (1968).
12. Zingirian, M., Gandolfo, E. and Orciuolo, M. Automation of the Goldmann perimeter. Doc. Ophthalmol. Proc. 35: 381–385 (1983).

Author's address:
Dott. A. Polizzi,
Department of Ophthalmology,
University of Genova,
Viale Benedetto XV, n°5,
16132 Genova, Italy

FUNDUS PERIMETRY AND OCTOPUS PERIMETRY FOR THE EVALUATION OF NERVE FIBER LAYER DEFECTS

KIYOSHI OKUBO and KUNIYOSHI MIZOKAMI

(*Kobe, Japan*)

ABSTRACT

Octopus F2 program and fundus perimetry were applied to evaluate visual sensitivity in nerve fiber layer defects of primary open angle glaucoma, low tension glaucoma and anterior ischemic optic neuropathy.

Some different patterns among the types or size of nerve fiber layer defect were detected. In diffuse atrophy, the depressed area extended to the optic disc while in wedge defects the abnormal areas are located within the area of NFLD, not extending to the optic disc. Around a scotoma the gradient was steep at the macular side, gradual at peripheral side. The uncertain area where the response was 0 dB in one of two measurements ranged from 0.5 to 1.0 degree around the scotoma. This indicates there are some influences of miniature eye movements even though high resolution projection perimetry was employed.

INTRODUCTION

A retinal nerve fiber layer defect (NFLD) is one of the most important signs of optic nerve diseases, such as glaucoma and anterior ischemic optic neuropathy. Various types of NFLDs can be seen clinically and depressed sensitivity is usually found in these NFLD using kinetic or static projection perimetry (2, 3, 7). However, sometimes no functional depression is detected in spite of the presence of a NFLD (8).

On the other hand, it is very difficult to make an accurate correlation between the depressed visual sensitivity detected by projection perimetry and the exact anatomical lesion on the fundus. This difficulty disturbs detailed analysis of functional impairments occompanied with NFLDs.

In this study, we applied the Octopus F2 program (1) for the detection and high resolution measurement of depression in visual sensitivity, and kinetic fundus perimetry, Quantitative Maculometry (4), for exact determination of the location in the fundus of the detected depressions. Based on these results, correlations between visual sensitivity and nerve fibre layer defect is various conditions were analysed.

Heijl, A. and Greve, E.L. (eds.), Proceedings of the 6th Int. Visual Field Symposium.
© *1985, Dr W. Junk Publishers, Dordrecht, The Netherlands. ISBN 978-94-010-8932-6*

Table 1. Cases and their types of NFLD

Case 1	POAG	26 M	R superior wedge-shaped
			L superior wedge-shaped and inferior slit-like
Case 2	POAG	69M	L inferior slit-like
Case 3	POAG	59M	L superior slit-like
Case 4	POAG	73M	R inferior wedge-shaped
			L inferior wedge-shaped
Case 5	LTG	65F	R inferior wedge-shaped
			L superior and inferior wedge-shaped
Case 7	LTG	39F	R inferior wedge-shaped ~ diffuse
Case 8	LTG	56F	R inferior wedge-shaped
			L superior and inferior wedge-shaped
Case 9	PION	54M	L superior slit-like
Case 10	PION	59M	R superior diffuse

MATERIALS AND METHODS

Four cases (7 eyes) of early stage perimary open angle glaucoma (POAG), 4 cases (6 eyes) of low tension glaucoma (LTG) and 2 cases (2 eyes) of anterior ischemic optic neuropathy (AION) with discernible NFLD were analysed.

Details of the conditions of NFLD, conformed to Hoyt et al. (3), were given in Table 1.

Black and white red-free NFL photographs using a Canon CF-60Z fundus camera with Kodak Wratten gelatin filter no. 58 were taken on all cases prior to perimetry. Octopus F2 program (1), which allows measurement of 31 linearly arrayed locations between two given points, was performed after testing with the 31 & 32 original program. Several lines of points were arranged to cross the corresponding NFLD discerned by photography. Quantitative Maculometry with dilated pupil (4) was performed kinetically under the following conditions; 198 asb. background illumination, 3, 19′ target and 1000 asb or 500 asb. test target brightness.

NFL photography, Octopus F2 program and Quantitative Maculometry were performed with interval of several days.

RESULTS

In this study, various types of NFLDs, such as slit-like NFLD, wedge-shaped NFLD and diffuse atrophy covering a quadrant were observed.

In *slit-like NFLDs*, the depressions of visual sensitivities were found at the distal portion far from blind spot (Cases 1L, 2, 3 and 9) (Fig. 1), while in diffuse atrophies covering one quadrant of the fundus (Cases 7 and 10) (Fig. 2), the deeply depressed areas extended to the blind spot from the distal depressed area. The depressed areas detected by Octopus F2 program and Quantitative Maculometry correlated well, and did not extend beyond the areas of the damaged NFL in diffuse atrophies.

In the cases of *wedge-shaped NFLD*, a shallower or no depression was

458

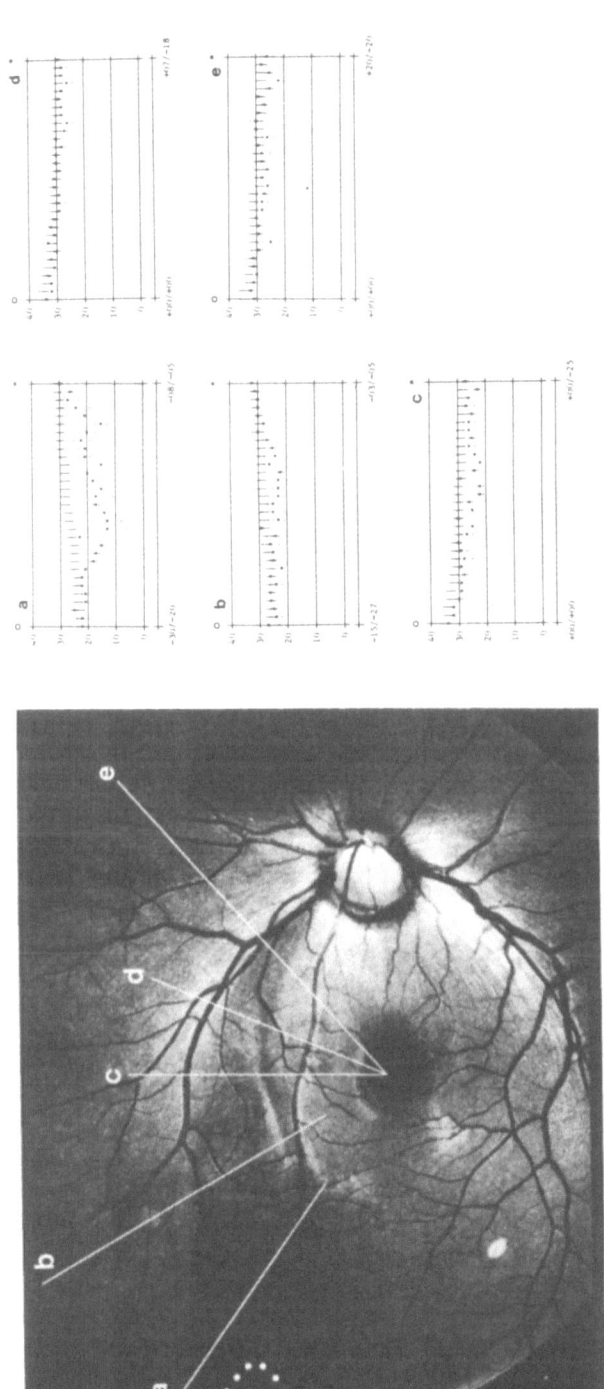

Fig. 1. Case 1 right eye. White and black circules indicate scotoma with 1000 asb and 500 asb respectively by Quantitative Maculometry. White bars (a–e) indicate examined lines using F2 program. Profiles on the right side.

459

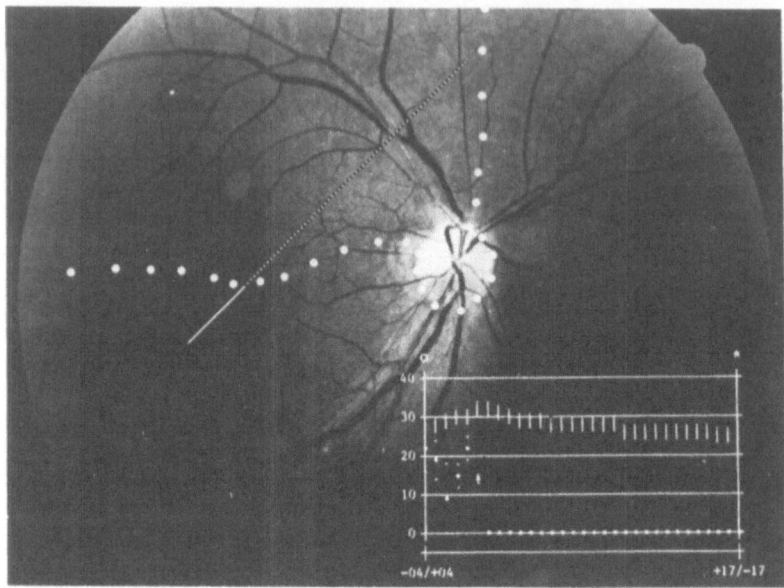

Fig. 2. Case 10. White circles indicate scotoma with 1000 asb using Quantitative Maculo-metry. White bar indicates examined F2 profile, dotted portion showed no response when tested twice.

detected near the blind spot, while deeper depressions were detected further away from blind spot (Figs. 3 and 4). The size of the depressed area defined by Quantitative Maculometry coincided well with that of the NFLD at distal portion of the NFLD. Near the blind spot the depression was smaller than NFLD.

The border of the deeply depressed area determined by Quantitative Maculometry completely coincided with the macular side margin of the NFLD at distally, but toward the optic disc the border dislocated inward of the margin of NFLD (Figs. 1, 3 and 4). In the Octopus F2 profiles, there were areas of uncertain visual sensitivy of about 0.5–1.0 degrees between areas with normal response and deeply depressed areas at macular side margin of the NFLD, (Figs. 3a–c, 4a–c). At the peripheral side margin of the NFLD, which was difficult to discern photographically, visual sensitivity fluctuated widely, gradually merging into the normal sensitivity area (Figs. 3a–c, 4a–d). At the distal portions of deeply depressed areas, actual profiles revealed mild depression of visual sensitivity within the NFLD.

DISCUSSION

Hoyt et al. (3) classified the NFLD, as follows; (1) slit-like (2) wedge-shaped (3) diffuse atrophy (4) total atrophy. The NFLD may occur with various optic nerve diseases and the type of functional impairment accompanying NFLD is supposed to be different according to its cause.

In our material, no differences of functional impairment were found between POAG, LTG and AION, but differences were found between different types of NFLDs. The functional impairment was influenced by the size of the NFLD but not by the cause of the NFLD.

On the other hand, for analysing the functional impairment accompanied with NFLD, it is very important to determine the accuracy of the correspondance of the fundus location and the test point of projection perimetry. A fully computerized automatic perimeter, Octopus, which allows to measure 0.2 degree resolution in F2 program, provides the highest resolution and reliability in all projecting type perimeters, available at present. But even using a high resolution method, it is very difficult to accurately determine the location in the fundus of the functional impairment and of the test target, when using projection perimetry. Kinetic fundus perimetry, Quantitative Maculometry, which can monitor the fundus directly and allows accurate positioning of the test target on the fundus was first applied to juvenile glaucoma cases with slit-like NFLD in our previous report (6).

In this study, we could find some differences between results obtained by Octopus F2 program and Quantitative Maculometry. The border detected by Quantitative Maculometry corresponded well to the macular side margin of NFLD, while Octopus F2 program provided some uncertain area, where measured the response was 0 dB in one of two measurements (0.5–1.0 degree between deeply depressed area and normal area at the macular side margin of NFLD). Maruo (4) reported about the possibility of minute eye movements ranging about 1.0 degree during fixation. Thus, there is possible influence of minute eye movements and there still remains some discordance of at least 0.5–1.0 degrees between retinal location and test point in projecting perimetry.

At the peripheral side and distal portion of the NFLD the fluctuating area, which accompanied the shallow depression measured by Octopus F2 program, was broader and gradually continued into the areas of normal sensitivity.

Red-free photography and ophthalmoscopy usually reveal the well demarcated macular side margin of NFLD while the peripheral and distal side is obscure. This is considered to be caused by the differences of density and thickness of nerve fibers. The visual sensitivities in the peripheral and distal portions of NFLD measured by Octopus F2 program indicate the presence of damaged and undamaged nerve fibers within NFLD.

In the present study, Quantitative Maculometry could determine the border of deeply depressed area but it was difficult to measure the shallower depression of visual sensitivity. Fundus perimetry would be clinically much more useful in the evaluation of less damaged NFL if brightness and illumination could be varied.

ACKNOWLEDGEMENTS

Our thanks are due to Prof. Dr. Y. Isayama and Dr. Y. Tagami for their valuable advice.

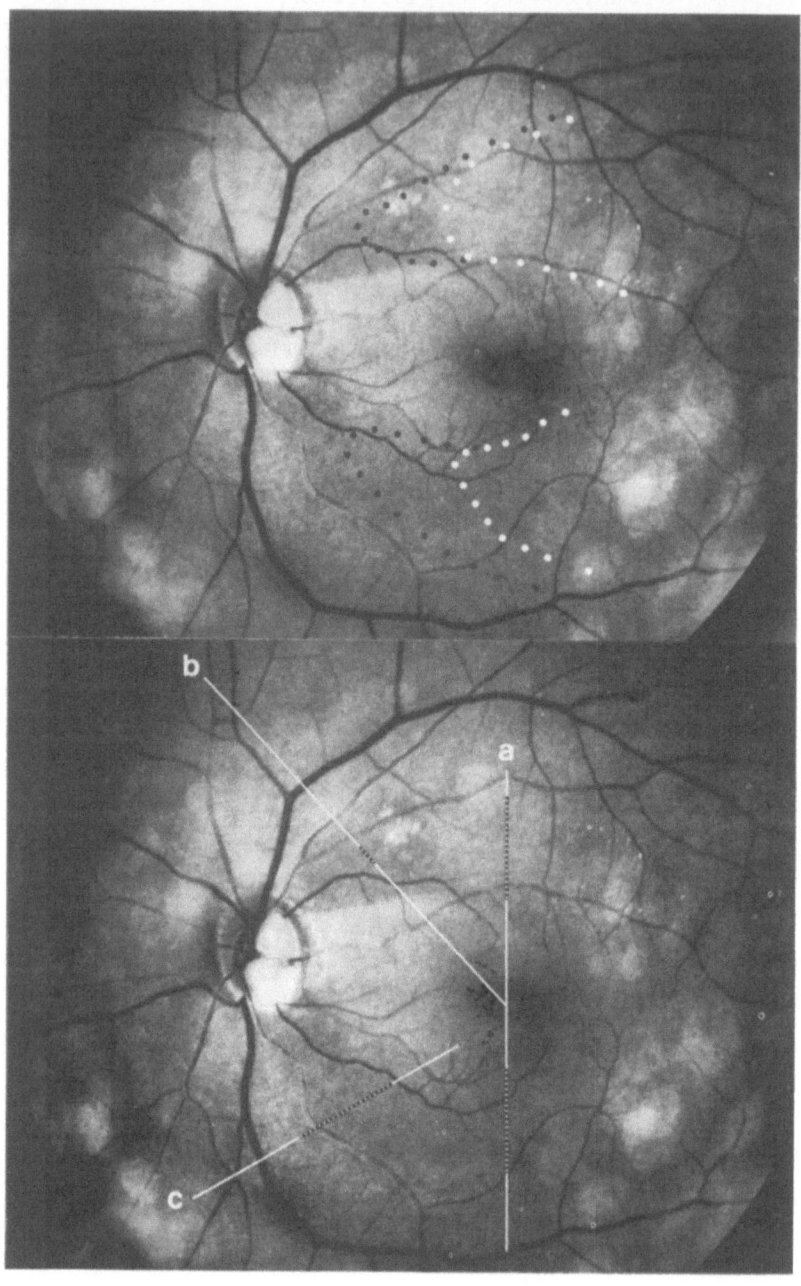

Fig. 3. Case 6. White and black circles indicate scotoma with 1000 asb, 500 asb respectively using Quantitative Maculometry. White bars (a–c) indicate by F2 profiles, dotted portion showed no response when tested twice. Actual profiles on the right side.

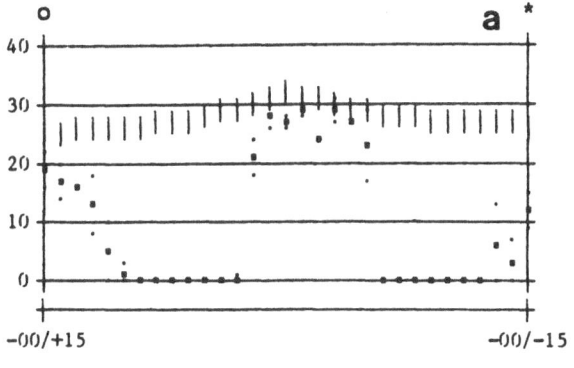

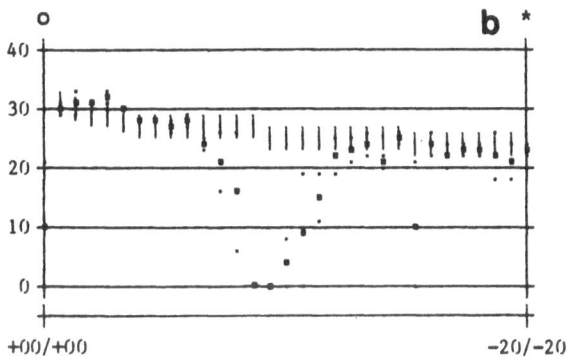

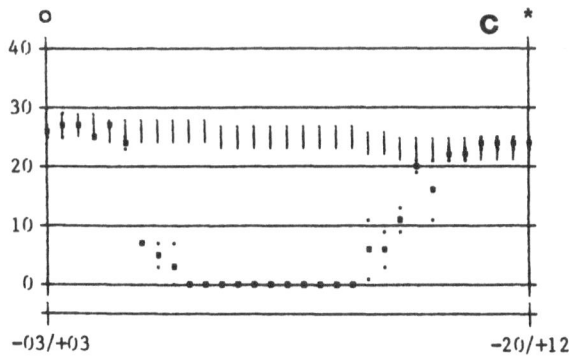

Fig. 3. Continued.

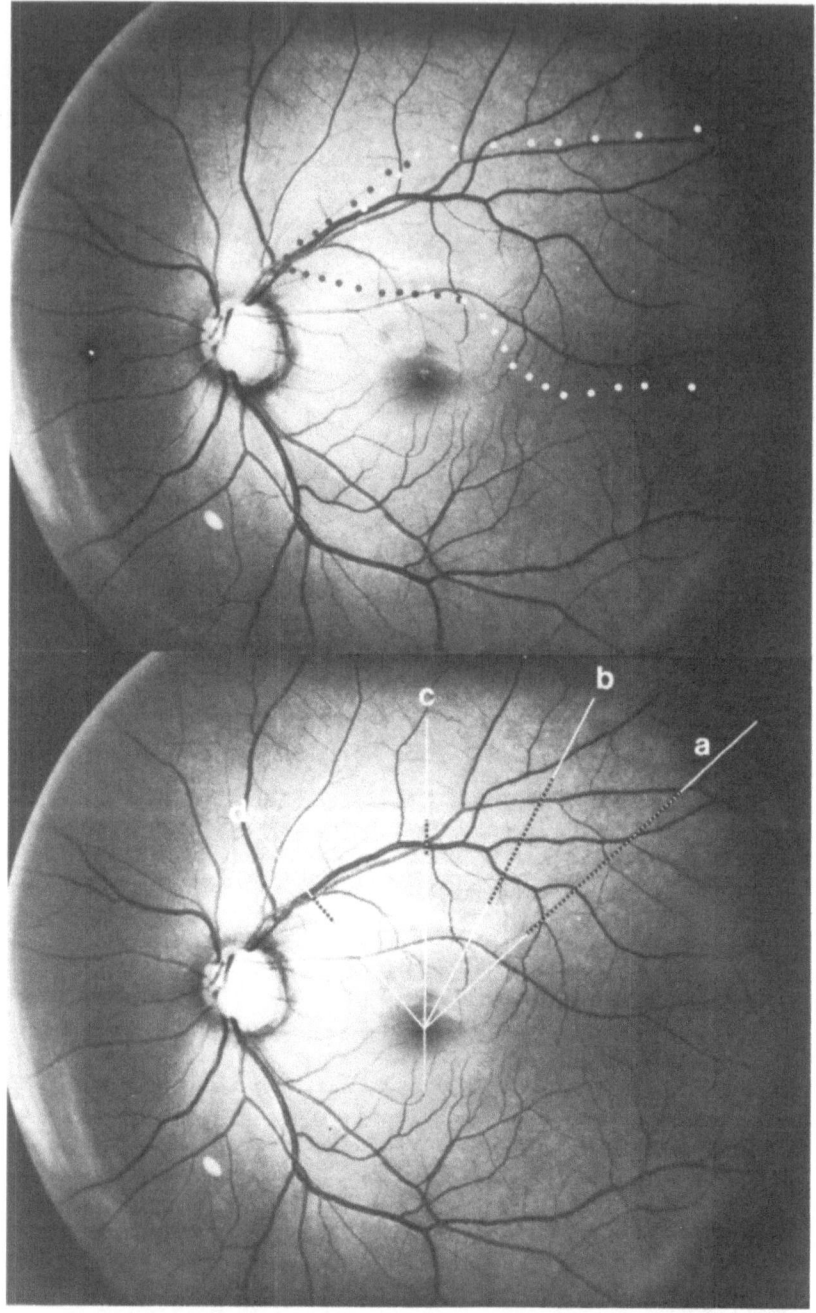

Fig. 4. Case 10. White and black circles indicate scotoma with 1000 asb, 500 asb respectively using Quantitative Maculometry. White bars (a–d) indicate F2 profiles, dotted portion showed no response when tested twice. Actual profiles on the right side.

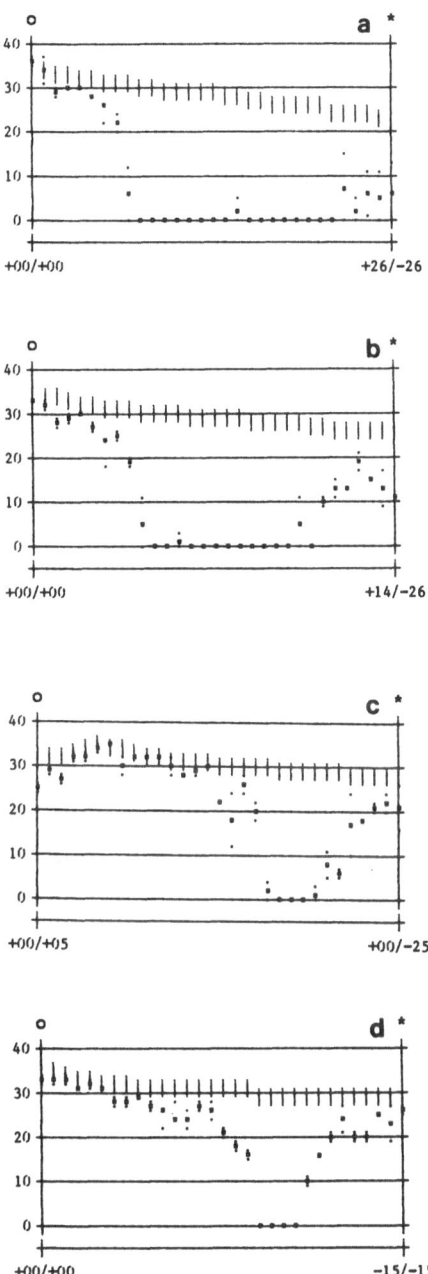

Fig. 4. Continued.

REFERENCES

1. Fankhauser, F., Haberlin, H. and Jenni, A. Octopus program SAPRO and F: Two new principles for the analysis of the visual field. Albrecht Graefes Arch. Klin. exp. Ophthalmol. 216: 155–165 (1981).
2. Heijl, A. and Airaksinen, P.J. Correlation between computerized perimetry and retinal nerve fiber layer photography after optic disc hemorrhage. Doc. Ophthalmol. Proc. Series. 35: 19–25 (1983).
3. Hoyt, W.F., Frisen, L. and Newman, N.N. Funduscopy of nerve fiber layer defects in glaucoma. Invest. Ophthalmol. 12: 814–824 (1973).
4. Isayama, Y. and Tagami, Y. Quantitative maculometry using a new instrument in cases of optic neuropathies. Doc. Ophthalmol. Proc. Series. 17: 237–242 (1977).
5. Maruo. T. The pattern of miniature eye movements made by normal persons during binocular fixation. Acta Soc. Ophthalmol. Jpn. 84: 2113–2120 (1980).
6. Mizokami, K., Tagami, T. and Isayama, Y. The reversibility of visual field defects in the juvenile glaucoma cases. Docum. Ophthal. Proc. Series, 19: 241–246 (1979).
7. Quigley, H.A., Miller, N.R. and George, T. Clinical evaluation of nerve fiber layer atrophy as an indicator of glaucomatous optic nerve damage. Arch. Ophthalmol. 98: 1564–1571 (1980).
8. Sommer, A., Pollock, I. and Maumenee, A.E. Optic disc parameters and onset of glaucomatous field loss. I. Methods and progression changes in disc morphology. Arch. Ophthalmol., 97: 1444–1448 (1979).

Author's address:
Dept. of Ophthalmology
School of Medicine
Kobe University
Kusunoki-cho, 7-chome, Chuo-Ku,
Kobe 650
Japan

STUDIES OF DRUSEN OF THE OPTIC NERVE HEAD

A. CENTARO, G.L. SAVAGE, J.M. ENOCH and N. NEWMAN

(*Modena, Italy*)

ABSTRACT

The etiology of drusen of the optic nerve head has never been established conclusively. Likewise, the functional consequences of this condition are difficult to explain. In this study, we further define and localize these alterations in function by using fundus photoperimetry and quantitative layer-by-layer perimetry.

The photoperimetric technique has confirmed that visual field defects often occur in areas which do not correspond with ophthalmoscopically visible drusen. Although this lack of correspondence has previously been noted, it has never been documented with such a precise and immediate method as we have used. Furthermore, in three of six patients studied, moderate to marked time-dependent losses in sensitivity have been found. The others demonstrate stable areas of visual loss expressed as enlarged blind spots and/or nerve fiber bundle anomalies.

Layer-by-layer perimetric analyses (as evolved in this laboratory) of areas within or adjacent to visual field defects, reveal abnormal inner retinal function in selected patients. These and other quantitative tests facilitate the localization of functional visual loss to retinal and/or optic pathway sites.

INTRODUCTION

The functional consequences of drusen of the optic nerve head (ONH) are poorly understood. For instance, it has never been explained why visual field defects typically occur in areas that do not correspond to ophthalmoscopically visible drusen. Damage to central nervous system axons, such as those of the optic nerve, produces retrograde as well as orthograde degeneration. Anatomical evidence of retrograde degeneration caused by ONH drusen has been observed by careful direct ophthalmoscopy and fundus photography of the retinal nerve fiber layer using red-free light (6). However, the functional extent of retrograde and orthograde degeneration has yet to be ascertained.

In this study we have attempted to further define and localize these alterations in visual function. We have utilized a fundus photoperimetric

Heijl, A. and Greve, E.L. (eds.), Proceedings of the 6th Int. Visual Field Symposium.
© *1985, Dr W. Junk Publishers, Dordrecht, The Netherlands. ISBN 978-94-010-8932-6*

technique allowing correlation between observed ONH drusen and field changes. Also, layer-by-layer perimetry (as evolved in this laboratory) has enhanced localization of anomalous responses. Sample data are provided here. A more complete report will be presented elsewhere.

MATERIALS AND METHODS

All subjects were given a thorough conventional eye examination including refraction. The Canon Fundus Photo Perimeter (model CPP-1) and Goldmann perimeter (Haag-Streit) were utilized to document sensitivity across the visual field. The Canon instrument enables the perimetrist to observe the patient's fundus and fixational stability on an infrared T.V. monitor while testing the patient. Since both the fundus image and the perimetric result can be photographed simultaneously, a very precise and immediate comparison is possible. The white background is standardly set at a luminance of 10 apostilbs. The test target size was set at the equivalent of a Goldman I and target luminance can be varied from 0.1 to 1000 apostilbs. Although the 45 degree fundus camera can be used in some patients without dilation, we found the photography easier if the patient was dilated with 1% Mydriacyl. Because the background luminance of the Canon instrument is less than one-third that of the standard Goldmann setting (10 vs. 31.5 asb), only qualitative comparisons are made in this study. Note that 10 apostilbs is actually the same luminance as the background of the Harms-Aulhorn Tubingen perimeter.

The Flashing Repeat Static Test (F.R.S.T.) is easily performed on the Goldmann perimeter. Prior to testing, the patient is instructed to close his eyes for five minutes. Upon opening the eye to be tested (the other eye being patched), static thresholds are measured repeatedly (from non-seeing to just detection) every 15 to 20 seconds at the same point in the visual field for a period of five minutes. Normal subjects show reasonably stable thresholds wih a typical loss of sensitivity of less than about 0.25 log units. Pathology affecting the optic nerve, i.e. the ganglion cell axons beyond the lamina cribrosa, may produce major losses of sensitivity. Such an abnormal response, which is often found in demyelinating disease such as multiple sclerosis, has been termed a visual fatigue or saturation-like effect (1, 3).

The Transient-like Function reflects the status of cells bordering on the inner plexiform layer. Likewise, the Sustained-like Function has been shown to be abnormal in disease processes which affect the inner and/or outer plexiform layers. These techniques have been described in detail previously (1, 3). Although the apparatus for these tests has been miniaturized into an attachment for the Goldmann perimeter (Haag-Streit), the results presented in this paper were obtained using a full scale apparatus.

RESULTS

Six patients were studied whose only known ophthalmic disorder was ONH drusen. Five of these showed ophthalmoscopically visible drusen, but the

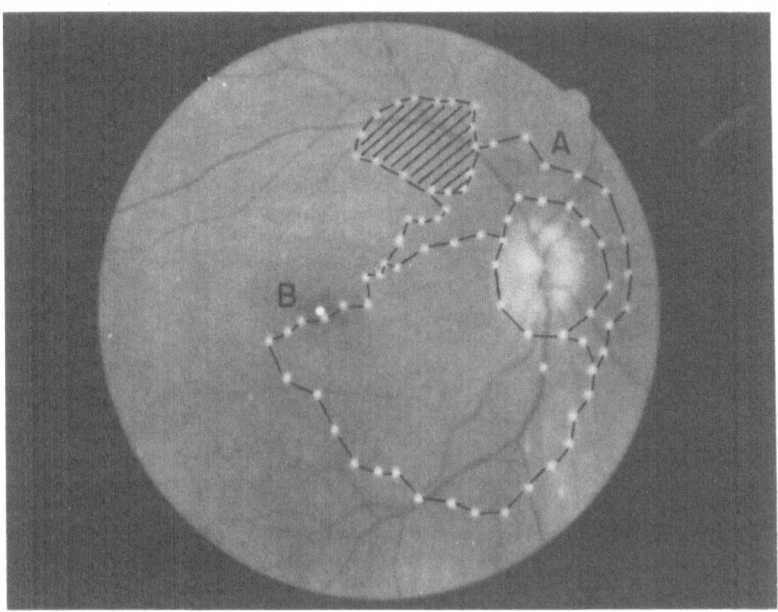

Fig. 1. Fundus photoperimetry on the right eye of patient E.W. Goldmann equivalents for the two isopters were: A = I/2e, B = I/2b. Note that isopter A demonstrated a mildly enlarged blind spot, revealed a relative scotoma (hatched area), and included all of isopter B.

remaining subject required ultrasound to verify the diagnosis. All patients demonstrated enlarged blind spots including the one with 'buried' drusen. Four of the six subjects had nerve fiber bundle defects confirmed by fundus photoperimetry which showed no particular relationship to visible disc drusen. For example, in Fig. 1 patient E.W. shows drusen on the nasal portion of the disc. However, the field loss corresponds to ganglion cell axons passing through the temporal part of the disc.

Half of our patients were shown to have abnormal results on the Flashing Repeat Static Test. Please see Fig. 2 which shows a graph of F.R.S.T. data for patient C.B. Note that the static threshold for the test point at 4 degrees eccentricity on the 135 degrees half meridian fluctuates only slightly; after five minutes, the sensitivity is virtually the same as at the start of the test. But at 15 degrees on the 255 degree half meridian, the patient was unable to see the test target at the highest luminance (4e) even though four minutes prior the 2c luminance was visible. This represents a decrease in sensitivity of *more than* 1.20 log units.

In three of four patients tested, markedly subnormal Transient-like Functions were recorded. Two of these three also showed reduced Sustained-like Functions. Figure 3 shows both functions for patient M.P. at abnormal and normal (control) points. In this patient the Sustained-like Functions are normal at both locations, but the Transient-like Function is almost non-existent at 3 degrees on the 210 degree half meridian. Figure 4 shows the

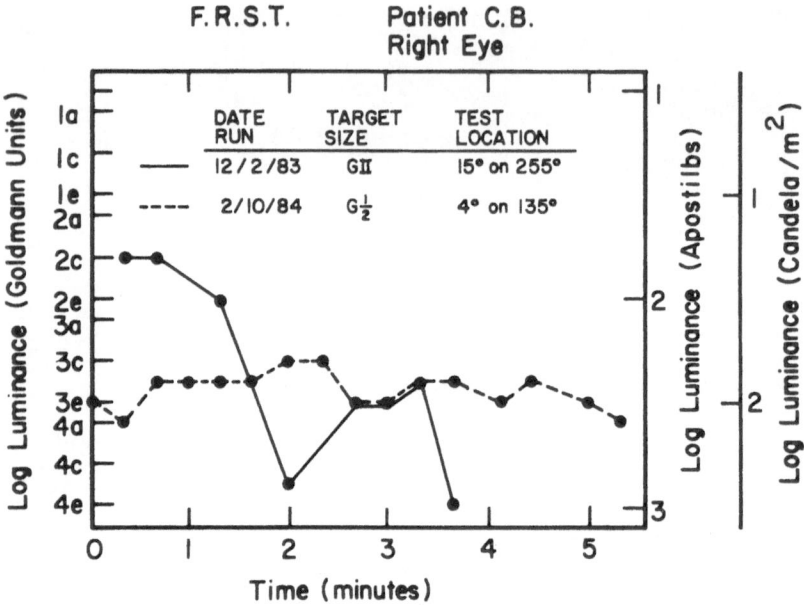

Fig. 2. The results of the Flashing Repeat Static Test for the right eye of patient C.B. At 4 degrees on the 135 degree half meridian, the static threshold after five minutes was identical to the initial threshold. At 15 degrees on the 255 degree half meridian, the patient was unable to see even the highest target luminance (4e) after less than four minutes despite an initial threshold luminance of 3e (Goldmann equivalents).

findings for patient C.B. Compared to the control point (4 degrees on 210) at 4 degrees eccentricity on the 135 degree half meridian both the Transient-like and the Sustained-like Functions are clearly abnormal.

DISCUSSION

The results of fundus photoperimetry and Goldmann visual fields confirm the lack of correlation between visible drusen and areas of reduced sensitivity. This seems to support the view that ONH drusen deposits themselves often represent effects of the disease process rather than the direct cause of the field defects.

Half of our subjects showed abnormal F.R.S.T. results, most probably indicating abnormal nerve fiber function beyond the lamina cribrosa. Since axoplasmic flow is presumably compromised beyond this point (5), this finding might have been anticipated. One might suppose that in a practical sense these areas of time-dependent sensitivity loss could cause contrast to fade under photopic conditions. This correlates nicely with 'obscurations' reported by some drusen patients (4).

Since most eyes with ONH drusen show loss of the retinal nerve fiber

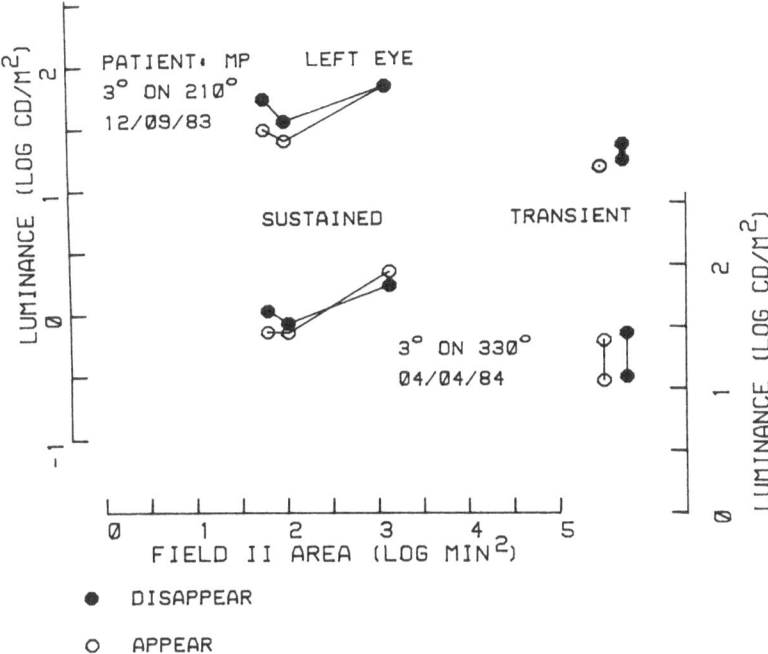

Fig. 3. Layer-by-layer perimetric findings for the left eye of patient M.P. at 3 degrees eccentricity. The sustained-like function is normal at both test points. The transient-like function, while within normal limits on the 330 degree half meridian, is almost completely attenuated on the 210 degree half meridian.

layer (vide ante), the discovery of an abnormal Transient-like Function in most of our patients and Sustained-like Function changes in some was expected. Recent evidence shows that damage to the overlying nerve fiber layer by juxtapapillary lesions can produce retrograde inner retinal dysfunction distal to the site of the lesion (2). Likewise in glaucoma, a disease whose direct effect is presumably in the region of the optic nerve head, similar functional anomalies of *the inner retina* have been found (1, 3).

The functional deficits of ONH drusen seem to correlate nicely with some of the neuroanatomical changes known to occur in this disease, except for the physical location of the visible drusen themselves. We plan to add other tests and more patients to our continuing study. The elucidation of the patho-physiological and anatomic changes associated with this condition, as revealed by psychophysics and other non-invasive techniques, may be of great value in understanding this and other diseases which affect the optic nerve head.

These data support the notion of two different sets of functional alterations occurring in anomalies of the nerve fiber bundle/optic nerve (1, 3). Similar effects have been show in radiation damage and in recent work by Enoch et al. (2). This unusual feature associated with optic nerve response needs further study and is important diagnostically.

471

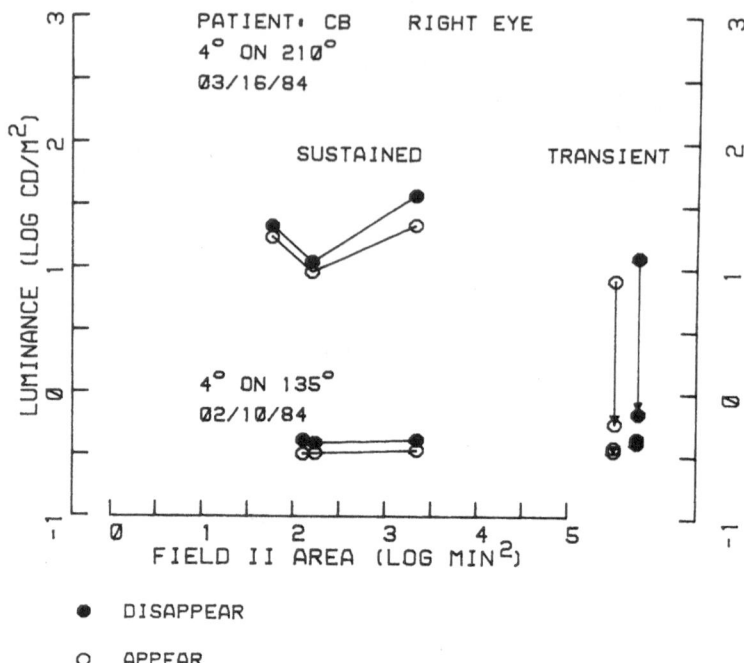

Fig. 4. Layer-by-layer perimetric results for the right eye of patient C.B. at 4 degrees eccentricity. Both sustained-like and transient-like functions are normal on the 210 degree half meridian and both functions are markedly abnormal on the 135 degree half meridian.

REFERENCES

1. Enoch, J.M. Quantitative layer-by-layer perimetry – Proctor Lecture. Invest. Ophthalmol. Vis. Sci. 17: 208–257 (1978).
2. Enoch, J.M., Essock, E.A., Williams, R.A. and Barricks, M. Functional visual effects of lesion located near the optic nerve head. Arch. Ophthalmol. (submitted 1984).
3. Enoch, J.M., Fitzgerald, C.R. and Campos, E.C. Quantitative Layer-by-Layer Perimetry, Grune and Stratton, Inc. New York (1981).
4. Lorentzen, S.E. Drusen of the optic disk – A clinical and genetic study. Acta Ophthalmol. Suppl. 90 (1966).
5. Spencer, W.H. Drusen of the optic disk and aberrant axoplasmic transport. Am. J. Ophthalmol. 85: 1–12 (1978).
6. Stevens, R.A. and Newman, N.M. Abnormal visual-evoked potentials from eyes with optic nerve head drusen. Am. J. Ophthalmol. 92: 857–862 (1981).

Author's address:
A. Centaro,
University of Modena,
Modena,
Italy

472

ABNORMAL INNER RETINAL FUNCTION IN GYRATE ATROPHY

JAMES O'DONNELL, MICHAEL FENDICK and JAY M. ENOCH

(*San Francisco, USA*)

ABSTRACT

Quantitative layer-by-layer perimetry provides a non-invasive, psychophysical means of evaluating the functional characteristics of human retina. By comparing the results obtained from normal, healthy subjects to those of patients exhibiting retinal abnormalities, insight may be gained into both the underlying pathophysiology of those abnormalities as well as their effects upon visual function.

Here, we report data obtained from a patient with gyrate atrophy of the retina and choroid. Evaluation of the spatial interaction properties of the fovea and two parafoveal areas of this patient's retina revealed a profound loss of spatial sensitization found in normal subjects. Testing performed at the same retinal locations, but using a stimulus which probed transient-like properties of the inner retina, revealed significant, though somewhat less dramatic deviations from normal. The foveal results showed no significant changes when retested 19 months after the initial evaluation. Thus, we conclude that this patient's visual loss was likely due to physiological effects whose influence was *not* limited to the outer retina, but included the inner retinal layer, as well.

Gyrate atrophy, first documented in 1888 by Jacobsohn (5), is a rare, (autosomal recessive) hereditary disease characterized by progressive degeneration of the choroid and retina. This degeneration begins in the outermost layers of the peripheral retina, slowly progressing, over the course of decades, towards the posterior pole (18). Ophthalmoscopy typically reveals sharply defined borders between the anatomically normal and atrophic retina (4). Yasuma et al. (21) using fundus photoperimetry, have recently demonstrated definite correspondence between these borders and the limits of visual field alterations in these patients. Other characteristic ophthalmic findings include night blindness, myopia, opacities of the lens and vitreous, and abnormal photoreceptor alignment (4), as well as abnormal EOG, ERG, and dark adaptation test results.

It has recently been established that gyrate atrophy is associated with a

Heijl, A. and Greve, E.L. (eds.), Proceedings of the 6th Int. Visual Field Symposium.
© *1985, Dr W. Junk Publishers, Dordrecht, The Netherlands. ISBN 978-94-010-8932-6*

deficiency of the mitochondrial matrix enzyme, L-ornithine: 2-oxiacid aminotransferase (OAT) (15, 17). Biochemical studies in which OAT deficiencies in cultured skin fibroblasts (8, 12–14, 19) and in transformed lymphocytes (7, 20) of gyrate atrophy patients have been demonstrated futher emphasize the systemic nature of the disease. Abnormalities have also been found in muscle (9, 10, 16), hair (6), and the EEG (10, 17), and in the structure of liver mitochondria obtained from human biopsies (1, 11).

Although observable fundus changes in the disease slowly progress from the mid-periphery towards the posterior pole, macular lesions are rarely found until quite late in the course of the disease, and the central 30° of visual field may be spared. Decreased visual acuity, however, may occur in the absence of observable macular abnormality, and the present study was undertaken to determine whether or not abnormal inner retinal function might account for some of this loss.

METHODS

Quantitative layer-by-layer perimetry consists of a battery of psychophysical tests designed to evaluate and distinguish between different aspects of human retinal function. Results of two of these tests are reported here. Both have been described elsewhere in considerable detail with respect to normal findings and those obtained from a variety of retinal abnormalities; therefore only a very brief review of the testing methods and normal results will be provided here. Readers desiring a more complete description are referred to the publications of Enoch (2) and Enoch et al. (3).

A 'sustained-like' response function, which reflects spatial interaction properties of the retina that are believed to be organized at the outer plexiform layer, is derived from responses of the patient to a small, flashing test spot superimposed upon larger, different sized, circular backgrounds. Having first measured the patient's threshold for detecting the test spot when presented alone upon a $10 \, cd/m^2$ evenly illuminated screen, the examiner then increases the test spot's luminance by 0.8 log units. Then, by successively superimposing upon the test spot each of three circular backgrounds whose sizes have been selected on the basis of extensive normative data, he proceeds to determine exactly how bright each background must be in order to lower the test spot's visibility to the level at which it can be just barely detected by the patient. Under such conditions, plotting these background luminance values as a function of background area invariably results in a V-shaped function when normal, healthy subjects are tested; the right-most arm of this function indicating the presence of sensitizing neural interactions known to exist in healthy vertebrate retinas. Anomalies of both the inner and outer plexiform layers cause characteristic alterations in the sustained-like function. Examples of normal findings of this test for each retinal location evaluated with our gyrate atrophy patient are shown by the dashed lines of Fig. 2.

By replacing the circular background with a windmill pattern and comparing the patient's sensitivity to the flashing test spot in the presence of

474

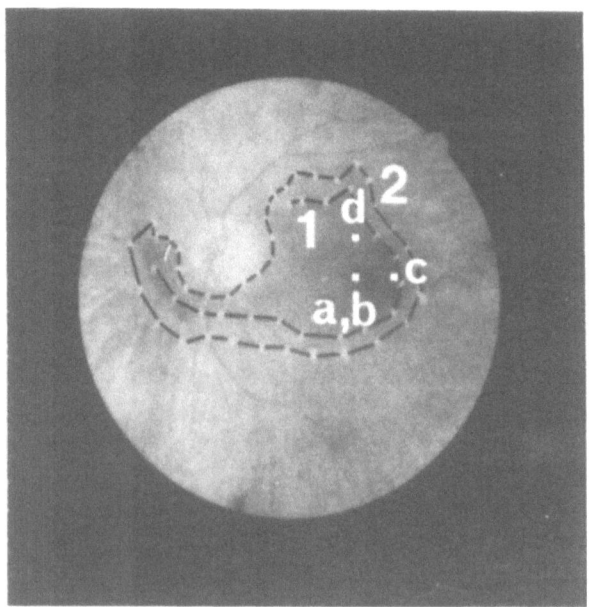

Fig. 1. Fundus photoperimetry (left eye) of the gyrate atrophy patient upon whom layer-by-layer perimetry was performed. Isopter '1' represents the limits of her visual field when plotted from non-seeing to seeing portions of the retina using a test stimulus corresponding to Goldmann I/4d against a 3.18 cd/m² background; isopter '2' was plotted from seeing-to-non-seeing areas under identical conditions. Points labeled a, b, c, and d mark the loci from which the corresponding layer-by-layer test results shown in Fig. 2 were obtained.

a rotating windmill as opposed to a stationary one, it is possible to assess the integrity of 'transient-like' properties of the inner retina. At the fovea, one typically finds that, to reduce an otherwise 0.8 log unit suprathreshold test spot to invisibility, a stationary windmill background needs to be about 0.4 log units brighter than a rotating one. In patients whose inner retina (more specifically, their inner plexiform layer) has been affected by retinal disease, either considerably less, or no such difference is found.

SUBJECT

The patient whom we tested is a 20 year old white female of Finnish ancestry whose best-corrected visual acuity was 20/100 (wearing $-4.50 + 1.25 \times 65°$) O.D., and 20/50 (with $-5.25 = + 1.25 \times 82°$) O.S. Her first complaints of decreased vision were at age 7 and there is no family history of consanguinity or ophthalmic disease. Apart from exhibiting blood plasma ornithine levels approximately 10 times that of normal subjects, other remarkable clinical findings included ophthalmoscopic evidence of gyrate atrophy, and abnormal electro-oculograms, electroretinograms, and dark adaptation curves. There

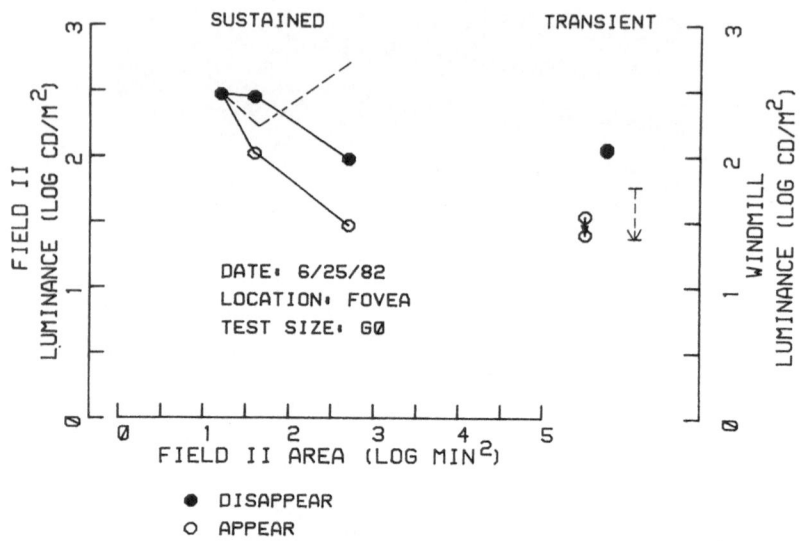

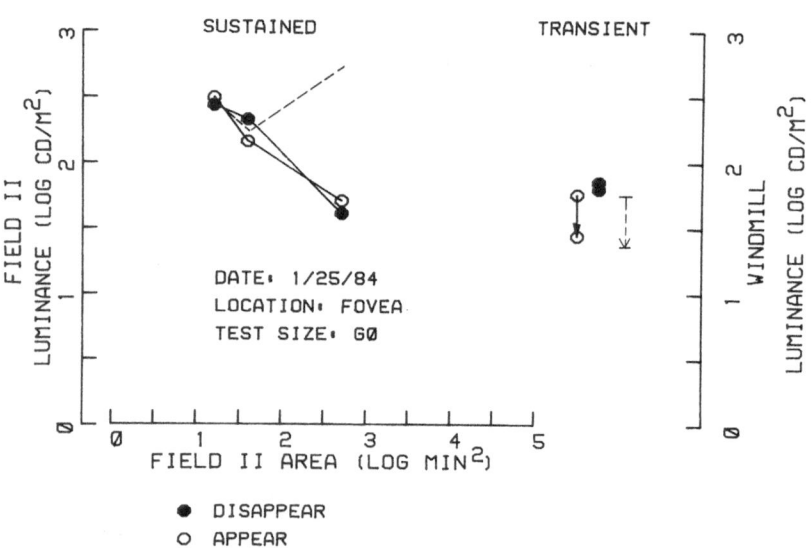

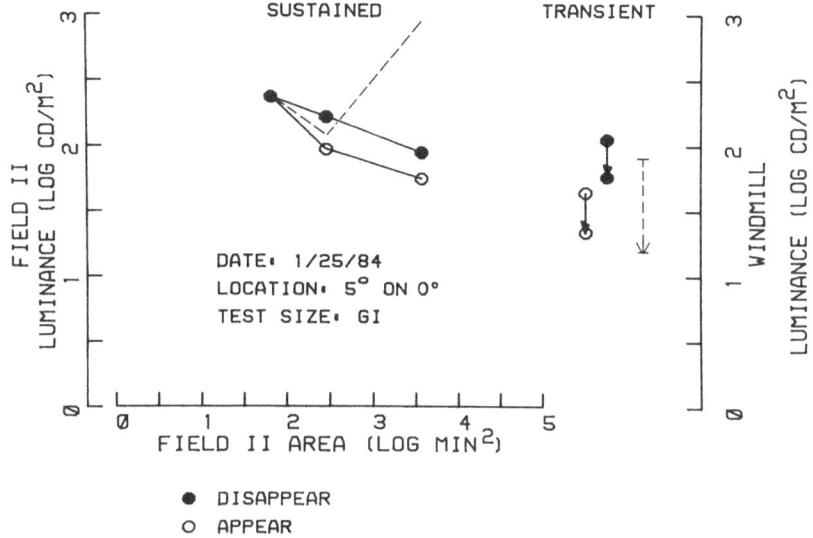

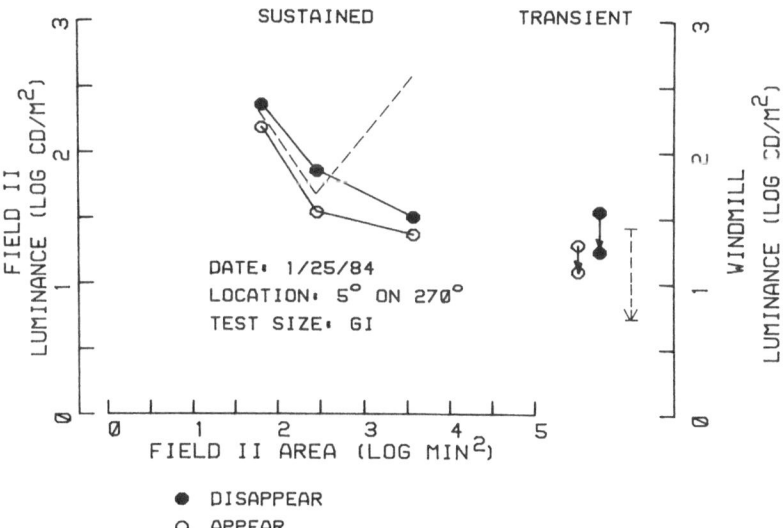

Fig. 2. Layer-by-layer perimetry test results obtained from the gyrate atrophy patient whose visual field is depicted in Fig. 1. Data obtained from testing a) at fixation in June, 1982; b) at fixation 19 months later, in January, 1983; c) 5 degrees nasal to fixation (1/83); 5 degrees superior to fixation (1/83). Dashed lines with each set of data depict typical results of normal subjects tested at the same retinal eccentricity. These have been shifted vertically on the graphs so as to facilitate comparison with our patient's data.

were only traces of cataracta complicata, bilaterally, and these were not sufficient to compromise the results of our evaluation.

RESULTS

Figure 1 is a fundus photograph of the patient's left eye on which is superimposed the limits of her visual field as measured on the Canon Fundus Photoperimeter (using a 3.18 cd/m² background with a test stimulus corresponding to Goldmann I/4d). Figure 2 depicts the results of the sustained-like and transient-like tests applied to the retinal locations marked a, b, c, and d on Fig. 1. Dashed lines in each panel depict the results obtained from normal subjects tested with stimuli presented at the same retinal eccentricities. The most remarkable characteristic of our patient's data is the obvious lack of any evidence of the normal surround sensitization response, suggesting inner retinal involvement in the disease process. Measures of the transient-like function reveal a diminished effect of windmill rotation upon the patient's sensitivity to a small, flashing, test spot, and thus provide additional evidence of abnormal inner retinal function.

The data obtained at fixation (Fig. 2a) were obtained on June 25, 1982, and Fig. 2b shows the results of retesting 19 months later, in January, 1984. No change in visual acuity was noted during this period and the two sets of data are essentially identical. Figs. 2c and 2d show the sustained-like and transient-like functions obtained with stimuli presented 5 degrees from fixation, projecting to the nasal and superior retina, respectively. Both indicate abnormalities of inner retinal function similar to those found at fixation.

DISCUSSION AND CONCLUSIONS

Visual system defects in gyrate atrophy generally have been thought to be restricted to the outer retina. The night blindness, and abnormalities of dark adaptation, EOG, ERG, and photoreceptor alignment that have been documented in affected patients all support the conclusion that the outer retina is indeed compromised. To our knowledge, this represents the first report of abnormal inner retinal function in a case of gyrate atrophy. Clearly, further study is indicated.

ACKNOWLEDGEMENTS

We would like to thank Edward A. Essock, Ph.D. and Rick A. Williams, Ph.D., both of whom have made significant contributions to this investigation.

REFERENCES

1. Arshinoff, S., McCulloch, J.C., Parker, J.A., Phillips, M.J. and Marliss, E.B. Ornithine (ORN) metabolism and liver pathology in hyperornithinaemia and gyrate atrophy of the choroid and retina (HOGA) (absract). Clin. Res. 25: 321A (1977).

2. Enoch, J.M. Quantitative layer-by-layer perimetry; Proctor Lecture. Invest. Ophthalmol. Vis. Sci. 17: 208–257 (1978).
3. Enoch, J.M., Fitzgerald, C.R., and Campos, E.C. Quantitative Layer-by-Layer Perimetry: An Extended Analysis. Grune and Stratton, Inc., New York, (1981).
4. Enoch, J.M., O'Donnell, J.J., Williams, R.A., and Essock, E.A. The relationship between observed retinal boundaries and the functional limit of vision in gyrate atrophy. Arch. Ophthalmol. (submitted).
5. Jacobson, E. Ein Fall von Retinitis pigentosa atypica. Klin. Monatsbl. Augenheilkd. 26: 202–206 (1888).
6. Kaiser-Kupfer, M.I., Kuwabara, T., Askanas, V., Brody, L., Takki, K., Dworestzky, I., and Engel, W.K. Systemic manifestations of gyrate atrophy of the choroid and retina. Ophthalmol. 88: 302–306 (1981).
7. Kaiser-Kupfer, M.I., Valle, D. and Del Valle, L.A. A specific enzyme defect in gyrate atrophy. Amer. J. Ophthalmol. 85: 200–204 (1978).
8. Kennaway, N.G., Weleber, R.G. and Buist, N.R.M. Gyrate atrophy of choroid and retina: Deficient activity of ornithine ketoacid aminotransferase in cultured skin fibroblasts. (correspondence) N. Engl. J. Med. 297: 1180 (1977).
9. Kennaway, N.G., Weleber, R.G. and Buist, N.R.M. Gyrate atrophy of the choroid and retina with hyperornithinemia: Biochemical and histologic studies and response to vitamin B$_6$. Amer. J. Hum. Genet. 32: 529–541 (1980).
10. McCulloch, C. and Marliss, E.B. Gyrate atrophy of the choroid and retina with hyperornithinemia. Am. J. Ophthalmol. 80: 1047–1057 (1975).
11. McCulloch, J.C., Arshinoff, S.A., Marliss, E.B. and Parker, J.A. Hyperornithinemia and gyrate atrophy of the choroid and retina. Ophthalmol. 85: 918–928 (1978).
12. O'Donnell, J.J., Sandman, R.P. and Martin, S.R. Deficient L-ornithine; 2-oxoacid aminotransferase activity in cultured fibroblasts from a patient with gyrate atrophy of the retina. Biochem. Biophys. Res. Commun. 79: 396–399 (1977).
13. Sengers, R.C.A., Trijbels, J.M.F., Brussaart, J.H. and Deutman, A.F. Gyrate atrophy of the choroid and retina and ornithine-detoacid aminotransferase deficiency (abstract) Pediat. Res. 10: 894 (1976).
14. Shih, V., Berson, E.L., Mandell, R. and Schmidt, S.Y. Ornithine ketoacid transaminase deficiency in gyrate atrophy of the choroid and retina. Am. J. Hum. Genet. 30: 174–179 (1978).
15. Simell, O. and Takki, K. Raised plasma ornithine and gyrate atrophy of the choroid and retina. Lancet 1: 1031 (1973).
16. Sipila, I., Simell, O., Rapola, J., Sainio, K. and Tuuteri, L. Gyrate atrophy of the choroid and retina with hyperornithinemia: tubular aggregates and type 2 fiber atrophy in muscle. Neurology 29: 996–1005 (1979).
17. Takki, K. Gyrate atrophy of the choroid and retina associated with hyperorni-thinaemia. Brit. J. Ophthalmol. 58: 3–23 (1974).
18. Takki, K.K. and Milton, R.C. The natural history of gyrate atrophy of the choroid and retina. Ophthalmol. 88: 292–301 (1981).
19. Trijbels, J.M.F., Sengers, R.C.A., Bakkeren, J.A.J.M., De Kort, A.F.M. and Deutman, A.F. L-ornithine-ketoacid-transaminase deficiency in cultured fibroblasts of a patient with hyperornithinaemia and gyrate atrophy of the choroid and retina. Clin. Chim. Acta 79: 371–377 (1977).
20. Valle, D., Kaiser-Kupfer, M.I. and Del Valle, L.A. Gyrate atrophy of the choroid and retina: Deficiency of ornithine aminotransferase in transformed lymphocytes. Proc. Natl. Acad. Sci. USA 74: 5159–5161 (1977).
21. Yasuma, Y., Hamer, R.D., Lakshminarayanan, V., Enoch, J.M. and O'Donnell, J.J. Directional sensitivity measured in a patient with gyrate atrophy: 1. Measurements in different parts of the remaining retina. Arch. Ophthalmol. (submitted).

Author's address:
James O'Donnell,
Department of Ophthalmology,
University of California,
San Francisco, CA, USA.

479

MEASUREMENT OF LAYER-BY-LAYER PERIMETRY RESPONSES USING DIRECT RETINAL PROJECTION BY THE SCANNING LASER OPHTHALMOSCOPE

ROBERT H. WEBB, EDWARD A. ESSOCK, JAY M. ENOCH and RICK A. WILLIAMS

(*Boston, USA*)

ABSTRACT

Two of the tests of layer-by-layer perimetry evaluate inner retinal function by measuring two types of local spatial interactions. The 'sustained-like' test (i.e., the 'sensitization effect') evaluates the effect of small concentric backgrounds on sensitivity to a small target. The 'transient-like' test evaluates the effect of introducing movement by rotating a windmill shaped background. Inner retinal anomalies can disrupt the normal spatial interactions measured by either of these tests. In the present applications of these tests, we take advantage of the simultaneous view of the retina and of the stimuli projected onto the retina provided by the Scanning Laser Ophthalmoscope (SLO). This method permits precise placement of test stimuli at desired retinal locations.

INTRODUCTION

The Scanning Laser Ophthalmoscope (SLO) and fundus camera/perimetric devices open a whole new era in the study of visual functions. These devices provide an immediate and referenceable correspondence between observed anatomical features and the non-invasive tests chosen for study. Here, we have applied the stimuli used in the quantitative layer-by-layer perimetry scheme (1) to the SLO developed at the Retina Foundation (3, 4). This allows far more effective control of each test and more meaningful response analysis relative to observed pathological lesions.

In this report we describe the initial results of the transfer of two layer-by-layer perimetric tests, to be described below, to the SLO. Responses measured on the SLO from a normal eye are virtually identical to previously reported results (1). Furthermore, the on-line view of the retina and visual stimuli that is provided by the SLO allows the direct observation of fixation stability (or instability) and generates an improved concept of the nature of the response obtained. Along these same lines, the relative sizes of the retinal areas contributing to a particular response at different degrees of eccentricity from fixation can be compared with visible retinal landmarks.

Heijl, A. and Greve, E.L. (eds.), Proceedings of the 6th Int. Visual Field Symposium.
© 1985, Dr W. Junk Publishers, Dordrecht, The Netherlands. ISBN 978-94-010-8932-6

In standard perimetry, simple light sense is quantitatively determined using a small spot of light (increment threshold). In tests of layer-by-layer perimetry (that is tests, each of which is specific to or biased towards a different layer of the visual system), a similar test spot is presented on carefully selected concentric backgrounds of different shapes and sizes. Two tests are used which evaluate the status of inner retinal function. In particular, the sustained-like test is a test of sensitization (5). In certain anomalies such as diabetic retinopathy, some cases of senile macular degeneration, and glaucoma, the sensitization by nearby backgrounds on increment threshold is lost. This test evaluates the status of inner and outer plexiform layer (IPL and OPL) function by determining whether this particular response has been disrupted locally. Similarly, in the transient-like test, a psychophysical effect of movement in a nearby background is evaluated. This response has been shown to be disrupted in cases of IPL layer anomoly. It was our goal in the present work to develop a means of presenting these special patterns to the eye for fundus perimetry using the SLO.

METHODS AND RESULTS

The experimenter begins the testing procedure by positioning the subject's eye by means of a forehead/chin rest. He/she then selects the retinal location to be tested by viewing an image of the retina with the stimulus on it. The eccentricity of the selected location is calculated automatically, along with the stimulus size appropriate for that test location. The threshold determination is then performed, also under computer control.

The sustained-like and transient-like tests require three stimulus fields: Field I is a small test probe flashed once per second for 150 msec. It is set to an intensity a criterion amount (usually 0.8 to 1.0 log units) above its increment threshold. Field II is a concentric background pedestal whose intensity is varied by the subject to bring the flashing test probe to threshold. Field III, a large outer background, is in this paradigm the raster used to illuminate the retina. The retinal illuminance of Field III ranged between 0.6 and 1.5 log trolands with a value of 1 log trolands typically selected for testing. The size of Field III (the raster) was 55 deg, 17 deg, or 19 deg depending on the magnification of the retinal image desired. The shape of Field II is a filled circle for the sustained-like test or radially-vaned pattern for the transient-like test. The size selected for these patterns is determined by retinal eccentricity (2). Figure 1 is an example of the video monitor image showing the stimulus configuration (large Field II disc background) for testing at 5 deg from fixation. Table 1 shows examples of the values used in the present study.

The sustained-like test consists of determing Field I threshold on a small, medium and large Field II. The transient-like test consists of determining this threshold on a static vaned pattern and on the same pattern rotating at about 8 on and off transitions per second. All thresholds, including the initial increment threshold obtained with Field II absent, were determined by a von Bekesey tracking procedure. The subject pressed a single button as long as the

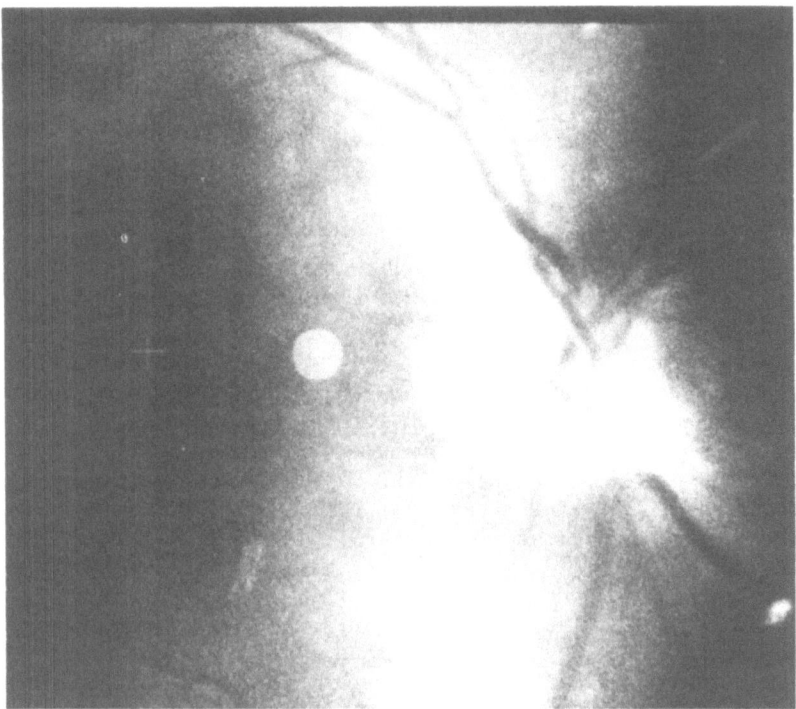

Fig. 1. SLO view of the retina and layer-by-layer stimulus as described in the text.

flashing test (Field I) was visible. Threshold was tracked with ascending and descending trials under computer control for a preset number of reversals (usually 6–8).

In a normal sustained-like test response, less light is required to bring the test spot (Field I) to threshold in the medium diameter Field II than in the large. The difference is typically as much as 1.5 log units, depending on eccentricity (1). In the transient-like test, a normal subject requires as much as one log unit less light in Field II when the vaned pattern is rotating than when it is static. Again this depends on eccentricity.

In anomalous cases, one or both of these effects are reduced or absent. The effects shown by normals with these raster-based stimuli are similar to those observed with the tangent-screen projection technique. An example of the results obtained from one of the five normals tested is shown in Fig. 2.

The Scanning Laser Ophthalmoscope presents a view of the retina as a television image. At the same time, the light falling on the retina may have computer-generated patterns impressed on it, so that psychophysical tests (such as perimetry) can be carried out at retinal loci identified – and observed – as they occur. A very weak laser beam (or beams, if a single color is to be avoided) is scanned over the retina at TV rates – fast enough so that pictures impressed on it appear to move smoothly, as they do on TV. Because the laser beam is so small, only about one mm of the eye's pupil is

Table 1.

Eccentricity = 2.5 deg			
Field I diam:	1.6 min		
Field II outer diam: Sustained-like:	4.8 min	11 min	40 min
Transient-like:			40 min
Eccentricity = 10 deg			
Field I diam:	19 min		
Field II outer diam: Sustained-like:	32 min	57 min	200 min
Transient-like:			200 min

used for its entrance. All the rest of the pupil is available for collection of light reflected or backscattered from the retina. Conventional ophthalmoscopes use the large area to get light into the eye, and must make do with the smaller area for viewing it. The inversion of exit and entrance pupils is what allows to SLO to function with so much less total light. The light emerging from the eye is detected by photomultiplier tubes (one for each laser color used) and processed as a TV signal for presentation. No true optical image is ever formed, and the electronic image is available for remote or group viewing, for videotape recording, or for computer processing.

The raster pattern falling on the patient's retina is just like that on a TV screen. So, by passing the beam through a modulator, the last beam can be turned on and off fast enough to put scenes on this view. Simple stimuli like perimetry dots and text require no more sophistication than normal computer graphics, but the stimuli of this study are animated and require 3 log units of gray scale. To achieve this, we have controlled the modulator with a graphics controller, supplied by Number Nine Computer Company, in an Apple IIe host. The controller allows storage of 250 000 picture elements (pixels) in 16 levels (4 bits). These 16 patterns may then be displayed with a modified analog 'palette' card as one of 4000 selectable intensities. We have, in fact, used only 256 intensities to map the modulator transport function onto 3 log units of optical intensity, with 0.025 log unit resolution. One memory level is used to store the fixation cross, another for Field III, and another for Field I. Twelve levels are used for 12 positions of the 4-bladed windmill pattern (Field II). Animation is achieved by strobing through these 12 patterns 350 times per second, so that the windmill appears to rotate at 7–8 on-off transitions per second. When Field II is a simple pattern only one level is needed. Again, any of the 256 intensities can be assigned to the pattern on display.

Calibration of the displayed intensity was possible without reliance on photometer of filter accuracy. Instead, we compared the photometer reading of N pixels illuminated at B intensity to the same reading when the number of pixels was $N + dN$ and the intensity was $B - dB$. Since we have 250 000 pixels available, this null technique made calibration to 0.025 log units simple and reliable. (The largest areal change is 13 984 pixels, and the smallest 14 pixels, though better precision is obtained by combining calibrations over smaller, overlapping ranges.)

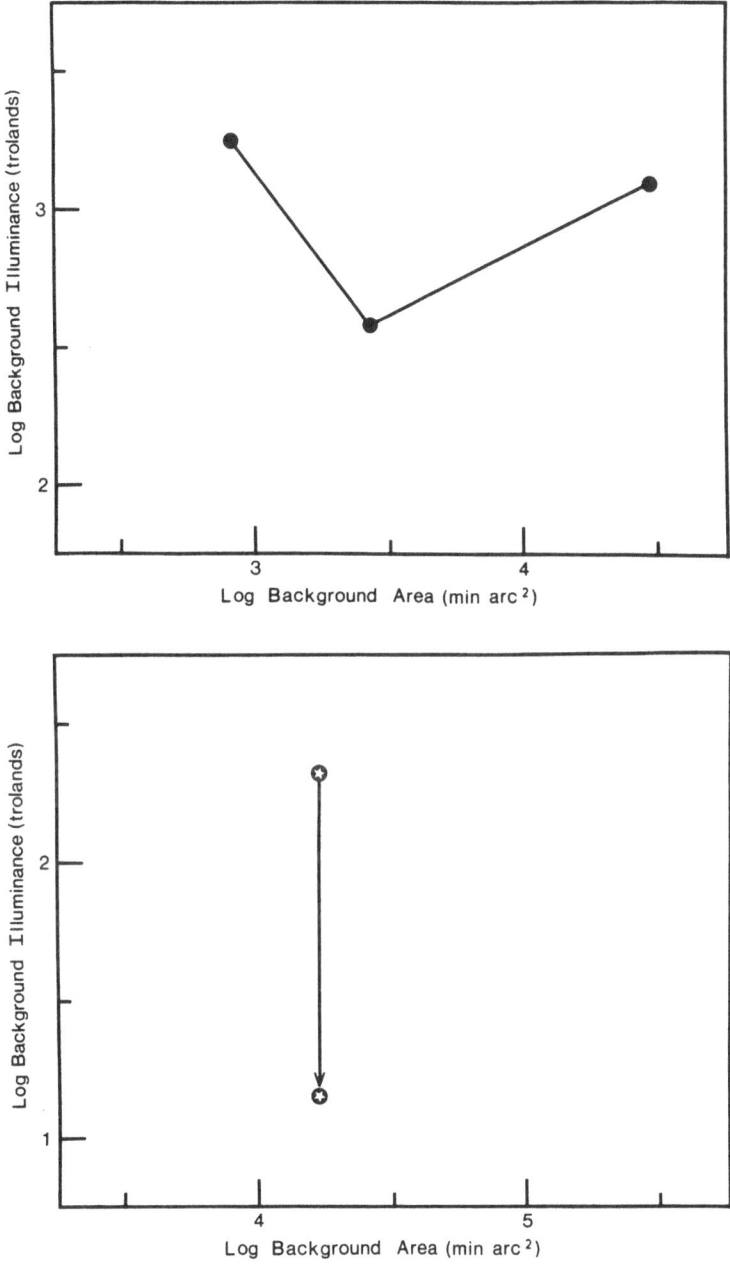

Fig. 2. Responses of a normal observer on the sustained-like test (a) and the transient-like test (b) measured on the SLO. In (b) the direction of the arrow indicates the reduction in sensitivity induced by rotation of the vaned pattern.

DISCUSSION

The methodology described here allows testing of layer-by-layer functions at visualized retinal points. Our present method allows us to view a good quality, real-time image of the retina as we choose our test loci. This enables us to place the test precisely, in relation to observed retinal anomalies and retinal vessels. On the view of the retina, we see the true location of the fixation target and of the test stimuli. Following selection of the test location, we dim the retinal illumination somewhat so that both the test increment and the Field II pedestal used in the tests can be presented. The resulting view of the retina allows for accurate, direct monitoring of fixation, although some detail is sacrificed if we are to reduce light levels to those approximating tangent-screen presentation.

The new methodology appears successful in this first feasibility test. Questions of gray scale and calibration have been raised and answered. These tests evaluate robust responses which we have shown to survive the transition to retinal projection, to raster presentation, to monochromaticity and to differing overall light levels. These differences should be explored further: higher light levels during test would be more convenient, and a change of parameters may maximize the size of the responses. The raster limits the ultimate spatial resolution of the patterns presented, and while new hardware is rapidly relieving this fact, and while we have seen no evidence of problems associated with it, we would like to know the point at which this sort of display is too coarse.

Ultimately, the value of any new methodology is in elucidating the older ways. We expect that this approach to layer-by-layer testing will give that process new dimension and allow us better to understand its results.

REFERENCES

1. Enoch, J.M. Quantitative layer-by-layer perimetry. Invest. Ophthal. Vis. Sci. 17: 208–257 (1978).
2. Enoch, J.M., Fitzgerald, C.R. and Campos, E.C. Quantitative Layer-by-Layer Perimetry: An Extended Analysis. Grune & Straton, Inc. New York (1981).
3. Timberlake, G.T., Mainster, M.A., Webb, R.H., Hughes, G.W. and Trempe, C.L. Retinal localization of scotomata by scanning laser ophthalmoscopy. Invest. Ophthal. Vis. Sci. 22: 91–97 (1982).
4. Webb, R.H., Hughes, G.W. and Pomerantzeff, O. Flying spot TV ophthalmoscope. Appl. Optics 19: 2991 (1980).
5. Westheimer, G.W. Spatial interaction in human cone vision. J. Physiol. 190: 139 (1967).

Author's address:
Robert H. Webb,
Eye Research Institute of the Retina Foundation
20 Staniford Street
Boston, MA 02114, USA

ANALYSIS OF THE BINOCULAR VISUAL FIELD OF STRABISMIC PATIENTS AND ITS OBJECTIVE CORRELATE

EMILIO C. CAMPOS and ROSANNA GULLI

(*Modena, Italy*)

ABSTRACT

Binocular visual field studies performed with fusable stimuli as test-targets demonstrate that a binocular single perception is present in patients with small angle concomitant strabismus all over the visual field considered (30°). This binocularity is sustained by anomalous retinal correspondence (ARC). No suppression scotomas are found. These perimetric results can be made objective by means of visual evoked responses (VER). VER show the existence of a binocular cortical integration in the same patients in which a binocular single preception was found with perimetry.

At the Tübingen IPS Symposium in 1977 Bagolini and Campos (1) showed that in patients with small angle-comitant esotropia and anomalous retinal correspondence (ARC) there is a binocular single perception all over the binocular visual field tested (30°). These results could be obtained using fusable stimuli as test-targets. In this way it was possible to demonstrate that the areas of single vision were not due to a suppression scotoma of the deviated eye, as previously thought, but were areas of anomalous binocular single vision sustained by ARC. It was also shown that red filters of increasing density anteposed to the fixing eye shrink the area of binocular single vision. This demonstrated that ARC is more deeply rooted in the center than in the periphery of the visual field. Subsequently it was shown that Visual Evoked Responses (VER) allow an objective evaluation of anomalous binocular vision in patients with strabismus and ARC (2–5).

In this paper results of binocular visual studies and VER recordings in the same group of patients with strabismus and ARC will be presented. The aim of this analysis is to provide a comparative evaluation of the two methods.

MATERIAL AND METHODS

Seven patients with small-angle comitant esotropia were examined. Five of them exhibited ARC as tested with Bagolini striated glasses. Two had suppression of the deviated eye with the same test. Pertinent data on the patients can be found in Table 1.

Heijl, A. and Greve, E.L. (eds.), Proceedings of the 6th Int. Visual Field Symposium.
© 1985, Dr W. Junk Publishers, Dordrecht, The Netherlands. ISBN 978-94-010-8932-6

Table 1. Patients data.

Patient	Sex	Age	Deviated Eye	Visual Acuity		Angle of Strabismus (in degrees)	Binocular Sensory status*
				OD	OS		
1	M	15	OD	6/9	6/6	4°	A.R.C.
2	M	14	OS	6/6	6/6	4°	A.R.C.
3	F	16	OS	6/6	6/7.5	8°	Supp. OS
4	M	12	OS	6/6	6/6	6°	A.R.C.
5	F	13	OD	6/7.5	6/6	5°	A.R.C.
6	F	10	OD	6/6	6/6	8°	A.R.C.
7	M	18	OD	6/9	6/6	6°	Supp. OD

*The binocular sensory status was measured with the Bagolini striated glasses test. A.R.C. = Anomalous Retinal Correspondence. Supp. = Suppression.

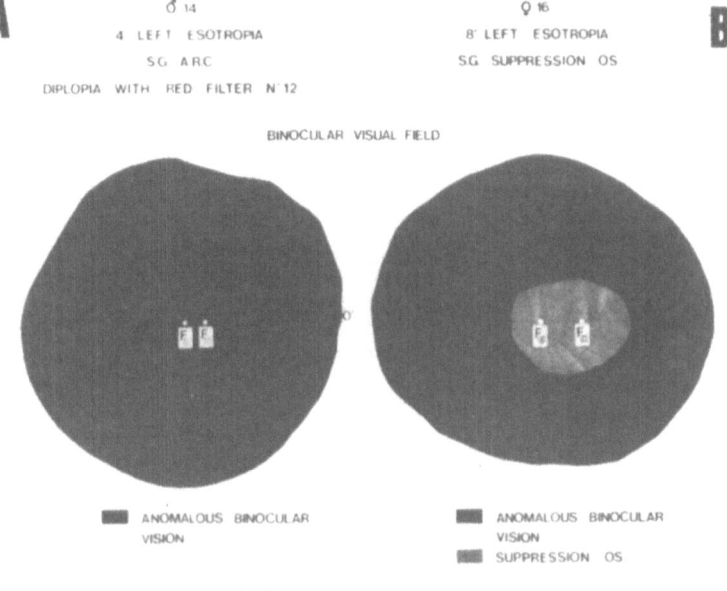

A
♂ 14
4 LEFT ESOTROPIA
S.G ARC
DIPLOPIA WITH RED FILTER N 12

♀ 16
8' LEFT ESOTROPIA
S.G SUPPRESSION OS
B

BINOCULAR VISUAL FIELD

ANOMALOUS BINOCULAR
VISION

ANOMALOUS BINOCULAR
VISION
SUPPRESSION OS

STIMULUS Ø 0.5 115   BACKGROUND 5

Fig. 1. Binocular visual fields. A: Patient with small-angle esotropia and anomalous binocular vision supported by anomalous retinal correspondence. No suppression scotomas are found in the tested area. B: Patient with small-angle esotropia and suppression scotoma, around which there is a wide area of anomalous binocular vision supported by anomalous retinal correspondence.

Binocular visual fields were examined with a modified von Graefe's technique described previously (1). Essentially, the patients wearing striated glasses looked at a white target screen (5 cd/m²). A white stimulus (0.3° in diameter, 115 cd/m² luminance) was moved perimetrically. The patients had to indicate whether they saw a disc crossed by two streaks (ARC), one streak only (suppression) or two discs each crossed by one streak (diplopia).

VER were recorded with a bipolar derivation, amplified and averaged with usual methods. A modified TV apparatus generating a pattern reversal at constant luminance was the stimulus (4). Spatial frequencies could be conveniently changed. Monocular and binocular VER were obtained in sequence. If the binocular VER was significantly larger than the mean of the two monocular ones, this indicated summation; the latter is considered to be an expression of binocular cortical integration (2–5). The absence of summation of the image of one eye.

RESULTS

All the five patients with strabismus and ARC showed an anomalous superimposition of the two visual fields without suppression scotomas (Fig. 1A). The same patients exhibited a VER summation (Fig. 2A). The two patients

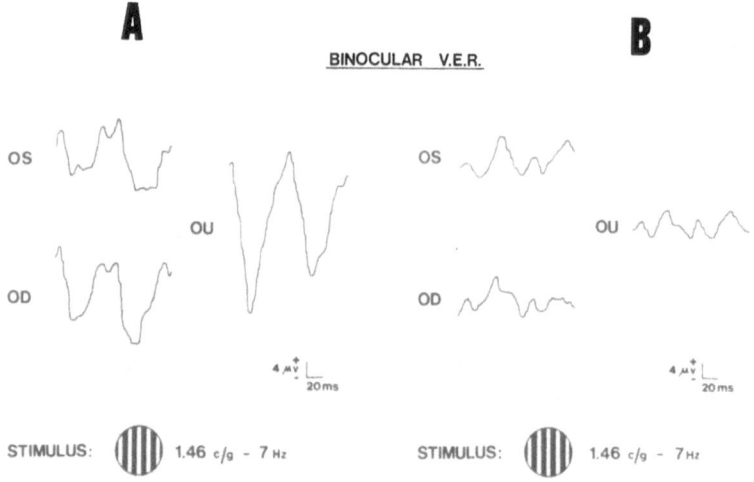

Fig. 2. Visual evoked responses (VER). A: In the patient, whose binocular visual field is presented in Fig. 1A, the binocular VER is larger than the two monocular ones, thus showing the existence of summation. B: No VER summation is found in this patient, who showed an extended suppression scotoma as can be seen in Fig. 1B.

with suppression at the striated glasses, showed a central area of the binocular visual field, where a suppression scotoma could be detected (Fig. 1B). No summation was found at the VER (Fig. 2B).

DISCUSSION AND CONCLUSIONS

In the same patients in which binocular visual field examinations revealed the presence of anomalous binocular vision, a VER summation could be detected as well. This is another argument in favour of the fact that VER summation is an expression of binocular cortical integration. In fact, in the presence of wide suppression scotomas in the binocular visual field, VER summation is absent.

It is therefore possible to state that in strabismus with ARC there is a quite sophisticated type of binocular cooperation in spite of the deviation. This cooperation can be detected also with electrophysiological techniques and shows characteristics similar to that one of normals.

It is important to stress the existence of this anomalous type of binocular vision in small-angle strabismus.

In fact, the latter is the most common end-result of surgery or other kinds of treatment. An objective demonstration of anomalous binocular vision by means of VER seems thus interesting because it substantiates previous peimetric results.

490

REFERENCES

1. Bagolini, B. and Campos, E.C. Binocular campimetry in small-angle concomitant esotropia. Second Int. Visual Field Symposium, Tübingen (1976). Docum. Ophthalmol. Proc. Series 14: 405–409 (1977).
2. Campos, E.C. Anomalous retinal correspondence. Monocular and binocular visual evoked responses. Arch. Ophthalmol. 98: 299–302 (1980).
3. Campos, E.C. Evaluation of binocularity by means of visual evoked responses. In: 'Strabismus' (M.C. Boschi and R. Frosini, editors). Proc. Int. Symposium in Strabismus, C.E.S.S.D., Florence, 119–140 (1982).
4. Campos, E.C. and Chiesi, C. Binocularity in concomitant strabismus. II Objective evaluation with visual evoked responses. Doc. Ophthalmol. 55: 277–293 (1983).
5. Chiesi, C. and Campos, E.C. Objective assessment of the strength of binocularity in normals and strabismics. In: 'Strabismus' (M.C. Boschi and R. Frosini, editors). Proc. Int. Symposium on Strabismus, C.E.S.S.D., Florence, 167–174 (1982).

Author's address:
Prof. Dr. Emilio C. Campos,
Clinica Oculistica dell'Università,
via del Pozzo 71,
41100 Modena,
Italy.

491

CRITICAL FUSION FREQUENCY IN AMBLYOPIA

OSAMU MIMURA, YUJI OKAMOTO, KAZUTAKA KANI, TAKASHI
UTSUMI and TOSHIO INUI

(*Nishinomiya, Japan*)

ABSTRACT

Critical fusion frequency (C.F.F.) in different retinal loci were measured in an amblyopic patients with eccentric fixation using a fundus perimeter. At the eccentric fixating retinal locus C.F.F. increased monotonically with stimulus intensity when the stimulus area was large. However, when the stimulus area was small, C.F.F. on the same retinal locus did not change with stimulus intensity. These results suggest that C.F.F. in amblyopia varies with the stimulus area.

INTRODUCTION

Numerous electrophysiological experiments for visual deprivation amblyopia have demonstrated the deterioration of both spatial and temporal frequencies in the visual system in amblyopia. In humans, several psychophysical studies analyzing the receptive field-like properties in amblyopia show spatial summation and lateral inhibition to be abnormal (3, 5). Isolated reports of abnormal as well as normal function of critical fusion frequency (C.F.F.) in amblyopia have appeared, but no systematic study of C.F.F. with reference to the intensity of the stimulus has been done.

In this study, the C.F.F. was measured in a patient with eccentric fixating amblyopia using a fundus perimeter with stimuli of different size and luminance.

MATERIAL AND METHODS

1. Subject

Subject T.U. was a 35-year-old man who had left-sided esotropia and subsequent muscle surgery twice at ages 6 and 10 years. His best corrected visual acuity was 1.5 in the right eye and 0.15 in the left eye. His ocular health appeared to be normal apart from a constant, comitant left esotropia.

Heijl, A. and Greve, E.L. (eds.), Proceedings of the 6th Int. Visual Field Symposium.
© *1985, Dr W. Junk Publishers, Dordrecht, The Netherlands. ISBN 978-94-010-8932-6*

The objective angle measured about 12 prisms at 30 cm and 18 prisms at 5 m on the prism cover test with correction for ametropia. The left fixation was eccentric 5 degrees nasally when measured monocularly by means of a projected ophthalmoscopic fixation target.

2. Apparatus

Trials were conducted on a new modified fundus perimeter which was originally designed by Kani and Ogita (4). This perimeter was composed of an infrared television fundus camera, a perimeter and a stimulator, generated by the insertion of a rotating sector disc in the stimulus light beam. Background and stimulus light beams were set up in a Maxwellian view arrangement. The light passed through the central 1.5 mm of the subject's pupil. The circular background subtended 30 degrees in diameter, and the luminance was 10 asb. The stimulus intensity could be changed with neutral-density filters (Kodak Wratten No. 96) in steps of 0.1 log unit. The principal experimental variables were stimulus size, stimulus luminance and retinal locus. The stimulus sizes used here were 4.5, 7.5, 9.3, 11.5 and 32 minutes in diamter. The C.F.F. determinations were made at 1) the eccentric fixating retinal locus of the amblyopic eye, 2) the fovea of the non-amblyopic eye, and 3) the retinal locus of the non-amblyopic eye, corresponding in the amblyopic eye to the eccentric fixating locus.

3. Procedure

The subject's pupil was dilated with a mydriatic, 0.5 percent tropicamide. The subject was allowed ten minutes for background adaptation. Prior to the experiment, the increment threshold for each stimulus size was determined by an up-down method in steps of 0.1 log unit. At the start of the experiment, the subject was instructed to press a buzzer-key if the flicker sensation disappeared and was replaced by the sensation of continuous stimulation. The subject was told to be sure that the fixation point was in good focus before initiating each session. Then the C.F.F. for each stimulus size and luminance in each retinal locus was determined. For every retinal locus 5 measurements were made.

RESULTS

The results of this experiment are illustrated in Figs. 1 and 2. Figure 1 shows the relationship between the C.F.F. and the stimulus intensity at the different retinal loci with the largest stimulus (32 minutes in diameter). The C.F.F. at the fovea in the non-amblyopic eye (open circles) and at the eccentric fixating retinal locus of the amblyopic eye (filled circles) monotonically increased with stimulus intensity. On the other hand, the C.F.F. at the reginal locus of the non-amblyopic eye, which corresponding to the eccentric fixating locus of the amblyopic eye (open triangles), showed no significant increase. Figure 2 shows the relationship between the C.F.F. and the stimulus intensity with a

494

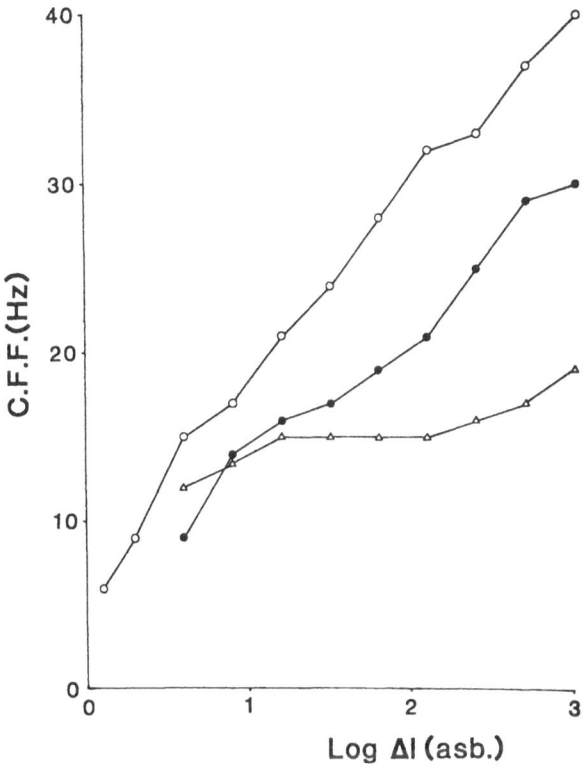

Fig. 1. Relationship between C.F.F. and stimulus intensity using the largest stimulus (32 minutes in diameter). Open circles: C.F.F. at the fovea of the non-amblyopic eye. Filled circles: C.F.F. at the eccentric fixating retinal locus of the amblyopic eye. Open triangle: C.F.F. at the eccentric retinal locus of the non-amblyopic eye, which corresponds to the eccentric fixating locus of the amblyopic eye.

smaller stimulus size (11.5 minutes in diameter). The C.F.F. at the fovea in the non-amblyopic eye increased monotonically with stimulus intensity. On the other hand, the C.F.F. at the eccentric fixating locus of the amblyopic eye and at the corresponding retinal locus of the non-amblyopic eye showed no marked change with stimulus intensity.

Using the smallest stimulus (4.5 minutes in diameter) we could not measure the C.F.F. at the eccentric fixating locus of the amblyopic eye in spite of the subject's great effort. Furthermore, it was quite difficult to reproduce a stable C.F.F. using the stimuli of 7.5 and 9.3 minutes in diameter.

DISCUSSION

Dissociation of central vision and the C.F.F. is so remarkable that a 'flicker test' can be used as an important and reliable test in the diagnosis of optic

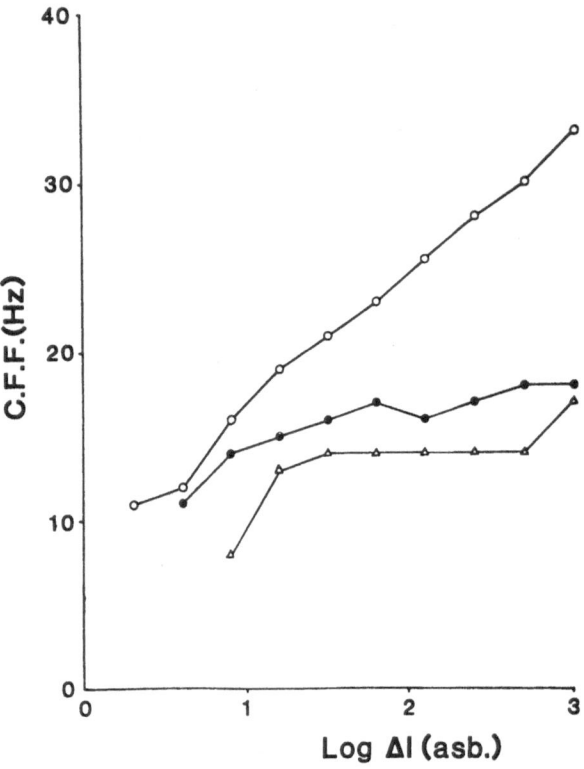

Fig. 2. Same relationship as in Fig. 1 but with a stimulus diameter of 11.5 minutes instead of 32 minutes.

nerve diseases (6). Furthermore, the deterioation of the C.F.F. has been shown to often precede the corresponding scotomata of classic perimetry (7). Several studies on the C.F.F. using small stimuli have been performed on normal subjects (1, 2, 7). A systematic study of the C.F.F. in amblyopia, however, has not been reported. The difficulties of studying the C.F.F. in amblyopia appear to be methodological. That is, the eccentric fixation in amblyopia is unstable and by using a classic stimulator the examiner cannot know where the stimulus falls on the subject's retina. In this study we applied a fundus perimeter (using an infrared television fundus camera) to the measurement of the C.F.F. in amblyopia. With this technique we can easily know where the stimulus falls and whether the eye moves or not during stimulation.

In this experiment, the C.F.F. at the eccentric fixating retinal locus of the amblyopic eye varied with the stimulus. Using a large stimulus the C.F.F. monotonically increased with stimulus intensity. However, the C.F.F. showed no significant increase with intensity when using a small stimulus. The C.F.F. for a large stimulus on the eccentric fixating retinal locus shows the same properties as in the central retina and for a small stimulus the same properties as in the parafoveal retina. These properties of the C.F.F on the eccentric fixating locus bear resemblance to those on the spatial summation and lateral inhibition, but more investigation is needed to draw further conclusions about the relationship of C.F.F. to amblyopia.

REFERENCES

1. Calabria, G., Gandolfo, E., Ciurlo, G. and Rossi, P. Flicker fusion in pericoecal area. Docum. Ophthal. Proc. Series, 26: 107–110 (1981).
2. Campos, E.C. and Jacobson, S.G. Receptive field-like properties tested with critical flicker fusion. Perimetric analysis. Docum. Ophthal. Proc. Series, 26: 103–106 (1981).
3. Kani, K., Inui, T., Haruta, R. and Mimura, O. Lateral inhibition in the fovea and parafoveal regions. Docum. Ophthal. Proc. Series, 35: 391–396 (1983).
4. Kani, K. and Ogita, Y. Fundus controlled perimeter – The relation between the position of a lesion in the fundus and in the visual field. Docum. Ophthal. Proc. Series 19: 341–350 (1979).
5. Mimura, O., Kani, K. and Inui, T. Spatial summation in the foveal and parafoveal region. Docum. Ophthal. Proc. Series 26: 139–146 (1981).
6. Otori, T., Hohki, T. and Nakao, T. Central critical fusion frequency in neuro-ophthalmological practice. Docum. Ophthal. Proc. Series. 19: 95–100 (1979).
7. Zingirian, M., Ciurlo, G., Rossi, P. and Burtolo, C. Flicker fusion and spatial summation. Docum. Ophthal. Proc. Series, 26: 127–130 (1981).

Author's address:
Osamu Mimura, M.D.
Department of Ophthalmology,
Hyogo College of Medicine,
1-1, Mukogawa-cho, Nishinomiya,
Japan, 663

DISTRIBUTION OF RETINAL SENSITIVITY IN AMBLYOPIA WITH ECCENTRIC FIXATION

KEIKO INOUE, OSAMU MIMURA, KAZUTAKA KANI and EMIKO OHMI

(*Nishinomiya, Japan*)

ABSTRACT

The distribution of the retinal sensitivity was measured using a fundus perimeter in 10 amblyopic patients with eccentric fixation. In 9 of 10 patients, the highest retinal sensitivity was detected in the eccentric fixation area. In no case was the peak sensitivity located in the fovea. These results suggests that the eccentric fixation develops in an attempt to fixate with a retinal locus having higher sensitivity, not visual acuity, than the fovea.

INTRODUCTION

Amblyopia with eccentric fixation has been one of the incurable diseases for ophthalmologists, thought recent electrophysiological experiments for visual deprivation amblyopia have gradually elucidated the basic mechanism of amblyopia. In order to elucidate the etiopathogenesis of amblyopia and to judge its prognosis for visual acuity, it is most important to conduct various examinations while monitoring its fixation behaviour.

In this study, a fundus perimeter was used to examine the distribution of the retinal sensitivity in amblyopia with eccentric fixation. The difference between the foveal sensitivity of the amblyopic eye and that of the fellow eye was also studied.

MATERIAL AND METHODS

1. Subjects

The experiments were carried out on 10 patients with eccentric fixation. All the patients had a thorough ophthalmologic examinations, and were shown to be free of other ocular or neurological diseases. The age of the patients ranged from 5 to 42 years, with a mean of 14.6 years. There were 4 males and 6 females.

Heijl, A. and Greve, E.L. (eds.), Procceedings of the 6th Int. Visual Field Symposium.
© *1985, Dr W. Junk Publishers, Dordrecht, The Netherlands. ISBN 978-94-010-8932-6*

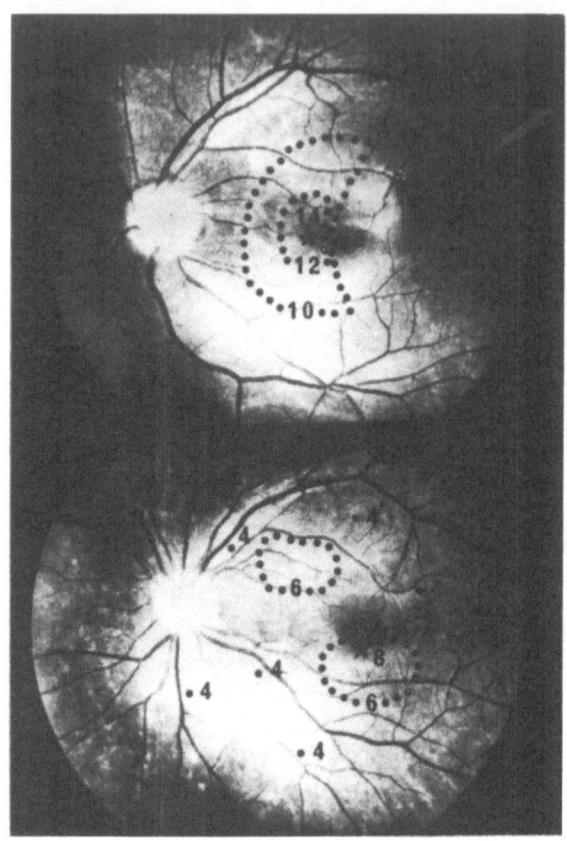

Fig. 1. Distribution of the retinal sensitivity in cases T.H. (top) and K.T. (bottom). Retinal sensitivity $S = (3 - \log \Delta I) \times 10$, $(0 = 1000 \, \text{asb}.,\ 10 = 100 \, \text{asb}.)$. Asterisk indicates the eccentrically fixating locus.

2. Apparatus

Trials were conducted with a fundus perimeter (Konan Camera Research Institute Inc., Nishinomiya). The fixation point at the center of the background was a red light spot, 7 or 20 minutes in diameter. The circular background subtended 30 degrees in diameter, and luminance was 10 abs. The stimulus was a white light spot, 7 minutes in diameter, and its intensity could be changed with neutral density filters in steps of 0.1 log unit. Exposure duration of the stimulus was 200 ms.

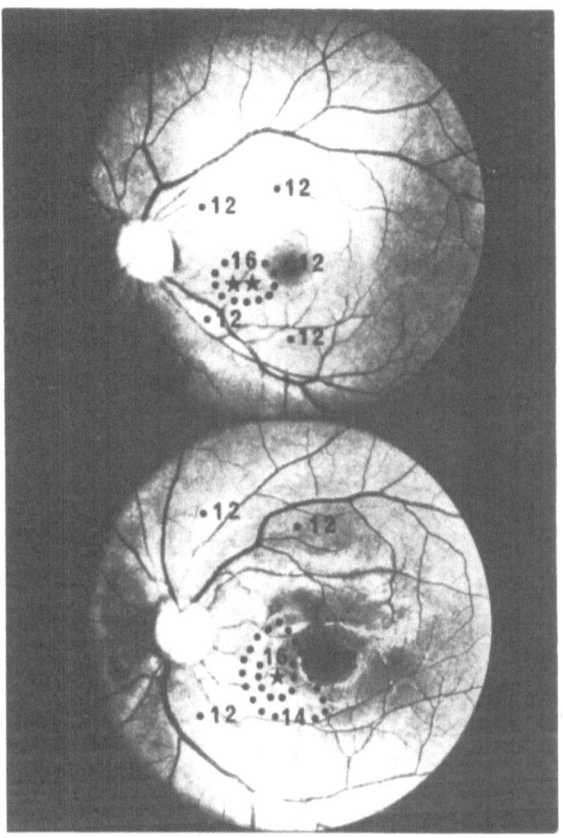

Fig. 2. Distribution of the retinal sensitivity in cases T.A. (top) and K.M. (bottom).

3. Methods

After the subject's pupil was dilated with 0.5 percent tropicamide, the subject was allowed 10 minutes for background adaptation. At the start of the experiment, the subject was instructred to press a buzzer-key if the stimulus was seen. The threshold was determined by the up-and-down method with 10 trials at each retinal locus. We measured the retinal sensitivity S which was defined as:

$$S = (3 - \log \Delta I) \times 10$$

Here, ΔI is an increment threshold. These experimental conditions were set up to facilitate comparison with the results using Tübinger perimeter.

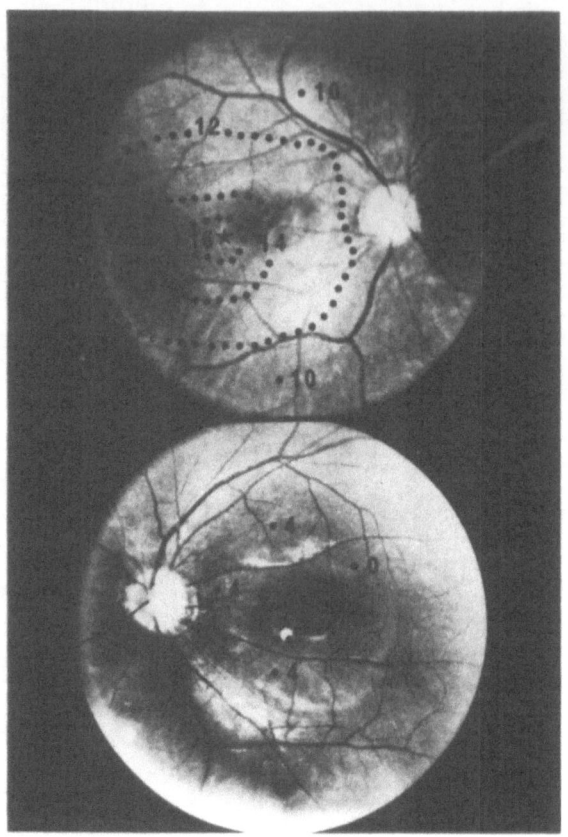

Fig. 3. Distribution of the retinal sensitivity in cases Y.N. (top) and H.K. (bottom).

RESULTS AND DISCUSSION

1. Distribution of retinal sensitivities

The results of these experiments are illustrated in Figs. 1 to 5. In 9 patients, the retinal sensitivity was highest in the eccentric fixation point. This finding might largely support the works of Aggarwal and Verma (1). In their report, however, the fovea of the amblyopic eye was more sensitive than the eccentric area of fixation and had predominance over all other retinal points in 7 of 25 cases (28%). In our study, the eccentric fixation area was identical to the point of peak retinal sensitivity in 9 of 10 patients, and in no amblyopic eye had the fovea predominance over all other retinal points. Thus, our findings strongly suggest that eccentric fixation develops in an attempt to fixate with an eccentric retinal locus having higher retinal sensitivity, not visual acuity, than the fovea.

502

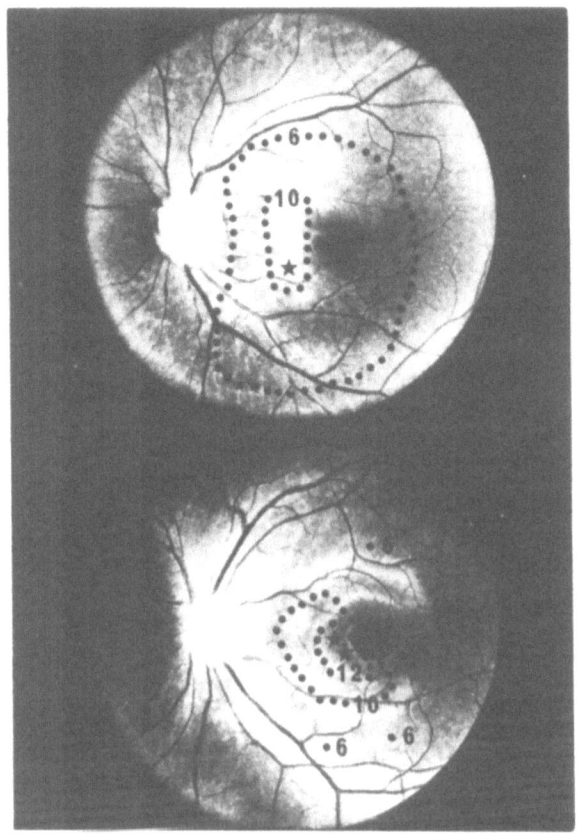

Fig. 4. Distribution of the retinal sensitivity in cases S.S. (top) and E.H. (bottom).

2. Retinal sensitivities of the amblyopic eyes and fellow eyes

In 6 of 10 amblyopic patients the retinal sensitivies of 1) the foveas in both eyes, 2) the eccentric fixation point in the amblyopic eye, and 3) the eccentric retinal locus of the same eccentricity in the fellow eye were measured. The results are shown in Table 1. The findings are in agreement with the traditional scotoma hypothesis for functional amblyopia (2, 3). The fovea of the amblyopic eye is located in the suppression scotoma proving that the suppression scotoma of the amblyopic eye exists even when the amblyopic eye views monocularly.

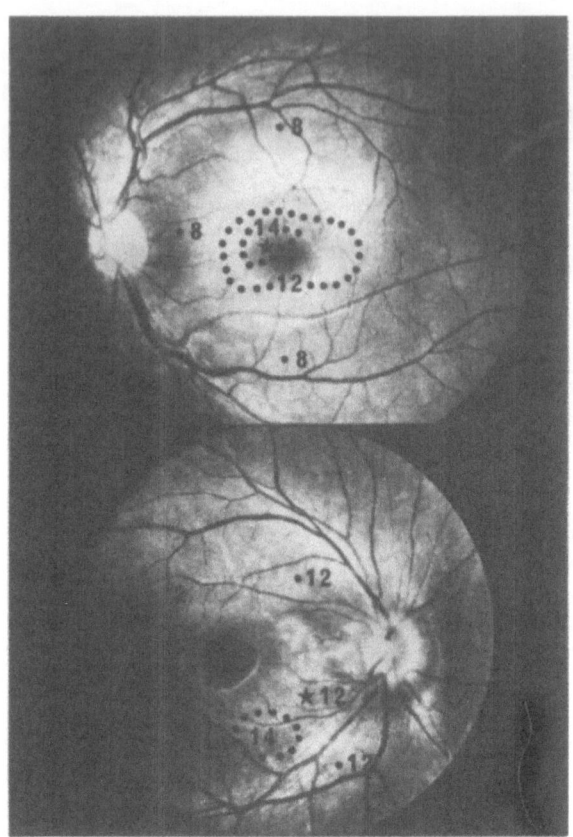

Fig. 5. Distribution of the sensitivity in case K.S. (top) and atypical case K.I. (bottom). In case K.I. the other retinal locus was more sensitive than the fovea and the eccentric fixation area.

Table 1. Retinal sensitivities at the various retinal loci in amblyopes. A: fovea in amblyopic eye, B: eccentric fixating retinal locus in amblyopic eye, C: fovea in non-amblyopic eye, D: the retinal locus of the non-amblyopic eye which corresponds in the amblyopic eye to the eccentric fixating locus.

	amblyopic eye		fellow eye	
Name	A	B	C	D
T.A.	12	16	17	16
K.M.	12	16	18	16
T.H.	6	14	18	14
K.T.	4	8	16	14
Y.N.	14	16	17	15
K.S.	12	14	16	14

REFERENCES

1. Aggarwal, D.P. and Verma, G. Static perimetry in the study of amblyopic scotomata. Br. J. Ophthalmol., 64: 713–716 (1980).
2. Higgins, K.E. Monocular performance of functional amblyopes: another look at the scotoma hypothesis. Am. J. Opt. Physiol. Opt., 55: 172–182 (1978).
3. Van Noorden, G.K. Etiology and pathogenesis of fixation anomalies in strabismus. IV. Role of supression scotoma and of motor factors. Am. J. Ophthalmol., 69: 236–245 (1970).

Author's address:
Keiko Inoue, M.D.
Department of Ophthalmology,
Hyogo College of Medicine,
1-1, Mukogawa-Cho, Nishinomiya,
Japan, 663

MONOCULAR AND BINOCULAR VISUAL FIELDS IN DIFFERENT TYPES OF STRABISMUS

RINI MAHENDRASTARI and GUY VERRIEST

(*Gent, Belgium*)

ABSTRACT

Monocular and binocular perimetry (without any dissociation between the two eyes) was performed by means of Goldmann kinetic perimetry in a group of normal subjects and in groups of subjects suffering from strabismus. The central region of the monocular field of the better eye is more sensitive in the strabismic groups than in the normal one. The binocular field is as sensitive in strabismus as normally; its extent is (nearly) normal.

The vast majority of the many studies concerning the binocular visual field in strabismus made use of dissociating techniques that permit to recognize at each moment which eye sees the target. In such conditions, and especially when dissociation is strong, the squinting eye does not see the target in extensive parts of the binocular field.

In this paper we consider the binocular visual field of the strabismic subjects not from the usual physiopathological point of view, but for estimating its functional value as compared with the normal binocular field. Accordingly we examined the binocular field without any dissociation between the two eyes: so we do not know exactly which eye sees the target, but we learn how far the squinting subject sees in daily life and in professional activities.

We examined 10 normal subjects (group 1), 6 subjects suffering from alternating convergent strabismus (group 2), 9 subjects suffering from not alternating strabismus (group 3) and 5 subjects presenting a divergent strabismus (group 4).

Age varied between about 15 years and about 50 years in all groups. Both sexes were represented. Visual acuity could be as low as <0.1 in the squinting eyes of groups 3 and 4. The strabismus angle ranged between $+8\Delta$ and $+65\Delta$ in group 2, $+20\Delta$ and $+60\Delta$ in group 3, -14Δ and -60Δ in group 4. We determined in group 1 which eye is dominant by means of the inversed prisma test (15Δ), and in the other groups which is the more fixating eye.

Each subject was submitted first in monocular vision of the right eye, subsequently in monocular vision of the left eye and finally in binocular

Heijl, A. and Greve, E.L. (eds.), Proceedings of the 6th Int. Visual Field Symposium.
© *1985, Dr W. Junk Publishers, Dordrecht, The Netherlands. ISBN 978-94-010-8932-6*

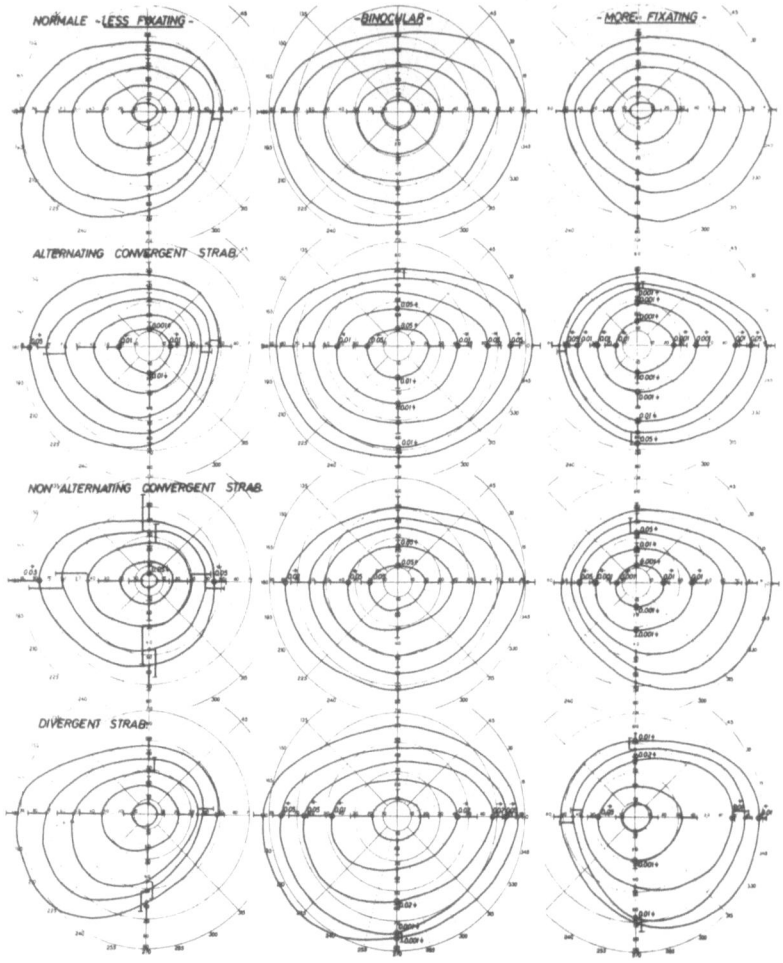

Fig. 1. Means and standard deviations of the perception eccentricities of the Goldmann targets V/4, I/4, I/3, I/2 and I/1 in the 4 groups of subjects. The arrows show the significative differences from the normal results; the figures give the value of *p*.

vision to cinetic perimetry by means of the white targets V/4, I/4, I/3, I/2 and I/1 of the Goldmann perimeter. These targets were moved centripetally along 12 meridians (successively 285°, 315°, 345°, 15°, 45°, 75°, 105°, 135°, 165°, 195°, 225° and 255°). The background luminance was 10 cd.m^{-2}. For the binocular test the head was placed in the middle of the bowl.

For the statistical evaluation of the results we calculated for each subject, for each monocular or binocular condition and for each target the temporal, superior, nasal and inferior perception eccentricities (from the observed eccentricities on the two neighbouring meridians). By inverting the graphs of the subjects in whom the right eye is weaker, we obtained artificially that the left eye is always the weaker one (not dominant eye in group 1, less frequently fixating eye in the other groups). Then, in each of the 4 groups, for each monocular or binocular conditions, for each target and for each of the 4 principal meridians we calculated the mean perception eccentricity and its standard deviation. Finally, we calculated the significancies of differences between group means using Student's t-test (the paired t-test when comparing results within a group).

As shown by Fig. 1, most perception eccentricities are greater in alternating convergent strabismus than in normal vision, the phenomenon being greater and more significative for the central isopters than for the outer ones, for the more fixating eye than for the less fixating eye, and also for the more fixating eye than for binocular vision.

In non alternating convergent strabismus, the perception eccentricities in the fixating eye are much greater than normally (just as in the most fixating eye of the group with alternating strabismus). The field of the amblyopic eye is narrower and the binocular field is nearly normal. We observe a diminution of the temporal extent of the monocular field of the amblyopic eye and also of the lateral extent of the binocular field at the side of the squinting eye.

In divergent strabismus we observe an augmentation of the perception eccentricities on the mid-periphery isopters as well in the best eye as in the binocular field.

We have also to observe that in the normal group the areas enclosed by the central isopters (I/1 and I/2) are greater in binocular vision than in monocular vision. The phenomenon is less marked or absent in the strabismus groups.

As tentative explanations for the observed facts we could argue (1) that in normal subjects monocular vision is an abnormal situation giving rise to inhibition, while in strabismus the vision of the best eye is maximally used and thus better than normally, (2) that binocular peripheral vision is better than monocular vision not only in the normal subjects but also in strabismus by lack of convergence, by (peripheral) anomalous correspondance and/or by monocular perceptions. In ergonomical contexts these facts signify that we may not consider strabismic subjects as having a constricted functional visual field.

We expected that the binocular visual field at the side of the squinting eye should be evidently narrower than normally in convergent squint and, on the contrary, wider than normally in divergent squint. We think that this was not clearly evidenced in our experiments because the Goldmann apparatus is not a choice perimeter for determining the most peripheral isopters.

ACKNOWLEDGEMENT

We thank Miss Sylvia De Bie for her help in the statistical analysis.

Author's address:
Dept. of Ophthalmology,
Akademisch Ziekenhuis,
De Pintelaan 185,
B-9000 Gent, Belgium.

PERIPHERAL ACUITY IN NORMAL SUBJECTS

PIERRE BLONDEAU and CHARLES D. PHELPS

(*Iowa, USA*)

ABSTRACT

We studied the influence of background brightness, stimulus presentation time, and stimulus orientation on peripheral visual acuity. Acuity is reduced at low background illumination but reaches a plateau with background illuminations brighter than 4.3 apostilbs. It is stable at presentation times greater than 1/8 second, but declines with briefer presentations. A slight reduction of acuity occurs with oblique stimulus pattern orientation; this oblique effect is more marked in the periphery than centrally, and is greater in the horizontal and vertical meridians than in the oblique meridians.

Intraindividual variation is minimal. Normal mean values and variance have been determined.

In a previous paper (2) we described an acuity perimeter, an instrument that tests visual acuity at any point in the visual field from fixation to 20 degrees eccentricity. Acuity is tested with a sine wave grating target one degree in diameter formed by laser interferometry.

The present study had three purposes. The first was to determine if acuity perimetry is a practical test that gives reproducible results when administered to untrained subjects. The second was to explore the effect on peripheral acuity of stimulus duration, background illumination, and stimulus orientation. The third was to determine normal values and interindividual variation at selected peripheral locations.

We used a forced-choice technique for each experiment. The subject was instructed to respond to the stimulus presentation by describing the orientation of the grating (vertical, horizontal, oblique right, or oblique left). He was requested to guess even if unable to see the striped pattern or if unsure of its orientation. Preliminary testing indicated that a forced choice technique provided a slightly better acuity and more consistent reponses than if the subject responded only when certain of the grating orientation.

The acuity threshold was obtained by presenting the stimulus several times at each spatial frequency. The acuity threshold was arbitrarily taken as the smallest visual angle at which the subject responded correctly to four of five

Heijl, A. and Greve, E.L. (eds.), Proceedings of the 6th Int. Visual Field Symposium.
© 1985, Dr W. Junk Publishers, Dordrecht, The Netherlands. ISBN 978-94-010-8932-6

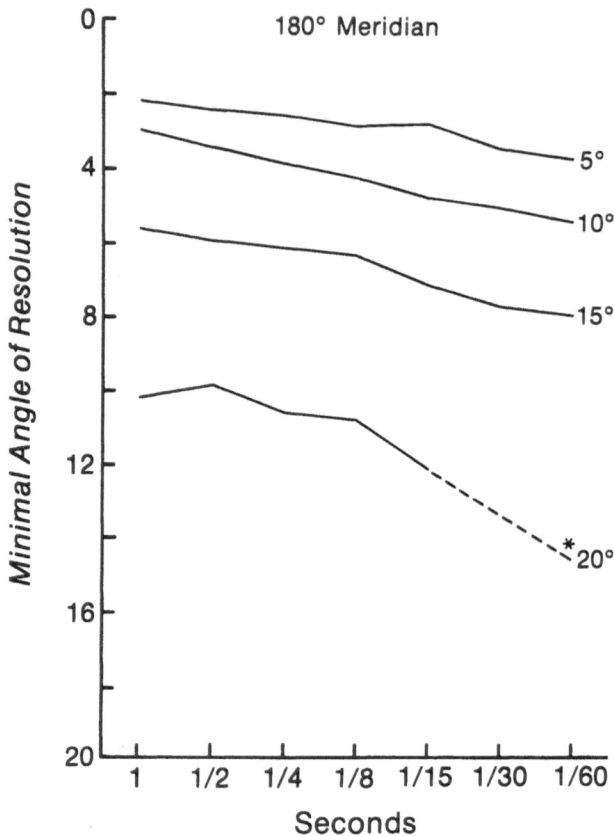

Fig. 1. Effect of stimulus duration on peripheral visual acuity. Mean of five observers at four eccentricities along the nasal horizontal meridian. (The data points connected by a dashed line are underestimated of the true mean resolution threshold; some observers were unable to resolve even the 20 minute grating at those loci and were arbitrarily assigned a value of 21 when the mean was calculated.)

stimulus presentations and (except for the experiment on the effect of stimulus orientation) to at least three of the four possible stimulus orientations.

1. EFFECT OF STIMULUS DURATION

(a) *Method*: A background illumination of 4.3 apostilbs was used. Five normal subjects ranging in age from 20 to 44 years were tested at twelve different positions in the visual field: at 5, 10, 15, and 20 degrees eccentricity along the 180, 270, and 225 degree meridians of the right eye. Seven stimulus presentation times were tested at each position: 1, 1/2, 1/4, 1/8, 1/15, 1/30, and 1/60 seconds.

(b) *Results*: The briefer the stimulus presentation, the poorer was the acuity for each subject at all locations tested (Fig. 1). The decline in acuity with decreasing presentation time was slight until the stimulus duration was less than 1/8 second. With presentation times shorter than 1/8 second, the decline became more precipitous, especially at the more peripheral locations. The decline of acuity with brief presentations was also more precipitous in the oblique and vertical meridians than in the horizontal meridian.

(c) *Comment*: One possible cause for the better acuity with long stimulus durations might be involuntary shifts in the subject's fixation. In two subjects we monitored eye movements during the testing sequence using the recording electrodes usually employed for electro-oculography. We detected no saccades, indicating good fixation.

In a related experiment, we told two subjects where the stimulus would be presented and asked them to purposely cheat: to look for the stimulus when it flashed on for 1/4 second. Their peripheral acuity was poorer when they looked for the target than when they maintained central fixation. This was true whether the target was presented at 5, 10, 15, or 20 degrees eccentricity.

We concluded that 1/4 second was the optimal stimulus presentation time. It was long enough for nearly maximal acuity at all locations but was too short to allow a refixation saccade.

2. EFFECT OF BACKGROUND ILLUMINATION

(a) *Method*: A stimulus presentation time of 1/4 seconds was used. Testing was done at the same field loci as in the experiments on stimulus duration. Five normal subjects ranging in age from 20 to 44 years were tested. Each subject was dark-adapted for 30 minutes. Peripheral acuity was first measured with no background illumination and with the fixation light at its minimum intensity. It was then measured with background illuminations of 1.5, 4.3, 8.9 and 15.1 apostilbs. The subject adapted to each new background for five minutes before testing began.

(b) *Results*: Peripheral acuity, particularly at the more eccentric loci, was poor at low background illuminations but rose rapidly as the background reached the dim illumination of 1.5 apostilbs (Fig. 2). It reached maximum between 4.3 and 8.9 apostilbs and remained fairly constant up to the maximum background illumination used in this experiment (15.1 apostilbs). The effect of background illumination was similar along each of the three meridians tested.

(c) *Comment*: These results demonstrate that the state of retinal adaptation does influence peripheral acuity and must be controlled during acuity perimetry. For clinical testing we wished to have some background illumination so that the patient's retina would be in a photopic state of adaptation. However, any background illumination decreases the contrast of the acuity target, which for laser interference fringes is 100% in the absence of background illumination. To obtain optimal acuity measurements, we needed a background illumination which would be just bright enough to give a photopic acuity profile, but no brighter, so that the target would have the highest possible contrast. For the remainder of our testing, we chose to use a background of 4.3 apostilbs.

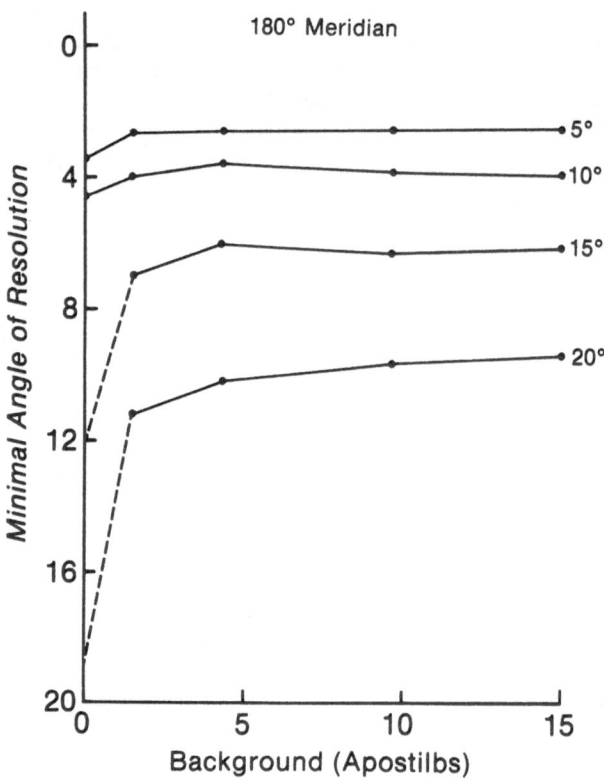

Fig. 2. Effect of background luminance on peripheral visual acuity. Mean of five observers at four eccentricities along the nasal horizontal meridian. (The resolution thresholds for zero apostilbs at 15 and 20 degrees eccentricity are underestimates; see legend for Fig. 1.)

3. THE EFFECT OF GRATING ORIENTATION

(a) *Method*: We conducted two experiments.

Experiment 1. The purpose of this experiment was to compare the acuity thresholds at different eccentricities of the two oblique orientations, taken in combination, with the combined thresholds of the vertical and horizontal orientations. We studied the right eye of a 28 year old experienced observer along the nasal horizontal meridian. Acuity was tested at one degree intervals from fixation to 20 degrees eccentricity. We presented the target eight times for each of the four possible orientations (32 presentations, in all) for each spatial frequency. We began with a slightly suprathreshold grating, for which the subject identified the orientation correctly in 100% of the presentations, and gradually increased the spatial frequency until the subject missed more than 50% of the oblique presentations. The spatial frequency was then further increased until the subject missed more than 50% of the combined

514

vertical and horizontal presentations. Threshold for each of the combinations was defined as the finest grating that could be seen during at least 50% of presentations. The standard 1/4 second presentation time and 4.3 apostilbs background was used. The experiment involved a total of 2496 target presentations and several test sessions.

Experiment 2. Five subjects ranging in age from 28 to 43 years were examined at test points located 15 degrees from fixation along the 45, 90, 135, 180, 225, 270, and 315 meridians. The 0 degree meridian was not examined because of the blind spot. Forty target presentations (ten of each of the four orientations) were made for each grating size. The procedure for defining threshold was the same as in Experiment 1, except that the threshold for each of the four orientations (vertical, horizontal, right oblique, and left oblique) was decided separately. This experiment entailed about 2000 target presentations per subject.

(b) *Results*:

Experiment 1. At all loci eccentric to two degrees, the acuity for vertical and horizontal presentations was slightly better than the acuity for oblique presentations (Fig. 3a). The identical results at fixation and at one degree of eccentricity are probably spurious, since our instrument is not designed to measure acuities with a minimal angle of resolution less than 0.75 (Snellen equivalent of 20/15). The difference between the two acuities tended to increase slightly with increasing eccentricity.

Experiment 2. The pooled results for the five subjects are displayed in Figure 3b. During the testing sessions, the subjects had the impression that a grating oriented parallel to the meridian was seen more easily than one perpendicular to the meridian. The results showed this impression to be true for all of the meridians tested except for the 225 degree meridian where acuities for the right and left oblique target orientations were equal. Either the vertical or the horizontal orientation was more easily perceived than the oblique orientations even along the oblique axes, with the exception, again, of the 225 degree meridian.

(c) *Discussion*: These results confirm that the oblique effect, described for central visual acuity by many investigators, is present for eccentric viewing as well. The orientation effect is important to recognize because it affects the measurement of acuity threshold when gratings are used as the target. However, the difference between the maximal and minimal acuities for different stimulus orientations at a given test locus is usually small, and if it is not necessary for the subject to correctly identify all four orientations, the variance induced by using several grating orientations during a testing sequence will be small. On the other hand, if only one stimulus orientation is used, differences in acuity from one meridian to another will, in part, result from the particular orientation selected.

515

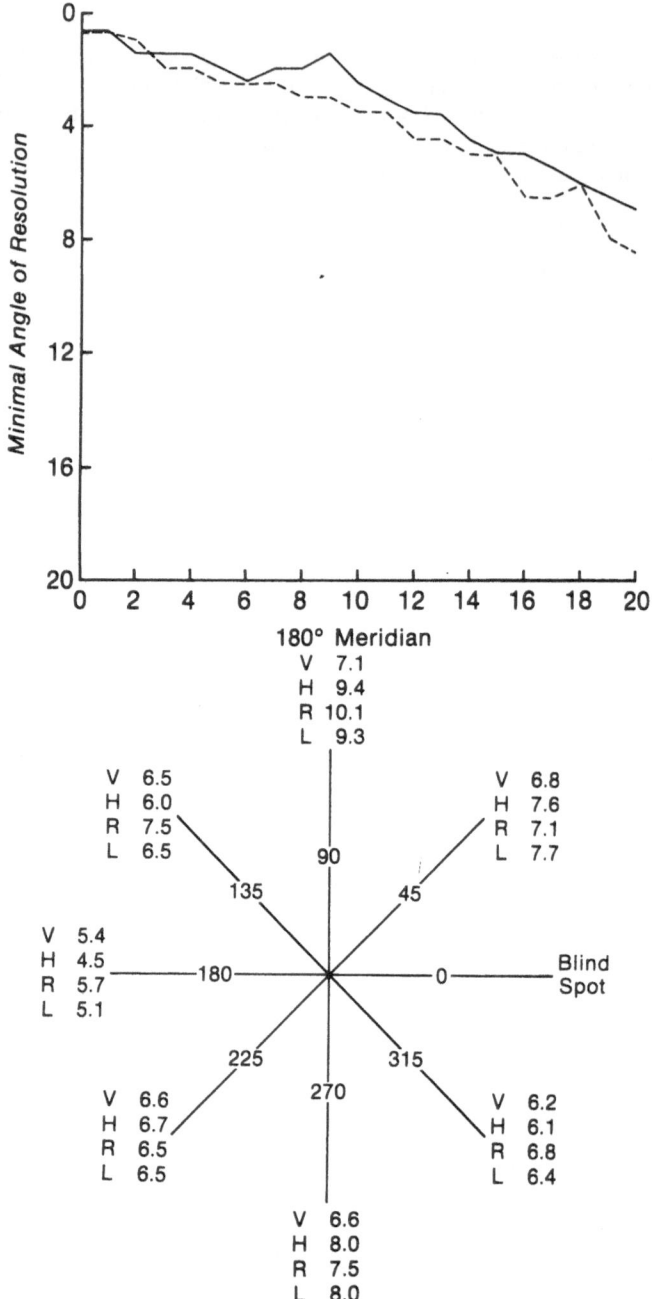

Fig. 3. Effect of stimulus orientation on peripheral visual acuity. (a) Acuity for ablique orientations (dashed line) and combined vertical and horizontal orientations (solid line) of a single normal observer tested along his nasal horizontal meridian. (b) Acuity for vertical (V), horizontal (H), oblique up-to-right (R), and oblique up-to-left (L) orientations. Mean of five normal observers at 15 degrees eccentricity.

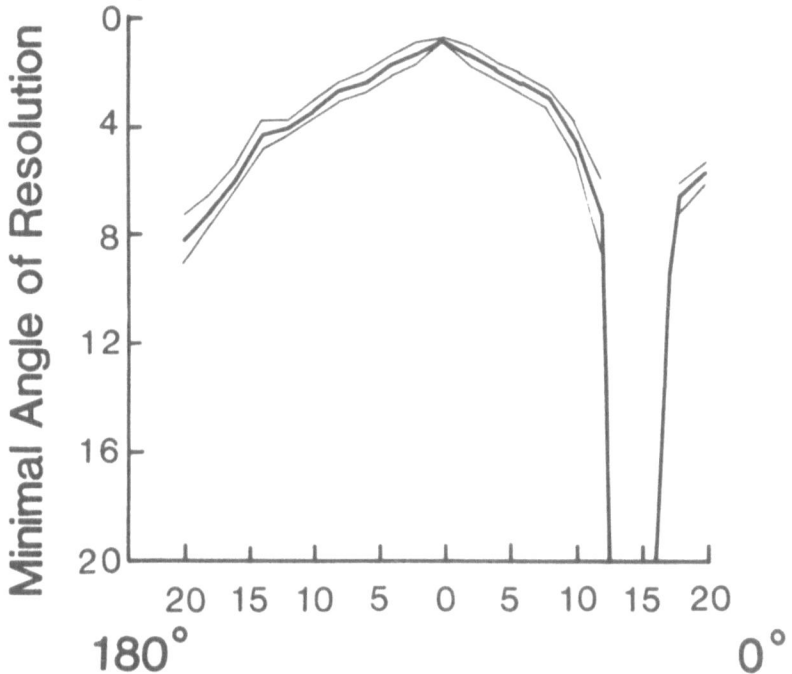

Fig. 4. Reproducibility of acuity perimetry. Mean (dark line) and one standard deviation (light line) of 10 determinations on separate days.

4. INTRAINDIVIDUAL VARIATION

(a) *Method*: Two subjects were tested along one meridian at every two degrees of eccentricity. The test was repeated on ten different days. Mean and standard deviation of the acuity thresholds were computed.

(b) *Results*: The results for the two subjects were similar; those for one subject, who was tested along the 0–180 degree meridian, are shown in Fig. 4. The absence of standard deviation at fixation is due to the fact that the subject had a better central acuity than could be tested with this instrument (0.75 minutes). There was a slight tendency for the variance to increase with increasing eccentricity. The standard deviation was small at all loci for both subjects.

(c) *Comment*: This experiment indicates that the measurement of peripheral acuity thresholds in normal subjects is quite repeatable from day to day. It suggests that acuity perimetry can be used to follow patients for stability, progression, or regression. In the absence of disease-associated changes, the measurements should be similar from examination to examination. However, further studies are needed of long-term variability of acuity thresholds in areas of abnormal acuity before stability can be assumed with certainty.

517

Table 1. Peripheral visual acuity (mean ± standard deviation) for 28 normal observers at 32 locations in the right visual field.

Meridian	Eccentricity			
	5 degrees	10 degrees	15 degrees	20 degrees
0 degrees	2.6 ± 0.4	4.3 ± 0.5	Blind spot	7.9 ± 1.7
45 degrees	2.9 ± 0.5	5.1 ± 0.9	8.2 ± 1.6	13.2 ± 3.7*
90 degrees	3.1 ± 0.8	5.8 ± 1.3	9.9 ± 2.9	18.2 ± 3.2*
135 degrees	2.9 ± 0.6	4.7 ± 0.8	7.6 ± 1.5	14.3 ± 3.6*
180 degrees	2.3 ± 0.5	3.8 ± 0.6	6.2 ± 0.9	10.1 ± 2.3
225 degrees	2.8 ± 0.5	4.7 ± 0.7	7.5 ± 1.2	14.6 ± 3.7*
270 degrees	3.6 ± 1.2	5.1 ± 0.8	8.0 ± 1.5	14.1 ± 3.9*
315 degrees	3.4 ± 1.0	5.0 ± 1.0	7.6 ± 1.4	11.5 ± 3.9*

*The minimal angle of resolution was greater than 20 minutes for some subjects. A value of 21 was then assigned arbitrarily.

5. INTER-INDIVIDUAL VARIATION AND NORMAL VALUES

(a) *Method*: We tested acuity thresholds of 28 normal subjects who ranged in age from 20 to 73 years. Acuity was measured at 5, 10, 15, and 20 degrees of eccentricity along the vertical, horizontal, and two oblique meridians. We calculated means and standard deviations of the thresholds at the different test loci. We also averaged the thresholds for the eight points at each eccentricity and looked for a relationship between peripheral acuity at each eccentricity and subject age.

(b) *Results*: The average acuity thresholds and the intraobserver variation at each locus are listed in Table 1. Acuity was better along the horizontal than along the oblique or vertical meridians. Except at five degrees eccentricity, it was better below than above fixation, confirming the results of previous investigators (1, 3, 4). At twenty degrees eccentricity along several of the meridians, some subjects were unable to see the largest target. Thus, the true average values and variances for these locations could not be calculated, and the displayed results (marked with asterisks) are underestimates. Little variation occurred between observers at eccentricities of 5, 10, and 15 degrees, but considerable variation occurred at 20 degrees.

The best acuities were found in the temporal field. The acuity at 20 degrees eccentricity on the temporal side of the blind spot was especially high (the average minimal angle of resolution was only 7.9), and consistently resembled the acuities at 15 degrees eccentricity along the other meridians tested.

No relationship was found between age and peripheral acuity at 5, 10, and 15 degrees eccentricity (Fig. 5). At 20 degrees eccentricity, age also had no obvious effect, but the failure of some individuals to see even the 20 minute target along one or more meridians makes the regression calculation for this eccentricity of dubious value.

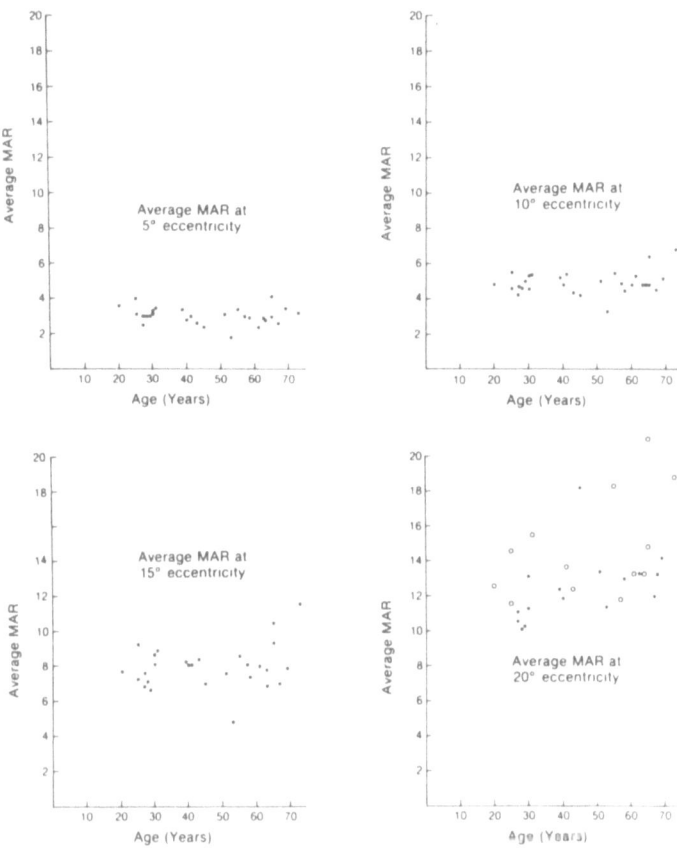

Fig. 5. Relationship between the minimal angle of resolution (M.A.R.) and age. Each point represents the average for one subject of acuity measurements along eight different meridians at that eccentricity. Open circles are probable underestimates because they include some locations for which a M.A.R. greater than 20 minutes was arbitrarily assigned a value of 21 when the mean was calculated.

6. INTRAOCULAR DIFFERENCE

(a) *Method*: Acuity was tested along the vertical meridian at 5, 10, and 15 degrees eccentricity in both eyes of 11 normal observers.

(b) *Results*: The mean difference between right and left eyes was greater at 15 degrees eccentricity than at 5 and 10 degrees eccentricity (Table 2). The variation from observer to observer also increased with increasing eccentricity.

(c) *Comment*: If the results from this small sample can be generalized, one should expect an acuity difference between eyes along the vertical meridian to exceed two minutes of arc at five degrees eccentricity in only 5% of normal individuals. The corresponding limit for 10 and 15 degrees eccentricity are 2.5 and 4.1 minutes of arc, respectively. These limits can be used to compare the acuity fields of the two eyes of a patient who is suspected of having unilateral or asymmetric optic nerve damage.

Table 2. Interocular difference in peripheral acuity along the vertical meridian (mean ± S.D. of 11 observers).

Meridian	Eccentricity	Interocular difference (minutes of arc)
90 degrees	15 degrees	1.3 ± 1.4
90 degrees	10 degrees	0.7 ± 0.9
90 degrees	5 degrees	0.7 ± 0.6
270 degrees	5 degrees	0.6 ± 0.7
270 degrees	10 degrees	0.8 ± 0.9
270 degrees	15 degrees	1.3 ± 1.4

7. EFFECT OF TRAINING

(a) *Method*: Ten of the 28 observers tested to establish normal values were experienced research subjects who had been tested repeatedly on the acuity perimeter over a several week period. The other 18 observers were undergoing the test for the first time. The mean and standard deviation for the acuity values at each test location were calculated separately for the two groups of observers.

(b) *Results*: The two groups had similar acuities at each test location. Thus, no learning effect could be detected in this experiment.

(c) *Comment*: This comparison does not prove the absence of a training effect for peripheral acuity. Perhaps one would be present if an individual was tested repeatedly during a brief time span. However, it suggests that no training occurs when an individual is tested at intervals ranging from days to weeks. Thus, acuity perimetry can be used for sequential testing of patients with little risk of spurious improvement from training.

ACKNOWLEDGEMENT

This research comprises part of a thesis accepted by the American Ophthalmological Society (Dr. Phelps) as part of the requirements for membership.

We are indebted to the National Eye Institute for their partial support of this research through NIH grant EY03330.

REFERENCES

1. Millidot, M. and Lamont, A. Peripheral visual acuity in the vertical plane. Vision Res 14: 1497–1498 (1974).
2. Phelps, C.D., Remijan, P.W. and Blondeau, P. Acuity perimetry. Doc. Ophthalmol. Proc. Series 26: 111–117 (1981).
3. Wertheim, T. Über die indirekte Sehscharfe, Ztsch. f. Psychol. u. Physiol. der Sinnesorg. 7: 172–187 (1894).
4. Weymouth, F.W., Hines, D.C., Acres, L.H., Raaf, J.E. and Wheeler, M.C. Visual acuity within the area centralis and its relation to eye movements and fixation. Am. J. Ophthalmol., 11: 947–960 (1928).

Author's address:
Charles D. Phelps, M.D.
Department of Ophthalmology
University Hospitals
University of Iowa
Iowa City, Iowa 52242
USA

VISUAL FIELD EXAMINATION BY ELECTRO-OCULOGRAPHY

G. VERRIEST, A. COLASANTI, R. FUSCO, A. MAGLI and G. TORTORA

(Ghent, Belgium)

ABSTRACT

The authors describe a method of objective assessment of the visual field by means of the electro-oculographic registration of the refixation eye movements. The first results are encouraging. Several possible improvements of the method are discussed.

INTRODUCTION

There are subjects, mainly children, elderly people, mentally handicapped and neurological patients, in whom the usual psychophysical (subjective) means of visual field testing provide no reliable results because of lack of attention or delayed communication of the response. For such cases objective perimetric techniques have been mainly based on pupillography, electro-retinography and recording of evoked occipital potentials. All these methods have drawbacks of technical difficulties absence of direct relationship with vision, lower peripheral sensitivity and especially lack of constant fixation.

Indeed, an often observed feature in subjective perimetry in the mentioned non cooperative subjects is that their gaze systematically leaves the fixation mark to looking at the just presented peripheral target.

Objective perimetry by means of direct observation of this refixaton reflex has been described by Lauber (7), Harrington (4), Verriest and Van de Casteele (9), Howe (5) and especially Futenma (3). The ocular movements can be registered by means of the reflexion on the cornea of a beam of (preferably infrared) light. Such methods of objective perimetry based on the refixation reflex and optical means of recording eye movements were achieved by Marvin and Jernigan (8) and by Whiteside (10). However, these methods imply a continuous accurate alignment of the light source, the eye and the light receptors, so that we preferred to record the eye movements by means of electro-oculography as this is simpler to make and sensitive enough for the purpose.

Heijl, A. and Greve, E.L. (eds.), Proceedings of the 6th Int. Visual Field Symposium.
© 1985, Dr W. Junk Publishers, Dordrecht, The Netherlands. ISBN 978-94-010-8932-6

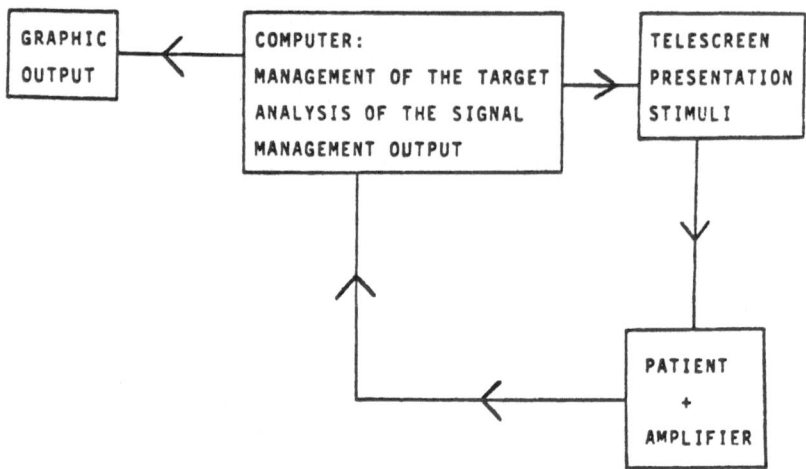

Fig. 1. Block diagram of our apparatus.

METHOD

Figure 1 is the block diagram of the aimed instrumentation (actually achieved except for analysis of the EOG signals by the computer).

The 37 stimuli (Fig. 2) are presented on a white-black 52 cm x 41 cm standard TV screen placed at 30 cm from the examined eye. The computer arranges that light alternatively appears for 4 sec in the central position and for 2 sec in a peripheral position in a pseudo-random sequence till all 36 peripheral positions have been used. In this way the subject expects the return in the center but cannot foresee the next peripheral position. Next with his spectacles in place the subject was encouraged to look towards every target. The stimuli were white dots of either 30' or 1°5 visual angle. Their luminance was 40 cd.m^{-2} (120 asb) and that of the background 5 cd.m^{-2} (15 asb). The examination was performed in a dimly lit room. It could be easily repeated for control.

A pair of Ag–AgCl electrodes was placed at the external and internal corners of the examined eye in order to record its horizontal movements. Another pair was placed above and beneath the orbit in order to record the vertical movements. A ground electrode was fixed on the ear lobe.

An EEG pen apparatus eliminated unwanted frequencies and amplified the electro-oculographic signals on two channels (one for the horizontal movements and the other for the vertical ones). A third channel recorded from the computer the beginning and the end of each stimulation.

In the first stage of our experiment the decision about the patient's seeing of a given stimulus was built either from the qualitative analysis of shape and sign of the electro-oculographic signals, or from the quantitative analysis of their amplitudes.

The shape analysis was based on the fact that, when the stimulus is seen, there are only two major eye movements, one bringing gaze from the central

522

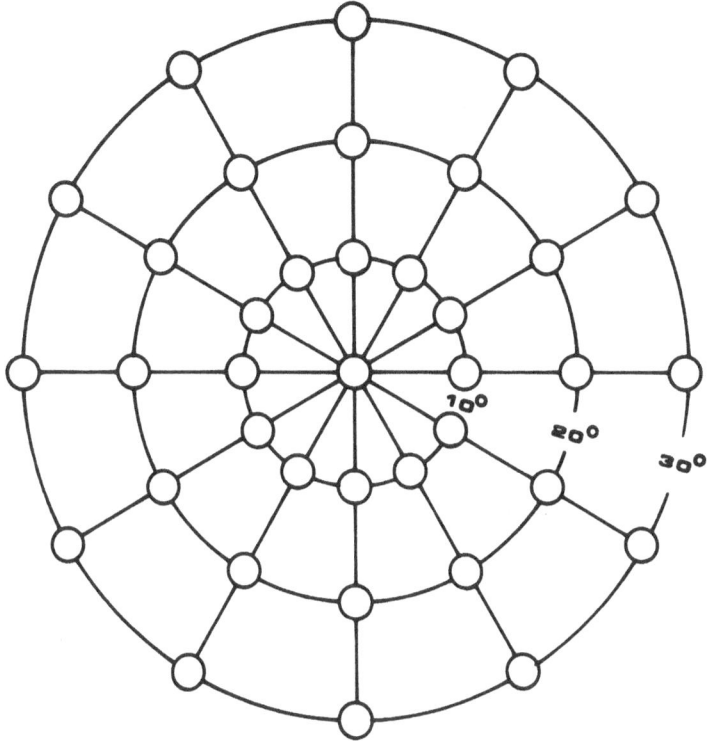

Fig. 2. Location of the 37 stimuli.

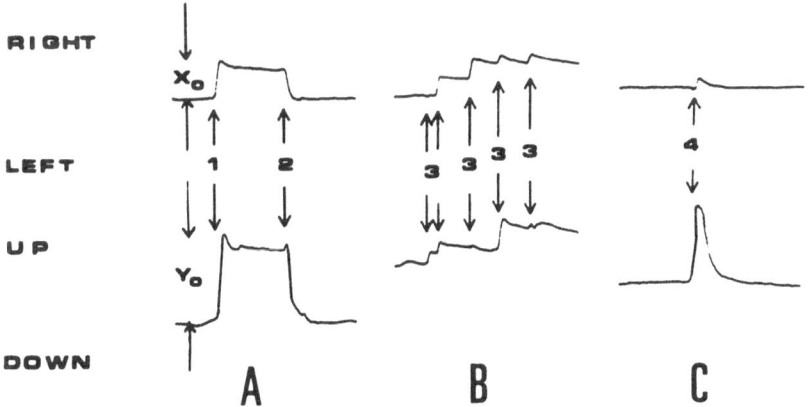

Fig. 3. Shape analysis. A: seen stimulus. B: not seen stimulus (search saccades). C: blinking movement.

position to the peripheral stimulus, and the other being the symmetrical return movement (Fig. 3A). On the contrary, when the stimulus is not seen, there are more searching saccades, a last one bringing gaze back to the center (Fig. 3B). Blinking can be distinguished from saccades by a special form, a short duration and a bigger vertical amplitude (Fig. 3C). The sign analysis was based on the fact that the combination of deflexion signs on the two channels is typical for each quadrant toward which the eye movement is directed. The stimulus was considered as not seen when the couple of signs did not correspond to the direction in which the stimulus was presented.

The amplitude analysis compared the recorded deflexions with the expected ones (on the basis of the law of Fenn and Hursh (2)). A stimulus was considered as not seen when the difference between the observed signal and the expected signal in one or in both derivations was greater than twice the correspondant standard deviation for signals seen according to shape analysis.

The duration of the examination was about 4 min. That of shape and sign analysis lasted about 10 min, and that of amplitude analysis about 30 min.

RESULTS

We examined first the right eye of a 22 year old normal subject. He saw all 30' targets as ascertained verbally. The shape and sign analysis of the ocular movements demonstrated also that all targets were seen. The amplitude analysis showed that all targets were seen except one.

Afterwards we examined two older subjects with pathology in whom usual psychophysical perimetry proved to be difficult. Figures 4 and 5 allow one to compare the outcomes of the two kinds of analysis of the EOG results with that of traditional kinetic perimetry. There is a good agreement, while the defect is obviously larger for the 30' target than for the 1°5 one.

DISCUSSION

The obtained results were encouraging so that we have now to improve the method. Of course analysis of the results by inspection and calculation is much too long and has to be replaced in the next stage by computer analysis: as in Jernigan's device (6), the computer should extract the necessary information to make an automatic objective decision. Another possible means of control of the movements is to amplify in DC the EOG signals and to combine them at right angles in such a manner that the point the subject is fixating appears as a spot on a second TV-screen (see Blaauw (1)) and can be directly compared with the expected location.

It has to be verified if it is better to use a constant central fixation mark that the patient should not deviate from when no peripheral stimulus is seen. But, on the other hand, it should also be possible to use no central fixation mark: once a stimulus is seen and fixated, the machine could present the next

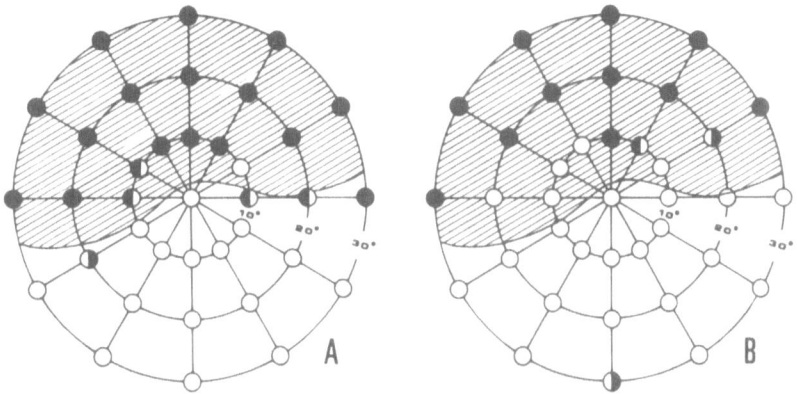

Fig. 4. Results in a right eye suffering from lower idiopathic retinal detachment (76 y old male subject). A black left half of a disk indicates that the stimulus was not seen according to shape and sign analysis, while a black right half indicates that the stimulus was not seen according to amplitude analysis. The continuous line gives the limit of the defect by usual kinetic perimetry. A: 30′ target. B: 1°5 target.

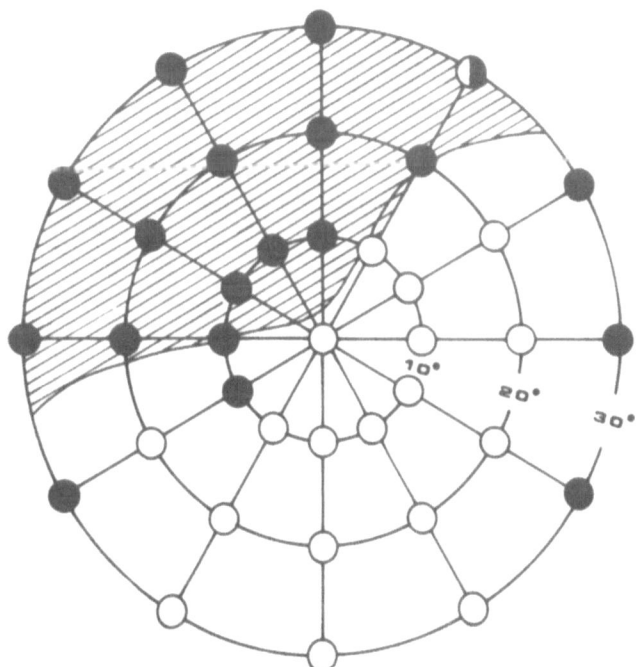

Fig. 5. Results in the right eye of a 64 y old male subject suffering from cerebral vascular pathology. See the legend of Fig. 4. 30′ target.

stimulus in the next position relative to the preceeding one (this was already done by Whiteside (10) but only along the horizontal meridian).

In our preliminary experiment we have put stimuli on the horizontal and vertical meridians for checking if a horizontal movement produced no deflexion on the vertical derivation and vice-versa. Such localisations could be avoided in the future. Another improvement to be realized is that the stimulus becomes stronger by increasing its size from center to periphery according to the normal sensitivity gradient. Moreover stimulation could be made near threshold, but we must not permit the examination to become too long.

REFERENCES

1. Blaauw, G.J. Drivers' scanning behaviour on some curved and straight road sections. 1er Congr. int. sur la Vision et la Sécurité Routière, 47–56 (1974).
2. Fenn, W.O. and Hursh, J.B. Movements of the eyes when the lids are closed. Am. J. Physiol. 118: 8–14 (1937).
3. Futenma, M. Perimeter for children or mentally handicapped. Acta Soc. Ophthalmol. Jap. 81: 1539–1548 (1977).
4. Harrington, D.O. The visual field. C.V. Mosby C°, St Louis (1956).
5. Howe, J.W. The causes and assessment of visual field defects in young children. Br. Orthopt. J. 34: 46–53 (1977).
6. Jernigan, M.E. Visual field plotting using eye movement response. IEEE Trans. Biomed. Eng. BME 26: 601–606 (1979).
7. Lauber, H. Das Gesichtsfeld, Untersuchungsgrundlagen, Physiologie und Pathologie. J.F. Bergmann, Munich/Springer, Berlin (1944).
8. Marvin, E. and Jernigan, M.E. A new technique for objectively plotting visual fields. Ann. Ophthalmol. 6: 335–341 (1974).
9. Verriest, G. and Van de Casteele, J. Le champ visuel clinique. Acta Belg. Arte Med. Pharmac. Milit. 18: 35–205 (1972).
10. Whiteside, J.A. Peripheral vision in children and adults. Child Development 47: 290–293 (1976).

Author's address:
Dept. of Ophthalmology,
University of Ghent,
Ghent, Belgium

INFLUENCE OF DIAZEPAM ON THE OUTCOME OF
AUTOMATED PERIMETRY

ANITA L. HAAS and JOSEF FLAMMER

(*Berne, Switzerland*)

ABSTRACT

In order to detect and follow up early functional defects in glaucoma, we are concerned with small changes which occur in quantitative perimetry. Changes due to a disease state must be differentiated from artificial changes, for example, those due to influence of drugs.

In order to satisfy a possible influence of tranquillizers on the visual field, we treated healthy volunteers with placebo, 5 and 10 mg diazepam, respectively. The visual fields were determined using program JO on the Octopus automated perimeter. We evaluated the effect of treatment on the differential light sensitivities, their scatter, the learning and fatigue phenomena as well as reaction times.

INTRODUCTION

In quantitative perimetry we are often interested to find changes over time. In chronic diseases such as glaucoma these changes might be small. We have therefore to separate real changes from long-term fluctuations as well as from artificial changes. The purpose of this study was to test whether diazepam could have such an artificial influence.

The assumption that diazepam could have an influence on the outcome of static perimetry was based on the fact that influences of psychopharmaca on visual function are already described (1, 3, 5). In addition to that benzodiazepine receptors have been found to occur in the retina.

MATERIAL AND METHODS

We tested thirty volunteers (nine females and twentyone males). They were mostly students with ages ranging between eighteen and twentyeight years. Individuals taking any kind of drugs were excluded from the study. Each individual was examined three times. In the first session they were introduced in the study and to the Octopus automated perimeter system. In the second

Heijl, A. and Greve, E.L. (eds.), Proceedings of the 6th Int. Visual Field Symposium.
© *1985, Dr W. Junk Publishers, Dordrecht, The Netherlands. ISBN 978-94-010-8932-6*

Mean (±SEM) of the differential light sensitivity

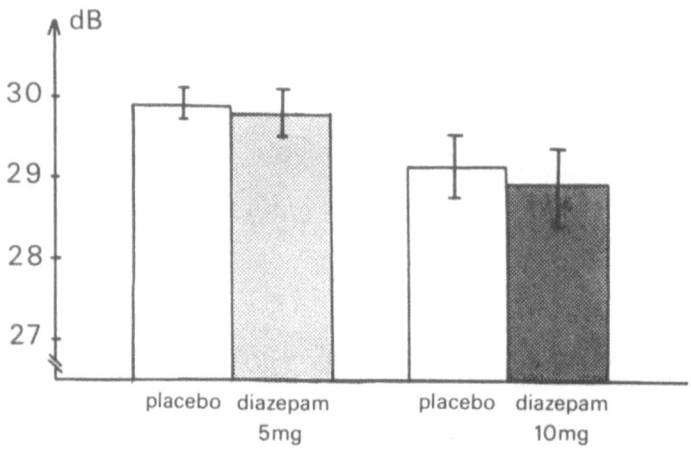

Fig. 1. The mean of the differential light sensitivity shows a slight, but statistically not significant decrease under diazepam treatment. SEM: Standard error mean.

and third sessions, the visual field test was carried out. Four hours before the test they took a tablet of placebo or diazepam in a randomized sequence. Seventeen subjects received five milligram diazepam and thirteen subjects ten milligram diazepam per os.

The time span between the two tests was two weeks. Twentyfour hours before the test alcohol was prohibited. The perimetry was done with program JO on the Octopus automated perimeter. This program is described elsewhere (3). We just like to emphasize here that the program JO provides a good estimation of fluctuation, since each test location is measured at least twice. It also enables us to recognize fatigue effects since at two test locations, the threshold is measured ten times distributed over the total visual field test. In addition, the program JO measures the reaction times.

The statistical analyses were done with paired T-Test and Mann-Whitney-U-Test. For the rate of false responses an arcine transformation was applied.

RESULTS

1. The differential light threshold: The differential light sensitivity was diffusely and slightly decreased in the total visual field after diazepam treatment. This could be observed with both dosages (5 and 10 mg diazepam). This slight change was not statistically significant, however. The mean values of each group are represented in Fig. 1.

528

Short–term fluctuation

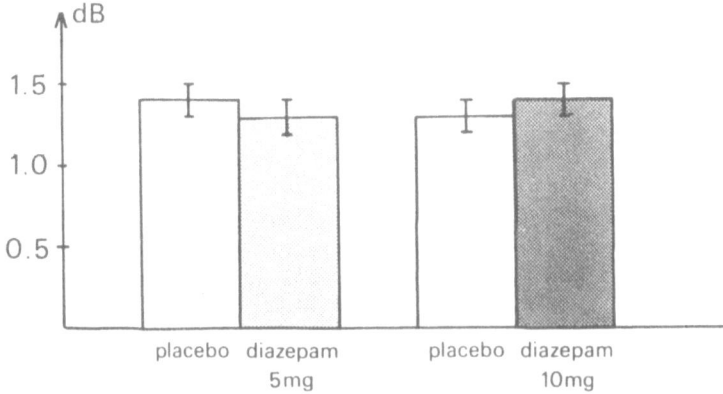

Fig. 2. The short-term fluctuation does not change significantly under treatment.

2. The short-term fluctuation was calculated as the root-mean-square of the local standard deviations. This scatter did not change statistically under treatment (Fig. 2).

3. The reaction time: We measured the time between the stimulus exposure and the response of the patient. The subjects were not instructed to respond as quickly as possible; rather they were to react in a normal way. They were not aware that we also measured the reaction time. Interestingly, this reaction time showed a slight tendency to decrease with treatment (Fig. 3).

4. False replies in catch trials: The Octopus perimeter has built in catch trials in which it tests for false positive and false negative replies. After diazepam treatment, the rate of false positive replies was smaller and the rate of false negative replies was larger than under placebo. But these changes also did not reach statistical significance (Fig. 4).

5. The fatigue effect: Under placebo, the sensitivity decreased slightly during the visual field test at the two locations tested ten times. This fatigue effect, however, was not increased after diazepam therapy.

6. The learning effect: The JO program measures the threshold at fortyseven test locations twice in separate phases. In the first visual field test, the mean sensitivity in the second phase was significantly ($p < 0.01$) higher than in the first phase. This is a well known learning effect (4). In the second visual field, the second phase was still slightly higher than in the first phase, but this difference was not significant anymore. Comparing the overall mean of the first visual field test with the overall mean of the second, we find further a significant ($p < 0.05$) difference, the sensitivity being higher in the second

Reaction time

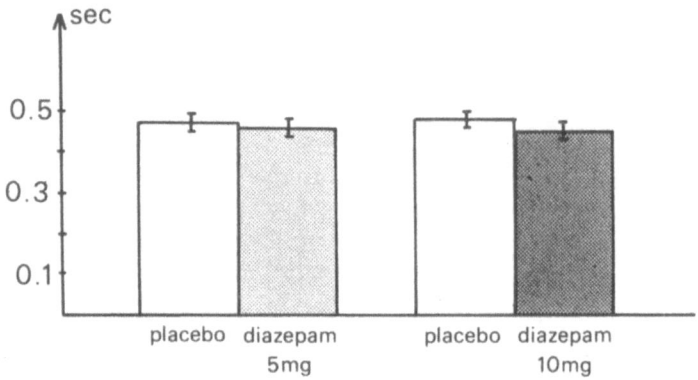

Fig. 3. The reaction time shows a slight tendency to decrease with treatment.

False positive replies   False negative replies

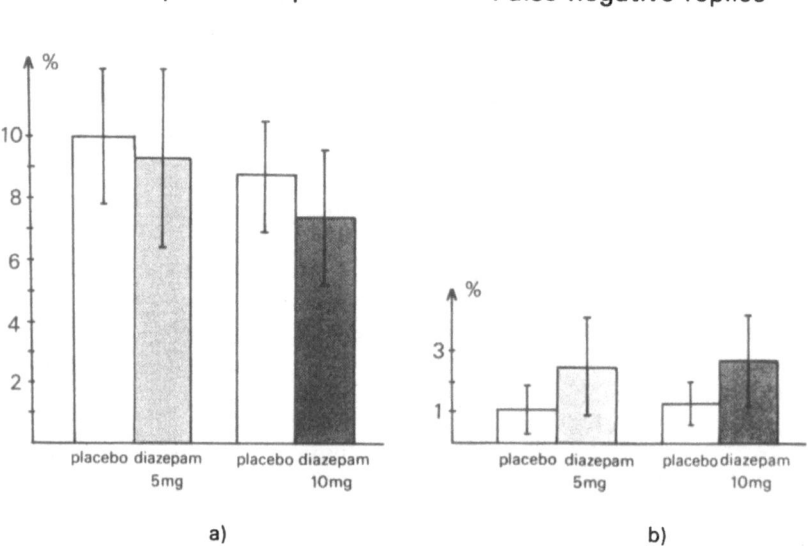

a)   b)

Fig. 4. After diazepam treatment, the rate of false positive replies was smaller and the rate of false negative replies was larger than under placebo.

visual field test. Breaking down this difference between the two phases as well as between the two visual field tests in placebo and diazepam treatment, we did not find any difference. This implies that diazepam had no detectable influence on the learning effect.

530

DISCUSSION

Our main concern is to separate true visual field changes from artificial changes such as influences of drugs. In our group of young volunteers, we did not find any sort of significant influence of diazepam after short-term treatment. We wish to emphasize that these results cannot be generalized. It is well possible that a long-term treatment or a treatment with older people might be different.

The overally sensitivity showed a slight tendency to decrease under diazepam treatment, but it was not significant and very little in comparison to the spontaneous fluctuation of the threshold.

It was very interesting, however, to observe that the short-term fluctuation did not increase at all. The short-term fluctuation is influenced by many factors, one main factor being the cooperation of the patient. The fact that it did not change is a good indication that the ability to cooperate during the visual field test did not change.

It is well known that the reaction time can increase under tranquillizer therapy. As mentioned before we did not instruct the volunteers to react as fast as possible. The natural reaction time was measured and this did not change under these conditions.

The decrease of false positive replies in catch trials and the increase of false negative replies is difficult to explain. Since it was not significant, it could be due to chance. A fatigue effect is described in retrolaminar processes, like for example after retrobulbear neuritis, but also in glaucoma patients. Interestingly we could observe such a fatigue effect already in normal subjects. This effect was very small, however. The diazepam therapy did not increase this effect at all as one could expect.

The learning effect was individually very different, but statistically significant and not influenced by diazepam.

We can conclude from our results that the outcome of automated static perimetry is not influenced by a short-term treatment with diazepam, at least not to young individuals. In perimetry we measure the differential light sensitivity which is a basic and elementary visual function. It is quite possible that higher and more complex visual functions are more sensitive to tranquillizers.

REFERENCES

1. Austen, D.P. and Gilmartin, B.A. The effect of chlordiazepoxide on visual field, extraocular muscle balance, colour matching ability and hand-eye coordination in man. The British Journal of Pharmacology (1971).
2. Fisch, H.U., Groner, M., Groner, R. and Menz, Ch. Influence of diazepam and methylphenidate on identification of rapidly presented letter strings: Diazepam enhances visual masking. Psychopharmacology 80: 61–66 (1983).
3. Flammer, J., Drance, S.M., Jenni, A. and Bebie, H. JO and STATJO: programs for investigating the visual field with the Octopus automatic perimeter. Can. J. Ophthalmol., vol. 18, no. 3 (1983).
4. Gloor, B. Die Computerperimetrie in der langfristigen Beurteilung des Glaucoms.

In Kriegelstein G.K. and Leydhecker, W. Medikamentöse Glaukomtherapie. J.F. Bergmann-Verlag, München 59–72 (1982).

5. Kamp, C.W. and Morgan, W.W. Benzodiazepines supress the light response of retinal dopaminergic neurons in vivo. European Journal of Pharmacology 77: 343–346 (1982).

Author's address:
University Eye Clinic
Inselspital
CH-3010 Berne, Switzerland

VOLUME OF THE THREE-DIMENSIONAL VISUAL FIELD AND ITS OBJECTIVE EVALUATION BY SHAPE COEFFICIENT: NORMAL VALUES BY AGE AND ABNORMAL VISUAL FIELD

HIROTAKA SUZUMURA, FUMIO FURUNO and HARUTAKE MATSUO

(*Tokyo, Japan*)

ABSTRACT

The distribution of visual field sensitivity was measured as a function of visual angle and expressed in polar coordinates. This procedure provides an accurate impression of the visual field and emphasises visual field sensitivity; additional coefficients are not necessary. As normal controls, 229 eyes of 145 cases were examined. The results of kinetic quantitative perimetry were calculated and three-dimensional visual field representations were plotted by a computer. The normal visual field is larger in the young (subjects from 10 to about 40 years of age). After the fourth decade the field size gradually reduces. The three-dimensional 'sensitivity loss' occurs first at the center, then at the peripheral regions. Further, glaucomas were classified into high tension glaucoma (HTG) and low tension glaucoma (LTG). LTG has a slightly different manifestation of visual field disturbance than HTG.

1. INTRODUCTION

Traquair's 'island of vision' is a visual field representation which appears as an island floating in a flat sea. It is useful in expressing a two-dimensional visual field, but does not correctly reflect the distribution of visual sensitivity. It is therefore not possible to evaluate visual function even though the volume may be determined directly. To take the sensitivity distribution as a function of visual angle into account, visual fields were expressed in three-dimensions by conversion into polar coordinates (1, 4). The results of this procedure are presented below.

2. MATERIALS AND METHODS

Patients were divided by age into one of eight groups ranging from 1 to 80 years of age. Grouping was in decade intervals. Thirty eyes of each age group with normal visual fields and with no abnormalities except anomalies of refraction were selected for study. For each age group, volume, isopter area

Heijl, A. and Greve, E.L. (eds.), Proceedings of the 6th Int. Visual Field Symposium.
© 1985, Dr W. Junk Publishers, Dordrecht, The Netherlands. ISBN 978-94-010-8932-6

and shape coefficient were determined. Fifty-five eyes with glaucoma were also examined. Difference glaucoma groups, high tension glaucoma (HTG) and low tension glaucoma (LTG) were compared. The category of 'LTG' consisted of those patients who presented with glaucomatous visual field change and glaucomatous optic disc change with a normal IOP ($\leqslant 22$ mmHg) but without known cause. These criteria included all types of LTG defined by Greve (2); impairment of control mechanism of IOP was not taken into consideration. The results of kinetic quantitative perimetry were converted into three-dimensional shapes based on the following criteria: the inverse number of the logarithm of target luminance of each isopter was assumed to be a sensitivity, and a three-dimensional form was constructed, assuming 0.5 log. units to be 50 mm. An isopter of V/4 with different target area from target I was excluded from the three-dimensional figure. Targets below I/4 were used to construct three-dimensional figures. The base point of a visual field was assumed to be on the surface of the eye and V/4 isopter was taken as the base point. The difference between V/4 and I/4 was assumed to be 2.5 log. units, and was placed so that it was 250 mm on a visual field chart. The sensitivity at the fixation point was assumed to be 0.5 log. units higher than the measured maximum sensitivity.

Based on the above, a program was constructed to measure individual visual fields, using a microcomputer. The area, circumference length and shape coefficient of each isopter were calculated and three-dimensional visual field figures were developed and their volumes were calculated.

For an objective evaluation of the visual field as an indicant of visual function, the volume referred to as 'modified volume' was calculated in addition to the original volume. The volume multiplied by the mean value of shape coefficients of each isopter was assumed to be a modified volume. It was considered that we mainly rely upon the shape of each isopter in our subjective evaluation and interpretation of visual field.

3. RESULTS

Mean values of volume by age and changes by aging in normal visual fields are presented in Table 1. The visual fields reaches a peak of 64 000–65 000 cm³ from age 10–39. The volume is gradually reduced after the age of 40. The rate of decay accelerates after the age of 60. The same tendency is seen with respect to modified volume. In a comparison of the visual field between normal and glaucomatous eyes, the volume of visual field was over 90% of the mean normal volume in 8 of 36 eyes with HTG, primary open angle glaucoma (POAG) or developmental glaucoma (DG) and 7 of 19 eyes with LTG. In 2 eyes with LTG with breakthrough, the volume was nearly the same as in normal eyes. In cases of DG and of middle stage and more advanced POAG, the severity of the decrease of visual field volume was greater than the severity of glaucomatous visual field change. Table 2 shows the volume and modified volume in patients with HTG and those with LTG, all of whom exhibited roughly the same degree of glaucomatous visual field changes.

The individual and mean volume were significantly greater in LTG with

Table 1. Mean values of volume and modified volume by age and standard deviation (cm³).

Age	Volume	Modified vol.
0–9	52850 ± 13701	39132 ± 10355
10–19	65349 ± 10506	49261 ± 9687
20–29	65128 ± 9199	49609 ± 7141
30–39	64757 ± 9919	48891 ± 7989
40–49	60636 ± 8805	46078 ± 7235
50–59	59265 ± 7665	44572 ± 6470
60–69	51316 ± 8963	38335 ± 7938
70–79	45710 ± 9846	34641 ± 8083

Table 2. Visual field volume in high tension glaucoma (POAG, DG) and low tension glaucoma in percentage to the mean normal value.

	POAG & DG		LTG	
	Volume	Modified vol.	Volume	Modified vol.
Only nasal defect Only arcuate defect	85.2 ± 30.9	78.9 ± 33.5	100	100
Nasal & arcuate defect Incomplete breakthrough	59.1 ± 19.9	46.3 ± 20.0	81.8 ± 32.0	68.2 ± 29.1
Complete breakthrough Temporal & central rest	48.6 ± 17.1	40.4 ± 13.7	42.2 ± 33.8	30.5 ± 28.0

middle stage, nasal and arcuate defects or incomplete breakthrough, than in HTG (t-test, $P < 0.05$). However, no significant difference was found between LTG with complete breakthrough or with temporal and central island and HTG with the same changes (t-test, $P < 0.05$). The same tendency was observed with the modified volume. LTG with early visual field changes was detected only in one case, which precluded comparison.

4. DISCUSSION

Figure 1 shows 3-dimensional visual field figures close to the mean normal volume grouped according to age. 'Sensitivity loss' starts at the upper part of the 3-dimensional visual field and then spreads towards the lower part. The reduction of volume of visual field due to aging, especially for accelerated reduction of volume of visual field at older ages may be due in part to delayed reaction time and reduced test comprehension. Deteriorating function of visual pathways and of transmission of media also may be cosidered. In our study on glaucomatous visual field disturbances, a significant difference between LTG and HTG was found. It has been generally believed that visual field change in LTG is identical with that in POAG. However, Levene (3), cited early dense field defect to within 5° of fixation, sudden visual field loss, early involvement of fixation and slow progression of visual field defect, as the characteristics of visual field change in LTG.

535

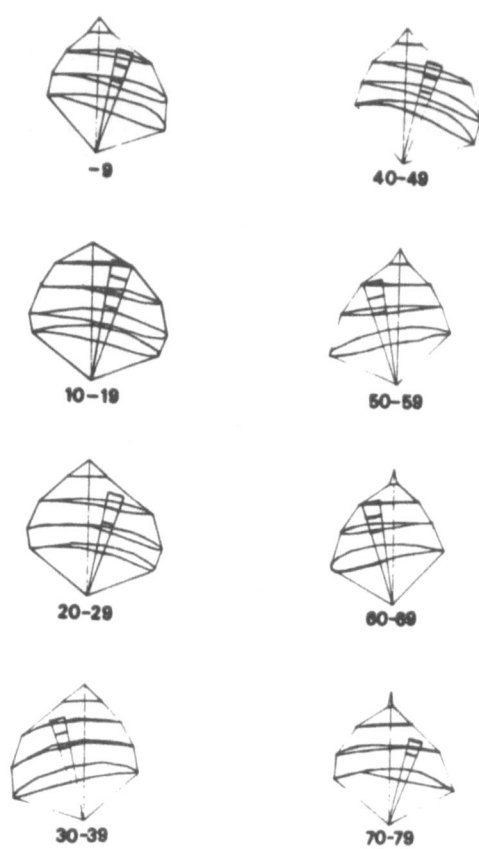

Fig. 1. Changes of 3-dimensional visual field by aging. The contraction of visual field with aging occurs firstly in the central area and gradually spreads towards the periphery.

Motolko (5) on the other hand, compared visual field change between LTG and POAG with the same degree of optic disc change, was found no difference in visual fields. There also seemed to be no difference between LTG and HTG in the pattern of defect in visual field change in our cases. In the present study involving the comparison of volume of visual field in patients with glaucomatous visual field change in the middle stage, it was confirmed that the volume of visual field was significantly greater in LTG than HTG. In LTG, it was significant that only the typical gluacomatous visual field defect was present and a general sensitivity loss was not detected. These results indicate that the difference between HTG and LTG on volume was caused by general sensitivity loss. That is, retinal sensitivity of the seemingly normal area in HTG is diminished in conjunction with typical glaucomatous visual field change. On the other hand, retinal sensitivity of the unaffected area remains nearly normal even if typical glaucomatous visual field change is considerably advanced in LTG.

Moreover, only one case of LTG showed early field defect. This, together with the fact that LTG is frequently discovered by chance during optic disc examination, suggests that visual field change already is advanced when LTG is detected. A retinal nerve fiber layer defect with sharp borders was frequently observed in LTG (6).

From the above findings, it is likely that susceptibility to elevated IOP and/or other factors in selected parts of optic disc, e.g. Bjerrum's area, is greater than in the other parts of the disc, and that visual field disturbance in LTG differs from that in HTG with respect to the mechanism of development.

The general sensitivity loss has not been given much attention in earlier studies of glaucomatous visual field change which have concentrated on the pattern of te visual field defect. However, clinical significance of the general sensitivity loss was revealed by the objective evaluation of visual field as based on volume estimates.

5. CONCLUSION

Our investigation suggests:

(1) The normal 3-dimensional visual field reaches maximum volume at the age of 10–39. 'Sensitivity loss' with aging occurs first at the central isopter. Thereafter 'sensitivity loss' spreads towards the peripheral area. 'General sensitivity loss' occurs in the visual field after 60 years of age.

(2) In the case of HTG, 'general sensitivity loss' in the visual field was observed together with localized glaucomatous visual field changes. In the cases of LTG, however, such 'general sensitivity loss' in the visual field was not observed until the late stage. We therefore believe that there may be some differences in the mechanism of the development of visual field disturbances in glaucoma.

REFERENCES

1. Furuno, F. Discussion in the Docum. Ophthalm. Proc. Series 35: 222–223 (1983).
2. Greve, E.L. and Geijssen, H.C. The relation between excavation and visual field in glaucoma patients with high and low intraocular pressures. Docum. Ophthalm. Proc. Series 35: 35–42 (1983).
3. Levene, R.Z. Low tension glaucoma. Glaucoma 4: 142–143 (1982).
4. Matsuo, H. On practice in perimetry. Jpn. J. of Clinical Ophthalmol. 37: 263–277 (1983).
5. Motolko, M., Drance, S.M. and Douglas, G.R. Visual field defects in low tension glaucoma. Arch. Ophthalmol. 100: 1074–1077 (1982).
6. Ogawa, T., Furuno, F., Seki, A., Miyamoto, T. and Ohta, Y. Kinetic quantitative perimetry of retinal nerve fiber layer defects in glaucoma by Fundus Photo-Perimeter. Docum. Ophthalm. Proc. Series 35: 27–34 (1983).

Author's address:
Department of Ophthalmology
Tokyo Medical Collega Hospital
6-7-1, Nishishinjuku,
Shinjuku-ku, Tokyo
Japan 160.

EFFECTS OF RANDOM PRESENTATION ON KINETIC THRESHOLD

E. GANDOLFO, P. CAPRIS, G. CORALLO and M. ZINGIRIAN

(*Genoa, Italy*)

ABSTRACT

The authors carried out perimetric tests to evaluate the influence of kinetic stimuli randomization on the threshold. The same target was presented first in a sequential manner (the examined subject knowing in advance the target direction) and afterwards in a randomized manner (the subject ignoring the stimulus direction). Both normal subjects (10 individuals) and patients suffering from visual field defects due to various pathological conditions (10 individuals) were tested. All tests were repeated five times in order to evaluate long term fluctuations of the kinetic threshold. The automated Goldmann Perimeter Perikon was employed to obtain good fixation control and consistency of the examination conditions. Stimuli randomization caused a significant isopteric contraction. On the other hand, sequential stimulus exposure seemed to assume more consistent results in repeated examinations, provided that the subjects showed a good attention level.

INTRODUCTION

In a recent paper, we have demonstrated that a random presentation of the kinetic perimetric stimuli caused an isopteric contraction compared to a visual field (v.f.) examination performed with sequentially arranged stimuli (1).

In order to increase our knowledge about this phenomenon and to verify what method (sequential or random) could give us more consistent results, we continued our studies. Our aim was to evaluate the influence of randomization on repeated kinetic tests both in normal and pathological fields.

MATERIAL AND METHOD

10 normal and 10 pathological subjects underwent our perimetric test. The normal people were young and healthy individuals without any refractive or

general disorder. The pathological subjects were 4 glaucomatous patients suffering from evident v.f. loss, 3 patients with neuro-ophthalmological disorders (optic neuritis, papilledema, hemianopia) and 3 patients affected by retino-choroidal diseases (diabetic retinopathy, pigmentary retinal degeneration, central artery branch occlusion).

Every subject underwent both sequential and random examinations repeated five times on different days and at different times of the day.

In the normal subjects the test was performed in the temporal v.f. of the right eye along the following meridians: $87°–60°–30°–5°–355°–330°–300°–273°$.

In the pathological individuals the test was performed along 8 meridians chosen in the v.f. sector in which the more evident alterations were present.

In all cases we used the I4e stimulus.

The entire study was performed utilizing the Automatic Goldmann Perimeter PERIKON (4).

We calculated for all subjects the validity coefficient (v.c.) as an index of the long-term fluctuation (see Table 1).

RESULTS

This study confirmed the negative effect of a random stimuli arrangement on the kinetic threshold. Both in normal and pathological cases randomization of the kinetic stimuli caused a significant isopteric contraction (normal v.f.: average contraction = $2°33'$; pathological v.f.: average contraction = $2°46'$) (Fig. 1).

The repetitive tests demonstrated that the long-term kinetic threshold fluctuation was higher in pathological than in normal cases: pathological cases: average variability coefficient (v.c.) = 8.7%; normal cases: average v.c. = 5.85%. The results in different pathological conditions were similar (glaucoma patients: average v.c. = 7.2%; neuro-ophthalmological cases: average v.c. = 11.1%; retino-choroidal disorders: average v.c. = 8.1%).

The comparison between the results obtained after sequential and random tests showed a better consistency of the first method in normal v.f. (average v.c. = 5.2 for sequential method; average v.c. = 6.5% for random method). On the other hand, in pathological cases, the threshold fluctuation was equal both in sequential and random tests (average v.c. = 8.7% for sequential method; average v.c. = 8.7% for random method).

CONCLUSIONS

The obtained results showed that kinetic stimuli randomization had noticeable effects on the eccentricity of the perception. This phenomenon was not due to fixation loss because our automated Goldmann perimeter possessed a precise computerized fixation control system.

In our opinion the role of attention was important. In fact the subject, knowing in advance the stimulus direction was psychologically stimulated to maintain better concentration. On the other hand the patient, ignoring the

Table 1. Statistical analysis carried out in all studied cases.

Name: D.F.
Right eye
Age: 29 years
Temporal visual field

Method Explored meridians	Sequential 87°	60°	30°	5°	355°	330°	300°	273°
Eccentricities of perceptions during kinetic perimetric tests	51	61	71	77	82	77	54	54
	51	59	75	81	78	79	68	59
	49	64	78	86	79	78	65	57
	60	51	67	78	77	57	54	48
	56	59	74	83	80	74	66	53
Mean	53.4	58.8	73	81	79.4	77	64	55.4
Standard deviation	4.28	4.82	4.18	3.67	2.24	1.87	4.18	2.51
Variability coefficient	8.01%	8.2%	5.73%	4.53%	2.82%	2.43%	6.53%	4.53%
Mean variability coefficient	5.347% (S.D. = 2.17)							

Name: D.F.
Right eye
Diagnosis: normal
Stimulus: I4E Perimeter: Perikon

Method Explored meridians	Random 87°	60°	30°	5°	355°	300°	300°	273°
Eccentricities of perceptions during kinetic perimetric tests	50	60	65	73	80	65	64	56
	52	53	70	76	79	76	70	58
	46	63	79	79	74	77	66	54
	48	49	69	83	70	69	55	56
	49	52	64	85	76	74	55	55
Mean	49	55.4	69.4	79.2	75.8	77.2	62	55.8
Standard deviation	2.24	5.86	5.94	4.92	4.05	5.07	6.74	1.48
Variability coefficient	4.57%	10.63%	8.56%	6.21%	5.34%	6.57%	10.87%	2.65%
Mean variability coefficient	6.914% (S.D. = 2.9)							

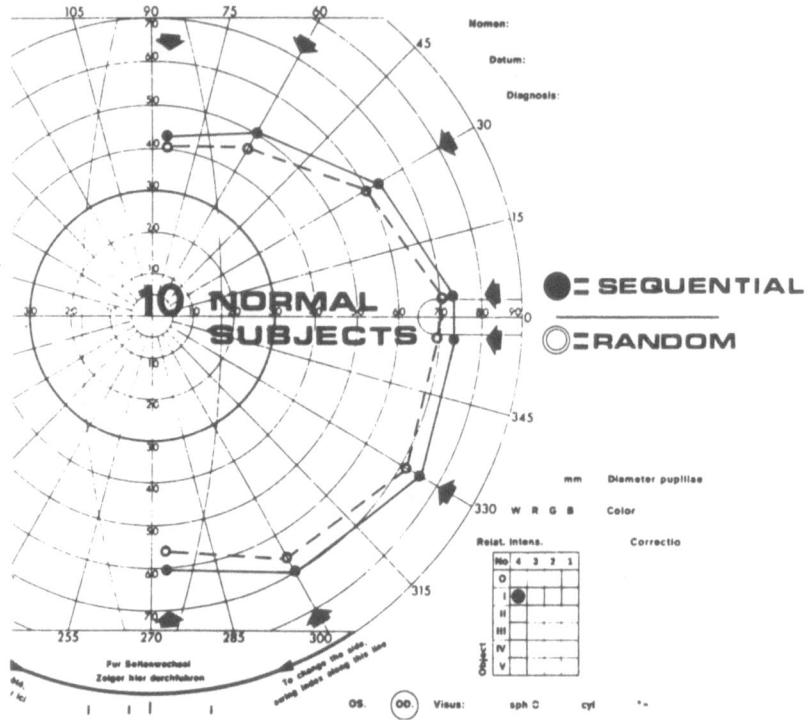

Fig. 1. Mean isopteric difference (in normal subjects) due to stimuli arrangement.

stimulus direction, often waited some time before pushing the button in order to ascertain real target presence: this fact practically increased the time in which the perception remained uncertain. The repetition of the tests showed that in normal field the results were more consistent when the stimuli were arranged in a sequential manner.

In pathological field, on the contrary, no relevant difference of the consistency of results was seen with the two methods.

On the basis of our results, we recommend the adoption of a sequential arrangement of the stimuli in automated kinetic perimetry since this method perimits a certain shortening of the examination and seems to guarantee more consistent results in normal subjects. All these consideration are valid only for subjects showing good cooperation and for perimeters with a precise system of automatic fixation control in order to avoid involuntary eye movements (2, 3).

In this phase of the research, we haven't tested the detection rates but we only looked for the best method for determining comparable isopters in successive examinations.

REFERENCES

1. Gandolfo, E., Corallo, G., Barabino, M. and Capris, P. Influenza della randomizzazione sulla percezione di stimoli cinetici. Boll. Oculist. (in press).

2. Heijl, A. and Krakau, T. A note on fixation during perimetry. Acta Ophthalmol. 5: 854–861 (1977).
3. Johnson, C.A. and Keltner, J.L. Automated suprathreshold static perimetry. Am. J. Ophthalmol. 89: 731–741 (1980).
4. Zingirian, M. Gandolfo, E. and Orciuolo, M. Automation of the Goldmann perimeter. Doc. Ophthalmol. Proc. 35: 381–385 (1983).

THE HILL OF VISION: A PREDICTABLE AGE
RELATED QUANTITY?

N. JACOBS and H. PATTERSON

(*Manchester, England*)

ABSTRACT

It has been assumed that the retinal threshold sensitivity profile is a standard which decreases predictably with age. On this bases, the significance of relative scotomata is decided on certain types of perimeter.

The Dicon perimeter measures the individual profile by simultaneous stimulation in 4 quadrants at equal eccentricity under photopic conditions. This circumvents possible error due to local field defects.

We measured this 'hill of vision' in 128 healthy eyes, and found that there is a large variation between individuals, with no relationship to age. The effects of refractive error were examined in 3 subjects.

INTRODUCTION

Automated static perimeters perform screening of the visual field at selected points. They may establish the threshold sensitivity at each point and compare it to an assumed age related value, as is the case with the Octopus (5). Otherwise a stimulus greater than the assumed normal threshold value is used, on the premise that any missed point shows a significant defect. This suprathreshold technique developed by Armaly (1) on the Goldmann perimeter, and later modified (6), has the advantages of speed and reproducibility in the hands of differing operators (3). It is used on many automated perimeters including the Fieldmaster (4), the Friedmann (2) and the Dicon. The Fieldmaster uses 2 levels of suprathreshold stimulus, the stronger one beyond $30°$ of eccentricity. In the case of the Friedmann, the threshold is not assumed but is determined for each patient, however the shape of the hill of vision is assumed. The Dicon measures the hill of vision in 4 quadrants, thereby avoiding artefact due to local field defects. Glaucoma screening is then performed at 0.4 Log Units (L.U.) suprathreshold.

Heijl, A. and Greve, E.L. (eds.), Proceedings of the 6th Int. Visual Field Symposium.
© *1985, Dr W. Junk Publishers, Dordrecht, The Netherlands. ISBN 978-94-010-8932-6*

Table 1. Description of age groups.

Group	Age Range	Visual Acuity Range	Number of Subjects
I	9–29 yrs	6/5–6/6	11
II	30–42 yrs	6/5–6/9	10
III	54–80 yrs	6/5–6/12	12

MATERIALS AND METHODS

The hill of vision was measured on the Dicon-2000 automated perimeter, with a background illumination of 31.5 Apostilbs (Asb) and a spot size Goldmann II. Threshold was determined by simultaneous stimulation in 4 quadrants along the 45°, 135°, 225° and 315° meridians at equal eccentricities of 2.5°, 5°, 15°, 25°, 40° and 60°. A bracketing technique is used where alternate stimulation above and below threshold in decreasing steps is concluded by a double confirmation to a resolution of 0.2 L.U.

Our 128 subjects were drawn from members of staff at the Manchester Royal Eye Hospital and patients attending its Accident and Emergency Department with a visual acuity of at least 6/12 in their healthy (tested) eye. Of these 33 were grouped according to age (Table 1). One representative from each group (Figs. 5 and 6) was tested to examine the effect of refractive error

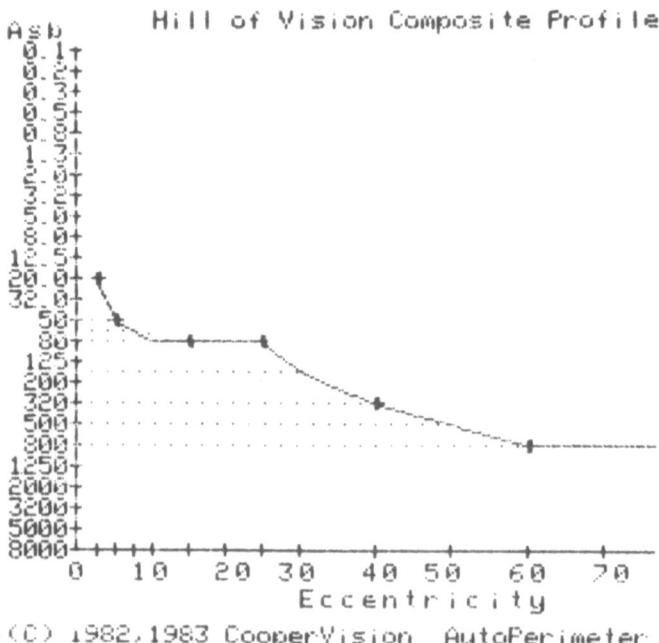

Fig. 1. A typical hill of vision described in 3 parts: the central peak, the mid-plateau from 15° to 25° and the peripheral decline.

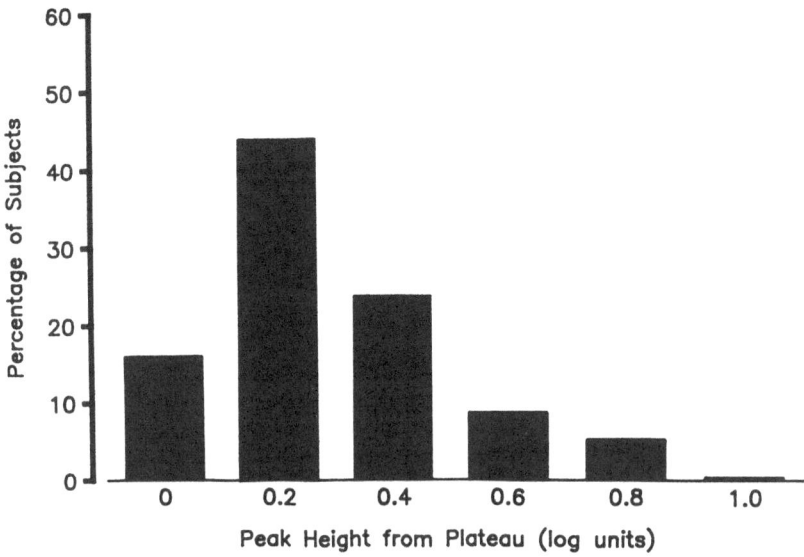

Fig. 2. The Central Peak – distribution according to height in 128 subjects.

over the range -7 to $+7$ dioptres. One eye per subject was tested, with a reading correction when applicable.

RESULTS

The hill of vision may be described in 3 parts: the central peak, the mid-plateau from $15°$ to $25°$ eccentricity and the peripheral decline. The components of 128 hills of vision were analysed with reference to the central peak height, the threshold sensitivity of the mid-plateau and the degree of peripheral decline.

The central peak height (Fig. 2): Its height was taken from the level of the mid-plateau at $15°$ eccentricity, and it showed a flat distribution over a range of 0 to 1.0 L.U. The largest group of 43% was found at 0.2 L.U.

The mid-plateau threshold sensitivity (Fig. 3): For this measurement we used the sensitivity at $15°$ in all cases. Although 37.5% of plateaus were sloping, only two fell by more than 0.4 L.U. The plateau sensitivity was concentrated, giving a sharp distribution with 89% of values found in the 50 and 80 Asb groups.

The degree of peripheral decline (Fig. 4): The drop in sensitivity from $25°$ skewed to the left over the range 0 to 1.8 L.U. Although the first group (0–0.4 L.U.) was the largest at 57%, 13% of declines were greater than 1.4 L.U. Only 4 subjects showed no decline.

The relevance of age to the hill of vision was assessed by comparing 3 groups (Table 1). The average peak height for each group was found to be highest in group II and lowest in group III (Table 2). Looking at the mean

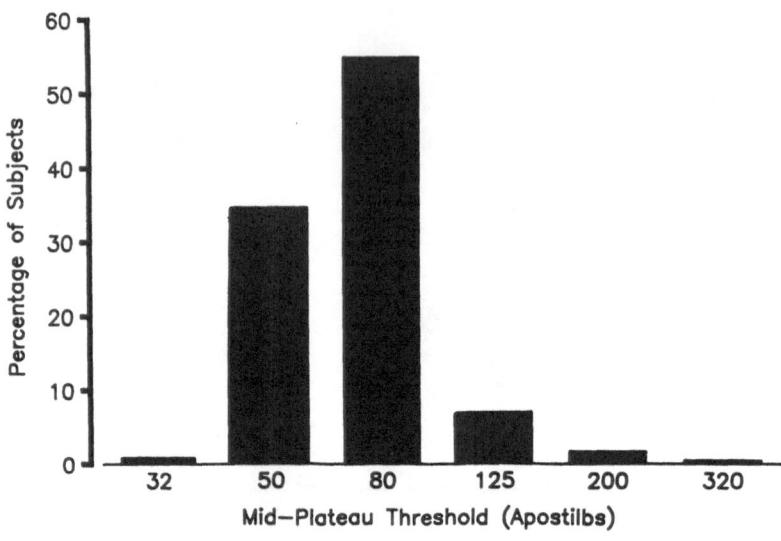

Fig. 3. The Mid-Plateau – distribution according to threshold sensitivity in 128 subjects.

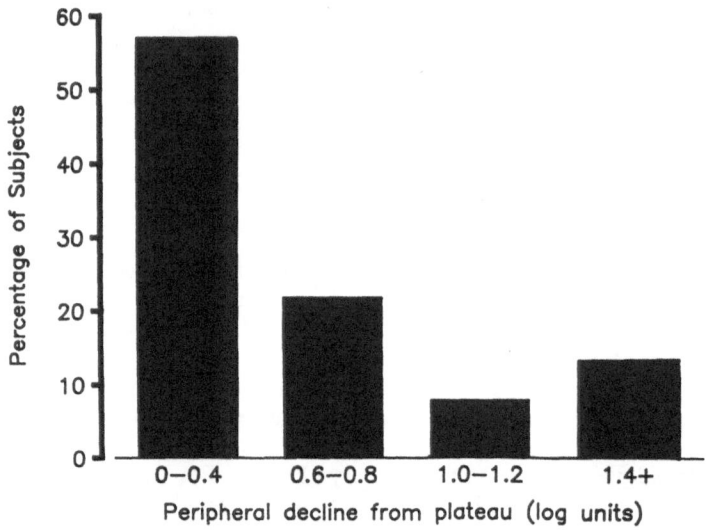

Fig. 4. The Peripheral Decline – distribution according to degree of fall in 128 subjects.

value of the mid-plateau threshold for each group, taken between the 15°
and 25° sensitivities, there was no significant difference between groups.
The highest value was found in group III. However, variation within groups
showed a decrease with age.

Refractive error (range $+7D$ to $-7D$) affected both the central peak
height and the mid-plateau threshold in 3 subjects of differing age groups
(Figs. 5 and 6). No direct correlation between changes in peak and plateau
value were noted. In the first 2 subjects plus error increments gave a stepwise

Table 2. The central peak height and mid-plateau threshold. Correlation with age.

Group	Average central peak height from plateau	Average mid-plateau threshold with standard deviation
I	0.35 Log Units	68.3 ± 23.5 Apostilbs
II	0.44 L.U.	66.5 ± 14 Asb
III	0.23 L.U.	75 ± 11 Asb

decrease in peak height, whereas minus increments gave no decrease in subject 1 and a sudden fall in subject 2. Subject 3 showed less variation, with no pattern evident. The plateau sensitivity was more predictable, being uninfluenced by moderate refractive error and symmetrically lowered at extreme error values.

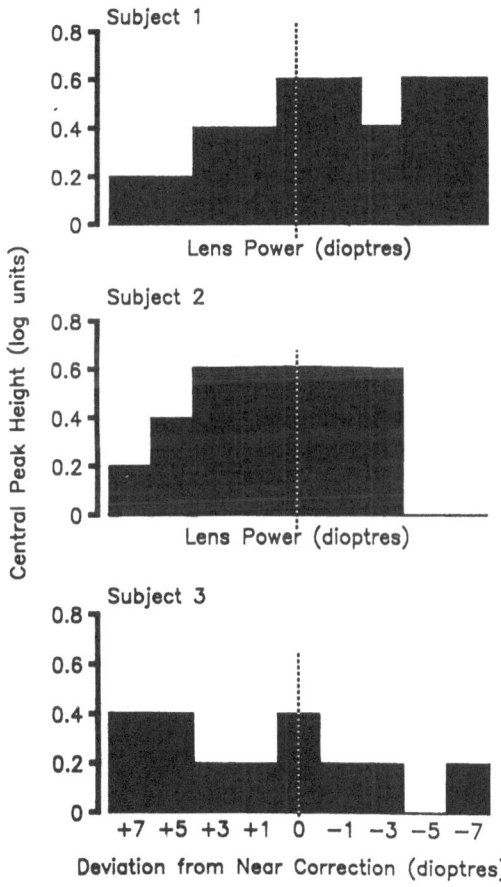

Fig. 5. The effect of refractive error on the central peak height in 3 subjects: Subject 1 – age, 25, VA 6/5; Subject 2 – age, 42, VA 6/5; Subject 3 – age, 64, VA 6/5.

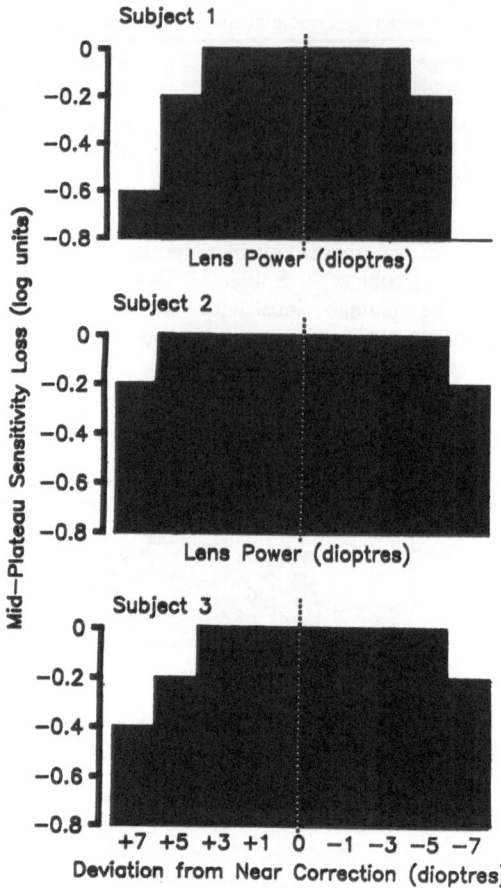

Fig. 6. The effect of refractive error on the mid-plateau sensitivity in the same 3 subjects as Fig. 5.

DISCUSSION

In deciding the significance of relative scotomata many automated perimeters must refer to standard values of threshold sensitivity and characteristics of profile deemed normal. Our findings show surprisingly large differences in both these respects amongst individual hills of vision. Both the central peak height and the degree of peripheral decline varied markedly (Figs. 2 and 4). Although the mid-plateau sensitivities showed less variation (Fig. 3), it was significant, especially in view of the fact that 37.5% of plateaus were sloping.

The results of subjects grouped by age (Table 2) failed to demonstrate any loss of sensitivity with increasing age. One subject aged 80 had a mid-plateau threshold of 50 Asb, whereas another aged 9 had one of 65 Asb.

Accommodation may have presented central peak height in subject 1 (Fig. 5) when minus refractive errors were used. As mid-plateau sensitivity fell

550

symmetrically with plus or minus errors (Fig. 6) perhaps accommodative effort was only initiated by central stimuli.

The concept of a hill of vision of uniform profile which decreases in sensitivity with increasing age is erroneous. Accurate perimetry depends on combining a high sensitivity (minimal false negatives) with a high specificity (minimal false positives). Variation from an assumed 'normal' in threshold related testing will give reduced specificity where threshold is above that expected and reduced sensitivity where it is below. In suprathreshold testing which assumed a 'normal' the degree of suprathresholdness can be increased to maintain specificity, at the cost of reducing sensitivity.

By tailoring the suprathreshold stimuli to the individual hill of vision, it should be possible to maintain a high specificity with a minimal degree of suprathreshold and hence a minimal loss of sensitivity.

ACKNOWLEDGEMENTS

We should like to extend our thanks to Mrs. Lynn Griffin for her secretarial assistance and to the Departments of Medical Illustration at the Manchester Royal Infirmary and at the Manchester Medical School.

REFERENCES

1. Armaly, M.F. Ocular pressure and visual fields. Arch. Ophthalmol. 81: 25−40 (1969).
2. Batko, K.A., Anctil, J.L. and Anderson, D.R. Detecting glaucomatous damage with the Friedmann analysis compared with the Goldmann perimeter and evaluation of steroscopic photographs at the optic disc. Am. J. Ophthalmol. 95: 435−447 (1983).
3. Johnson, C.A., Keltner, J.L. and Balestrery, F.G. Suprathreshold static perimetry in glaucoma and other optic nerve disease. Ophthalmology 86: 1278−1286 (1979).
4. Keltner, J.L., Johnson, C.A. and Balestrery, F.G. Suprathreshold static perimetry. Initial clinical trials with the Fieldmaster automated perimeter. Arch. Ophthalmol. 97: 260−272 (1979).
5. McCrary, J.A. and Feighton, J. Computerised perimetry in neuro-ophthalmology. Ophthalmology 86: 1287−1301 (1979).
6. Rock, W.J., Drance, S.M. and Morgan, R.W. A modification of the Armaly visual field screening technique for glaucoma. Canad. J. Ophthalmol. 6: 283−292 (1971).

Author's address:
N. Jacobs
Manchester Royal Eye Hospital
Manchester
England
H. Patterson
Coopervision
San Diego
USA

551

FUNCTIONAL PERIMETRY USED TO EVALUATE LASER TREATMENT IN DIABETIC MACULAR DISEASE

G.M. GRECO, R. FUSCO, A. GRECO and G.De CRECCHIO

(*Naples, Italy*)

ABSTRACT

34 patients with diabetic macular disease were examined by static and kinetic perimetry before and after Argon-laser photocoagulation.

Focal photocoagulation was used to treat exudative macular disease; grid-photocoagulation of the macula was used for oedematous disease.

After treatment 80% of cases with exudative macular disease showed increased retinal sensitivity while 20% were unchanged.

50% of oedematous cases showed increased retinal sensitivity, 38.5% were unchanged, 11.5% became worse.

There are reports in the literature of studies using perimetry to evaluate the effects that Argon-laser photocoagulation may have on the visual field (5, 6, 10, 11).

Hitherto most consideration has been given to the damage which photocoagulation therapy, especially if it is confluent causes to the visual field and so to the appearance of relative and/or absolute scotomas. Instead we have used static and kinetic perimetry as a parameter for evaluating functional recovery. Following photocoagulation treatment, especially in diabetic macular disease, visual acuity remains unaltered whilst in a significant percentage of cases there is an overall increase in retinal sensitivity.

MATERIALS AND METHODS

We examined 14 affected eyes (with diffuse leakage of fluorescein at the whole area of the macula) and 20 with exudative disease of the macula both before and after Argon-laser photocoagulation therapy.

In selecting the patients we considered: their degree of co-operation; the absence of opacities of the refractive mechanism; the absence of preretinal haemorrhages; visual acuity was never less than 2/10.

We performed perimetry, by a Harms hemispherical perimeter, using both standard kinetic and static meridian methods. Patients were examined before and at least three months after photocoagulation.

Heijl, A. and Greve, E.L. (eds.), Proceedings of the 6th Int. Visual Field Symposium.
© *1985, Dr W. Junk Publishers, Dordrecht, The Netherlands. ISBN 978-94-010-8932-6*

Table 1. Results.

	Cases	Improved	Unchanged	Worse
Oedematous maculopathy	14	7(50%)	6(38.5%)	1(11.5%)
Exudative maculopathy	20	16(80%)	4(20%)	–(–)

In exudative types treatment was focalized onto affected capillaries and micro-aneurysms with spots of $100-250\mu$ of medium-high intensity.

In oedematous types the photocoagulation method consisted of treating the macula directly using spots of $100-250\mu$ of medium intensity placed along a grid as described by English authors. In some cases a panretinal method was added due to the presence of large areas of capillary non-function.

RESULTS

In all, we examined 14 patients with oedematous macular disease and 20 with exudative macular disease (Table 1).

Positive results were shown by a global increase of retinal sensitivity of several logarithmic units (Fig. 1) and by the appearance on perimetry in photopic adaptation of a typical shape with a central point (Fig. 2).

The improvement was less brilliantly successful for the other eyes. In the only case in which the visual fields worsened there were recurrent episodes of bleeding into the vitreous.

Of the 20 patients with exudative macular disease treated, 16 showed improved retinal function and four were unchanged.

DISCUSSION AND CONCLUSIONS

In order to evaluate the results of Argon-laser photocoagulation in diabetic macular disease it is important to study central retinal sensitivity which, we believe, is a far more sensitive parameter than simply measuring visual acuity.

In exudative types (localised leakage) it is universally accepted that medium-high intensity impact be used to photocoagulate directly anomalous capillaries which give rise to exudates or local oedema.

There is still uncertainty, however, as to the efficacy of photocoagulation therapy for cases with diffuse oedema at the macula and consequently many methods have been described by the various authors. Since we had not previously obtained satisfactory results with indirect methods (horseshoe, paravenous, etc.), in 1979 we began to use the grid treatment as described by English authors for this type of case.

As was to be expected, the response differed in the two types of macular disease studied.

The best functional results were achieved in the exudative type, which the greatest success the earlier treatment was started.

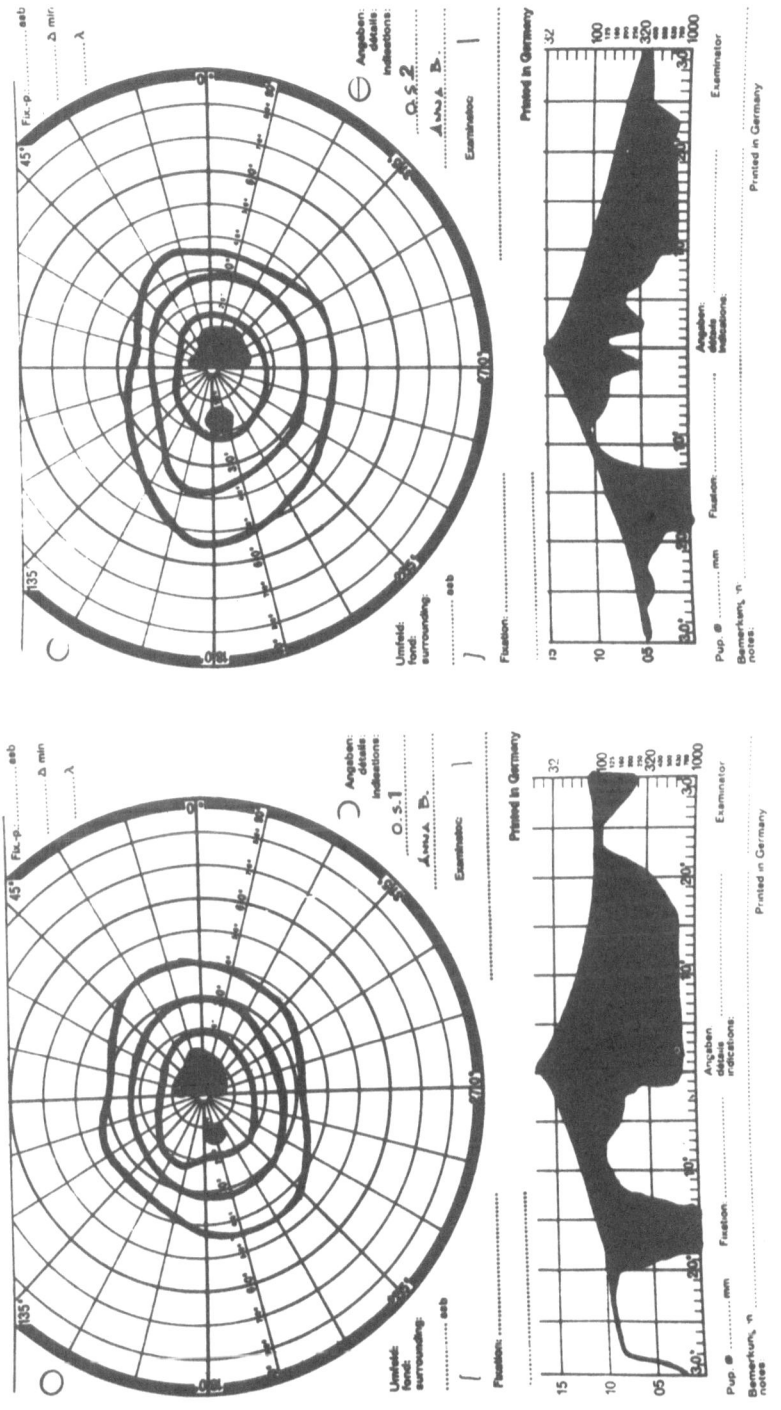

Fig. 1.

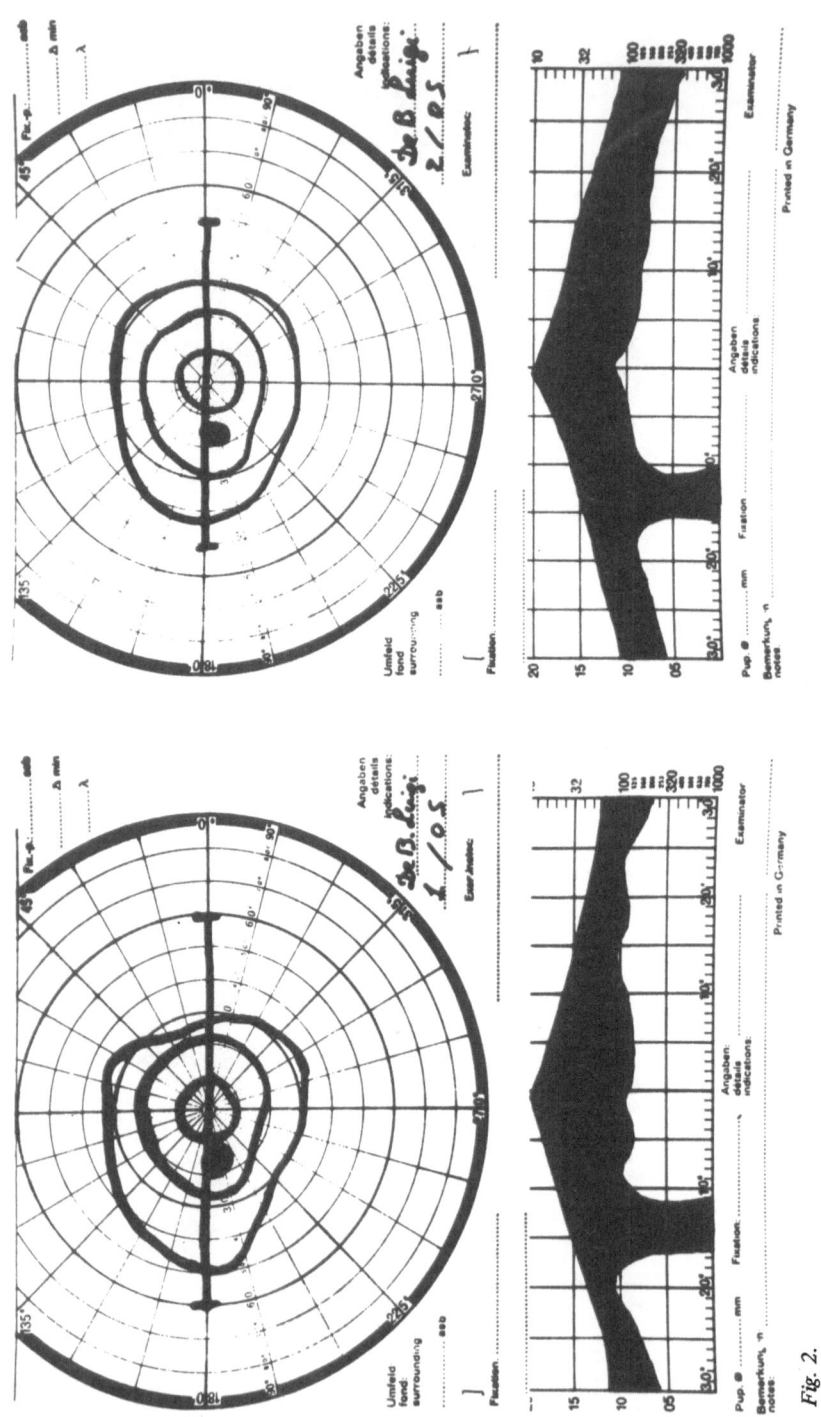

Fig. 2.

556

The method employed gave improvement in central retinal sensitivity in 50% of cases of the oedematous type (even though visual acuity remained unchanged).

Given the length of follow-up (four years) even in the latter, we feel able to confirm the validity of the method of photocoagulation used.

REFERENCES

1. Brancato, R., Sparavier, A. and Piscitelli, M. Modificazioni perimetriche in pazienti con retinopatia diabetica dopo trattamento Argon-laser. Ann. Ott. 105: 771–776 (1979).
2. Costantinides, G., Hache, J.C. and Francois, P. Aspect fontionnel de la Pan-photocoagulation retinienne Bull. Soc. Ophtal. Fr. 78: 603 (1978).
3. Diabetic Retinopathy Study Research Group. Preliminary report on effects of photocoagulation therapy. Amer. J. Ophth. 81: 483 (1976).
4. Francois, J. and De Laey, J.J. Natural history and preoperative evaluation of diabetic retinopathy. Symposium on light-coagulation. Doc. Ophthal. Proc. Series 1: 67 (1972).
5. Frank, R.N. Visual fields and electroretinography following extensive photo-coagulation. Arch. Ophthal. 93: 591 (1975).
6. Greco, G.M., Fusco, R., Greco, A. and de Crecchio G. Esame del campo visivo in soggetti affetti da retinopatia diabetica prima e dopo fotocoagulazione con Argon-laser. Relazione al 60° Congresso S.O.I. Roma (1980).
7. Grignolo, A., Tagliacco, V. and Zingirian, M. L'esame del campo visivo: stato attuale e prospettive. Relazione al 58° Congresso S.O.I. (1975).
8. Little, H., Zweng, H.C., Jack, R.L. and Vassiladis, A. Techniques of Argon-laser photocoagulation of diabetic disk new vessels. Amer. J. Ophth. 82: 675 (1976).
9. Meuer, G. Le caractere des deficits périmétrique dans les affections rétiniennes. J. Fr. Ophthalmol. 1: 163 (1978).
10. Zingirian, M. Danni perimetrici provocati dal trattamento fotocoagulativo della retinopatia diabetica. Bull. Ocul. 55: 451 (1976).
11. Zingirian, M., Pisano, E. and Gandolfo, E. Visual field damage after photo-coagulative treatment for diabetic retinopathy. Docum. Ophthalmol. Proc. Ser. Second International Visual Field Symposium, Tubingen (1976).

Author's address:
University of Naples,
Naples,
Italy.

STATIC AUTOMATED PERIMETRY IN THE FOLLOW-UP
OF LENS OPACITIES

G. CALABRIA, E. GANDOLFO, G. CORALLO and C. BURTOLO

(*Genova, Italy*)

ABSTRACT

Modern perspectives of cataract medical therapy have induced researchers to study objective methods for the evaluation of lens transparency. Visual acuity determination, slit-lamp examination, photographic and densitometric methods have poor reliability. In this study computerized static perimetry was tested and our strategy was based on two automatic perimeters: Peritest (Rodenstock) and Perikon (Optikon). Peritest was very useful in the static analysis of cataract-induced threshold changes in the central visual field. Static meridional perimetry by Perikon was utilized to study peripheral threshold changes. This method, tested in 50 patients (25 under therapy with anti-cataract drugs) appeared to be reliable, rapid, easily standardized and well-accepted by patients.

INTRODUCTION

Modern perspectives of cataract medical therapy have induced many researchers to study objective methods for measuring lens transparency variation. Cataract evolution is usually followed by checking visual acuity and by slit-lamp examination. The visual acuity examination is a subjective test that does not give us information concerning lens opacity variations that outside of the lens axis. With this method, morphoscopic discrimination is evaluated without considering differential light sensitivity which can show important modifications even without appreciable visual acuity variations. Slit-lamp microscopy should be integrated with photographic documentation, which, however, is not yet reliable due to the intrinsic variability in development and print procedures (1, 2, 4). Modern electronic instruments (densitometer, reflectometer, colorimeter, etc.) appear to be the most promising methods, but are not available on the medical instrument market at this time and are difficult to use in clinical practice (6, 7). In order to study the usefulness of static perimetry in evaluating cataract evolution with currently available equipment, we used two computerized instruments: Peritest (Rodenstock) and Perikon (Optikon).

Heijl, A. and Greve, E.L. (eds.), Proceedings of the 6th Int. Visual Field Symposium.
© *1985, Dr W. Junk Publishers, Dordrecht, The Netherlands. ISBN 978-94-010-8932-6*

MATERIAL AND METHOD

Fifty patients with incipient cataract formation were examined and followed. Twenty-five of these patients were under treatment with non-steroid, anti-inflammatory agents.

Each patient underwent a complete ophthalmological examination with determination of the natural and corrected visual acuity. During slit-lamp examination, a photograph of the lens was taken by retroillumination according to the technique described by McLean (5). The Peritest and Perikon unit were used for static perimetery (using the techniques described by Greve and Zingirian, (3, 8). For homogeneous opacities, 40 points of the visual field, within 10° eccentricity, were examined with the Peritest, while the 0°−180° meridian was examined by statically using the Perikon.

Besides central visual field examination with the Peritest unit for sectorial opacities, selected static perimetry along the meridian corresponding to the opacified region of the lens was also performed with the Perikon unit.

These tests were repeated every two months for a period of eight months.

RESULTS

In the 50 patients (78 eyes) examined a subcapsular posterior opacity was present in 66% of the cases (52 eyes) and nuclear sclerosis in 12.8% (10 eyes). In the remaining 20.5% (16 eyes) isolated or associated opacities of different characteristics and position were seen.

In 32 eyes the opacities worsened, while 12 improved and 34 remained stationary during the 8 months study when evaluated by visual acuity and slit-lamp examination.

In all the cases in which the lens opacity worsened a corresponding threshold regression was seen.

Also, in 10 of the 12 cases in which the opacity appeared reduced, this improvement was confirmed through perimetric testing.

In those cases in which the opacities remained stationary only modest variations in the perimetric results were demonstrated.

In all cases with homogeneous opacities in the central lens area, the Peritest revealed an alteration in the threshold which corresponded to the density of the opacity. Perikon perimetry showed an irregular deflection of the static perimetry curve in sectorial opacities (Fig. 1).

DISCUSSION

The validity of static automatic perimetry in the evaluation of lens transparency variation was demonstrated when comparing the data obtained by traditional method with the results of computerized static perimetry. Both the central lens area by evaluation of the sensitivity in the central portion of the visual field, and the lens paracentral area through examination of the peripheral visual field can easily be checked with this method.

560

PERIKON   STATIC   DIAGRAM

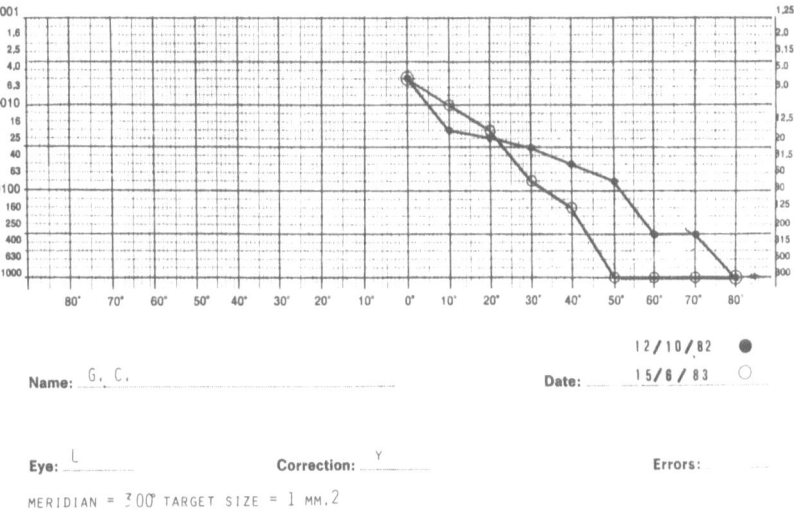

Name: G. C.

Date: 12/10/82 ●
      15/6/83 ○

Eye: L   Correction: Y   Errors:

MERIDIAN = 300° TARGET SIZE = 1 MM.2

Fig. 1. Perimetric curves demonstrated by the Perikon unit in a sectorial cataract opacity tested eight months apart. The static curve of the 300° meridian, already altered at the time of initial observation, shows further deflection corresponding to increased opacity.

The most peripheral stimuli capable of producing visual sensation pass through a portion of the paracentral lens measuring about 3 mm on the anterior lens surface and 0.5 mm on the posterior surface. Threshold determination according to the Peritest strategy can give fairly precise indications on opacity progression in homogeneous opacities. This technique gives reliable results for partial or incipient cataracts only. It is of course necessary that retinal function should not be altered, and perimetric alteration of different nature must be absent.

This technique is easily performed in clinical practice, well accepted by the patients, and a useful adjunct to traditional examination methods.

ACKNOWLEDGEMENTS

This study was supported from a grant of the Consiglio Nazionale delle Ricerche, Progetto Finalizzato Medicina Preventiva e Riabilitativa, Sotto-progetto Malattie Degenerative, Obiettivo n. 47a, Rome, Italy.

REFERENCES

1. Brown, N. Quantitative slit image photography of the lens. Trans. Ophthalmol. Soc. U.K. 92: 303–307 (1972).

2. Dragorimescu, V., Mockwin, O., Koch, M.R. and Sasaki, K. Development of a new equipment for rotating slit image photography according to Scheimpflug's prinicple. Interdiscip. Top. Gerontal. 13: 1–13 (1978).
3. Greve, E.L., Dannheim, F. and Bakker, D. The Peritest, a new automatic and semi-automatic perimeter. International Ophthalmology. 5–3: 201–214 (1982).
4. Hayashi, N. Transillumination photography of the lens-utilisation of slit lamp microscopic photography. Ophthalmo. (Japan) 12: 788–792 (1970).
5. McLean, M. The Melbourne Catalin trial. Current protocol and some early results. Austr. J. Ophthal. 5: 183–187 (1977).
6. Marcantonio, S.M., Duncan, G., Davies, P.D. and Busmeil, A.R. Classification of human senile cataract by nuclear colour and sodium content. Exp. Eye Res. 31: 227–237 (1980).
7. Sigelman, J., Trokel, S.L. and Spector, A. Quantitative biomicroscopy of lens light back scatter. Arch. Ophthalmol. 92: 437–442 (1974).
8. Zingirian, M., Gandolfo, E. and Orciuolo, M. Automation of the Goldmann Perimeter. Soc. Ophth. Proc. Series 35: 365–369 (1983).

Author's address:
Giovanni Calabria
University Eye Clinic,
Viale Benedetto XV n. 5
I-16132 Genova, Italy

THE EFFECT OF BLUR UPON STATIC PERIMETRIC
THRESHOLDS

MARCUS D. BENEDETTO and MARSHALL N. CYRLIN

(*Gainesville, Florida*)

ABSTRACT

Emmetropes with no ocular disease were cyclopleged and corrected for cupola distance. Following the induction of from -2.5 to plano to $+10.0$ diopters of spherical blur the subjects were tested on an Octopus 201 Automated Perimeter.

The differential effect on thresholds with respect to retinal location will be explored. The clinical significance of the effect of hyperopic or myopic blur and its potential influence on perimetric findings in the investigation of ocular disorders will be discussed.

INTRODUCTION

It has generally been stressed that in order to obtain valid results, in the perimetric evaluation of visual function, one must carefully correct for refractive error as well as cupola distance.

This study evaluates the effect of low to high levels of spherical blur on retinal thresholds, as tested by the Octopus Automated Perimeter, in normal individuals and one subject with a small paracentral scotoma of presumed macular origin. Evaluation of the central 12 degrees and the central 30 degrees as tested with programs 31 and 61, respectively, was performed. The clinical and diagnostic significance of the findings will be discussed.

METHODS

Three emmetropes underwent complete ophthalmologic examinations and were found to have no ocular disease. Retinal thresholds on these subjects were determined on an Octopus Automated Perimeter (Model # 201). Background cupola luminance was constant throughout the experiment at 4 asb. The cupola to eye distance was 0.5 M. All three subjects were dioptrically corrected for cupolar distance following maximum cycloplegia with the topical application of 2% cylcopentalate hydrochloride drops.

Heijl, A. and Greve, E.L. (eds.), Proceedings of the 6th Int. Visual Field Symposium.
© *1985, Dr W. Junk Publishers, Dordrecht, The Netherlands. ISBN 978-94-010-8932-6*

Thirteen blur conditions were used; $-2.5, -2.0, -1.5, -1.0, 0.0, +1.0,$ $+1.5, +2.0, +2.5, +3.0, +5.0, +7.5, +10.0$ diopters of spherical blur. This optical blur was induced with a set of corrected curve trial lenses.

The subjects were tested across all blur conditions on 2 visual field examination programs. Program 31 and program 61 with test stimulus size 3 (Goldmann III equivalent) were employed. Program 31, which tests a 30 degree field with 6 degrees resolution centered at fixation, was used to determine changes in sensitivity with eccentricity. Program 61, which tests 12 degrees of field with 3 degrees resolution centered at fixation, was used to yield greater definition of the more central versus peripheral areas of the 30 degree field with respect to blur.

Following maximum cycloplegia each subject was seated at the Octopus Perimeter. The subjects were corrected with 2.0 diopters for cupola distance which was added to the positive or negative spherical correction for each test condition.

RESULTS

Figure 1 contains a summary of the data for three subjects. The graphs on the top represent the mean sensitivity loss in decibels for 0 and 30 degrees (filled and unfilled circles, respectively). The graphs on the bottom represent the mean sensitivities in decibels for 0, 6, and 12 degrees (filled circles, filled, and unfilled triangles, respectively). Examination of the top three graphs reveals that the loss of sensitivity at fixation is greater than at 30 degrees. Additionally, the loss of sensitivity with increased blur is more acute centrally than peripherally. For the subject on the left, discovered to manifest a small paracentral scotoma, the 30 degree sensitivity from -2.5 to 0.0 D.S. was superior to that of 0 degrees. For the center and right subjects sensitivity decreases with increases in eccentricity and also with increases in blur. For the subject on the left, 12 degrees shows better sensitivity with high amounts of blur than for the lesser degrees of eccentricity.

Figure 2 shows a greyhard printout of Program 31 with 0.0 D.S. for the first subject. Also shown are greyhard printouts of Program 61 with -1.5 and $+2.5$ D.S. blur for comparison. The small paracentral scotoma is manifested more under the $+2.5$ D.S. blur condition than the -1.5 D.S. blur condition. This magnification continues to spread with further increases in blur.

DISCUSSION

Analysis of the mean sensitivites of high resolution testing of the central 12 degrees with program 61 reveals no statistically or clinically significant alteration in the range of $+/-2.0$ D.S. of blur. For blur of $+3.0$ D.S. and greater there is a rapid loss of central sensitivity. This generalization applies to normal individuals and may not apply to persons with glaucoma, retinal disease, high astigmatism, or other ocular disorders associated with visual field loss. This may be inferred from the differential effect of low degrees of blur

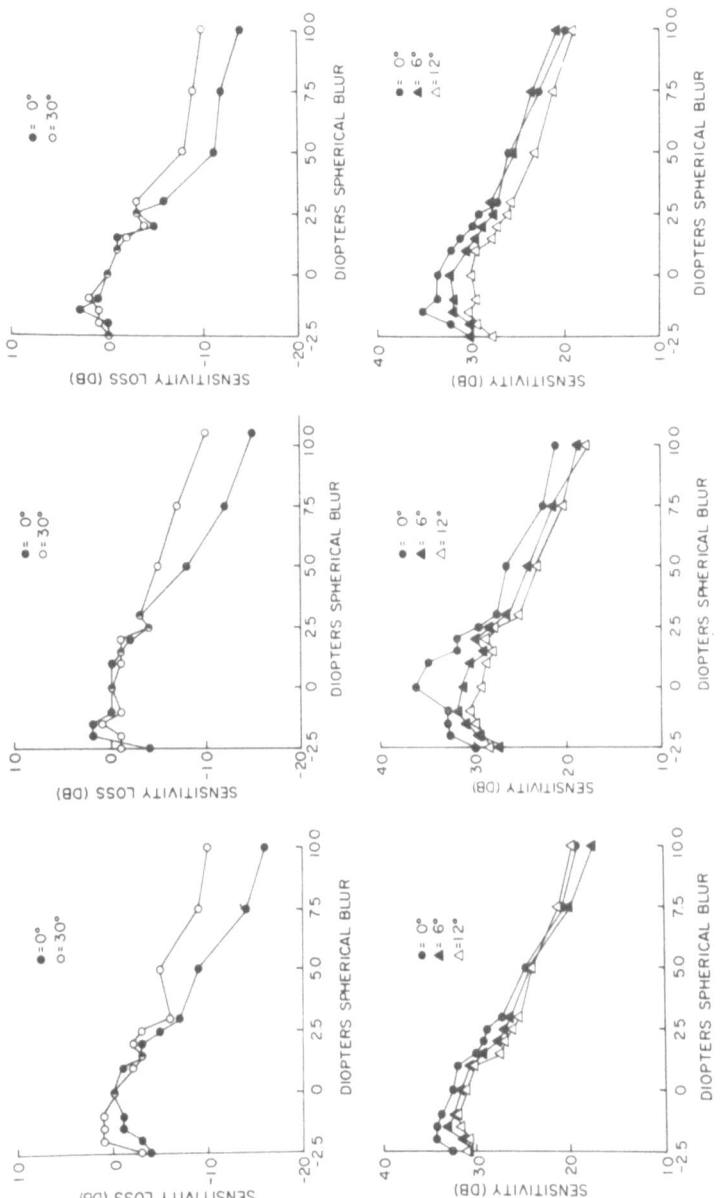

Fig. 1. The top graphs represent the loss of sensitivity with change in amount of blur for 0 and 30 degrees (filled and unfilled circles, respectively). The bottom graphs represent the change in sensitivity with change in amount of blur for 0, 6, and 12 degrees (filled circles, filled, and unfilled triangles, respectively).

565

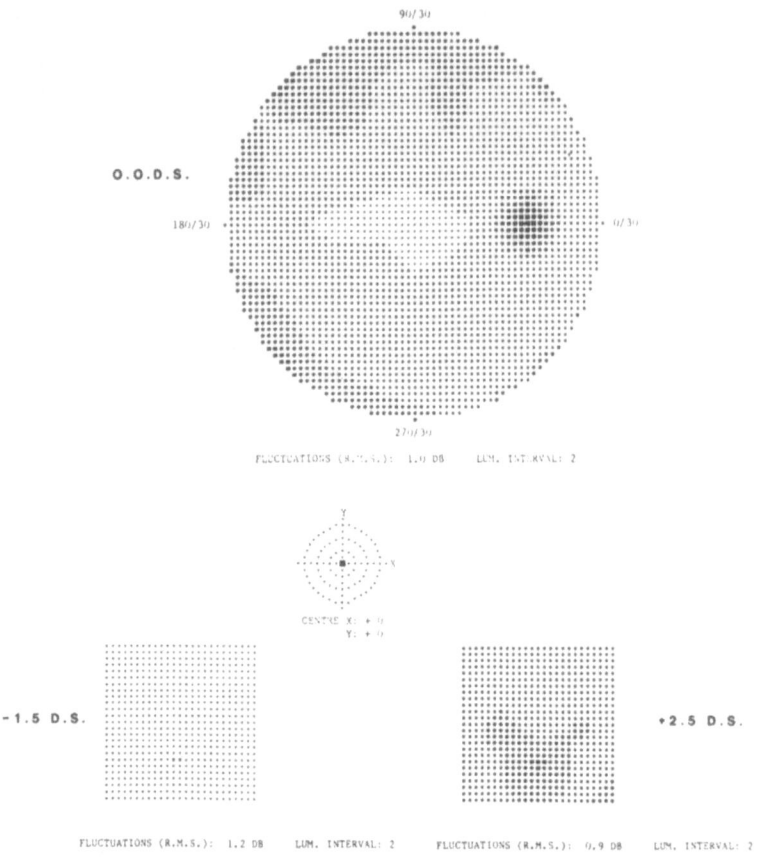

Fig. 2. Top – 0.0 D.S. Greyhard printout of Program 31 for subject #1. Center – representation of location of testing for Program 61. Bottom – Greyhard printout of Program 61 for a comparison of −1.5 D.S. versus + 2.5 D.S. blur.

in the subject with the subtle paracentral scotoma (Fig. 2). When changes in retinal threshold with programs 31 are compared with program 61 for + 3.0 D.S. and greater blur it was found that there is a more rapid drop of sensitivity in the central 12 degrees as compared with the entire central 30 degrees. Thus it appears that the island of vision 'sinks' more rapidly in the center than it does in the more peripheral regions.

Preliminary data for kinetic visual field testing to be reported further elsewhere reveals similar changes induced by spherical blur.

SUMMARY

For small amounts of blur +/−2 D.S., there are small changes in retinal sensitivity which result in a slight reduction of the central sensitivity. For larger amounts of blur, a loss is recorded peripherally as well as centrally. However, the central loss is more acute. Hence, with blur we see an overall 'sinking' of the island of vision as well as an acute falling of the central peak. This is also seen in kinetic perimetry.

Although it is not advocated that central field testing be performed without correction for cupola distance, the induced change in retinal sensitivity may not be clinically significant in the normal patient. In patients ocular disease simple errors in correction for near and distance may become significant.

Author's address:
Department of Ophthalmology,
University of Florida,
Gainesville, Florida, USA.

APPLICATION OF HYPERACUITY TO ASSESS VISION THROUGH MEDIA AND RETINAL OPACITIES: METHODOLOGY

JAY M. ENOCH, RICK A. WILLIAMS, EDWARD A. ESSOCK and SYLVAN RAPHAEL

(*Berkeley, CA, USA*)

ABSTRACT

The development of a new test methodology for evaluation of visual function through media opacities is described. Two version of a vernier acuity task, the 'gap test' and the 'perimetry test', provide an esimtate of the functional effect of the opacity and a profile of central visual response. Results from a group of otherwise normal cataract patients establish a normal data base for clinical application. The effects of a cataract are simulated in several patients with retinal anomalies to demonstrate the utility of hyperacuity perimetry in detecting retinal disease through opacities. Finally, a means of compensating for modest amounts of image defocus is discussed.

INTRODUCTION

Our laboratory has recently developed a series of tests which are designed to detect retinal functional anomalies in the presence of opacities (1–6). These non-invasive, psychophysical tests of vision are based upon a patient's ability to *compare the locations* of two visual stimuli rather than upon the ability to *individually resolve* them. There is no restriction on the type of opacity which may be present, including corneal leukomas, vitreous hemmorhages, *etc*.

The purpose of this paper is to describe the rationale behind the development of this test battery including: the use of the hyperacuity gap test to differentiate optical from non-optical components of visual loss; and the use of a perimetric version of the test for assessment of visual function at a variety of points across the central retina. The minimization of the effects of modest image defocus is also dicussed. Clinical trials utilizing this new methodology are reported in a companion paper (7).

The term 'hyperacuity' refers to a group of tasks, each of which involves the discrimination of very fine differences in the spatial locations of two or more visual stimuli, differences of a magnitude much less than the center-to-center spacing between individual photoreceptors in the retina (thus the term 'hyper'-acuity). Vernier acuity, or the appreciation of a relative offset

Heijl, A. and Greve, E.L. (eds.), Proceedings of the 6th Int. Visual Field Symposium.
© *1985, Dr W. Junk Publishers, Dordrecht, The Netherlands. ISBN 978-94-010-8932-6*

between two lines or spots of light, is one member of this group of tasks. Common to all hyperacuity responses is an extremely low spatial threshold, on the order of 3 to 10 sec of arc.

Selected hyperacuity configurations possess the property of being relatively resistant to image degradation (1, 6). Thus, the spatial offset between two spots of light viewed through a cataractous lens may still be appreciated even though the spots are seen as 'blobs' of light, if a sufficiently large separation or *gap* is present between the spots. This resistance to optical degradation is illustrated in Fig. 1. The observer's task is simply to indicate whether the upper spot is displaced to the right or to the left of the lower spot. A hand-held response box with two buttons (one for 'right' and one for 'left') provides a means of recording the response. A small computer may be programmed to first present large offsets which are easily seen, and proceed to smaller and smaller offsets with each correct response, until the observer cannot tell for sure whether the spot is displaced left or right. Patients are provided feedback relative to the accuracy of their individual judgements. In this way, the vernier acuity for a specific gap size can be determined in two to three minutes.

1. The Hyperacuity 'Gap Test'

Figure 2 shows the average vernier acuity *vs.* gap results obtained from a group of 15 otherwise normal cataract patients. These pre-operative results were grouped according to the gap size that provided best vernier acuity. The averaged gap function for each group is shown, and the shaded area on each group depicts the range of each group's data. The Snellen acuities of the patients in each of the four groups fall into four distinct ranges, as indicated on the figure. This relation between optimum gap and Snellen acuity allows the shape of the gap curve to be used to infer the degree of optical visual loss caused by the cataract. For example, if a cataract patient's gap curve shows a 4' optimum gap size (group 1), we would expect their Snellen acuity to be 20/40 or better. Poorer acuity is suggestive of an additional disease process distinct from the cataract that must be further reducing vision.

The hyperacuity perimetry test which is described next provides a quantitative determination of both central and para-central visual response that can be applied in the presence of cataracts.

2. The Hyperacuity Perimetry Test

On the basis of clinical experience, it seemed to us that a perimetric profile of visual performance across the central field would be valuable in evaluating probable surgical outcome. By assessing a patient's hyperacuity at both central and eccentric locations in the visual field, it is possible to directly assess central vision in the presence of an opacity (2). Normally better performance will be achieved with foveal viewing than when the stimuli are presented to any other retinal location.

In Fig. 3 results of both standard Goldmann perimetry and hyperacuity perimetry for a patient with a macular hole are compared to the normal

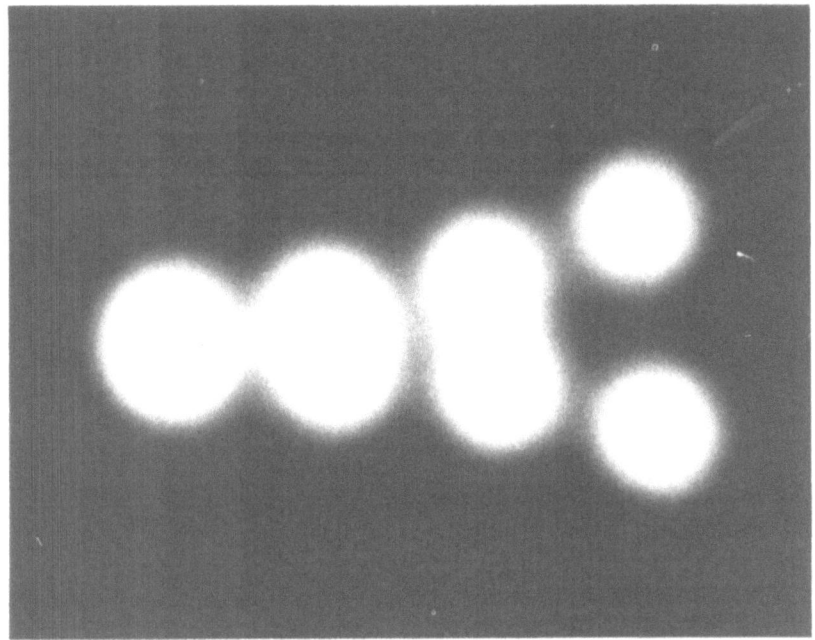

Fig. 1. Photograph, taken through a sheet of ground glass, of four examples of the two-dot vernier stimulus to illustrate the image that might be seen by a cataract patient. The gap size increases by successive factors of two from the left image to the far right image.

case. This patient (59 year old, while male) had suffered a persistant superior retinal detachment in the right eye. Two successive scleral buckle operations eventually resulted in the development of a preretinal membrane over the macula and a macular hole, with best vision of 20/200. Static perimetry results (0°−180° meridian) are shown in Fig. 3a, and the results of vernier acuity perimetry testing are shown in Fig. 3b. The static perimetry indicates a functional loss extending to about 4 degrees to either side of fixation. The hyperacuity perimetry data suggest a similar visual loss relative to the normal curve (dashed) which is obvious even when the stimulus was artificially degraded by interposing a sheet of ground glass to simulate a cataract for this patient (filled symbols).

The next case demonstrates that other topographic patterns of visual loss across the central retina can also be documented in the presence of media opacities using hyperacuity perimetry (2). This patient (51 year old, white male) had a 10 year history of diabetes mellitus. He had received panretinal laser photocoagulation in both eyes over the course of two years. Vision in the tested eye (OD) eventually fell to 20/40, and fluorescein angiography demonstrated capillary drop-our in the fovea (Fig. 4a). Figure 4b shows the hyperacuity perimetry curves measured both with a simulated opacity (20/200 level, filled circles) and with totally clear media. In both cases, vernier acuity *could not be measured* in the areas indicated by shading on the

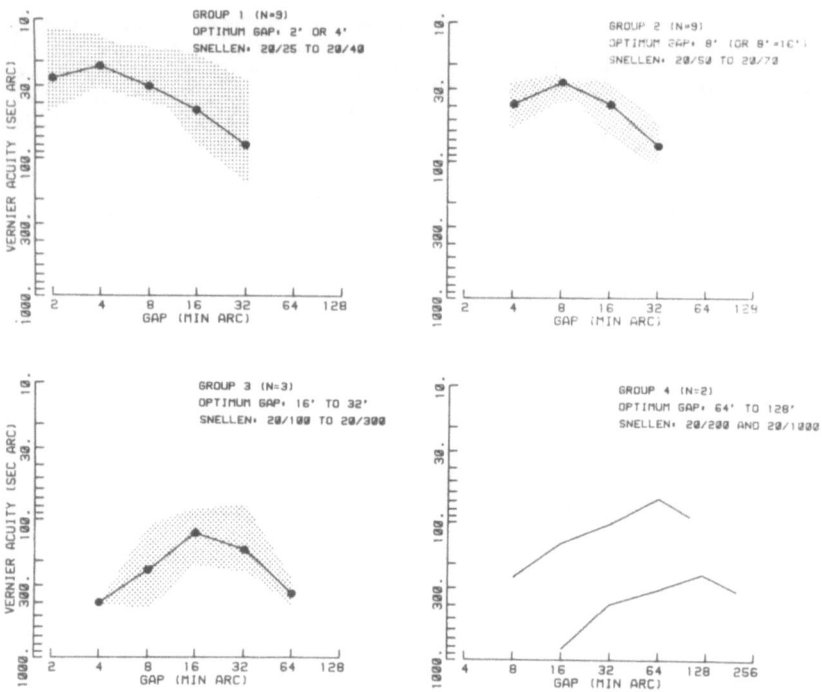

Fig. 2. Averaged vernier acuity-versus-gap size curves of four groups of cataract patients: a) Group 1, b) Group 2, c) Group 3, d) Group 4. Optimum gap sizes and Snellen acuity ranges as indicated on graphs. The shaded regions indicate the range of gap functions for each group.

graph, since the patient could not see the stimuli in these areas. Vernier measurements obtained at other stimulus locations were very close to the normal data (dashed curve). Despite the relatively good acuity which this patient exhibited, the paracentral defects, located by hyperacuity perimetry to either side of the fovea, make normal reading particularly difficult for him.

Hyperacuity perimetry therefore provides an excellent means for the analysis of central retinal function in cases where the retinal image has been substantially degraded. In a companion paper, the initial clinical trials of the joint application of the gap and perimetry tests are discussed.

3. Image Defocus

In our clinical applications of the hyperacuity tests, each patient is carefully refracted before testing is initiated. This ensures that the best possible Snellen acuity is measured and that vernier measurements will be minimally affected by lens defocus. It is our experience that lens defocus is much more detrimental to vernier performance than is image degradation caused by a ground glass screen or by nuclear cataracts. Controlling the variable of defocus is therefore important in these studies. In addition to spectacle

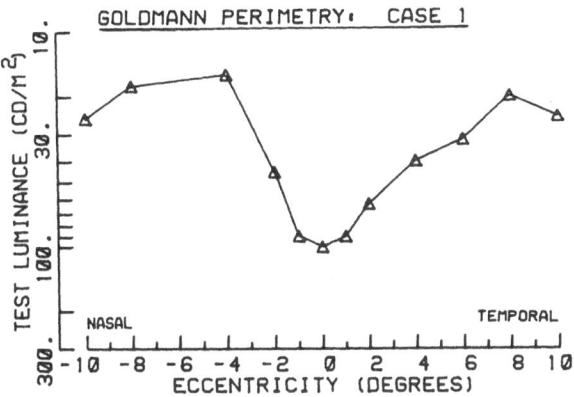

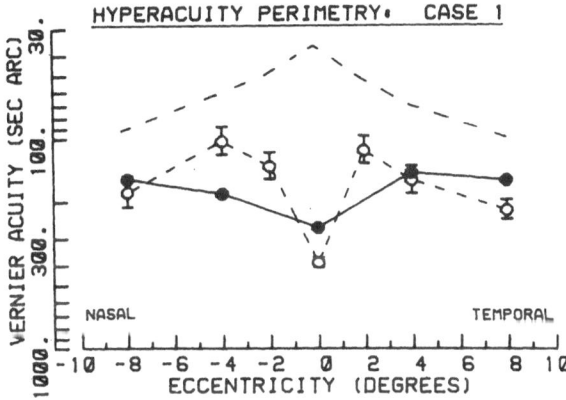

Fig. 3. Example of a patient with a macular hole. (a) Static increment sensitivity (OD), 0°–180° meridian (Goldmann Perimeter). (b) Hyperacuity perimetry (OD): no simulated opacity (open circles), with ground glass stimulating a 20/100 opacity (filled circles).

correction as a means of minimizing the effects of defocus, we have found that slightly degrading (via the ground glass screen) the stimulus viewed by a defocused eye enhances vernier performance (8). For example, when an emmetropic observer viewed the vernier stimulus through a +2.5 D spectacle lens, vernier acuity with a 16 min arc gap size was about 30 sec arc. When the stimulus was slightly degraded with the ground glass screen (to about the 20/100 level) and then viewed by the defocused eye, vernier performance improved on about 15 sec arc. This was true for other spectacle lenses and gap sizes and for other observers. Apparently, the ground glass screen filters out the stimulus components that give rise to 'spurious resolution' in the defocused image thereby enhancing performance.

In terms of analyzing patients with relatively uniform cataracts, these results suggest that modest uncorrected refractive errors in these cases will

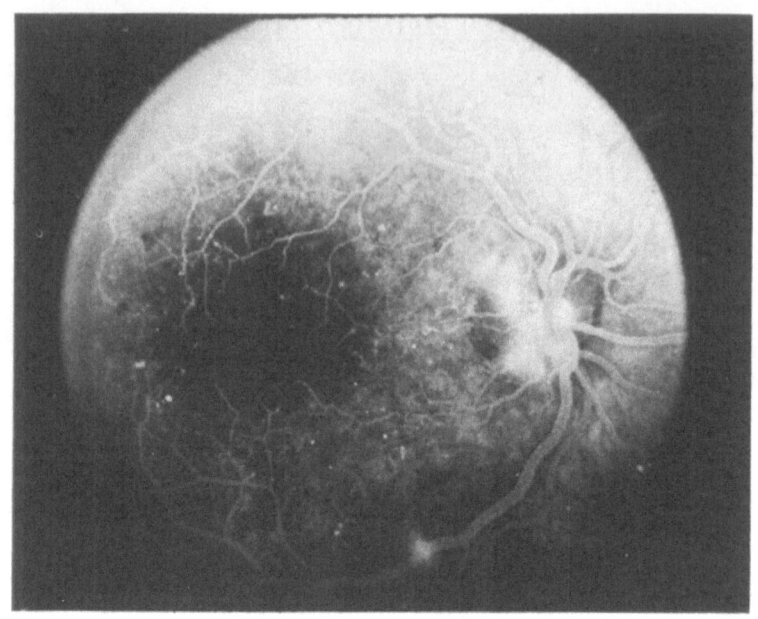

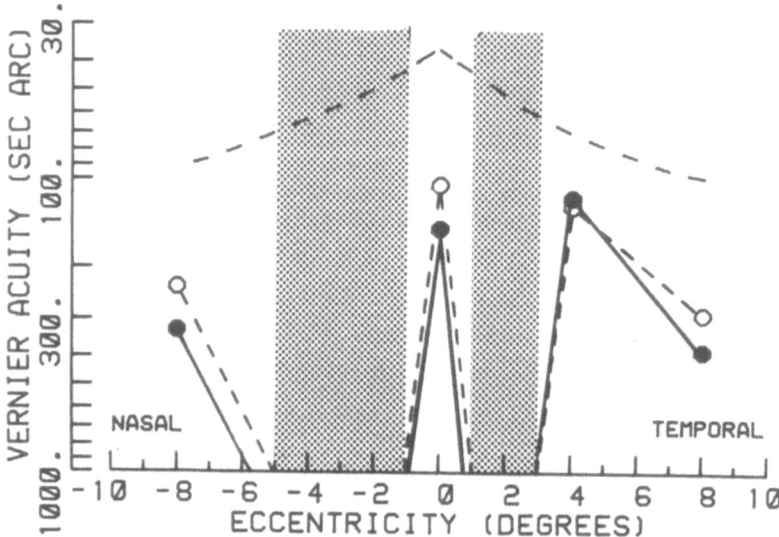

Fig. 4. Example of a patient with diabetic retinopathy and capillary dropouts in the macula. (a) Fluorescein angiogram of the right eye (note areas of capillary loss). (b) Hyperacuity perimetry results, right eye: no simulated opacity (open circles), with a 20/200 simulated opacity (filled circles). The dashed curve is from a normal observer with a 20/400 simulated opacity.

probably have little effect on hyperacuity performance, since the cataract will have filtered out the high spatial frequency components that are most

574

influenced by lens defocus. However, for postoperative testing, when the filtering effects of the cataract are no longer present, it is crucial to achieve optimum refraction.

CONCLUSIONS

We have described the background and development of two clinical tests which have the potential to parcel out optical from non-optical visual loss in cases where media opacities prevent the formation of an optical retinal image, and where a clear view of the macula is impossible. In our companion paper, we describe clinical trials of this methodology (7). The key point is that a single visual measurement (e.g. interference acuity) may not be an accurate predictor of a post-surgical functional capability of the patient. A profile of visual performance is more useful in evaluating the suitability of surgical intervention.

REFERENCES

1. Enoch, J.M. and Williams, R.A. Development of clinical tests of vision: Initial data on two hyperacuity paradigms. Percept. Psychophys. 33: 314–322 (1983).
2. Enoch, J.M., Williams, R.A., Essock, E.A. and Barricks, M. Hyperacuity perimetry: assessment of macular function through ocular opacities. Arch. Ophthalmol. (in press) (1984).
3. Enoch, J.M., Williams, R.A., Essock, E.A. and Fendick, M.G. Hyperacuity: A promising means of evaluating vision through cataracts. In Progress in Retinal Research, Neville Osborne, ed. (in press) (1984).
4. Essock, E.A., Enoch, J.M., Williams, R.A., Barricks, M.A. and Raphael, S. Joint application of hyperacuity perimetry and gap tests to assess visual function behind cataracts: Initial trials. Arch. Ophthalmol. (submitted) (1984).
5. Essock, E.A., Williams, R.A., Enoch, J.M. and Raphael, S. The effects of image degradation by cataracts of vernier acuity. Invest. Ophthal. Vis. Sci. (in press) (1984).
6. Williams, R.A., Enoch, J.M. and Essock, E.A. The relative resistance of selected hyperacuity configurations to retinal image degradation. Invest. Ophthal. Vis. Sci. 25: 389–399 (1984).
7. Williams, R.A., Enoch, J.M., Essock, E.A. and Barricks, M. Application of hyperacuity to assess vision through media and retinal opacities: Clinical trials. Doc. Ophthal. Proc. Ser. (IPS, in press) (1984).
8. Williams, R.A., Essock, E.A., Enoch, J.M. and Raphael, S. Spatially filtering a blurred hyperacuity stimulus may enhance spatial localization performance. Invest. Ophthalmol. Vis. Sci. (Suppl) 24: 92 (1983).

Author's address:
Jay M. Enoch, Dean
School of Optometry
University of California
Berkeley, CA 94720
USA

APPLICATION OF HYPERACUITY TO ASSESS VISION THROUGH MEDIA AND RETINAL OPACITIES: CLINICAL TRIALS

RICK A. WILLIAMS, JAY M. ENOCH, EDWARD A. ESSOCK, and MICHAEL A. BARRICKS

(*Berkeley, CA, USA*)

ABSTRACT

The clinical application of the hyperacuity 'gap test' and 'perimetry test' for the analysis of visual function in the presence of cataracts is described. A series of three cases illustrate how the vernier testing first provides an estimate of the extent to which the cataract is responsible for the observed acuity loss, and then provides a profile of visual function across the central visual field that can be measured through the opacity. The hyperacuity methods predict normal function in two cases and additional functional loss in a third case.

INTRODUCTION

Two psychophysical tests, based upon a vernier acuity judgement (Fig. 1), can be applied in cases of ocular media opacities in order to parcel out optical from retinal-neural visual loss (1, 3). The development of these new tests was the topic of a companion paper presented at this symposium (2). The joint application of these two tests in the analysis of visual function in actual cataract patients is described in the present paper.

The value of the gap test is that the functional consequences of the stimulus degradation produced by a cataractous lens can be estimated, relatively independently of any additional retinal disease which may be present, by comparison to normal baseline data. Hyperacuity perimetry (i.e. vernier acuity as a function of eccentricity from fixation) provides a profile of visual function over the central visual field. Normally, vernier acuity at fixation (i.e. the fovea) is far superior to that measured at any other visual field location. Anomalous visual function is indicated by central or paracentral vernier acuity loss. The results of these two tests taken together provide a powerful, preoperative analysis of visual function in cases of media opacities. In practice, we have found no limit to the type, severity or density of opacity which may be penetrated. The following series of clinical cases demonstrates the vernier testing procedure and the potential utility of the results.

Heijl, A. and Greve, E.L. (eds.), Proceedings of the 6th Int. Visual Field Symposium.
© *1985, Dr W. Junk Publishers, Dordrecht, The Netherlands. ISBN 978-94-010-8932-6*

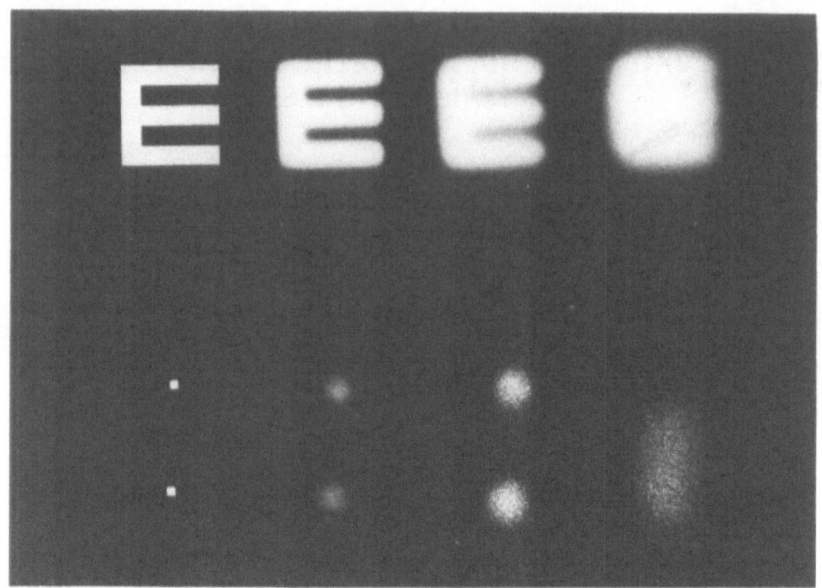

Fig. 1. Photograph of two-dot vernier stimulus and Snellen 'E' taken through increasing degrees of image degradation produced by ground glass.

RESULTS

Case 1: Bilateral Cataracts with Suspected Macular Dysfunction

This case illustrates a particularly common clinical situation; i.e., the patient who demonstrates both cataracts and some signs of macular degeneration.

This patient (66 year-old, white woman) presented with bilateral cataracts, both lenses showing evidence of nuclear sclerosis and anterior defects (more pronounced OD). Snellen acuities were 20/50 OD and 20/25 OS. Ophthalmoscopy revealed macular drusen in the right eye. Laser interferometry indicated acuities of 20/40 (16.5 lines/degree) OU. The right fundus was more distinctly visible than might be expected given the 20/50 acuity.

The gap test results (i.e. vernier acuity as a function of the gap separating the two spots) obtained from this patient's right eye are shown in Fig. 2a. Recall from the previous paper (2) that the patient must merely judge whether the upper of two small spots of light is to the right or left of a fixed lower spot (i.e. a two-dot vernier task). The shaded area on the graph indicates the range of gap functions measured in a group of otherwise normal cataract patients, all of whom showed best vernier performances for gap sizes of 8 min arc. The Snellen acuities of these patients ranged from 20/50 to 20/70. The shape of the preoperative gap function for patient 1 (filled symbols) fits within this normal group and her Snellen acuity matches that of the normal group. The gap test therefore indicates that the cataract alone can account for the 20/50 acuity and suggests that the maculopathy was probably not affecting central visual function at the time of testing.

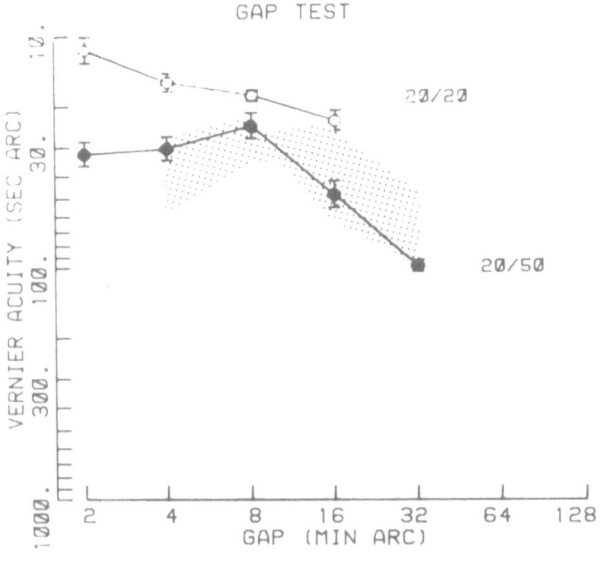

GAP TEST

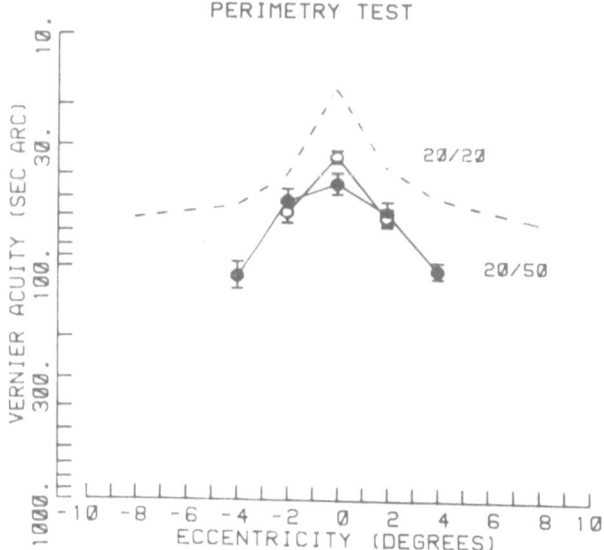

PERIMETRY TEST

Fig. 2. (a) Pre- (filled symbols) and postoperative (open symbols) gap functions for Patient 1. Shaded area indicates range of gap curves from normal group as described in text. (b) Pre- (filled symbols) and postoperative (open symbols) perimetry functions for Paitnet 1. Dashed curve is result obtained from normal observer with clear media.

Direct evidence that the macular drusen were not contributing to central visual loss is provided by the hyperacuity perimetry results (Fig. 2b). The preoperative perimetry function revealed a central vernier sensitivity peak that corresponds very closely to that obtained from normal, healthy subjects (dashed curve). Thus, the vernier testing indicates that the macular anomaly is mild relative to the functional consequences of the cataract.

After removal of the cataract, the patient was able to demonstrate 20/20 Snellen acuity with the right eye. Consistent with this level of acuity, her postoperative gap function (Fig. 2a, open symbols) showed improvements in vernier acuity for all gap sizes and optimum performances at the smallest gap tested. Her post-op perimetry profile was essentially identical to the preoperative one. This, of course, would be expected in the absence of retinal dysfunction.

Thus, preoperative vernier acuity testing correctly predicted a normally functioning visual system behind the opacity.

Case 2: Unilateral Posterior Subcapsular Cataract

This case is illustrative of the problem of testing vision through a relatively dense posterior subcapsular cataract, a variety which is often visually devastating for the patient.

The patient (64 year-old while female) presented with unilateral cataract. VA (with correction) was 20/400 OD and 20/30 OS. There was mild nuclear sclerosis with dense, central posterior subcapsular opacities in the right lens which did not appear sufficiently dense to account for the entire visual loss. Laser interference acuity suggested the potential for 20/50 vision OU.

The results of the gap test are shown in Fig. 3a. The shaded region indicates the range of gap functions with optimum 16 min gap measured in a group of otherwise normal cataract patients. The Snellen acuities of these patients ranged from 20/100 to 20/300. The preoperative gap function measured in patient 2 (filled symbols) fits within this normal group, suggesting that the cataract accounted for most of the 20/400 visual loss. However, since the patient's acuity is slightly worse than that exhibited by the normal group, additional evidence of functional normality was sought in the form of the hyperacuity perimetry test.

The perimetry function measured preoperatively (Fig. 3b, filled symbols) indicated superior vernier sensitivity at fixation, and the shape of the function matches that of normals. Both the gap and perimetry tests suggest that, behind the cataract, central visual function is relatively normal.

One month following surgery for cataract removal and intraocular lens implantation, the patient exhibited 20/20 vision in the right eye. The gap function (Fig. 3a, open circles) showed improvement at all gap sizes commensurate with 20/20 vision. The perimetry function also showed improvement at all eccentricities tested, but the shape of the function demonstrated preoperatively remained the same (e.g. peak performance at fixation).

Thus, the hyperacuity testing successfully predicted good postoperative vision and normal central field profile despite the rather dense cataract.

580

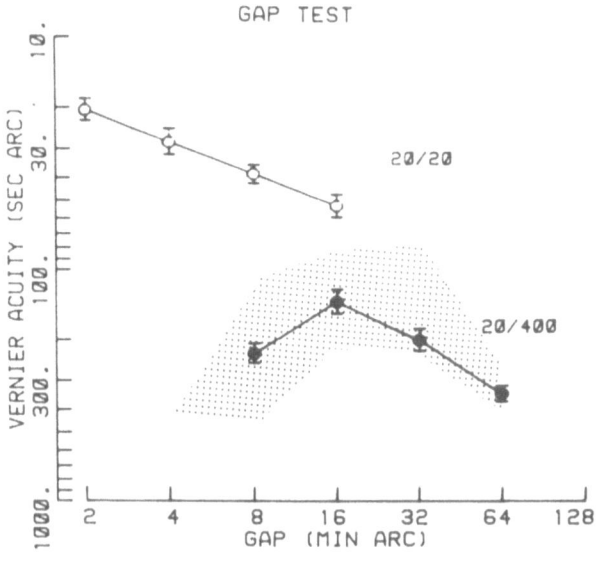

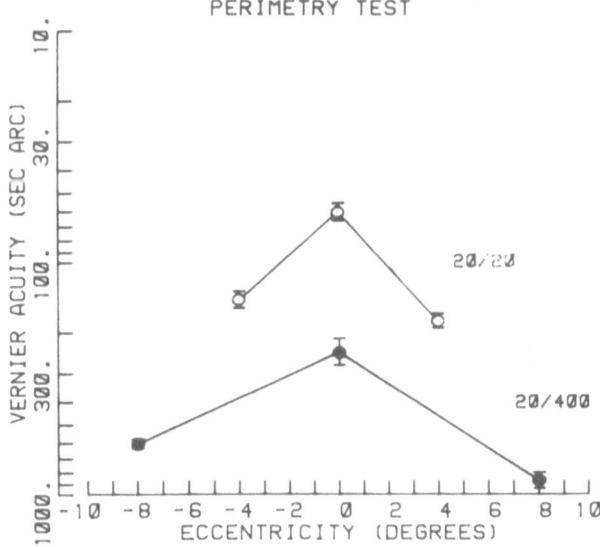

Fig. 3. (a) Pre- and postoperative gap data for Patient 2 (symbols as in Fig. 1). Shaded area indicates normal range as described in text. (b) Pre- and postoperative perimetry data for Patient 2 (symbols as in Fig. 1).

Case 3: Diabetic Reintopathy

This patient (74 years old, white female) had suffered from diabetes mellitus for 29 years and had developed bilateral proliferative diabetic

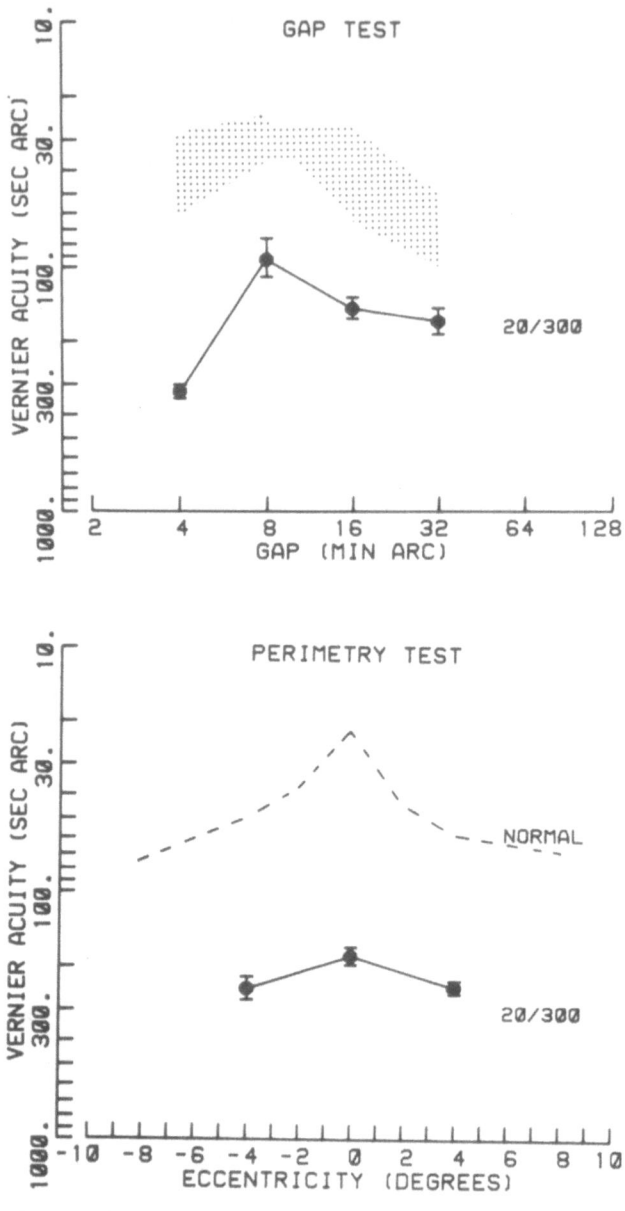

Fig. 4. (a) Preoperative gap results for patient 3. Shaded area as in Fig. 2. (b) Preoperative perimetry data for patient 3 and normal (dashed curve) with comparable amount of induced image degradation.

retinopathy. Her left eye, having received laser therapy 10 years ago, had developed a hemorrhage 4 years later. After subsequent cyclocryotherapy, vision in this eye ultimately deteriorated to NLP (no light perception).

The right eye (which we tested) had been treated with panretinal photo-coagulation. There was moderate nuclear sclerosis and 1+ posterior sub-capsular opacification in the right lens; visual acuity was 20/300. The eye subsequently developed neovascular glaucoma and was treated with panretinal cryotherapy. At the time of testing, visual acuity had fallen to 20/400.

This is a case for which the ocular history indicated probable macular dysfunction. The question was, how much improvement in vision could be expected upon removal of the cataract? The gap test results for this patient are shown in Fig. 4a. The *shape* of the gap curve (8 min optimum gap) very closely matches that of the group of otherwise normal cataract patients with Snellen visual acuities between 20/50 and 20/70 (shaded area). However, vernier *sensitivity* is reduced relative to the normal range, and Snellen acuity is considerably worse (20/400) than the group norm. This patient's gap test results therefore suggest that the opacity might be expected to drop Snellen acuity to about 20/50 or 20/70, and that the remainder of the visual loss is probably due to the retinal anomaly.

The hyperacuity perimetry test confirmed that the retinopathy was affecting *central* visual function. Figure 4b compares the patient's hyperacuity perimetry profile to that of a normal subject for whom the effects of a comparable cataract were simulated by ground glass stimulus degradation. The patient failed to show the enhanced vernier acuity normally found at fixation, indicating that function in the central visual field was indeed reduced.

Taken together, the hyperacuity gap and perimetry tests were able to distinguish between the moderate loss of visual function due to the cataract and the loss attributed to the pathology within the central retina. Our pre-operative predictions were subsequently verified by the patient's ophthal-mologist who later informed us that, following cataract removal (which was accomplished with 'no particular complications'), the best visual acuity that could be obtained was 20/200 and a 'macular lesion was present'.

DISCUSSION

The three cases presented illustrate the clinical application of the two vernier acuity tests in the analysis of visual function through cataracts. Each test in itself provides an independent evaluation of the relative contributions of the opacity and of retinal/neural anomalies to preoperative vision. The two tests applied conjointly provide a powerful methodology for preoperative evaluation of vision in the presence of ocular opacities. Further studies are in progress to extend the application of these techniques to other forms of media opacities (e.g. corneal leukomas, vitreous opacities), and to further streamline the clinical testing procedures, based on previous experience, to provide maximum information from a relatively small time investment.

REFERENCES

1. Enoch, J.M., Williams, R.A., Essock, E.A. and Barricks, M. Hyperacuity perimetry: Assessment of macular function through ocular opacities. Arch. Ophthalmol. (in press) (1984).
2. Enoch, J.M., Williams, R.A., Essock, E.A. and Raphael, S. Application of hyperacuity to assess vision through media and retinal opacities: Methodology. Docum. Ophthalmol. Proc. Ser. (International Perimetric Society, in press) (1984).
3. Essock, E.A., Williams, R.A., Enoch, J.M. and Raphael, S. The effects of image degradation by cataracts on vernier acuity. Invest. Ophthal. Vis. Sci. (in press) (1984).

Author's address:
Jay M. Enoch, Dean
School of Optometry
University of California
Berkeley, CA 94720
USA

LIGHT THRESHOLD AND TEMPORAL RESOLUTION IN THE CENTRAL VISUAL FIELD

P.L. ROSSI, R. TERRILE, C. BURTOLO and G. CIURLO

(Genoa, Italy)

ABSTRACT

A target flickering at a constant speed presented at different points of the central visual field is fused at luminancies that are directly related to the light threshold of the tested point.

Previous works have reported that threshold stimuli are fused at a constant flickering frequency throughout the central visual field (C.V.F.) (2, 3). The finding highlights the relationship between temporal resolution and light threshold and defines the standard values of flicker fusion frequency (F.F.F.) in this area; further assessment of its validity therefore appears justified.

If the former statement is true, then its reverse should also be true and target flickering at a constant frequency, presented in different points of the C.V.F., should be fused at luminances that are directly related to the light threshold of each point.

This work evaluates and discusses the latter assumption.

MATERIALS AND METHODS

Seven eyes of four normal individuals, ranging in age from 19 to 27, were studied. All had normal visual acuities and fields.

A Goldmann perimeter, equipped with a previously described flickering device was used (1). The examination was carried out in the following manner:

(a) The light threshold for targets of 1/4, 4 and 64 mm^2 was determined at the fixation point, and at 3, 5 and 10 degrees of nasal and temporal eccentricity.

(b) The threshold luminance at the fixation point for each target was increased by 0.4 L.U. and the F.F.F. determined with a descending technique. Five measurements were taken for each target and the average value calculated.

(c) The flickering frequency was kept constant and the eccentric points

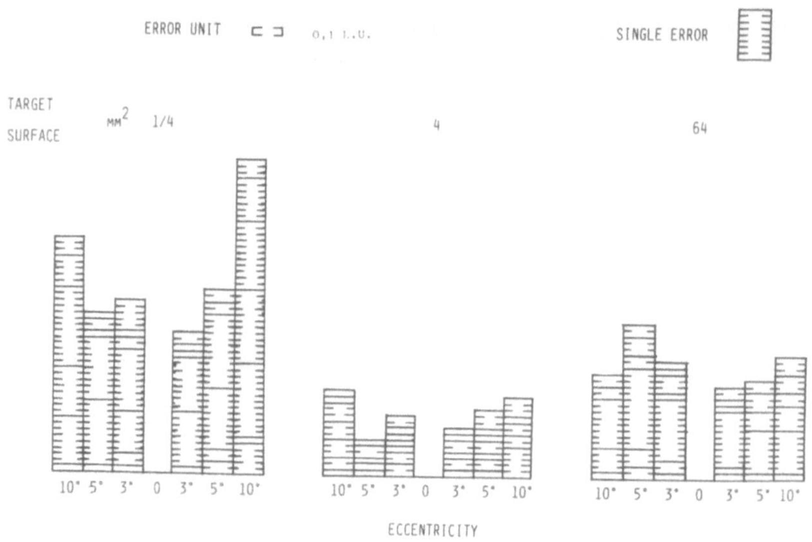

Fig. 1.

tested. In each point the target luminance was progressively increased to determine the lower luminance level at which the target was seen as a continuous stimulus. A sampling presentation method was used.

(d) The obtained light value was compared with the light threshold at this point. Any difference of O.I.L.U. or greater was considered significant.

RESULTS

Of the 126 measurements, 17 showed a correspondence between the light threshold and target luminance at the flicker fusion frequency.

Figure 1 reports the number and degree of errors according to the target diameter and the eccentricity of the tested point.

CONSIDERATIONS

The overall agreement between the light threshold and target luminance at the F.F.F. was 13.49%. The agreement remained low (65.98%) even when a 0.3 L.U. physiological fluctuation of the threshold was allowed.

The error frequency is not related to eccentricity of the tested point, nor target diameter. On the contrary, the amount of error is significantly related to target diameter. Over 97% of the errors within the $4 \, mm^2$ target fall within the physiological threshold fluctuation, while only 61.23% with the $1/4 \, mm^2$ target and 83.68% with the $64 \, mm^2$ fall within these limits. Result scattering was also high with these latter targets. Errors greater than 0.6 L.U. were 30.6% for the smaller and 12.24% for the larger target.

586

Therefore, only the results obtained with the 4 mm² target are reliable and support the statement that threshold stimuli are fused at a constant F.F.F. thoughout the C.V.F.

The data obtained with the 1/4 and 64 mm² targets point to the same conclusion, but their scattering is too large to make them reliable and conclusive.

The explanation of the inaccuracy of these measurements does not rely on the photometric features of the stimuli, since, using threshold stimuli of these same surfaces constant F.F.F. value was found in previous reports (2, 3). This inaccuracy is likely related to the difficulties of completing the task required when very large or very small stimuli are used. However, this does not seem to invalidate the assumption that threshold stimuli are fused at a constant frequency throughout the central visual field, but may perhaps suggest that the 1/4 and 64 mm² targets are less suitable for testing the F.F.F.

CONCLUSIONS

A target flickering at a constant frequency is fused at a luminance that is directly related to the light threshold of the tested point. A good agreement between the two values is found with targets of 4 mm², while a less significant relationship is found with 1/4 and 64 mm² targets.

REFERENCES

1. Ciurlo, G., Rossi, P. and Suetta, G. Nuovo apparecchio per flicker-perimetria. Min. Oftalmol. 20: 61–68 (1978).
2. Rossi, P. Ciurlo, G., Burtolo, C. and Calabria, G. Temporal resolution and stimulus intensity in the central visual field. Doc. Ophthalmol. Proc. Series, 28: 439–441 (1983).
3. Zingirian, M., Ciurlo, G., Rossi, P. and Burtolo, C. Flicker fusion spatial summation. Doc. Ophthalmol. Proc. Series 26: 127–130 (1981).

Author's address:
Rossi Pietro
University Eye Department
Viale Benedetto XV, 5
Genoa
Italy

THE ROLE OF RETINAL GANGLION CELL DENSITY AND RECEPTIVE-FIELD SIZE IN PHOTOPIC PERIMETRY

JYRKI ROVAMO, ANTTI RANINEN and VEIJO VIRSU

(*Helsinki, Finland*)

ABSTRACT

The invariance of visibility across the visual field, obtained by magnifying the stimulus (in inverse proportion to the human cortical magnification factor) and reducing its luminance (in inverse proportion to Ricco's area) with increasing eccentricity, provides a novel method for clinical investigation of visual fields. In this optimal perimetry normal thresholds as a function of visual field location are horizontal lines called perimetrograms. Conseqently, visual field defects are readily recognized as pits, as in an audiogram.

INTRODUCTION

In photopic vision the number of visual cells analysing one solid degree of visual field decreases with increasing eccentricity. This inhomogeneity of visual sampling is principally determined by the retinal ganglion cells.

To study visual information processing in retinotopically different parts of the central nervous system we have developed a method, called M-scaling (10), that is designed to bypass the effect of ganglion cell sampling. This paper reviews our recent results (3–11) concerning the information transfer from various parts of the human visual field.

METHOD

Contrast sensitivity. Sinusoidal gratings were generated under computer control on a white cathode-ray screen (10). Contrast sensitivity (the inverse of contrast threshold) was determined in a detection task using a computer controlled, two-alternative forced-choice method that indicated the contrast required for a probability of 0.84 of correct choices.

Critical flicker frequency. Sinusoidal flicker with a modulation of 30% at 20–70 Hz was generated on a green cathode-ray screen with a linearized luminance response (5). Critical flicker frequency was determined with the

Heijl, A. and Greve, E.L. (eds.), Proceedings of the 6th Int. Visual Field Symposium.
© *1985, Dr W. Junk Publishers, Dordrecht, The Netherlands. ISBN 978-94-010-8932-6*

method of adjustment: six, alternatingly ascending and descending trials were averaged.

The human cortical magnification factor. Visual field is represented topographically in the striate cortex but the central parts have a much larger representation than peripheral regions. The scale of the map, called cortical magnification factor (M), indicates the length, in millimetres along the cortical surface, that corresponds to one degree of arc in the visual field. In monkeys, the cortical magnification factor squared is directly proportional to the retinal ganglion cell density corrected for the foveal displacement. Using this relationship and previously published data on human ganglion-cell and cone density we have estimated the values of the human cortical magnification factor along the principal meridians of the visual field (6).

RESULTS

Contrast sensitivity and grating acuity (cut-off frequency at 100% contrast) decreased rapidly with increasing eccentricity (Fig. 1A) when the test gratings had constant retinal area at different eccentricities.

In Fig. 1B grating acuity became independent of visual field location when the contrast sensitivity functions of Fig. 1A were replotted (4) as a function of cortical spatial frequency, calculated as f/M where f is the retinal spatial frequency in c/deg of the visual field (11). This means that grating acuity is directly proportional to the human cortical magnification factor (10). Our recent results suggest that even the local anisotropy of monocular M within ocular dominance columns (7) is reflected in the resolution of gratings oriented along and across meridians in peripheral vision (8).

Despite replotting, contrast sensitivity did not become independent of eccentricity but was found in Fig. 1B to increase with cortical projection area (10) calculated as M^2A where A is the retinal grating area in deg^2 of the visual field (11). This indicates that, although replotting compensates for the variation of cortical spatial frequency with eccentricity, this partial M-scaling, as such, is insufficient for equalizing contrast sensitivity.

However, as Fig. 1C shows, contrast sensitivity functions became almost identical at different eccentricities when the test gratings were M-scaled (10) to produce similar spatial representations in cortical projections originating from different retinal locations: with increasing eccentricity, grating area was increased in inverse proportion to the cortical magnification squared and consequently, the range of test frequencies was extended towards lower spatial frequencies (9).

Figure 1C also illustrates the superiority of complete over partial M-scaling: in addition to spatial frequency (cf. Fig. 1B) stimulus area must be scaled too. Similarly, if two stimuli, moving at different visual field locations, are to be compared, their cortical translation velocities must be the same (11).

In Fig. 1D some of the contrast sensitivity functions of Fig. 1C are replotted as a function of retinal spatial frequency (10); the retinal grating areas used in the experiment of Fig. 1C are also indicated.

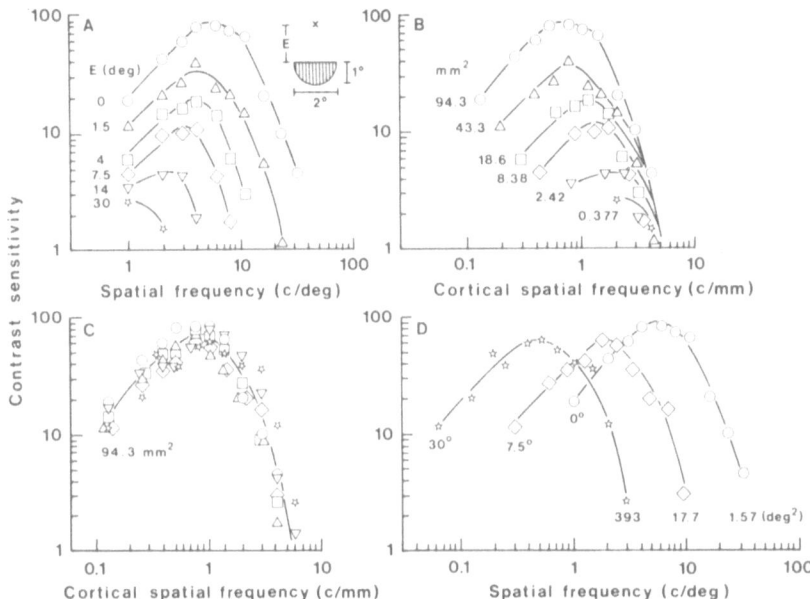

Fig. 1. Spatial contrast sensitivity functions at various eccentricities (E). The inset depicts the stimulus geometry; X is the fixation point. Modified from (9).

In comparison with Fig. 1A, contrast sensitivity in Fig. 1D increased markely at low retinal spatial frequencies and maximal sensitivity reached almost the foveal peak level in the periphery. Also, the shapes and spatial bandwidths of the contrast sensitivity functions were similar at all visual field locations tested, indicating a corresponding amount of low-frequency attentuation, but the functions as a whole were shifted along the spatial frequency axis towards lower spatial frequencies at larger eccentricities because resolution was not much affected by M-scaling.

In addition, M-scaling has been found to apply to luminance-modulated chromatic gratings, to colour contrast, to pattern-reversal evoked potentials, to temporal integration, to fine-grain movement illusion, to the detection of coherent movement in random-dot patterns, to differential motion detection and velocity discrimination, and to the slowest velocity needed for perceiving movement (see ref. 5 for review).

Critical flicker frequency (CFF) was not independent of eccentricity but first increased and then decreased with increasing eccentricity (Fig. 2A) when the stimulus field had constant retinal area and illuminance (3, 5) at different eccentricities.

In Fig. 2B, the stimulus area was M-scaled (10): when eccentricity increased from 0 to 100 deg, the stimulus area increased from 0.209 to 369 deg^2 of the visual field. Despite M-scaling, CFF increased monotonically with eccentricity. The result means that CFF cannot be made independent of visual field location by M-scaling the spatial stimulus parameters. In addition, there are (see ref. 4 for review) other measures (e.g. Vernier acuity,

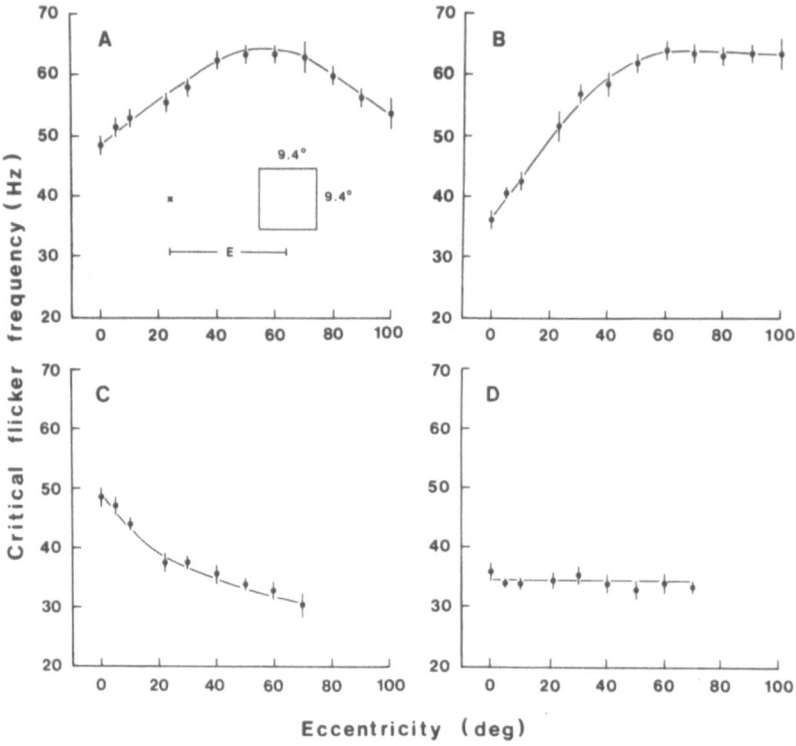

Fig. 2. Critical flicker frequency (Mean ± SD) as a function of eccentricity (E). The inset depicts the stimulus geometry; X is the fixation point. Modified from (5).

orientation discrimination, stereoacuity, fusional vergence response, and temporal order detection) that evidently cannot be made independent of visual field location by M-scaling. In agreement with (10), these complications indicate that M-scaling, as such, is incomplete.

The human cortical magnification factor has been estimated (6) by assuming that cortical magnification is directly proportional to the square-root of retinal ganglion-cell receptive-field density. Thus, M-scaling of spatial stimulus parameters compensates only for the decrease of sampling density of ganglion cells with increasing eccentricity. On the other hand, CFF of single feline ganglion cells increases with flux (1) defined as retinal illuminance multiplied by the area of receptive field centre. This suggests that the monotonical increase of CFF with eccentricity in Fig. 2B results from the increase of receptive field size towards the retinal periphery because retinal illuminance and the number of ganglion cells stimulated were constant. This hypothesis can be tested by reducing retinal illuminance in inverse proportion to the area of receptive field centre (F-scaling).

Ricco's area provides an estimate for the area of receptive field centre in man: by pooling together the results of Inui et al. (2) and Wilson (12) we found, in agreement with (10), that the radius R of Ricco's area, in degrees, is linearly related to the inverse of cortical magnification: $R = 0.0263$ $(1 + 3.15/M)$. This suggests that, when expressed in cortical millimetres, the size and overlap of receptive fields are largest in foveal vision and decrease with increasing eccentricity. Our previous results (e.g. 3, 11) indicate, however, that the spatial frequency producing the maximal contrast sensitivity is at all eccentricities directly proportional to the human cortical magnification factor.

In Fig. 2C the area of the stimulus field was constant at all eccentricities but retinal illuminance was F-scaled: stimulus luminance was reduced with increasing eccentricity in inverse proportion to Ricco's area. Thus, when eccentricity increased from 0 to 70 deg, retinal illuminance decreased from 2510 to 40.2 photopic td. CFF decreased now monotonically with increasing eccentricity. The decrease evidently results from the decrease of cortical projection area and retinal ganglion cell density with increasing eccentricity, because retinal illuminance was F-scaled.

In the experiment of Fig. 2D both the stimulus area and retinal illuminance were scaled, i.e. M-scaling and F-scaling were combined to produce MF-scaling. Now, CFF became independent of visual field location.

DISCUSSION

Our results support the view that spatiotemporal information processing is qualitatively similar for stimuli presented at different locations of the visual field and that quantitative differences result from retinotopical differences in the density, size and overlap of sampling apertures, i.e. ganglion-cell receptive-fields. Also, eye movements and ocular optics evidently contribute to quantitative differences. For example, during steady fixation peripheral stimuli are more stabilized than foveal stimuli because receptive field size grows with increasing eccentricity. On the other hand, peripheral image quality exceeds the requirements of neural sampling which may result in aliasing distortions.

The invariance of visibility across the visual field obtained by magnifying the stimulus (M-scaling) and reducing its luminance (F-scaling) with increasing eccentricity provides a novel method for clinical investigation of visual fields. In this optimal perimetry normal thresholds as a function of visual field loation are horizontal lines called perimetrograms. Consequently, visual field defects are readily recognized as pits, as in an audiogram.

REFERENCES

1. Enroth-Cugell, C. and Shapley, R.M. Flux, not retinal illumination, is what cat retinal ganglion cells really care about. J. Physiol. 233: 311–326 (1973).
2. Inui, T., Mimura, O. and Kani, K. Retinal sensitivity and spatial summation in the foveal and parafoveal regions. J. Opt. Soc. Am. 71: 151–154 (1981).
3. Rovamo, J. Cortical magnification factor and contrast sensitivity to luminance-modulated chromatic gratings. Acta Physiol. Scand. 119: 365–371 (1983).
4. Rovamo, J., Leinonen, L., Laurinen, P. and Virsu, V. Temporal integration and

contrast sensitivity in foveal and peripheral vision. Perception, in press.

5. Rovamo, J. and Raninen, A. Critical flicker frequency and M-scaling of stimulus size and retinal illuminance. Vision Res., in press.
6. Rovamo, J. and Virsu, J. An estimation and application of the human cortical magnification factor. Expl. Brain Res. 37: 495–510 (1979).
7. Rovamo, J. and Virsu, V. Isotropy of cortical magnification and topography of striate cortex. Vision Res. 24: 283–286 (1984).
8. Rovamo, J., Virsu, V., Laurinen, P. and Hyvärinen, L. Resolution of gratings oriented along and across meridians in peripheral vision. Invest. Ophthalmol. Vis. Sci. 23: 666–670 (1982).
9. Rovamo, J., Virsu, V. and Näsänen, R. Cortical magnification factor predicts the photopic contrast sensitivity of peripheral vision. Nature 271: 54–56 (1978).
10. Virsu, V. and Rovamo, J. Visual resolution, contrast sensitivity, and the cortical magnification factor. Expl. Brain Res. 37: 475–494 (1979).
11. Virsu, V., Rovamo, J., Laurinen, P. and Näsänen, R. Temporal contrast sensitivity and cortical magnification. Vision Res. 22: 1211–1217 (1982).
12. Wilson, M.E. Invariant features of spatial summation with changing locus in the visual field. J. Physiol. 207: 611–622 (1970).

Authors' addresses:
Jyrki Rovamo & Antti Raninen
Department of Physiology
University of Helsinki
Siltavuorenpenger 20 J
SF-00170 Helsinki 17
Finland

Veijo Virsu
Department of Psychology
University of Helsinki